Sustainable Protein Sources

Sustainable Protein Sources

Edited by

Sudarshan R. Nadathur
Givaudan Flavors, Cincinnati, OH, United States

Janitha P. D. Wanasundara
Agriculture and Agri-Food Canada, Saskatoon SK, Canada

Laurie Scanlin
Colorado State University, Fort Collins, CO, United States

AMSTERDAM • BOSTON • HEIDELBERG • LONDON • NEW YORK • OXFORD • PARIS
SAN DIEGO • SAN FRANCISCO • SINGAPORE • SYDNEY • TOKYO

Academic Press is an imprint of Elsevier

Academic Press is an imprint of Elsevier
125 London Wall, London EC2Y 5AS, United Kingdom
525 B Street, Suite 1800, San Diego, CA 92101-4495, United States
50 Hampshire Street, 5th Floor, Cambridge, MA 02139, United States
The Boulevard, Langford Lane, Kidlington, Oxford OX5 1GB, United Kingdom

Copyright © 2017 Elsevier Inc. All rights reserved.

No part of this publication may be reproduced or transmitted in any form or by any means, electronic or mechanical, including photocopying, recording, or any information storage and retrieval system, without permission in writing from the publisher. Details on how to seek permission, further information about the Publisher's permissions policies and our arrangements with organizations such as the Copyright Clearance Center and the Copyright Licensing Agency, can be found at our website: www.elsevier.com/permissions.

This book and the individual contributions contained in it are protected under copyright by the Publisher (other than as may be noted herein).

Notices

Knowledge and best practice in this field are constantly changing. As new research and experience broaden our understanding, changes in research methods, professional practices, or medical treatment may become necessary.

Practitioners and researchers must always rely on their own experience and knowledge in evaluating and using any information, methods, compounds, or experiments described herein. In using such information or methods they should be mindful of their own safety and the safety of others, including parties for whom they have a professional responsibility.

To the fullest extent of the law, neither the Publisher nor the authors, contributors, or editors, assume any liability for any injury and/or damage to persons or property as a matter of products liability, negligence or otherwise, or from any use or operation of any methods, products, instructions, or ideas contained in the material herein.

British Library Cataloguing-in-Publication Data
A catalogue record for this book is available from the British Library

Library of Congress Cataloging-in-Publication Data
A catalog record for this book is available from the Library of Congress

ISBN: 978-0-12-802778-3

For Information on all Academic Press publications
visit our website at https://www.elsevier.com

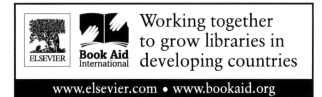

Publisher: Nikki Levy
Acquisition Editor: Megan Ball
Editorial Project Manager: Karen Miller
Production Project Manager: Susan Li
Designer: Mark Rogers

Typeset by MPS Limited, Chennai, India

This book is dedicated to the memory of my father,
Dr. N.R. Ranganthan,
who instilled in me the desire to aim high and
to make a difference for the greater good ∼ Nadathur

And to the memory of
Dr. Amanda Minnaar of the University of Pretoria,
who devoted her life to improving the nutrition of the people of Africa

And to those who work to sustain the earth ∼ Nadathur,
Wanasundara, Scanlin

Contents

List of Contributors xv
Preface xvii
Acknowledgments xix
Introduction xxi

1. **Proteins in the Diet: Challenges in Feeding the Global Population**
   S.R. Nadathur, J.P.D Wanasundara and L. Scanlin
   1.1 Introduction 1
   1.2 Proteins and Their Role in Food and Diet 1
     1.2.1 Defining Proteins: Structure Levels and Existing Classification Systems 2
     1.2.2 Protein as a Macronutrient in Food 4
     1.2.3 Protein as a Macromolecule in Food Systems 5
     1.2.4 Overview of Plant-Derived Protein and Alternate Protein Sources 7
   1.3 Sustainable Sources of Proteins 8
     1.3.1 Dietary Patterns Around the Globe 8
     1.3.2 Health and Wellness Trends 9
     1.3.3 Product Trends 9
   1.4 Reasons to Consume Plant and Alternate Proteins 10
     1.4.1 Living on the Earth in 2050 10
     1.4.2 Natural Resources for Agriculture: Land, Water, Nitrogen 12
     1.4.3 Global Warming and Climate Change 14
     1.4.4 Quality of Life 15
   1.5 Meat Consumption: Why We Are on the Current Path 15
   1.6 Role of the Consumer for the Greater Good 16
   References 16

Part I
Plant Derived Proteins

2. **Soy Protein: Impacts, Production, and Applications**
   M. Thrane, P.V. Paulsen, M.W. Orcutt and T.M. Krieger
   2.1 Introduction 23
   2.2 Production 23
   2.3 Soybean Protein Recovery: Protein Isolation 24
   2.4 Types of Soy Proteins and Protein Products 26
   2.5 Sustainability 26
     2.5.1 Two Life Cycle Inventory Models 27
     2.5.2 Cradle-to-Gate Life Cycle Impact Assessment 28
     2.5.3 Other Perspectives on Sustainability of Soy 31
   2.6 Nutritive Value 33
     2.6.1 Protein Nutrition 33
     2.6.2 Muscle Health 34
     2.6.3 Weight Management and Satiety 35
     2.6.4 Cardiovascular Health 36
     2.6.5 Nutritional Relevance of Other Seed Constituents 37
     2.6.6 Protein Allergies 38
     2.6.7 A Good Source of Protein Across the Lifespan 39
   2.7 Uses and Functionality 39
   2.8 Application and Current Products 40
   2.9 Potential New Uses, Issues, and Challenges 40
     2.9.1 Generational Flavor Improvements 41
     2.9.2 Genetic Modified and Identity Preserved 42
   2.10 Concluding Remarks 42
   References 43

3. Rice Protein and Rice Protein Products

H. Hoogenkamp, H. Kumagai and J.P.D. Wanasundara

3.1 Introduction 47
3.2 Production of Rice 48
  3.2.1 Land Use 48
  3.2.2 Water Use 48
  3.2.3 Energy Use 49
3.3 Processing of Rice and Rice Proteins 49
  3.3.1 Proteins in Rice 51
  3.3.2 Production of Rice Protein 53
3.4 Functional Properties and Applications 55
3.5 Allergenicity, Off Tastes, and Antinutritional Factors 55
  3.5.1 Allergenicity 55
  3.5.2 Flavor Compounds and Off Tastes 57
  3.5.3 Antinutritional Factors 58
3.6 Potential New Uses and Emerging Health Benefits 59
  3.6.1 Reduction of Cholesterol and Triacylglycerol Levels 59
  3.6.2 Suppression of Hyperglycemia 59
  3.6.3 Antioxidative Activity 59
  3.6.4 Reduction in Hypertension 60
  3.6.5 Ileum-Contracting, Antiopioid, and Phagocytosis-Promoting Activities 60
3.7 Concluding Remarks 60
References 61

4. Proteins From Wheat: Sustainable Production and New Developments in Nutrition-Based and Functional Applications

M. Flambeau, A. Redl and F. Respondek

4.1 Introduction 67
  4.1.1 Agricultural Production 67
  4.1.2 Land Use 67
  4.1.3 Water Use 68
  4.1.4 Energy Use 68
  4.1.5 Sustainability of Wheat 68
4.2 Proteins From Wheat 69
  4.2.1 Gluten Extraction From Wheat 70
  4.2.2 Protein Hydrolysis 70
4.3 Nutrition and Digestibility, Allergen, and Antinutritive Aspects 71
  4.3.1 Amino Acid Composition 71
  4.3.2 Digestibility Data and Mechanism 72
  4.3.3 Allergenicity and Intolerance Mechanism 73
  4.3.4 Antinutritive Factors 73
4.4 Protein Functionality 74
  4.4.1 Solubility 74
  4.4.2 Foaming 74
  4.4.3 Emulsification 74
  4.4.4 Satiety 74
4.5 Applications in Food and Feed 74
  4.5.1 Gluten in Bread Application 74
  4.5.2 Animal Nutrition 75
  4.5.3 Breakfast Cereals and Pasta 75
  4.5.4 Protein-Enriched Foods 75
  4.5.5 Uses in Vegetable-Based Meat Alternatives 75
  4.5.6 New Product and Technology for Wheat-Based Meat 76
4.6 Conclusion 76
References 77

5. Proteins From Sorghum and Millets

J.R.N. Taylor and J. Taylor

5.1 Introduction 79
5.2 Sorghum and Millet Production: Land, Water, and Energy Use 79
  5.2.1 Production 79
  5.2.2 Land-Use Efficiency 82
  5.2.3 Water Efficiency 82
  5.2.4 Cultivation With Legumes 83
  5.2.5 Sustainable Agriculture 83
  5.2.6 Cost of Grains 83
5.3 Protein Nutritive Quality 83
  5.3.1 Protein Quality 84
  5.3.2 Antinutrients 84
  5.3.3 Protein Toxicity 86
  5.3.4 Other Nutrients, Phytochemicals, and Nutritional Quality Issues 86
5.4 Protein Types, Composition, and Structure 87
  5.4.1 Prolamin Proteins 87
  5.4.2 Protein Isolation and Functionality 87
  5.4.3 Potential Applications for Kafirin 92
5.5 Sorghum and Millet Processing 92
  5.5.1 Effects of Cooking on the Proteins 92
  5.5.2 Milling 93
  5.5.3 Malting 93
  5.5.4 Lactic Acid Fermentation 94
  5.5.5 Brewing and Bioethanol Production 95
  5.5.6 Compositing With Legumes 96
5.6 Developments in Improving Sorghum and Millet Protein Quality 97
  5.6.1 Sorghum 97
  5.6.2 Millets 99
5.7 Conclusion 99
References 99

6. **Protein From Oat: Structure, Processes, Functionality, and Nutrition**

   O.E. Mäkinen, N. Sozer, D. Ercili-Cura and K. Poutanen

   6.1 Introduction 105
   6.2 Oat as a Protein Crop 105
      6.2.1 Land Use 105
      6.2.2 Water Use 106
      6.2.3 Energy Use 106
      6.2.4 Health Aspects of Oats 106
   6.3 Localization and Structure of Oat Proteins 107
      6.3.1 Protein in the Oat Grain 107
      6.3.2 Oat Protein Fractions 107
      6.3.3 Nutritional Properties and Suitability for Celiac Patients 109
   6.4 Manufacture of Oat Protein Isolates and Concentrates 111
      6.4.1 Wet Methods 111
      6.4.2 Dry Methods 111
   6.5 Functionality and Potential Uses 112
      6.5.1 Functional Characteristics of Oat Protein 112
      6.5.2 Applications of Oat Protein 114
   6.6 Future Outlook 115
   References 115

7. **Hemp Seed (*Cannabis sativa* L.) Proteins: Composition, Structure, Enzymatic Modification, and Functional or Bioactive Properties**

   R.E. Aluko

   7.1 General Overview 121
      7.1.1 Growing Regions and Yield 121
      7.1.2 Land Use 122
      7.1.3 Water Use 122
      7.1.4 Energy Use and Cost 122
      7.1.5 Plant and Seed 122
      7.1.6 Seed Composition and Protein Quality 123
   7.2 Major Seed Proteins 123
      7.2.1 Globulin 123
      7.2.2 Albumin 124
      7.2.3 Sulfur-Rich Proteins 124
      7.2.4 Allergenicity 125
   7.3 Functional Properties of Hemp Seed Protein Products 125
      7.3.1 Defatted Flour 125
      7.3.2 Protein Concentrates 126
      7.3.3 Protein Isolates 127
   7.4 Bioactive Properties of Hemp Seed Proteins and Peptides 128
      7.4.1 Renal Disease Modulation 128
      7.4.2 Antioxidant 129
      7.4.3 Antihypertensive 129
   7.5 Concluding Remarks 131
   References 132

8. **Protein From Flaxseed (*Linum usitatissimum* L.)**

   H.K. Marambe and J.P.D. Wanasundara

   8.1 Introduction 133
      8.1.1 Plant and Seeds 133
      8.1.2 Chemical Composition 134
   8.2 Sustainability of Flax: Land, Water, and Energy Use 134
      8.2.1 Land Use 134
      8.2.2 Water Use 135
      8.2.3 Energy Use 135
   8.3 Processing of Proteins and Types of Products From Flaxseed 135
   8.4 Nutritive Value of Flaxseed Proteins 138
      8.4.1 Amino Acids and Proteins 138
      8.4.2 Allergenicity of Flaxseed Proteins 139
   8.5 Uses and Functionality of Flaxseed Protein 139
   8.6 Application and Current Products 140
   8.7 Potential New Uses, Issues, and Challenges 141
   8.8 Concluding Remarks 142
   References 142

9. **Pea: A Sustainable Vegetable Protein Crop**

   M.C. Tulbek, R.S.H. Lam, Y.(C.) Wang, P. Asavajaru and A. Lam

   9.1 Introduction 145
      9.1.1 Cultivation 145
      9.1.2 Cultivars 146
   9.2 Sustainability, Energy, and Water Use 146
   9.3 Processing of Peas 147
   9.4 Nutritive Value of Peas 150
      9.4.1 Major Components 150
      9.4.2 Minerals and Vitamins 152
      9.4.3 Antinutritive Factors 152
      9.4.4 Bioavailability 153
      9.4.5 Allergenicity 154
      9.4.6 Off-Tastes 154
   9.5 Uses and Functionality 155
      9.5.1 Whole Peas 155
      9.5.2 Split Peas 156

9.5.3 Pea Flour 156
9.5.4 Pea Proteins 156
9.5.5 Pea Starch 157
9.5.6 Pea Fiber 158
9.6 Applications and Current Products 159
9.6.1 Baked Goods 159
9.6.2 Pasta and Noodle 159
9.6.3 Extruded Snacks 160
9.6.4 Meat and Meat Analogs 161
9.7 Health Benefits of Peas 161
9.8 Conclusion 161
References 162

10. **Lupin: An Important Protein and Nutrient Source**

    M. van de Noort

    10.1 Introduction 165
    10.1.1 Cultivation of *Lupinus* Species 165
    10.2 Sustainability 166
    10.2.1 Land Use 166
    10.2.2 Water Use 166
    10.2.3 Energy Use 167
    10.3 Food (Protein) Dependence of the EU 168
    10.4 Processing of Lupin 168
    10.4.1 Flour 168
    10.4.2 Concentrate 168
    10.4.3 Isolates 169
    10.5 Nutritive Value 169
    10.5.1 Protein 170
    10.5.2 Fats 170
    10.5.3 Carbohydrates 170
    10.5.4 Minerals and Vitamins 171
    10.5.5 Evaluation of the Protein Quality and Digestibility of Lupin 171
    10.6 Antinutritive Factors and Allergenicity 172
    10.6.1 Antinutritive Factors 172
    10.6.2 Off-Tastes 174
    10.6.3 Allergenicity 174
    10.7 Uses and Functionality 174
    10.7.1 Lupin Flour 174
    10.7.2 Lupin Protein Concentrate 175
    10.7.3 Lupin Protein Isolate 175
    10.8 Application/Current Products 175
    10.8.1 Bakery Applications 175
    10.8.2 Egg Replacement in Baked Goods 175
    10.8.3 Application of Lupin Protein Concentrate in Batters 176
    10.9 Current Food Products 176
    10.9.1 Nutritional Applications 176
    10.10 Health Aspects of Lupin 177
    10.10.1 Cholesterol 178
    10.10.2 Bowel Function 178
    10.10.3 Satiety and Glucose Blood Level 178
    10.10.4 Blood Pressure 179
    10.10.5 Other Health Effects 179
    10.11 Conclusion 179
    References 180

11. **Lentil: Revival of Poor Man's Meat**

    A. Samaranayaka

    11.1 Introduction 185
    11.2 Sustainability 185
    11.2.1 Land Use 185
    11.2.2 Water Use 186
    11.2.3 Energy Use 187
    11.2.4 Diseases Affecting Lentil Plant 187
    11.3 Lentil Proteins: Characterization and Processing Into Concentrates and Isolates 187
    11.3.1 Characterization 187
    11.3.2 Processing Into Protein Concentrates or Isolates 187
    11.4 Nutritional Value, Antinutrients, and Allergenicity 188
    11.4.1 Nutritive Value 188
    11.4.2 Phytochemicals 189
    11.4.3 Protein Quality 189
    11.4.4 Antinutritional Factors and Protein Digestibility 190
    11.4.5 Allergenicity 191
    11.5 Applications and Current Products 191
    11.6 Protein Functionality 192
    11.7 Health Properties 192
    11.7.1 Bioactive Peptides 192
    11.7.2 Chronic Diseases 193
    11.8 Off-Flavors Associated With Lentil Flour and Lentil Protein Ingredients 193
    11.9 Conclusion 193
    References 194

12. **Underutilized Protein Resources From African Legumes**

    M. Gulzar and A. Minnaar

    12.1 Introduction 197
    12.2 Marama Beans 197
    12.2.1 Introduction (Land, Water, Sustainability) 197
    12.2.2 Composition of Marama Beans 199

    12.2.3 Composition of Marama Proteins   199
    12.2.4 Protein Isolation   199
    12.2.5 Nutritive Value, Allergenicity, and Antinutritive Factors   200
    12.2.6 Current and Future Uses and Applications   201
    12.2.7 Off-Tastes Associated With Marama Beans   202
    12.2.8 Issues and Challenges   202
12.3 Bambara Groundnut   202
    12.3.1 Introduction (Land, Water, Sustainability)   202
    12.3.2 Composition of Bambara Groundnut   203
    12.3.3 Composition of Bambara Proteins   203
    12.3.4 Protein Isolation   203
    12.3.5 Nutritive Value, Allergenicity, and Antinutritive Factors   204
    12.3.6 Current and Future Uses and Applications   204
    12.3.7 Off-Tastes Associated With Bambara Groundnut   205
    12.3.8 Issues and Challenges   205
12.4 Conclusion   206
References   206

13. Peanut Products as a Protein Source: Production, Nutrition, and Environmental Impact

H.N. Sandefur, J.A. McCarty, E.C. Boles and M.D. Matlock

13.1 Introduction   209
13.2 Environmental Impact and Sustainability   209
    13.2.1 Climate Change Impacts   209
    13.2.2 Water Use Impacts   211
    13.2.3 Land Use Impacts   212
13.3 Peanut Cultivation and Production   213
    13.3.1 Production Regions   213
    13.3.2 Cultivation Techniques   213
13.4 Peanut Processing   214
    13.4.1 Peanut Drying   214
    13.4.2 Grading   214
    13.4.3 Shelling   215
    13.4.4 Product Processing   215
13.5 Uses, Functionality, and Current Products   215
13.6 Nutritional Value   216
    13.6.1 Calories, Fats, Protein, Carbohydrates   216
    13.6.2 Amino Acids and Protein   217
    13.6.3 Micronutrients   218
    13.6.4 Taste Profiles and Allergenicity   219
13.7 Conclusions   219
Acknowledgments   220
References   220

14. Quinoa as a Sustainable Protein Source: Production, Nutrition, and Processing

L. Scanlin and K.A. Lewis

14.1 Introduction   223
14.2 Production of Quinoa   224
    14.2.1 Growing Regions and Yields   224
    14.2.2 Land Use   225
    14.2.3 Water Use   225
    14.2.4 Energy Use and Cost   225
14.3 Morphology   225
14.4 Nutritional Quality   226
    14.4.1 Protein Content   226
    14.4.2 Protein Quality   226
    14.4.3 Protein Digestibility   228
    14.4.4 Macro- and Micronutrients and Phytochemicals   229
    14.4.5 Antinutritional Factors and Allergenicity   230
14.5 Processing Methods   230
    14.5.1 Quinoa Seed From "Farm to Fork"   230
    14.5.2 QPCs and Isolates   231
14.6 Quinoa Protein Functionality, Off-Tastes, and Challenges   233
14.7 Concluding Remarks and Future Research Needs   234
References   235

15. Amaranth Part 1—Sustainable Crop for the 21st Century: Food Properties and Nutraceuticals for Improving Human Health

D. Orona-Tamayo and O. Paredes-López

15.1 Introduction   239
15.2 Nutritional Components in Amaranth   240
15.3 Amaranth Proteins and Amino Acids for Human Nutrition   242
15.4 Bioactive Peptides Related to Antihypertensive Functions   244
15.5 Antioxidant Capacities of Amaranth Peptides   247
15.6 Potential Uses of Amaranth Proteins in the Food Industry   248

- 15.7 Genetic Engineering of Amaranth Proteins 249
- 15.8 Concluding Remarks 251
- Acknowledgments 251
- References 251

16. Amaranth Part 2—Sustainability, Processing, and Applications of Amaranth

D.K. Santra and R. Schoenlechner

- 16.1 Sustainability of Amaranth Production 257
  - 16.1.1 Origin and Distribution 257
  - 16.1.2 Production and Yield 257
  - 16.1.3 Land, Water, and Energy Uses 258
  - 16.1.4 Harvesting 259
  - 16.1.5 Postharvest Processing (Cleaning and Storage) 259
  - 16.1.6 Production Cost 260
- 16.2 Processing of Amaranth 260
  - 16.2.1 Milling and Fractionation 260
  - 16.2.2 Wet Milling for Production of Starch-Rich, Fiber-Rich, or Protein-Rich Fractions (Protein Concentrates and Isolates) 261
- 16.3 Food Applications 262
- References 263

17. Chia—The New Golden Seed for the 21st Century: Nutraceutical Properties and Technological Uses

D. Orona-Tamayo, M.E. Valverde and O. Paredes-López

- 17.1 Introduction 265
- 17.2 Sustainability of Chia 265
  - 17.2.1 Production 265
  - 17.2.2 Land Use 266
  - 17.2.3 Water Use 266
  - 17.2.4 Energy Use 267
- 17.3 Consumption of Chia 267
- 17.4 Nutritional Value 268
  - 17.4.1 Fiber 268
  - 17.4.2 Lipids 268
  - 17.4.3 Phenolic Compounds 268
  - 17.4.4 Protein Content and Amino Acids 269
  - 17.4.5 Polyphenols, Oil, and Peptides With Antioxidant Capacity 274
- 17.5 Chia Compounds Significant to the Food Industry 275
  - 17.5.1 Antioxidant Properties 276
  - 17.5.2 Health Benefits 276
  - 17.5.3 Functional Benefits 276
- 17.6 The Future of Chia Seeds: Molecular Engineering and Gene Editing 277
- 17.7 Concluding Remarks 278
- Acknowledgments 278
- References 278

Part II
Upcoming Sources of Proteins

18. Proteins From Canola/Rapeseed: Current Status

J.P.D. Wanasundara, S. Tan, A.M. Alashi, F. Pudel and C. Blanchard

- 18.1 Introduction 285
- 18.2 Production of C/RS 285
  - 18.2.1 Land Use 286
  - 18.2.2 Water Use 286
  - 18.2.3 Energy Use 286
- 18.3 Proteins of C/RS 286
  - 18.3.1 Chemical Composition of the Seed 286
  - 18.3.2 Protein Types of C/RS 288
- 18.4 Processes of Protein Product Preparation 289
  - 18.4.1 Significant Considerations 289
  - 18.4.2 Involving Aqueous Alkaline Conditions 290
  - 18.4.3 Processes Targeting Specific Seed Protein Types/Fractions 291
  - 18.4.4 Combination of Chemical and Physical Methods 292
- 18.5 Nutritional Value 292
  - 18.5.1 Amino Acid Composition 292
  - 18.5.2 Digestibility in Human and Animal Models and the Processing Effects 293
- 18.6 Antinutritional Factors of C/RS 294
  - 18.6.1 Glucosinolates 294
  - 18.6.2 Phytates 295
  - 18.6.3 Phenolics 295
  - 18.6.4 Carbohydrates and Fiber 295
- 18.7 Allergenicity of C/RS Proteins 296
- 18.8 Functional Properties of Protein Products 296
  - 18.8.1 Solubility 296
  - 18.8.2 Emulsifying Properties 296
  - 18.8.3 Heat-Induced Gel Formation Ability 297
  - 18.8.4 Foaming Properties 297
- 18.9 Applications and Current Products 297

18.9.1 Potential Food Applications as Protein Supplements or Bulk Proteins 297
18.10 Potential New Uses, Issues, and Challenges 298
  18.10.1 New Uses 298
  18.10.2 Issues and Challenges 299
18.11 Off-Tastes Associated With Using Oilseed Proteins 299
18.12 Concluding Remarks 300
References 300

19. Mycoprotein: A Healthy New Protein With a Low Environmental Impact

T. Finnigan, L. Needham and C. Abbott

19.1 Origins and Discovery of Mycoprotein 305
19.2 Food Safety and the Regulatory Framework 305
19.3 Cultivation and Processing of Mycoprotein 306
  19.3.1 Fungal Fermentation Technology 306
  19.3.2 Mycoprotein and the Creation of Meat-Like Texture 309
  19.3.3 Process Variables That Impact Quality 312
  19.3.4 Creation of Granular Comminute Texture 313
  19.3.5 Fat Mimetics 313
19.4 Nutritional Characteristics of Mycoprotein 313
  19.4.1 Nutritional Properties 313
  19.4.2 Nutrition Research 316
19.5 Mycoprotein and Environmental Impact 317
  19.5.1 Environmental Impact 318
  19.5.2 How Low Can We Go? 322
References 323

20. Heterotrophic Microalgae: A Scalable and Sustainable Protein Source

B. Klamczynska and W.D. Mooney

20.1 Introduction 327
20.2 *Chlorella* Classification 327
20.3 Production 328
20.4 Sustainability Profile 329
  20.4.1 Case Study: TerraVia Inc. 329
  20.4.2 A Low Environmental Impact 330
  20.4.3 Climate Change Adaptation and Resilience 333
20.5 Nutritional Value and Safety 333
  20.5.1 Nutritional Value 333
  20.5.2 Safety 335
20.6 Properties and Applications of Whole Algae Protein 335
20.7 Consumer Acceptance 336
20.8 Future Developments 337
20.9 Conclusion 338
References 338

21. Edible Insects: A Neglected and Promising Food Source

A. Van Huis and F.V. Dunkel

21.1 Introduction 341
21.2 Ethno-Entomology 342
21.3 Environment 343
21.4 Farming Insects 344
21.5 Nutrition 345
  21.5.1 Protein Content and Amino Acids 345
  21.5.2 Fats and Fatty Acids 346
  21.5.3 Chitin 346
  21.5.4 Minerals 346
  21.5.5 Vitamins 346
21.6 Consumer Attitudes 347
21.7 Food Safety 348
21.8 Processing and Marketing 349
21.9 Legislation 350
21.10 The Way Forward 351
References 352

Part III
Consumers and Sustainability

22. Meat Reduction and Plant-Based Food: Replacement of Meat: Nutritional, Health, and Social Aspects

M. Neacsu, D. McBey and A.M. Johnstone

22.1 Transition Towards Plant-Based Protein Supplementations 359
22.2 Plant Protein Sources: Nutritional Adequacy Aspects 360
22.3 Plant-Based Protein Sources: Health and Wellbeing Aspects 363
  22.3.1 Systemic and Gut Health Impacts 363
  22.3.2 Satiety and Weight Management 364
22.4 Meat Replacement: Social Aspects 367
  22.4.1 The Complexity of Food Choice 367

         22.4.2 Changing the Diet of a Nation 368
         22.4.3 Decreasing Meat Consumption 369
    22.5 Overall Concluding Remarks 370
    References 370

23. **Flavors, Taste Preferences, and the Consumer: Taste Modulation and Influencing Change in Dietary Patterns for a Sustainable Earth**

    S.R. Nadathur and M. Carolan

    23.1 Consumers: Dietary and Purchase Habits 377
    23.2 Flavor and Taste 378
         23.2.1 Physiology of Taste 378
    23.3 Why We Eat What We Eat: Taste Preferences and Influences 379
         23.3.1 Genetics and Food Choices 380
         23.3.2 Our Upbringing and Cultural Influence on Food Choices 380
         23.3.3 Affording a Healthy Diet 382
         23.3.4 Ice Cream, Broccoli, or Nuts? 382
    23.4 Sustainable Protein Sources in Foods and their Challenges 383
         23.4.1 Off-Tastes Associated With Plant Proteins 383
         23.4.2 Role of Flavors in Modulating Off-Notes in Protein-Based Products 384
         23.4.3 Binding of Flavors by Proteins 384
    23.5 Introduction of New Foods and Changing Consumer Habits 385
    23.6 Conclusions 386
    Disclaimer 386
    References 386

24. **Food Security and Policy**

    M. Carolan

    24.1 Introduction 391
    24.2 Livestock: Facts and Trends 392
    24.3 Rethinking Food Security 395
    24.4 Growing Homogeneity in Global Food Supplies 398

    24.5 Sociological Pathways for More Sustainable Protein Options 399
    24.6 Conclusion 405
    References 406

25. **Feeding the Globe Nutritious Food in 2050: Obligations and Ethical Choices**

    S.R. Nadathur, J.P.D. Wanasundara and L. Scanlin

    25.1 Closing Commentary 409
    25.2 Sustainable Protein Sources 409
         25.2.1 Current State of Protein Production 409
         25.2.2 Change in Consumption Patterns, Especially Meat and the Western Diet 411
         25.2.3 Are We Consuming Too Much Protein? 412
         25.2.4 Diet Change, Consumers, and Policies 412
         25.2.5 Challenges With Diet Change 413
    25.3 Environmentally Friendly Food Options 413
         25.3.1 Meat Alternates 413
         25.3.2 Newer Sources of Protein 414
    25.4 Relevance of Big Food Manufacturers 415
    25.5 Production of More Food From the Same Land (and Alternate Farming Methods) 415
         25.5.1 Agriculture and Climate Change: Crop Adaptation 416
         25.5.2 Are GMO's Necessary to Feed the World? 416
    25.6 Reduction in Food Waste 417
    25.7 Using Microbiomes to Our Advantage 417
    25.8 Sustainable Future Populations 418
    25.9 Moral Obligations and Questions People Need to Debate 419
    Disclaimer 420
    References 420

Index 423

List of Contributors

C. Abbott, Quorn Foods, North Yorkshire, United Kingdom

A.M. Alashi, University of Manitoba, Winnipeg, MB, Canada

R.E. Aluko, University of Manitoba, Winnipeg, MB, Canada

P. Asavajaru, AGT Foods, Saskatoon, SK, Canada

C. Blanchard, ARC ITTC for Functional Grains, Charles Sturt University, Wagga Wagga, NSW, Australia

E.C. Boles, Paradigm Sustainability Solutions, Fayetteville, AR, United States

M. Carolan, Colorado State University, Ft. Collins, CO, United States

F.V. Dunkel, Montana State University, Bozeman, MT, United States

D. Ercili-Cura, VTT Technical Research Centre of Finland, Espoo, Finland

T. Finnigan, Quorn Foods, North Yorkshire, United Kingdom

M. Flambeau, Tereos, Marckolsheim, France

M. Gulzar, University of Pretoria, Hatfield, Pretoria, South Africa

H. Hoogenkamp, RiceBran Technologies Inc., Scottsdale, AZ, United States

A.M. Johnstone, University of Aberdeen, Aberdeen, United Kingdom

B. Klamczynska, TerraVia Holdings Inc., South San Francisco, CA, United States

T.M. Krieger, DuPont Engineering Research & Technology, Wilmington, DE, United States

H. Kumagai, Nihon University, Fujisawa-shi, Japan

A. Lam, AGT Foods, Saskatoon, SK, Canada

R.S.H. Lam, AGT Foods, Saskatoon, SK, Canada

K.A. Lewis, Food Industry Professional Consultant, Littleton, CO, United States

O.E. Mäkinen, VTT Technical Research Centre of Finland, Espoo, Finland

H.K. Marambe, Agriculture Research Branch, Saskatchewan Ministry of Agriculture, Regina, SK, Canada

M.D. Matlock, University of Arkansas Office for Sustainability, Fayetteville, AR, United States

D. McBey, University of Aberdeen, Aberdeen, United Kingdom

J.A. McCarty, University of Arkansas, Fayetteville, AR, United States

A. Minnaar, University of Pretoria, Hatfield, Pretoria, South Africa

W.D. Mooney, TerraVia Holdings Inc., South San Francisco, CA, United States

S.R. Nadathur, Givaudan Flavors, Cincinnati, OH, United States

M. Neacsu, University of Aberdeen, Aberdeen, United Kingdom

L. Needham, Quorn Foods, North Yorkshire, United Kingdom

M.W. Orcutt, Solae, LLC, St. Louis, MO, United States

D. Orona-Tamayo, Centro de Investigación y de Estudios Avanzados del IPN, Irapuato, Mexico

O. Paredes-López, Centro de Investigación y de Estudios Avanzados del IPN, Irapuato, Mexico; Université Pierre et Marie Curie, Paris, France

P.V. Paulsen, Solae, LLC, St. Louis, MO, United States

K. Poutanen, VTT Technical Research Centre of Finland, Espoo, Finland

F. Pudel, Pilot Pflanzenöltechnologie Magdeburg e.V., Magdeburg, Germany

A. Redl, Tereos, Marckolsheim, France

F. Respondek, Tereos, Marckolsheim, France

A. Samaranayaka, POS Bio-Sciences, Saskatoon, SK, Canada

H.N. Sandefur, University of Arkansas, Fayetteville, AR, United States

D.K. Santra, University of Nebraska-Lincoln, Scottsbluff, NE, United States

L. Scanlin, Colorado State University, Fort Collins, CO, United States

R. Schoenlechner, University of Natural Resources and Life Sciences, Vienna, Austria

N. Sozer, VTT Technical Research Centre of Finland, Espoo, Finland

S. Tan, ARC ITTC for Functional Grains, Charles Sturt University, Wagga Wagga, NSW, Australia

J. Taylor, University of Pretoria, Hatfield, South Africa

J.R.N. Taylor, University of Pretoria, Hatfield, South Africa

M. Thrane, DuPont Nutrition Biosciences ApS, Brabrand, Denmark

M.C. Tulbek, AGT Foods, Saskatoon, SK, Canada

M.E. Valverde, Centro de Investigación y de Estudios Avanzados del IPN, Irapuato, Guanajuato, Mexico

M. van de Noort, MFH Pulses, Rotterdam, The Netherlands

A. Van Huis, Wageningen University, Wageningen, The Netherlands

J.P.D. Wanasundara, Agriculture and Agri-Food Canada, Saskatoon SK, Canada

Y.(C.) Wang, AGT Foods, Saskatoon, SK, Canada

Preface

Do we eat to live or live to eat? Our diets are not only a source of pleasure but essential for our health and well-being. Thus, food and health are vital aspects of our lives that are closely interwoven. A well-balanced diet is a necessity for the growth phases of human development and the maintenance of proper adult health. Diets also support the proper functioning of all organs and systems, intracellular components, and the body's ability to fight off diseases. Every culture has specific foods and diets that aid in improving health issues ranging from minor ailments to systemic issues (http://greatist.com/health/healthy-habits-from-around-the-world), with examples found deeply rooted in many Asian countries (http://www.journalofethnicfoods.net/article/S2352-6181(15)00043-8/pdf; http://www.theguardian.com/life-andstyle/2013/jun/19/japanese-diet-live-to-100). Foods cooked in herbs and spices may ward off regular colds, lower fevers, reduce risk of influenza, and address hepatitis. As such, traditional foods have been a source of health as well as to savor. In the last century, the more developed and industrialized countries have become, the more links between traditional foods and health have been lost. Can consumers return to past practices and restore traditional dietary patterns?

Most of us who live in developed countries take for granted the nutrients supplied from the meal as vital. At the same time, highly processed foods that were meant to save time, have become a source of high caloric intake and are a cause of many of the noncommunicable diseases associated with affluent nations. The lack of critical nutrients or the improper balance of protein, fat, and carbohydrate are linked to the development of chronic and systemic diseases and even cancer. In fact, epidemiological studies show that one-third of all cancers are related to our diets (http://www.ncbi.nlm.nih.gov/pubmed/24374225). With global trade, meat consumption and high-caloric diets have spread to emerging economies, which can ill afford the high cost of associated medical issues. Should nutrition be sacrificed to support our fast-paced lives or should it aid our health?

As people in developed economies shop at supermarkets, sometimes they forget the numerous factors involved in moving food from the farm to our table. As the global population increases, the question of feeding people nutritious food, especially protein, was a fundamental thought in proposing this book. Can we feed the 30% increase in population that is expected by 2050 (http://www.un.org/apps/news/story.asp?NewsID=45165#.VubDcKRViuc)? Probing deeper into this topic has raised issues of cultivating crops for humans or for animals. It became clear to us that meat consumption has driven the production of crops that are suitable for animal feed, although meat protein produced from livestock fed plants is via an inefficient process. Should people care about this current environment we live in? Should those in the Western societies worry about the food supply in emerging economies? Such complex issues raised several ethical and moral questions on the total food supply around the globe, further shaping the content of this book.

How do we define food sustainability? Sustainability may be defined as our ability to perform tasks in a continued manner without affecting the equilibrium. Yet, sustainability is complex and affected by several dynamics. For the purpose of this book, we will restrict the definition of the term sustainability to mean food availability and maintenance of the earth for future generations. Is it enough if those in the developed economies consume more soy or meat alternates? Can the planet be sustainable for future generations if people switch from fossil energy-fueled cars to zero-emission electric cars? What happens to the rest of the people living in the developing economies? Can one part of the globe have more access to food and infrastructure while the majority subsists on less nutrition and inadequate necessities? Will food security, or lack of it, affect our future generations?

This book was born at the interface of these two vital aspects that affect our future state of the planet and how humans can continue to thrive in a soon to be overcrowded earth. Our food choices affect our health and those same choices will likely influence the future state of agriculture and the environment. Protein is an important nutrient that is critical for our development and bodily functions (https://www.nlm.nih.gov/medlineplus/ency/article/002467.htm), the lack of which affects many adults, juveniles, and infants around the globe. Do plant proteins provide similar nutrition to animal-derived proteins? Are plant-based diets better for the environment? Answers to these questions will be critical to persuade people to change their diets.

Originally, this book sought to identify sustainable protein sources that would aid the nutrition of consumers in reducing animal-derived protein. As the team delved into the topic of plant-based protein versus animal protein, larger questions came into the forefront. These included questions regarding the role of agriculture in contributing to climate change and the concern of feeding 30−40% more people from the same amount of land. Furthermore, questions that arose provided a stark reminder of the inequalities that exist between populations on the planet.

A number of professionals will benefit from this book including agriculturists, food product developers, application technologists, food scientists, nutritionists, and especially those involved in sustainability. Information and analysis provided on protein sources in this book will benefit researchers, food formulation scientists, and product managers, where they can focus on promoting these sources for new products that can sustain future protein demands. Farmers may consider growing some of the cited crops should those fit the regional climate. Food processors may consider reformulating some of the protein-rich products with these alternative, sustainable sources.

Experts from around the globe in academia, government, and industry have joined to help support this publication. It was clear that the topics of sustainability and health were front of mind for all contributors, which has led to a pursuit to make a difference. Regardless of your profession, we hope that the discussions within this book will provide a mechanism for transformation and allow at least one small step towards a sustainable planet. The food supply chain cannot change instantaneously, nor can dietary habits. Yet, continuous and steady positive progress will make a difference and will need to come from all of us—together—making a collective modification for a sustainable earth for future generations to come.

Acknowledgments

I would like to acknowledge and genuinely thank my wife, Priya Nadathur and children Meera, Govind, and Hari, for their complete support and enduring patience during these past 24 months to enable the pursuit of this larger goal. I am extremely grateful to my sister-in-law, Mrs. Maithreyi Nandakumar, for her insightful comments to develop and shape the Introductory, Taste, and Conclusion chapters. In addition, I wish to thank my mother, my in-laws, family, and friends for their constant encouragement.

This book would not have been possible without the astute insight of Dr. Janitha Wanasundara and Dr. Laurie Scanlin. In addition to the time spent pouring over the numerous chapters, their recommendations and input have been invaluable for the completion of this book and sorting out various issues along the way. Contributions from academic, government, and industry experts from around the globe are the centerpiece of this book and are greatly appreciated. The authors not only offered their expertise in various aspects of food proteins but shared in common goals to improve human nutrition concurrently with sustaining the planet for our future generations. We are also deeply honored and fortunate to have the experiences and wisdom of Dr. Amanda Minnaar, who worked to bring global attention to underutilized beans of Africa, shared with the readers. This book is a tribute to her dedication in completing the chapter while challenged with serious health issues before her passing.

A salute to Givaudan for their strong commitment to sustainability and many thanks to my colleagues: Dr. Jay Slack, Mr. Mark Yates, Dr. Jeff Spencer, Mr. Scott Harris, Dr. Chad Hansen, Mr. Gabriel Wickizer, Mr. Jeff Peppet, Mr. Michael Peters, Mr. Pablo Krawec, Ms. Jennifer Haggard, and Dr. Sarah Kirkmeyer for reviewing manuscripts, providing needed recommendations, and inspiration. I am also very grateful to the Institute of Food Technologists (IFT) for providing leadership opportunities in supporting their Sustainability Program. Involvement with this program in various capacities guided me to a deeper understanding of the challenges facing the planet, especially feeding the global population. These opportunities and associations inevitably led to a book proposal and acceptance from Elsevier, for which I am enormously thankful.

Nadathur

First and foremost, we wish to express sincere gratitude to our spouses, friends, and family who supported us with love, encouragement, and understanding during the many family hours that were postponed to dedicate to this book endeavor. Our sincere appreciation goes to the organizations we are affiliated with for their wholehearted endorsements. We thank the members of the production team at Elsevier for their advice, proficiency, and patience throughout this process. We wish to also thank the following people for their inspiration and wisdom: Dr. Udaya Wanasundara, Dr. Rachel Cheatham, Sergio Nuñez de Arco, Dr. Ken Foster, Cristina Munteanu, Dr. Klaus Lorenz, and Dr. Dave Sampson. Together, we have been able to see this first-of-its-kind book effort come to fruition from its initial conception by Dr. Sudarshan Nadathur.

Scanlin and Wanasundara

Introduction

The global population is currently 7.4 billion, which is already twice the number of people that the earth can sustainably support (http://www.footprintnetwork.org/en/index.php/GFN/page/world_footprint/). A majority of this populace lives in underdeveloped economies with only modest access to necessities. In addition, the greater number of people in these regions consume at most one-third of their required caloric intake or go hungry (http://www.fao.org/news/story/en/item/161819/icode/; http://www.wfp.org/hunger/stats). In stark contrast, most citizens in developed economies have an overabundance of food and necessities.

Human activities, including agriculture, have become a contributory factor for higher greenhouse gases (GHG) leading to a warmer planet. The consequences of warmer temperatures have affected weather patterns and areas of rainfall in many parts of the globe. Exploitation of water aquifers has greatly reduced our reserve supplies for irrigation.

Now imagine possible scenarios as our earth's population is on track to reach 9.7 billion by 2050 and nearly 11 billion by 2100—numbers that are 30—50% higher than at present. The overall food supply will need to increase by 70%, while meat consumption is predicted to climb by 80% (http://www.meatpoultry.com/articles/news_home/Trends/2011/12/Global_meat_consumption_to_ris.aspx?ID = %7B3E8D6C8C-B2D4-4055-A1FE-33AFB54CDD21%7D). At the same time, rising global temperatures have led to the melting of polar caps and altered weather patterns. This combined with the tapping of aquifers will likely affect fresh water availability—a critical requirement for agriculture.

Scenario 1: Meat consumption rises as expected, requiring large tracts of land to be set aside for growing animal feed. This will further require significant use of precious natural resources (land, water, and fossil energy) to provide food for a smaller proportion of the global populace. Consequently, current trends in caloric inequality will be further exacerbated and an increasing number of inhabitants will subsist on very little nutritious food. With rising inequalities in other facets of society (education, income, employment, infrastructure), those groups residing predominantly in emerging countries will live in crowded cities with few necessities, most likely leading to strife. Conversely, high-caloric food consumption in the developed and affluent countries will lead to high rates of chronic diseases and soaring healthcare costs. All of which would result in an unsustainable state of affairs for future generations.

Scenario 2: Diets have shifted to becoming more plant-based, while meat consumption has remained steady or declined. Land originally dedicated to animal feed can now be cultivated with a variety of plant-based protein sources, with an overall reduction in water use. Alternating pulse crops enables fixing of nitrogen in the soil, reducing the demand for fertilizers. Since protein-rich crops would be produced for direct human consumption, switching corn and other feed crops to a combination of pulses and other protein sources can also aid in the supply of valuable nutrition to the undernourished. Plant-based foods provide proteins and a variety of phytonutrients and minerals, thus promoting better health. This is reflected in a reduction in the incidence of chronic diseases, positively benefiting human health and healthcare costs. In addition, as we deal with the effects of climate change, a number of opportunities arise leading to developments in science and technology that aid agriculture, food and nutrition, policy, and governmental decisions. All of this can culminate in a more sustainable planet.

Which is the scenario that you would want for our planet? How can each of us play a role in this effort as we confront the challenges acknowledged above? How will a warming planet affect agriculture in the coming decades? How can our food choices shape what farmers cultivate for our consumption? Can developed societies make the right dietary choices and in turn, aid those in developing regions? The following chapters provide a combination of scientific and ethical content to initiate discussions that can create debates and action. As the reader of this book, we hope that you will join the editors and authors in helping to support a sustainable earth.

Chapter 1

Proteins in the Diet: Challenges in Feeding the Global Population

S.R. Nadathur[1], J.P.D Wanasundara[2] and L. Scanlin[3]
[1]Givaudan Flavors, Cincinnati, OH, United States, [2]Agriculture and Agri-Food Canada, Saskatoon SK, Canada, [3]Colorado State University, Fort Collins, CO, United States

1.1 INTRODUCTION

Food is essential for sustenance and, in particular, consumption of protein is critical for maintaining our body and various cellular functions. With the projected increase in population growth over the next two to three decades, the concern of feeding 30% more people is on the minds of many, including governments, policymakers, and those involved in agriculture. Producing food (and adequate protein) for the projected 10 billion people by 2050 cannot be the responsibility of the few. Vast amounts of resources are spent in meat production, which has become the major source of protein globally. In order to provide adequate protein in the diet for much of the global populace, a shift in dietary pattern from animal-derived protein to plant-based protein needs to occur soon, especially in the developed economies. We will discuss the need for protein in the diet and its role in food systems, challenges we face in the quest to feed the global population, sources of protein that can be produced in a sustainable manner, and the trends that are shaping changes in people's dietary patterns. The discussion of this topic has interlinks with scientific, economic, social, and political aspects. The onus is on consumers to play a major role in altering their diet and activities for the greater good of the planet.

1.2 PROTEINS AND THEIR ROLE IN FOOD AND DIET

Proteins are vital for life, essentially found in all living organisms, and are an important nutrient that is required for critical functions in the cell, tissues, organs, and systems. Our food is derived from animal and plant tissues, thus by default the proteins of these tissues become food proteins. However, for practical reasons, proteins that are digestible by the human body and provide nutrition, are nontoxic, have usable functionalities in food applications, are available in abundance, and can be produced sustainably are considered food proteins. Among the chemical components of food, protein is one of the three macromolecules, besides lipids and carbohydrates, that are integral to food systems. Therefore, food proteins satisfy our body requirement (human nutrition) as well as the requirements in creating food systems (food functionalities).

In 1816, the French physiologist Francois Magendie pointed out the need for nitrogenous food in the diet in order to maintain life; and later in 1838 the term "protein" (in Greek "proteios" means primary) was coined by Gerard J. Mulder with the suggestion of Jöns J. Berzelius to designate a complex N-containing radical found in both animal and plant materials. With the discovery of amino acids (AAs) in the early 19th century, an understanding of their release due to acid or enzymatic hydrolysis, along with evidence of their arrangement in linear "peptide" formation, laid the foundation to consider protein as vital constituents of food required to maintain life. There are 20 AAs found in nature (Fig. 1.1); they are similar in carboxylic- and amino- functional groups, differ in side chain attachments, and are assembled in numerous combinations to form proteins. Naturally occurring polymers of AA (L-form) that have a defined three-dimensional (3-D) structure are referred to as a protein, while a polypeptide refers to any polymer of AA, and a peptide is a short oligomer of AA without stable conformation. Proteins vary in size; among the smallest known is the subunit of an enzyme called 4-oxalocrotonate tautomerase (~10 kDa in size and composed of ~62 AAs)

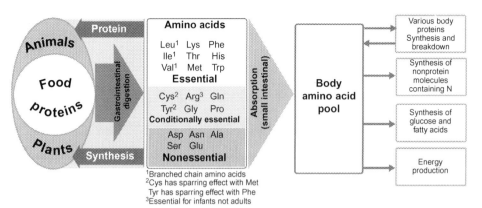

FIGURE 1.1 Depiction of amino acid and dietary protein flow. Food proteins are from the animal and plant kingdoms, which are made of the same amino acids required in the synthesis of proteins and various biochemical activities in our body.

(http://bionumbers.hms.harvard.edu/default.aspx), while the largest known protein is found in the human body called titin (isoform of 3816.19 kDa molecular mass and 34,350 AA) (Titin—*Homo sapiens* (Human), Universal Protein Resource, UniProt Consortium; ExPASy Proteomics Server. Swiss Institute of Bioinformatics, Accessed 10.07.15).

1.2.1 Defining Proteins: Structure Levels and Existing Classification Systems

The design and architecture of proteins are to enable them to participate in an extraordinary number of tasks within living organisms, for example: to regulate enzymatic reactions in entire biological pathways; to bind to chemicals from simple ions to complex molecules; to act as biological sensors and switches that amplify and transduce signals, cause motion, and control genes. This incredible array of diverse tasks depends on the accurate synthesis of protein molecules, a process that is highly regulated in all organisms.

1.2.1.1 Structural Levels

Construction of proteins is initiated in the ribosomes by covalently linking AAs via an amide (peptide) bond and arranging according to the sequence provided by the genetic code. This unbranched, sequentially arranged polypeptide forms the base or the primary structure of a protein molecule. The spatial arrangement of AA residues is not considered at this level (Fig. 1.2). Certain sections of the polypeptide chain assume different spatial arrangements due to H-bonding. These form the secondary structure consisting of α-helices, β-turns and sheets, and random coils (Fig. 1.2). Hydrophobic interactions between the nonpolar side chains of the AA of a polypeptide chain that has assumed a secondary structure, and the disulfide bonds between cysteine residues form a compact internal scaffold that stabilizes the overall 3-D arrangement (conformation) of the polypeptide. This 3-D structure is the tertiary-level arrangement of the protein and contains "domains" or regions that are tightly folded and compact, providing specific structural or functional feature(s) of a protein. Multimeric proteins can also exist in a quaternary structure (Fig. 1.2), which refers to the spatial relationship of polypeptides (or subunits) within the protein (eg, hemoglobin). The AA sequence of a protein determines the tertiary structure which in turn determines its chemical, biological, and physical function, that is, protein function is derived from structure, and the structure is derived from the sequence, linking the genetic code of protein expression to its functional role.

1.2.1.2 Classification of Proteins

Due to the enormous diversity of proteins, several classification systems exist and are in use for categorizing food proteins (Fig. 1.2). Some systems pertain to technological application, while some are based upon chemical and biological properties. The oldest protein classification system, still in use today, is based on the solubility of proteins in various solutions first identified by Thomas B. Osborne (1859–1929). Over the years, the Osborne classification system evolved and has identified five protein groups: (1) the albumins, are readily soluble in water and dilute salt solutions do not have specific AA composition, but are abundant in the acidic AAs (albumins are widely found in body fluids and plant storage organs such as seeds); (2) the globulins, are poorly soluble in water, but readily soluble in dilute salt solutions, usually rich in glutamates and aspartates (globulins are abundant in animal and plant cells); (3) the histones, are soluble in acidic salt solutions and rich in basic AAs with a small amount of *S*-containing AA (histones make complexes with nucleic acids and are components of the nuclei of eukaryotic cells); (4) the prolamins, are insoluble in water

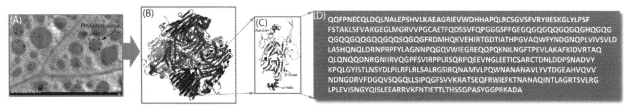

FIGURE 1.2 Proteins have well-organized and complex structure and there are several classification systems in use adding more complexity. Components (A)–(D) illustrate protein structure hierarchy using major globulin seed storage protein cruciferin of canola/rapeseed: (A) 11S cruciferin is one of the proteins stored in protein storage vacuoles of crucifer oilseeds; (B) according to crystal structure data six subunits (monomers) form cruciferin quaternary structure and the dotted circle outlines one cruciferin subunit; (C) tertiary structure of a cruciferin subunit showing secondary structure components of the composing two (acidic and basic) polypeptide chains; (D) primary structure or amino acid (AA) sequence of the two polypeptide chains that fold and form cruciferin CRUA subunit (466 AAs are found in the acidic and basic polypeptides without signal peptide); and (E) a list of commonly used protein categorization schemes.

and absolute ethanol, but soluble in ethanol–water mixtures, and commonly have high arginine, proline, glutamate, and asparagine levels; and (5) the scleroproteins, are insoluble in water and salt solutions, and include fibrous proteins of animal connective tissues rich in glycyl, prolyl, and alanyl residues. The solubility-based classification is most relevant to food processing and commercial manufacturing of food proteins.

Another classification system distinguishes proteins as simple or conjugated (or complex). Simple proteins generate only AA upon hydrolysis. Conjugated proteins have nonprotein chemical (prosthetic) groups attached to the molecule. Conjugation with prosthetic groups generates proteins with multiple functions, further increasing the diversity of proteins. Conjugated proteins are categorized according to the non-AA component of the molecule such as phosphoproteins, glycoproteins, lipoproteins, metalloproteins, and nucleoproteins.

Proteins are also classified according to their shape as fibrous or globular. Fibrous proteins are composed of extended polypeptide chains that are rod-shaped, fibrous, or thread-like. Globular proteins are folded and the molecule is compact, spherical, or ellipsoidal in shape. The shape and hydrodynamic parameters of the molecule are used in isolating food proteins. The sedimentation coefficient or "$S_{20,w}$" in Svedberg units measures how fast a molecule moves in a concentration gradient, assuming the proteins are spherical in shape. For example, in the protein repertoire of soybean seeds, 11S globulin glycinin (~360 kDa), 7S globulin β-conglycinin (150–200 kDa), and 2S albumin (8 kDa) Bowman–Birk trypsin inhibitor are found (Lakemond & Vereijken, 2003).

Proteins are also classified specific to their function as catalytic, structural, regulatory or hormonal, transport, genetic, immune, contractile, and storage. One of the oldest examples of this type of classification system is the Enzyme Commission, a hierarchical classification that defines six principal classes of enzymes based on their function.

Food proteins can be classified according to nutritional value. Complete proteins contain essential AAs (Fig. 1.1) in the proportion required by the human body, whereas incomplete proteins are those that are deficient in one or more essential AAs. Most proteins of animal origin and some plant proteins are complete, whereas some animal proteins (such as collagen) and most plant proteins fall into the incomplete protein category.

Structure-based classification systems have evolved with the growing knowledge and accumulating information on primary and tertiary structure of the proteins and allow protein to merge into structural classes and families based on molecular similarity. This classification is useful in many scientific areas, including the study of food allergens (Gendel, 2004; Gendel & Jenkins, 2006). Protein databases (examples are: Protein Data Bank, http://www.rcsb.org/pdb/home/home.do and structural classification of proteins, http://scop.mrc-lmb.cam.ac.uk/scop/) are available that identify different hierarchies when proteins are merged and compared; the common ones being family, superfamily, and folds. When the biological activities of food proteins are considered (including allergenicity, enzyme activity, antimicrobial activity, etc.), protein structure-based classification is highly relevant. Identification of the biochemical function can be obtained through homology-based structure modeling (Laskowski, Watson, & Thortonton, 2005). For example, the studies of Barre et al. (2005, 2007) and Cabanos et al. (2010) showed the possibilities of predicting allergenicity of peanut proteins Ara h1, Ara h2, Ara h3, and profilin using in silico homology modeling of the 3-D structure. This technique is also useful in screening potential allergenicity of novel proteins.

High-throughput, molecular biology technologies have generated enormous amounts of information about protein structure and function, and evolution of genes and gene products of several food crops. Databases such as UniProt or the Universal Protein Resource (http://www.uniprot.org) are comprehensive resources for protein sequences and their biological functions. Aligning biochemical and technological aspects of food protein with structure-based protein classifications become highly relevant to link food protein advances with genomics; simultaneously increasing learning among users.

1.2.2 Protein as a Macronutrient in Food

Protein is one of the three macronutrients that we need to obtain from our food. As a source of energy, food proteins generate 4 kcal/g. Upon consumption, food proteins are deconstructed to an absorbable form, single AAs or peptides of two or three AAs (Fig. 1.1). Proteolytic enzymes of gastric and intestinal fluids catalyze hydrolytic reactions that generate medium and small peptides and reach the lumen of the small intestine. The end products of protein digestion are transported to the intestinal bloodstream via specific transporters. Absorption of intact proteins is rare because intestinal epithelial cells are bound together by tight junctions making a polymer-impermeable membrane (except, in the first few days after birth to allow absorption of immunoglobulins in colostrum to build a temporary immune system). However, certain disease conditions, such as celiac disease and immature barrier functions of intestinal mucosal layer, can allow intact proteins and large peptide fragments to escape normal barriers and enter into the bloodstream. Some of the food proteins that are absorbed intact have the ability to elicit an initial IgE response and then elicit a clinical response on subsequent exposure to the same or similar protein; the basis of gastrointestinal allergenicity of proteins.

As depicted in Fig. 1.1, the AAs acquired from food protein digestion are also the same AAs needed for protein synthesis in the human body. In nutritional terms, AAs are grouped according to their metabolic demand, which is the flow of AAs through metabolic pathways that together maintain structure and function of the body. The AAs that cannot be synthesized in our body are essential (indispensable) AAs (EAA; Fig. 1.1) and must be obtained from food sources. Effective utilization of digestible dietary proteins occurs with a balance of those EAAs and ones that are nonessential or dispensable. Nonessential or dispensable AAs (Fig. 1.1) are also obtained through dietary sources and somewhat adequate amounts are available in the body AA pool. Conditionally essential AAs (Fig. 1.1) are those that can be limited under special pathophysiological conditions (such as individuals in severe catabolic distress).

The basic concepts of AA requirements for growth and maintenance were understood since the time (1916) of experiments of Thomas B. Osborne and Laffayette E. Mendel, who systematically studied many food sources. Digestibility of a food protein is not a fixed attribute of the food, but rather reflects the interactions between food and the person eating it. Therefore, digestibility is subjected to individual variation. The bioavailability of AAs from food protein digestion is considered under the following three criteria: (1) net absorption of AAs; (2) chemical integrity (the proportion of AA that is absorbed and utilized); and (3) freedom of interference from other components that limit AA utilization. The AAs that are not used in peptide or protein synthesis are deaminated and the C-unit is used for energy or synthesis of glucose or fatty acids. Many of the proteins in our body serve specific functions in the maintenance of life; any loss in body proteins is a loss of cellular function. The human body has no true reserves of protein (in contrast to lipids or carbohydrates), therefore, dietary protein insufficiency is compensated by catabolizing some, but not all, tissue proteins of our body. The pool of protein that is irreversibly catabolized in the course of a body's metabolism is the recommended daily protein intake, which varies when considering age, physiological status, and gender. According to WHO/FAO/UNU (2002) recommendations, assuming a mean total protein requirement of 0.66 g/kg per day for a healthy adult, in order to maintain body N homeostasis, intakes of about 0.18 and 0.48 g/kg per day of indispensable and dispensable AAs, respectively, are estimated. The quality of protein is determined by how well it is digested and absorbed. Indices and measurements that are developed to assess and compare protein nutritional quality include protein efficiency ratio (PER), protein digestibility corrected amino acid score (PDCAAS) and most recently the digestible ileal amino acid score (DIAAS) (FAO, 2013).

The AAs that are released from food proteins, enter into the body's AA pool from which all cells withdraw the AAs for synthesis of biologically valuable proteins, peptides, and AA derivatives. The peptides are hormones or cytokines of the various signaling systems of our body. Food-protein-derived bioactive peptides (mainly di- and tripeptides) once absorbed in sufficient amounts can elicit systemic responses providing a physiological benefit, such as blood pressure regulation, inhibition of cancer cells, cholesterol reduction, appetite suppression, and improved respiration (Rutherfurd-Markwick, 2012).

1.2.2.1 Allergenicity and Food Protein

About 6–8% of newborns to 3-year-olds and ~4% of adults in the United States show adverse immune responses to certain food proteins. Proteins that induce an allergic response must be present in substantial amounts in the food supply, stable during processing, and resistant to heat and digestion in the gastrointestinal tract. Most of the allergenic proteins have common structural features, such as multiple, linear IgE-binding epitopes, multiple disulfide bonds, repetitive motifs, and glycosylation; however, it is not possible to point out any structural motif or conformational sequence pattern common to all allergenic proteins (Gendel, 2002).

Almost all plant food allergens known are either protective (eg, lipid transfer proteins and profilins) or seed storage proteins, and those that trigger development of an allergic response through the gastrointestinal tract belong to either the cupin or prolamin superfamilies (Shewry, Beaudoin, Jenkins, Griffiths-Jones, & Mills, 2002). However, according to the molecular basis of cross-reactivity, sharing of structural determinants and sequence similarities has been observed in a limited number of protein families (Pfam). According to allergenic protein database ALLFAM (http://www.meduniwien.ac.at/allergens/allfam) only 2% of known domains, consisting of 1043 proteins from 180 Pfam (which is a small subset of 12,273 Pfam) are identified as allergens (Hoffmann-Sommergruber & Mills, 2009; Radauer, Bublin, Wagner, Mari, & Breiteneder, 2008). Processing-induced structural changes in the protein molecule can substantially reduce allergenicity of proteins, an essential factor in food processing. An example is hydrolytic cleavage of the epitope region during protein hydrolysate preparation (Sen et al., 2002; Terracciano, Isoardi, Arrigoni, Zoja, & Martelli, 2002).

1.2.3 Protein as a Macromolecule in Food Systems

Besides providing required AAs, proteins provide several useful properties (functional properties) that are central to make our food desirable and pleasurable to consume. After all, we eat food rather than nutrients. Therefore, we utilize the functionality of proteins to satisfy many nonnutritional needs of eating food. Moreover, the nutritional value and functional properties go hand-in-hand when making a protein-rich food more desirable to eat. The functional properties are related to the multitude of chemical and physical properties that protein can assume. The functionality of food proteins was first defined by Kinsella (1976), "any physico-chemical property which affects the processing and behavior of protein in food systems, as judged by the quality attributes of the final product." This broad definition includes complex interactions of the protein molecules with other food components, and the nature of the environment in which these interactions occur (Kinsella, 1976). Protein has an effect on the following three main acceptability factors of food: (1) appearance (color, size, shape); (2) taste and flavor (aroma, smell, taste); and (3) texture (all perceptions that occurs through tactile, kinesthetic, visual, and hearing senses). Table 1.1 lists some examples of physicochemical properties of protein molecules and the functional and sensory properties they provide in food systems to show their integral relationships. It is important to mention that protein functional properties vary with the source, the environment (eg, pH, temperature, solvent and solute concentration, ionic strength, dielectric constant of the medium, and other macromolecules such as lipids and carbohydrates), and the treatment used during commercial protein processing (eg, modification of side chain residues, controlled denaturation and hydrolysis, drying, agglomeration). Similar to biological properties, the domains (eg, hydrophobic patches) and residues (eg, charged residues) on the protein molecule surface are the determining factors of how the protein will respond to its environment (eg, pH, temperature, other molecules), any number of possibilities it may be subject to during food processing. Therefore, manifestation of physicochemical properties of the protein molecules is dictated by the structural attributes of the protein molecule and the interaction with the environment.

TABLE 1.1 Examples of Functional Properties and Their Relationships With Physicochemical Properties of Proteins and Sensory Properties Provided in Foods

Functional Property	Mechanism and Physicochemical Property of Protein	Example Food System	Example Protein	Sensory Property
Solubility	Hydrophilicity, charge and ionization of surface residues, H-bonding	Milk, protein-rich beverages, nondairy milks	Dairy, soy, almond, rice, proteins	Flavor, taste, mouthfeel, turbidity
Viscosity	Hydrodynamic size and shape, H-bonding	Soups, gravies, salad dressings, desserts	Gelatin, soy, egg	Taste, consistency, mouthfeel
Water binding	H-bonding, ionic hydration	Comminuted meats, low-fat meat products, bakery products	Muscle, egg, cereal, soy proteins	Texture, consistency
Gelation (heat-induced)	Water entrapment and immobilization, network formation, thermal aggregation	Emulsified meat products, bakery products, puddings	Muscle, egg, dairy, and many seed proteins	Mouthfeel, texture, grittiness, smoothness
Cohesion and adhesion	Hydrophic-, ionic- and H-bonding	Emulsified meats, pasta and noodles, bakery products, extruded snacks	Muscle, egg, dairy, and several seed proteins	Stickiness, chewiness, particulate
Elasticity	Hydrophobic bonding, disulfide cross-linking	Meat products, leavened bakery products, extruded products	Muscle proteins, gluten protein, casein	Texture, crispiness, chewiness
Emulsification	Adsorption and film formation in oil–water interface, hydrophobicity and hydrophilicity	Comminuted meats, cakes, soups, salad dressings, nondairy milks, desserts	Muscle, egg, dairy, and several seed proteins	Mouthfeel, flavor, smoothness
Foaming	Adsorption and film formation in air–water interface, hydrophilicity and hydrophobicity	Ice cream, cakes, whipped toppings, mousses, desserts	Dairy, egg, and certain seed proteins	Mouthfeel, smoothness, frizziness
Fat and flavor binding	Hydrophobic bonding, entrapment	Flavored milks, protein-rich beverages, emulsified meats, bakery products, sauces and gravies	Dairy, egg, muscle, and many seed proteins	Flavor, odor, smoothness

Source: Adapted from Damodaran, S. (1997). Food proteins: An overview. In: S. Damodaran & A. Paraf (Eds.), *Food proteins and their applications* (pp. 1–24). New York, NY: Marcel Dekker Inc (Damodaran, 1997).

Proteins from different sources manifest different functionalities. One example is the gluten proteins of wheat, which are known for extensibility which is useful in dough formation by trapping air and CO_2, which increase dough volume and create a porous structure in baked bread. Another example is that of egg white proteins, well-known to coagulate into a soft or firm solid with heat, and are capable of stabilizing air–water interfaces that create stable foams upon whipping. It is possible to relate essential functionalities of food proteins to the molecular structure and the interactions of protein with solvent and other molecules under given conditions. Establishing structure–function relationships of food protein enables us to relate or categorize proteins in relation to food functionalities. The structure–function relationship of food proteins for the nonbiological functions was first modeled by Nakai and group (Nakai, 1983; Nakai & Li-Chan, 1993) for various animal proteins. Later, Kumosinski, Brown, and Farrell (1991a,b) using casein (κ- and α s-1) showed that primary sequences of these proteins can be employed in modeling unrefined secondary and 3-D structures and prediction of structure–function relationships relevant in food applications. Use of bioinformatics data of food crops to predict functionality of seed storage proteins was recently (Withana-Gamage & Wanasundara, 2012) demonstrated by modeling and examining the structure of five known soybean glycinins (a 11S seed storage protein) using their primary sequences. Such investigations into protein structure—function relationships at a fundamental structure level show divergence may occur into a small number of groups, when food protein functionality is concerned. Such understanding is helpful in creating new food systems as well as finding sustainable proteins that can provide similar functions in replacement of costly proteins, such as animal muscle or milk protein. The functional properties of food proteins can be considered as the determining factors when using protein-containing ingredients for our "plate" and "palette." The food industry today uses functional properties to assess suitability of new protein sources/ingredients to create new food systems and also to reengineer existing foods with alternative protein sources.

1.2.4 Overview of Plant-Derived Protein and Alternate Protein Sources

Main dietary protein sources of prehistoric humans were animal-based. Modern humans may have started cultivating plants and domesticating animals, due to the associated variations in the climate in the early Holocene period (c. 10,000 years ago). Adoption of agriculture as a means of subsistence, during the "Neolithic revolution," has led to an increase in population, sedentism, and associated urbanization, which has led to a general decline in health and stature (Bar-Yosef & Belfer-Cohen, 1992; Richards, 2002). Furthermore, industrial agriculture has led to an emergence of nutritional disorders and disease conditions such as malnutrition, infectious disease, in addition to social inequalities (Armelagos, 2014). Diversity of food encompasses a variety of plants and living organisms, and is evident from cuisines of different world cultures. Although agricultural intensification continues to limit the number of plants and animal species in our diet, there are highly nutritious protein sources not yet mass produced. A few examples include indigenous pulses and root crops, ancient grains, lower organisms (eg, microalgae, fungal mycelia, yeasts, and insects in different stages of the life cycle). Most of these are supplemental protein sources depending on culture and geography.

One of the objectives of agriculture is to produce digestible N for humans from animal and plant protein sources. According to Prescott-Allen and Prescott-Allen (1990), only 103 plant species provide 90% of today's per capita supply of food by weight, calories, protein, and fat. The share of land area for feed production (to generate animal protein) is about 37% of cultivated land worldwide (Manceron, Ben-Ari, & Dumas, 2014). Cereals including rice, corn, wheat, barley, and oats, are staple foods in many cultures accounting for a major source of plant protein in the diet. Protein-rich legumes or pulses (eg, soy, lentil, chickpea, beans, peanut) and tree nuts (eg, almond, cashew, hazelnut, pecan) comprise major protein sources of vegan diets while supplementing dietary protein intakes. Existing protein sources are converted to food products based on traditional knowledge (eg, tofu and milk from soy, seitan from wheat) or through new technological interventions (eg, textured vegetable proteins from soy, chicken meat alternatives from pea). Legumes and oilseeds have become the major plant protein sources that generate nonanimal-derived counterparts to those of dairy (eg, milk, cheese, ice cream, yogurt-like desserts), and meat (burger-, frankfurter-, cutlet-like products).

When considered as a nutrient, proteins of animal sources differ from plant protein sources in their AA profile and the rate at which the absorbed AA are utilized in our body. Plant proteins are somewhat compromised by their limitation of one or more AA, therefore restoration of the deficient AAs is needed to reach the response rate equivalent to animal protein. The combination of plant protein sources improves protein quality of the blend due to their complementary AA profiles. A good example is that most of the pulses rich in lysine and deficient in S-AA provide complementary AA profile when combined with lysine-limited cereals such as corn, finger millet, rice, sorghum, and wheat. Scientific evidence is available to confirm that consumption of plant protein sources as a whole provides substantial health benefits, such as reducing cardiovascular disease and improved blood lipid profiles (Hu, 2003; Huang et al., 2014), circumventing type 2 diabetes (Trapp & Barnard, 2010), providing bone health (Massey, 2003), and diversifying gut microbiota (Glick-Bauer & Yeh, 2014). Lipids associated with plant protein sources are without cholesterol and composed of healthy fatty acid profiles. The associated cell walls of plants comprise the dietary fiber fraction and its minor components, such as phenolics and pigments, and the digestible carbohydrates, particularly starches, become slow in releasing glucose (low glycemic) due to matrix component association. Among the macronutrients, protein is the most satiating and fiber is effective in inducing the satiating effect (Bonnema, Altschwager, Thomas, & Salvin, 2015), therefore foods rich in both these provide dual activities by controlling appetite and food intake and, consequently, body weight. In contrast, meat proteins are associated with lipids with limited fatty acid diversity, comprised mainly of saturated fayy acids and also contain cholesterol, cell walls, and indigestible connective tissue (rich in collagen) has completely different composition than dietary fiber. The minor components, except vitamin B1 associated with animal tissues, are much more different than plant foods.

The unfolding chapters on different plant protein sources show a myriad of chemical components associated with those proteins and the multistep processes required in obtaining purified protein, subsequently employed in meat-like or animal protein-like product development. The components that will be eliminated through these processes are part of the whole nutritional package of the particular source. Separating protein fractions of cereals or legumes which are already part of our diet may remove valuable nutrients and reduce the wholesomeness of food. Rather, the focus ought to be on obtaining concentrated protein forms from crops that have less value as wholesome foods. A good example is canola/rapeseed meal. Canola/rapeseed meal is not a current food ingredient (compared to lentil or chickpea), which places it as a suitable candidate for protein ingredient production that may support the sustainability of this valuable oilseed crop as well as advance the alternate protein supply. Thorough understanding of chemical, biological, and physical properties of plant proteins, together with advances in engineering, food technology, and human nutrition can create food products that provide digestible N that are produced more economically and sustainably than animal protein.

1.3 SUSTAINABLE SOURCES OF PROTEINS

Plant-based diets including grains, nuts, seeds, pulses, and vegetables provide nitrogen. In fact, animals consume plant-derived protein to produce meat or milk. Plant proteins are produced more efficiently, and require less water, land, nitrogen, and fossil energy to produce a given amount of protein relative to animal-derived protein. The conversion of plant-based protein to meat is inefficient, and will be discussed later in the chapter. From the same amount of land, 20 times the amount of soy protein can be grown compared to a given quantity of beef (http://www.soyfoods.org/good-for-the-planet/soy-and-sustainability). In addition, the same land can produce 10 times the amount of beans and legumes or 13 times the amount of rice. In other words, consumption of a plant-based diet can feed 10–20 times more humans than if crops were cultivated for animal feed (http://www.greencommon.com/food-sustainability). This would translate to using fewer natural resources to produce food meant directly for human consumption.

There are several plant-based protein sources that have been consumed widely around the globe for many centuries. Grains (wheat, rice, millets, sorghum), seeds (chia, hemp), nuts (almond, walnut), pulses (beans, lentils, peas, lupins), and leaves (moringa, duckweed) are sources of proteins which can be sustainably produced. In addition to providing nitrogen, plant-based foods provide phytonutrients, vitamins, minerals, and fiber, which are essential for the body. Hemp and chia provide omega-3 fats, while pulses provide fiber for normal health and functioning. People in many parts of the globe have consumed such diets for centuries, and such diets have been found to benefit in a variety of ways including prevention of chronic diseases (Tuso, Ismail, Ha, & Bartolotto, 2013). Different trends are encouraging the shift in diets from meat-based to plant-based diets. Consumers are choosing diets based on locally produced foods, to support the environment and reduce the carbon footprint. In addition, consumers are aware of the health benefits of such diets. The following section discusses the trends that are shaping consumer shifts in dietary patterns.

1.3.1 Dietary Patterns Around the Globe

Two-thirds of the world's population lives primarily on plant-based diets, while a third lives primarily on meat-based diets. In the 21st century, a Western diet that is high in calories, animal products, refined fats and oils, sugars, and processed food, has spread in tandem with a global economy. A Western diet is associated with chronic Western diseases such as obesity, type 2 diabetes, coronary heart disease, and cancers of the breast, prostate, and bowel. What is even more alarming is that over a billion people remain undernourished and malnutrition is the single largest underlying cause of death worldwide and associated with over a third of all childhood deaths (WHO, 2010). Surely, the two extreme states of affairs are distressing and resolutions are intertwined in today's global economy.

In areas of the world such as China and Taiwan where Western diets have replaced traditional plant-based diets, increases in Western diseases have been found and higher consumption of animal-based foods has been implicated (Segelken, 2001). Following a 20-year epidemiological study (known as the China-Cornell-Oxford Project), authors of the China Study deduced that avoiding animal products altogether will eliminate, reduce, or reverse the evolution of Western diseases (Campbell & Campbell, 2005). Although opposition exists to the authors' conclusions, the China Study (one of the US's best-selling books about nutrition) has inspired a movement away from the current Western diet toward more plant-based nutrition.

On one hand, the Western diet has spread with a global economy. It evolved decades ago in the United States when demand rose for easy-to-prepare foods. New products were easily compared on market shelves for taste, convenience, and cost, and more often than not, at the expense of adequate nutrition. A competitive marketplace is a strong driver for high-yielding industrial food production; and highly processed foods that offer more volume for less money are a significant result of this competitiveness. As the world becomes increasingly technological in the 21st century, a Western diet that provides taste, convenience, and perceived value is attractive. As a result, multinational food companies have expanded rapidly to provide food products for a global economy. On the other hand, at its origin, is a movement away from a Western diet with its high consumption of animal products, processed foods, and impending health consequences.

1.3.2 Health and Wellness Trends

In spite of misperceptions that may exist that plant-based diets do not provide adequate protein for proper health; vegetarian, pescetarian, vegan, and predominantly plant-based Mediterranean diets, have all been shown to reduce the risk of obesity, type 2 diabetes, cancer, and coronary mortality, as well as, provide essential AAs to sustain life. Indeed, a majority of the world's people are nourished mainly by plant-based diets and benefit from optimal health and wellness compared to those on Western diets.

Resulting Western diseases have initiated public interest in the United States in food labels and food industry production practices, as well as an abundance of food and ingredients promoted as "good-for-you" such as plant protein powders, whole grains, ancient grains, sprouted grains and seeds, tree nuts, peanuts, pulses, and "superfoods" designated for being nutrient-dense. One of the "good-for-you" items, whole grains, contains all the essential components and naturally occurring nutrients of their intact seed or kernel. Studies support that eating one to three servings per day of whole grains (typically 16–48 g dry weight) instead of refined flours or refined grains as customary, lowers the risk of many chronic Western diseases. As a result, the amount of whole grain in a product has been promoted on thousands of labels, delivering on consumer interest in plants for improved health and wellness.

Other health-related catalysts that have sparked interest in the wholesomeness of the food supply include food safety outbreaks and food allergen awareness. The Food Allergen Labeling and Consumer Protection Act (FALCPA) is a US law that requires all food labels to list ingredients that may cause allergic reactions from the top eight food allergens identified in the United States. After implementation of FALCPA on Jan. 1, 2006, what has been coined "allergen warning labels", there has been a steady rise in "free-from" foods, for instance, gluten-free; wheat-free; soy-free; dairy-free; lactose-free; casein-free; animal-free; and "free-from" saturated fats, trans-fatty acids, and cholesterol.

Gluten-free foods, above all other "free-from" foods, have paved the way for interest in ancient grains (Blumenfeld, 2014). Ancient grains are loosely defined as cereals and pseudocereals that have not been repeatedly bred as modern day crops have been. Compared with commodity crops, in general, ancient grains are genetically diverse and can thrive in extreme environments using lower levels of pesticides, fertilizers, and irrigation, favoring a reduced carbon footprint. Ancient grains are also compared against conventional refined, bleached wheat flour, white rice, and corn, and praised for being more nutritious, higher in protein, micronutrients, and phytochemicals. Ancient grains that have the most consumer awareness are typically gluten-free and include sorghum, millet, quinoa, amaranth, and teff. However, other ancient grains in the wheat family are recognized such as einkorn, farro/emmer, khorason/Kamut, and spelt. Ancient grains have also gained public interest in efforts to protect biodiversity of heirloom and indigenous crops, as well as to support production of alternative crops relative to the world's dominant production of corn, wheat, and rice. Although ancient grains have been used at minor levels in many foods, they played major roles on consumer-facing labels, ancient grains have crossed over from niche into global food products with unique stories that appeal to consumers and at the same time satisfy demand for healthy, plant-based alternatives.

1.3.3 Product Trends

Plant proteins may also fit into "freedom foods," as stated by Christopher Shanahan, Global Program Manager for Frost & Sullivan (Gelski, 2015). In particular, "freedom foods" are not constrained by worries pertaining to human disease, animal welfare, and food safety concerns specific to animal-based proteins. In fact, plant proteins from pulses, seeds, and grains have significant roles within "freedom foods," "free-from," and "good-for-you" foods. Five to ten grams or more of plant protein per serving are often promoted on many foods, beverages, and healthy snacks. Plant proteins are regularly associated with energy; and labels may include wording such as "plant-powered protein," "powered by," "energized," and "fueled by." Plant proteins have been marketed to offer a "boost" of protein for energetic workouts, as well as for good breakfasts and most important part of the day to keep you moving. Plant proteins that have been recently highlighted in this manner include pea and other pulses, sunflower and pumpkin seeds, cashews, almonds, amaranth, quinoa, macadamia nuts, sesame seeds, hazelnuts, and walnuts. Above all accounts, soybean protein has been directly linked to heart health. According to US Code of Federal Regulations, Title 21, 101.82 the following health claim can be made on a food product containing at least 6.25 g soy protein per reference amount of that food item: "As part of a diet low in saturated fat and cholesterol, 25 g soy protein per day may reduce the risk of heart diseases." On a product such as this, one may also find the label adorned with wording such as "heart health" and "heart healthy protein."

Many plant-based powders, beverages, and meal replacements today have advertisements on consumer-facing labels such as "plant-based protein," "organic plant protein," "vegan," "green protein powder," "super-food," "complete and balanced protein," and/or "healthy alternative." Plant-based foods are also marketed to break down potential consumer barriers to entry. For example, plant-based foods draw special attention to calcium comparisons to dairy milk or omega levels relative to salmon. In addition, plant proteins in the form of sprouted grains and seeds with increased enzyme activity are increasing in popularity because of an association with disease healing, aid in digestion, nutrient absorption, and increased protein and nutrient density. Sprouted seeds include but are not limited to pumpkin, watermelon, chia, flax, hemp, and sunflower. On websites and in the media, plant protein is marketed as the future of protein. Although leading this movement are lentils, grains, and nuts in whole or minimally processed forms, there is some consideration spent on meat and dairy analogs (in general, analogs are highly processed plant ingredients made to simulate animal products). Often, manufacturers of plant-based meat analogs have heavy marketing campaigns that call out the meat industry on animal welfare and slaughterhouse issues, food safety concerns, environmental downsides with livestock, climate change and water scarcity, use of antibiotics and growth hormones, and negative health impacts of cholesterol and saturated fats.

A correlation has been discovered between Western diets high in meats, refined sugars, and fats, that is both unhealthy for humans as well as the planet (Tilman & Clark, 2014). Ecologists Tilman and Clark estimate that by 2050 food production for such diets will lead to an 80% increase in agriculture-based global greenhouse gas emissions. Production for Western-style diets has already caused damage, including deforestation in underdeveloped countries. The current increasing demand for Western foods will drive an escalation of land cleared for meat production and major oil crops soya and palm. Tilman and Clark's study unfolded quickly in media articles targeting Western diets as bad for human health and the environment (Healy, 2014; Skirble, 2014). Therefore, replacing traditional diets by Western-style diets is not sustainable. This dietary shift has accompanied a rise in type 2 diabetes, coronary heart disease, and other chronic Western diseases. A global trilemma of poor diet, health, and environment will require dietary, policy, and business solutions. This trilemma is likely to be exacerbated by the projected increase in the global population by 30% in the next 30 years and a further 10% by the turn of the century. Growing nutritious food for this large number of people will become vital. Below we will discuss how humanity can tackle this situation, and prepare to make critical choices.

1.4 REASONS TO CONSUME PLANT AND ALTERNATE PROTEINS

1.4.1 Living on the Earth in 2050

Nutritious food is one of the main requirements for human existence, along with water. As the population increases, a number of challenges loom for current residents in the years ahead. Various human activities, including agriculture, require exploitation of our natural resources such as land, water, and energy at high rates. The result is the emission of a large amount of greenhouse gases (GHG) contributing to climate change (Fig. 1.3). Much of this large population will reside in packed urban areas and will be affected by many inequalities in living standards. We will discuss these challenges in detail, and identify potential solutions, which can alter our path forward for a better life on earth. We can choose to stay on our current path until an overburdened earth is unable to support our current way of living, leaving

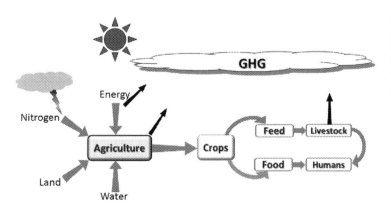

FIGURE 1.3 Production of food and consequences. Food chain produces GHG at prefarm, farm, and postfarm stages. Dairy and meat products account for approximately half of food-generated GHG emissions and 18% of global GHG emissions (FAO, 2006; Garnett, 2009). *GHG*, greenhouse gases.

future generations with an unpredictable and difficult planet to reside on. An alternate path exists, where humanity will be required to make hard choices. This would comprise collective sacrifices for the greater good. Some of these choices may not be appealing to current residents, such as reducing our appetite for animal-derived protein, altering our lifestyle for tackling global warming, or having stricter controls on population growth. Without these sacrifices, we face a grim future on this planet. "I believe that to meet the challenge of our times, human beings will have to develop a greater sense of universal responsibility. We must all learn to work not just for our own self, family, or nation but for the benefit of all humankind. Universal responsibility is the key to human survival. It is the best foundation for world peace, the equitable use of natural resources, and through concern for future generations, the proper care of the environment" (The 14th Dalai Lama, Tibet). The choice for a more hospitable earth is ours to make.

1.4.1.1 Population Increases and Their Effects

Our biggest challenge is a predicted swell in inhabitants adding to the current populace, which will likely affect every single aspect of life. The global population is growing by large numbers, and expected to peak around the beginning of the 22nd century (United Nations, 2015). It was only in 1804 that the world population reached 1 billion (Living Green, 2013). By 1960, the number had risen to 3 billion, and currently the earth supports 6.7 billion people. Numerous projections indicate that the global populace will swell to 9.6 billion by 2050, and expand to 11 billion by 2100 (Fig. 1.4).

"Some of these (Asian) countries, like India, far from needing a bigger population, would be better off with fewer people" (Jawaharlal Nehru, 1889—1964, India). This would have been a defining moment had India switched to a different path, and strongly advocated for smaller families.

Rather, India and China are the most populous countries, adding about 2.6 billion people. Over the next 30—50 years, India will become the most inhabited country in the world, and peak at 1.7 billion citizens, before gradually stabilizing with a population of 1.6 billion people. Although birth rates are declining in India, advances in health care, and medicine, have reduced infant mortality and aided the increase in new inhabitants. China's population, with stricter population controls over the last few decades, will increase marginally by 25 million over the same period. Some of the major increases in new inhabitants will be in Africa, where an additional 2 billion people will be born in the next several decades as birth rates edge up. The population of the United States, Canada, Japan, and parts of Western Europe will see minor increases or remain steady. One of the reasons is that birth rates in the developed economies are stagnant or declining.

This large influx in population over the next three decades will exacerbate several critical issues that confront us right now. People require certain necessities such as food, housing, education, healthcare, and jobs. In addition, infrastructure such as roads, power, and transportation are essential for a reasonable quality of life. Some countries have more access to these necessities than others. A repetitive theme would be the disparities between the developed

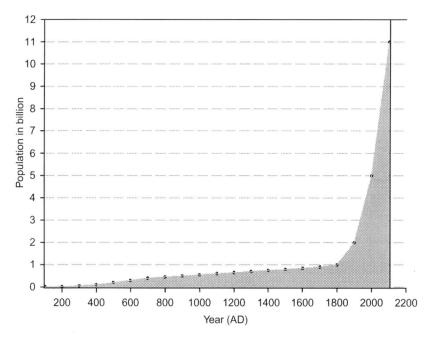

FIGURE 1.4 World population growth and projection for year 2100. *Adapted from United Nations, http://www.unfpa.org/world-population-trends.*

economies of the West versus emerging economies of South Asia, parts of South America and sub-Saharan Africa. Large pockets of people in parts of Asia and Africa go hungry or lack safe water. For the context of this book, we will focus on what we believe is our principal task, which would be to grow, and provide food for the 10 billion inhabitants of the earth in the next 30 years.

1.4.2 Natural Resources for Agriculture: Land, Water, Nitrogen

1.4.2.1 Land for Food, Feed, or Fuel?

Outside of the polar regions, agricultural land makes up about half the available vegetated land (World Res. Inst., 2013) and a third of this land is cultivated for crops. Another 30% is forested land, while the rest is arid/semiarid. Forested land is cleared for numerous needs, including agriculture, infrastructure, and natural resources. Each year, more than 10 million hectares of forested land make way for what we deem progress (FAO, 2012). "Any fool can destroy trees. They cannot run away; and if they could, they would still be destroyed,—chased and hunted down as long as fun or a dollar could be got out of their bark hides, branching horns, or magnificent bole backbones. Few that fell trees plant them; nor would planting avail much toward getting back anything like the noble primeval forests. During a man's life only saplings can be grown, in the place of the old trees—tens of centuries old—that have been destroyed" (John Muir, 1838–1914, USA).

Meat-based diets require large tracts of land dedicated to growing significant amounts of animal feed. Corn is predominantly grown, and used around the globe for animal feed. In the United States alone, over 80 million acres of land are utilized for growing and harvesting corn (USDA, 2015). Food production needs to increase 70% from current levels to support the 9.6 billion global inhabitants by 2050 (FAO, 2011), while meat consumption is projected to rise by 80%. Affluence and Western influence are driving food choices in many parts of the globe, including China where meat consumption is increasing. Meat production requires that livestock consume plant-based protein sources for conversion to animal protein. A contrary view from the cattle industry is that livestock consume roughage, which humans cannot digest. However, this land use for animal feed comes at the expense of growing other more nutritious and valuable grains, seeds, pulses, and vegetables. With its recent affluence, China is now able to purchase lands in other countries, especially southern Africa for growing its required crops at the cost to native farmers (National Geographic, 2014). Hence, it is irresponsible for consumers to increase meat consumption at the expense of the poor. More importantly, it is vital that we cultivate and utilize nonanimal protein sources directly for the benefit of all.

Current food supply in the Western societies is dominated with large mechanized farms producing corn, soy, wheat, and potato. A majority of the corn and soy crops go toward animal feed for meat and milk production. Although these mainstay crops have other uses besides animal feed, they have become globally entrenched in our food supply. Yields of crops are also reducing at the same time our world faces pressures from new inhabitants (FAO, 2012). This is due to several reasons including nutrient depletion, weather changes, and water stress. In addition, development of these seeds, especially corn and soy, originates from multinational organizations. Breeding and genetic engineering are techniques used to increase resistance to certain known pests. There is concern that a new type of pest could destroy some of these crops as they originate from the same monoculture. This would have a devastating effect on our food supply. At the same time, indigenous crops like millets, sorghum, marama beans, amaranth, and pulses have lagged behind in their uses, though that trend is reversing due to the plant protein boom. These sources provide valuable proteins and other nutrients, which can assist the global food supply.

1.4.2.2 Will Water Become a Commodity?

Water is one of our most precious resources, and distinguishes the earth from other planets. "Thousands have lived without love, not one without water" (William Auden). Water is critical for life to exist and in fact forms over 80% of our bodies. Without water, we will not be able to survive on this planet, nor can plants grow and produce all the things we enjoy. Lack of clean water supply leads to spread of diseases, and affects our long-term health. Six to eight million people die each year due to waterborne illness or other water-related disasters (UN World Report, 2013). Parts of Asia and Africa have acute water scarcity, and around 800 million inhabitants do not have a source of clean water (McDonald et al., 2011). Ensuring a clean water supply is an important step for a sustainable planet.

Though 70% of the earth's surface is covered with water, most of it is salty and present in seas and oceans. Most of the fresh water falls as precipitation, and accounts for about 2% of all available water. Fresh water is present in lakes, reservoirs, as snow on mountains, and as polar ice. Some regions of the earth receive a large amount of rainfall, while other regions are extremely dry. Assam in northeast India receives over 500 cm of rain during the monsoon, while the

Chilean desert has seen less than 0.1 cm of rain. Rainwater requires building of large reservoirs to prevent run-offs and enable providing for various uses. Though the Great Lakes in North America have a large supply of fresh water, it is not viable to supply this water across the states. Careful utilization and reusing of our locally available fresh water supplies in a sensible manner is even more critical.

Water classification into several types is based on its usability. These include blue water (present in water bodies such as lakes, reservoirs, and aquifers), green water (rainfall), and gray water (water from washing machines and baths). Blue water is widely used for agriculture via irrigation canals. Tapping of this source occurs, especially in areas of limited rainfall or in places where agriculture would otherwise not be possible. One of the main nonfood uses of blue water is in the maintenance of golf courses. This use of land and water for the benefit of a few should be a topic of discussion in a warming planet. Plants and their roots use green water, which falls as precipitation. This water is also lost to the atmosphere via transpiration. Since agriculture depends on green and blue waters, choosing optimum plants for that region is crucial.

With an unpredictable weather pattern in recent times, it is increasingly important that we reuse gray water, which does not include sewage water. Soapy water from kitchens and baths will be tolerated by plants, and this would be a primary use of gray water. However, any use of chemicals or solvents will likely affect the plant negatively. The reuse of gray water is helpful for the environment, especially in areas of reduced rainfall or during times of drought. Awareness of trapping rainfall (rain harvesting) is increasing around the globe as people recognize that water supply is precious. Desalination is another important process to provide clean water, and is used primarily in the Middle East due to its high cost and need.

Water stress, or the lack of sufficient water availability, is expected to increase in the next several years. In rainfall-deficient areas, we have been tapping into ground water supplies to nourish our crops. Aquifers (blue water) are our reserve supply of fresh water and require a long time to accumulate. In fact, in the plains of India, China, and now California, deep wells are tapping into aquifers for agriculture. Water stress affects crop yields and this reduction in yields correlates to climate change data. Higher temperatures affect the amount of rainfall, and a lack of rainfall creates a drier weather pattern. Wheat cultivars showed changes in overall plant growth and lower yields with reduced water availability (Akram, 2011). Similar results were observed when the common bean (*Phaseolus vulgaris* L) was subjected to water stress (Manjeru, Madanzi, Makeredza, Nciizah, & Sithole, 2007). The authors proposed that seeds would need planting much earlier in times of dry weather to ensure that the plants can mature, and be ready for harvest. Other techniques, such as drip irrigation or growing plants with shorter maturity times, will become necessary. More farmers and planners will require adaptation to these situations in the coming decades.

Water is critical for agriculture and consumes 70% of the available fresh water (Clay, 2004). Water footprint or the amount of water used per capita is highest in developed countries. Countries with a meat-based diet require more water use, while the footprint is low in the emerging economies consuming a plant-based diet. Water consumption is high in developed economies partly due to the greater availability of clean water, but also due to the use of water to grow crops meant for animal feed, and ultimately for meat production (Hoekstra & Mekonnen, 2012). Data from the FAO and United Nations indicate that it takes 15,000 L of water to produce 1 kg of beef, which is seven times the amount needed to produce 1 kg of rice or soybeans. Those consuming meat should understand that the resources needed to satisfy their plates could support numerous people in other parts of the globe. A variety of plants, grains, and pulses utilize less water, yet provide much higher usable protein per acre. Aligning our diets with the goals ahead will ensure that current water supplies last for our future generations.

1.4.2.3 Fossil Energy, Nitrogen, and Proteins

Nitrogen is the next important component in food production. While nitrogen is plentiful in the atmosphere, it requires conversion to soluble forms such as ammonium, and its salt, or as nitrates for use by the plants. Natural sources of soluble nitrogen form during lightning storms. The intense thermal energy in lightning creates nitrates from nitrogen, which fall to the ground during precipitation. A preferred mode would be the fixing of nitrogen to the soil by bacteria. Rhizobia aid in the conversion of nitrogen to ammonia, which the crops absorb to form proteins (Dixon & Wheeler, 1986). In addition, pulses and other leguminous crops also fix nitrogen in the soil (Herridge, Peoples, & Boddey, 2008). This process helps the soil retain its fertility and improve the yields of the following crop. There is a symbiotic relationship between Rhizobia and leguminous plants. The legumes provide energy to the bacteria, while the bacterium fixes the nitrogen for the plant to take up (Brewin, 2010).

To increase yields, farmers began to add fertilizers in the 1960s. These fertilizers contain soluble forms of nitrogen, which begin with the formation of ammonia by the Haber–Bosch process. This process is energy-intensive and highly dependent on fossil fuels. Ubiquitous addition of fertilizers is common nowadays and farmers depend on their use to boost crop yields. Global demand for fertilizers is expected to surpass more than 200 million tons, and is expected to increase in the next couple of decades as farmers face pressure to produce more crops from each hectare of arable land (FAO, 2015). It is worth noting that a study found that plants absorbed only a portion (15—20%) of the nitrogen added (UNEP, 2007). Thus, the addition of nitrogen as fertilizers far exceeds the amount required by crops, creating an imbalance in the nitrogen cycle (Fields, 2004). The low cost of fertilizers relative to the need for increasing food production is leading to this situation. Unused nitrogen dissolves in water and ends up in water bodies, leading to undesirable environmental effects such as algal blooms. Furthermore, fertilizers release nitrous oxide through denitrification by anaerobic bacteria in the soil (Bremner & Blackmer, 1978). Nitrous oxide is a potent GHG and a contributory factor to the warming of the planet. Continued addition of fertilizer will create additional nitrous oxide and the likelihood of a warmer planet.

1.4.3 Global Warming and Climate Change

Increased population, their needs, and the advent of industrialization have played a role in the warmer temperatures the earth has observed in recent times. The resultant increases in temperatures have occurred throughout the globe with various effects. GHG, such as carbon dioxide (CO_2), methane, and nitrous oxide, have increased due to a variety of human activities, such as power generation, transportation, and agriculture (Fig. 1.3). CO_2 levels have increased from 280 ppm in the preindustrial era to near 400 ppm currently (Climate Central, 2014). GHG trap heat radiation, reducing the earth's ability to reflect heat, causing temperatures to rise. Global warming has caused temperatures to increase by about 1°C over the last 100 years (UCAR, 2015). Melting of polar ice caps or drying up of glaciers are examples of the effects of global warming. The consequences of warmer temperatures include a projected rise in sea levels, which may submerge coastal lands over the next century. In addition, rising temperatures are likely to make storms or weather events stronger as heat increases moisture availability from water bodies. Unpredictable changes in weather patterns may also affect or change areas of precipitation. Therefore, droughts or floods may occur in regions unaccustomed to these events in recent times.

"What nature does in the course of long periods we do every day when we suddenly change the environment in which some species of living plant is situated" (Lamarck, 1809). Removal of forests releases large amounts of stored CO_2 and about a quarter of the CO_2 increase is due to deforestation which is currently >10 million hectares annually (FAO, 2012). Forests not only help to temper the weather but also to utilize and store carbon while helping to prevent erosion. The replacement of forested land for agriculture or infrastructure results in irreparable damage to the environment. This includes run-offs and landslides after heavy rainfall, while the lack of trees affects wildlife habitats. A new study shows that a mass extinction of animals is ongoing (Ceballos et al., 2015). The authors point out that this sixth mass extinction has higher rates than the prior five extinctions and that many more species may vanish. "Wilderness is not a luxury but a necessity of the human spirit, as vital to our lives as water and good bread" (Edward Abbey, 1927—48, USA).

Vegetation is classified as C3 or C4 depending on the type of molecule formed during photosynthesis. Thus, C3 plants form a 3-carbon moiety, while C4 plants form a 4-carbon molecule (Smithsonian Environmental Research Centre (SERC) CO_2 Lab, http://www.serc.si.edu/labs/co2/c3_c4_plants.aspx). The majority (about 95%) of all vegetative growth is C3 plants. They include many of the common vegetables and grains we consume such as beans, potato, rice, and wheat. C3 plants capture CO_2 during daylight by opening their pores. This process can increase evaporation from the leaves and make C3 plants more susceptible to heat and vagaries in weather. C4 plants include corn, amaranth, sugarcane, and most grasses. These plants can absorb CO_2 during the night, when the weather is relatively cooler, and are less affected by drier weather. C4 plants have a more efficient method to absorb CO_2 and can open their stomata for a shorter time.

A number of studies have determined the effects of projected high CO_2 levels in the atmosphere. Increased CO_2 levels led to faster growth of C3 plants, but less nutritious produce. Increased photosynthesis caused more leaf growth and higher starch to protein levels (Weigel, 2014). C3 grains and legumes also contained lower levels of iron and zinc, while C4 plants were less affected (Myers et al., 2014). High CO_2 levels also reduced nitrogen in the air and C3 plants had lower protein content (Pleijel & Uddling, 2011). Wheat, rice, and soybeans had lesser protein levels, and addition of fertilizers did not help counter this reduction. Thus, producing nutritious food will likely become a challenge in a warmer environment.

1.4.4 Quality of Life

"Excessive (population) growth may reduce output per worker, repress levels of living for the masses and engender strife" (Confucius, 551–479 BC, China). Humanity has always tried to come up with solutions for inequality that has long existed. There is a growing disparity between the developed and developing countries. Population levels affect several indicators including resource availability, incomes, food, education, jobs, and access to health care. A lower population in the Western world aids in a higher percapita expenditure for other needs, while high populations in the emerging economies negatively affect many quality of life indicators.

A sustainable development should include a variety of support structures for these inhabitants. Over the last several decades, farming has declined significantly, and fewer people own larger farms in developed countries. In the emerging economies, including parts of Asia and sub-Saharan Africa, small farms are still the norm. Wealthier nations like China are now acquiring these farms to cover their appetite for natural resources (National Geographic, 2014). Agriculture and the growing of crops require a lot of capital, including equipment, fertilizers, and seeds. Fair trade helps farmers receive a reasonable compensation for their efforts. Farmers need to ensure that they are practicing sustainable cultivation methods, and supporting the environment. This relationship ensures that both farmers and the consumers receive a good product and are supportive of the environment.

By 2050, about 65% of the global population or 6.25 billion will be living in urban locations (UN World Report, 2013). Cities or urban dwellings have been a magnet for migrants in several countries due to the available opportunities for a better life. However, with the projected urban swell of 6 billion people, planners are finding that income inequality, inadequate resources, and declining budgets have contributed to this inability to provide an equitable quality of life. This portends an increase in slum dwelling in the developing world with less access to opportunities (Awasthi, 2011). Food security is a major concern now, and in the future. "An imbalance between rich and poor is the oldest and most fatal ailment of all republics" (Plutarch, 46–119 AD, Ancient Greece). Food security, lack of socioeconomic mobility, and an increased population are all the ingredients of a tinderbox waiting to explode. In addition, lack of healthcare may lead to endemic diseases and exacerbate an already inflamed state of affairs. Hence, not only providing food, but assisting people with support in their personal situations including talking jobs, education, and healthcare will alleviate some of the concerns that are central to this issue (Clover, 2003).

1.5 MEAT CONSUMPTION: WHY WE ARE ON THE CURRENT PATH

A central theme in the challenges we face in tackling global hunger is the consumption of meat. Meat consumption is a mainstay of Western diets, and increasing in other parts of the globe. The United States consumes 325 g of meat per person per day, which is the equivalent of three hamburger patties. Consumption of meat and milk is increasing in the developing economies, driven by urbanization and affluence (Delgado, 2003). China now consumes more meat than the United States. Though pork is the meat of choice, beef consumption has steadily risen to about 4 k/capita. This is still a very large number as the Chinese population is four times that of the United States.

Meat consumption by itself is not the issue, but rather the large requirement of dedicated land, water, nitrogen, and fossil energy. Crops for animal feed cover greater than 90 million acres of land in the United States. The primary use of corn is animal feed, while other uses include biofuel, food ingredients, and products (USDA-ERS). Contributing factors for dependence on grain include the long winter in much of North America and Europe, and its low cost. The resources required in converting plant matter to animal-derived protein, such as meat or milk, is very poor and inefficient. The feed conversion ratio (FCR) determines the amount of feed required to produce 1 kg of meat or milk. Typical FCR is 7:1, while the figures range from 5 to 20 kg of dry feed matter (National Research Council, 2000). Some studies from the meat industry also indicate that the FCR is much smaller. The meat industry contends that if the fact that cows consuming matter unsuitable for human digestion is taken into consideration, meat production is not unsustainable.

Feed requirements are different for pigs and chicken compared to cows and sheep. The presence of multiple stomachs and a variety of microorganisms aid cows, goats, and sheep to breakdown plant matter. Rumen microorganisms produce volatile fatty acids from carbohydrates for energy. Enteric fermentation also breaks down plant protein into AAs, which are then converted into animal protein, either meat or milk. A result of the rumen microorganisms' metabolism is the production of methane, which is a GHG 20 times more potent than CO_2.

Methane, nitrous oxide, and other hydrofluorocarbons, are grouped together as short-lived climate pollutants (SLCPs). Livestock release methane mainly by belching and about 10% via the excreta. In addition, nitrous oxide is released via the excreta, though most of the nitrous oxide present in the atmosphere develops from fertilizer denitrification. Together with CO_2, methane and nitrous oxide add to GHG produced from agriculture. New studies have found that CO_2 still ranks as the main GHG, whose emissions we need to control (Ramanathan & Feng, 2008). Though SLCPs are several times more potent than CO_2, they last for a decade in the atmosphere, while CO_2 lasts for centuries. Therefore, warming-induced changes to our planet can be longlasting with unpredictable changes to our weather and living traditions.

1.6 ROLE OF THE CONSUMER FOR THE GREATER GOOD

We have discussed why proteins are important for human nutrition, the challenges we face in providing nutrition for 9.7 billion people, the consequences of staying on a meat-based diet, and trends moving consumers to change dietary patterns. Several plant-based and alternate protein sources have provided sustenance for people around the globe for centuries in addition to supporting health. The following chapters will discuss the sustainability of each protein source, their benefits and applications. The presence of allergens or antinutritional factors may limit the use of some proteins. Methods to mitigate and broaden this source will follow, along with a comparison of the AA profiles relative to animal-derived protein. The book will conclude with a discussion on consumer's taste preferences and ways of influencing those on a meat-based diet to consider a plant-based diet. Besides, food security will become important as the population reaches 10 billion and many critical issues will require spirited debate and action.

"The hungry world cannot be fed until and unless growth of its resources and the growth of its population come into balance. Each man and woman and each nation must make decisions of conscience and policy in the face of this great problem" (Lyndon Johnson, 1903–73, USA). There is a consequence if we continue to increase meat consumption, which would result in our using much of the natural resources (land, water, energy) in the near future. The resultant GHG emission would create an earth that is increasingly warmer and with a very different environment for future generations. It is imperative we choose an alternate path, modify our diets, and work to reduce our population growth. In either situation, we may have to deal with certain unpredictable or unintended consequences. The second path will require sacrifices from current inhabitants to ensure that the planet is habitable for the future. We can choose this second path ourselves by making a conscious choice to reduce meat consumption, food waste, and decrease future population growth. If each of us fails to adhere to this choice, policy changes may be required to affect this change. This would mean that we have crossed a tipping point, where someone else forces us to change our food habits and daily activities or commit to a one-child policy.

"You must be the change you wish to see in the world" (Mahatma Gandhi, 1869–1948, India). For every aspect of life that we will change, there will be opportunities to find better solutions. For example, inclusion of grains, legumes, and other produce will positively affect the health of many in Western societies, such as the reduction in chronic and systemic diseases like cardiovascular and diabetes. Various branches of science will get a boost as we try to find better methods to grow, preserve, and package foods to reduce wastage. New research into agriculture, biotechnology, and other related sciences will require understanding and the creation of seeds for a new type of weather pattern, such as those that withstand drier climates or more types of plants that can fix nitrogen. Greater understanding of the microbiome may present opportunities to alter our diets and shift to a healthier lifestyle. The potential reduction in population forecasts may assist in preserving our resources. In addition, with the needed scientific advances required to make our future, new types of job opportunities may arise, perhaps providing a better socioeconomic climate. Ultimately, the seemingly dire situation ahead of us may require greater cooperation for resources between various nations. If approached in an appropriate manner, these challenges may create a common bond, bringing people together and create a more hospitable planet. "The greater the obstacle, the more glory in overcoming it" (Molière, 1622–73, France). The choices for the future of our planet are ours to make.

REFERENCES

Akram (2011). Growth and yield components of wheat under water stress of different growth stages. *Bangladesh Journal of Agricultural Research, 36* (3), 455–468.

Armelagos, G. J. (2014). Brain evolution, the determinates of food choice, and the omnivore's dilemma. *Critical Reviews in Food Science and Nutrition, 54*, 1330–1341.

Awasthi, P. (2011). Socio-economic challenges and sustainable development in developing countries. *SMS Management Insight, 7*(2), 56–63.

Barre, A., Borges, J.-P., & Rougé, P. (2005). Molecular modelling of the major peanut allergen, Ara h1 and other homotrimeric allergens of the cupin superfamily: A structural basis for their IgE-binding cross-reactivity. *Biochimie, 78*, 499–506.

Barre, A., Jacquet, G., Sordet, C., Culerrier, R., & Rougé, P. (2007). Homology modelling and conformational analysis of IgE-binding epitopes of Ara h3 and other legumin allergens with a cupin fold from tree nuts. *Molecular Immunology, 44*, 3243–3255.

Bar-Yosef, O., & Belfer-Cohen, A. (1992). From foraging to farming in the Mediterranean Levant. In A. B. Gebauer, & T. D. Price (Eds.), *Transition to agriculture in prehistory* (pp. 21–48). Madison: Prehistory Press.

Blumenfeld, J. (2014). New love for ancient grains and what it means for the future of food. *Nutrition Business Journal*, November-December, 38–41. http://www.newhope360.com/nbj.

Bonnema, A. L., Altschwager, D., Thomas, W., & Salvin, J. L. (2015). The effects of beef-based meal compared to a calorie matched bean-based meal on appetite and food intake. *Journal of Food Science, 80*, H2038–H2093.

Bremner, J. M., & Blackmer, A. M. (1978). Nitrous oxide: Emission from soils during nitrification of fertilizer nitrogen. *Science, 199*, 295–296.

Brewin, N. J. (2010). *Root nodules (legume–rhizobium symbiosis). eLS*. Chichester: John Wiley & Sons Ltd.

Cabanos, C., Tandang-Silvas, M. R., Odijk, V., Brostedt, P., Tanaka, A., Utsumi, S., & Maruyama, N. (2010). Expression, purification, cross reactivity and homology modelling of peanut profilin. *Protein Expression and Purification, 73*, 36–45.

Campbell, T. C., & Campbell, T. M. (2005). *The China study: Startling implications for diet, weight loss and long-term health* (1st ed.). Dallas, TX: BenBella Books.

Ceballos, G., Ehrlich, P. R., Barnosky, A. D., García, A., Pringle, R. M., & Palmer, T. M. (2015). Accelerated modern human–induced species losses: Entering the sixth mass extinction. *Science Advances, 1*(5), e1400253. Available from http://dx.doi.org/10.1126/sciadv.1400253.

China-Cornell-Oxford Project. Accessed May 20, 2015. <http://web.archive.org/web/20090223222003/http://www.nutrition.cornell.edu/ChinaProject>.

Christiansen, S., Ryan, J., Singh, M., Ates, S., Bahhady, F., Mohamed, K., ... Loss, S. (2015). Potential legume alternatives to fallow and wheat monoculture for Mediterranean environments. *Crop and Pasture Science, 66*, 113–121.

Clay, J. (2004). *World agriculture and the environment: A commodity-by-commodity guide to impacts, and practices*. Washington, DC: Island Press.

Climate Central. New CO2 Milestone: 3 Months Above 400 PPM. (2014). <http://www.climatecentral.org/news/co2-milestone-400-ppm-climate-17692>.

Clover, J. (2003). Food security in sub-Saharan Africa. *African Security Review, 12*, 5–15.

Damodaran, S. (1997). Food proteins: An overview. In S. Damodaran, & A. Paraf (Eds.), *Food proteins and their applications* (pp. 1–24). New York, NY: Marcel Dekker Inc.

Delgado, C. L. (2003). Rising consumption of meat and milk in developing countries has created a new food revolution. *Journal of Nutrition, 133*(11 Suppl. 2), 3907S–3910S.

Dixon, R. O. D., & Wheeler, C. T. (1986). *Nitrogen fixation in plants*. Glasgow: Blackie.

FAO. (2006). *Livestock's long shadow—Environmental issues and options*. Rome: Food and Agriculture Organisation.

FAO. (2011). The state of the world's land and water resources for food and agriculture. Managing Systems at Risk. <http://www.fao.org/nr/water/docs/solaw_ex_summ_web_en.pdf>.

FAO. (2012). State of the world's forests. <http://www.fao.org/docrep/016/i3010e/i3010e.pdf>.

FAO. (2013). *Dietary protein quality evaluation in human nutrition. FAO Food and Nutrition Paper 92. Report of an FAO Expert Consultation*. Rome: Food and Agriculture Organization of the United Nations.

FAO. (2015). Fertilizer use to surpass 200 million tonnes in 2018. <http://www.fao.org/news/story/en/item/277488/icode/>.

Fields, S. (2004). Global nitrogen: Cycling out of control. *Environment and Health Perspective, 112*, A556–A563.

Fukao, T., Yeung, E., & Bailey-Serres, J. (2012). The submergence tolerance gene *SUB1A* delays leaf senescence under prolonged darkness through hormonal regulation in rice. *Plant Physiology, 160*, 1795–1807.

Garnett, T. (2009). Livestock-related greenhouse gas emissions: Impact and options for policy makers. *Environmental Science & Policy, 12*, 491–503.

Gelski, J. (2015). Dialing into plant-based protein. *Food Business News*. April 9. <http://www.foodbusinessnews.net>

Gendel, S. M. (2002). Sequence analysis for assessing potential allergenicity. *Annals of the New York Academy of Sciences, 964*, 87–98.

Gendel, S. M. (2004). Bioinformatics and food allergens. *Journal of AOAC International, 87*, 1417–1422.

Gendel, S. M., & Jenkins, J. A. (2006). Allergen sequence databases. *Molecular Nutrition and Food Research, 50*, 633–637.

Glick-Bauer, M., & Yeh, M.-C. (2014). The health advantage of a vegan diet: Exploring the gut microbiota connection. *Nutrients, 6*, 4822–4838.

Healy, M. (2014). Western diet's spread bad for health, climate? It doesn't have to happen. *Los Angeles Times*. November 12. <http://www.latimes.com/science/sciencenow/la-sci-sn-western-diet-climate-health-20141112-story.html>

Herridge, D. F., Peoples, M. B., & Boddey, R. M. (2008). Global inputs of biological nitrogen fixation in agricultural systems. *Plant and Soil, 311*, 1–18.

Hoekstra, A. Y., & Mekonnen, M. M. (2012). The water footprint of humanity. *Proceedings of National Academy of Sciences, 109*, 3232–3237.

Hoffmann-Sommergruber, K., & Mills, E. N. C. (2009). Food allergen protein families and their structural characteristics and application in component-resolved diagnosis: New data from the EuroPrevall project. *Annals of Bioanalytical Chemistry, 395*, 25–35.

Hu, F. B. (2003). Plant-based foods and prevention of cardiovascular disease: And overview. *American Journal of Clinical Nutrition, 78*, 544S–551S.

Huang, Y.-W., Jian, Z.-H., Chang, H.-C., Nfor, O. N., Ko, P. C., Lung, C. C., ... Liaw, Y.-P. (2014). Vegan diet and blood lipid profiles: A cross-sectional study of pre- and post menaposal women. *BMC Women's Health, 14*, 55.

Jacobsen, R. (2014). The top-secret food that will change the way you eat. *Outside Live Bravely*. December 26. <http://www.outsideonline.com/1928211/top-secret-food-will-change-way-you-eat>.

Kenong, X., Xu, X., Fukao, T., Canlas, P., Maghirang-Rodriguez, R., Heuer, S., ... Mackill, D. J. (2006). *Sub1A* is an ethylene-response-factor-like gene that confers submergence tolerance to rice. *Nature, 442*, 705–708.

Khoury, C. K., Bjorkman, A. D., Dempewolf, H., Ramirez-Villegas, J., Guarino, L., Jarvis, A., ... Struik, P. A. (2014). Increasing homogeneity in global food supplies and the implications for food security. *Proceedings of National Academy of Sciences, 111*, 4001–4006.

Kinsella, J. E. (1976). Functional Properties of proteins in foods: A survey. *CRC Critical Reviews in Food Science and Nutrition, 7*, 219–280.

Kumosinski, T. F., Brown, E. M., & Farrell, H. M., Jr. (1991a). Molecular modelling in food research: Technology and techniques. *Trends in Food Science and Technology, 2*, 110–115.

Kumosinski, T. F., Brown, E. M., & Farrell, H. M., Jr. (1991b). Molecular modelling in food research: Applications. *Trends in Food Science and Technology, 2*, 190–195.

Lakemond, C. M. M., & Vereijken, J. M. (2003). Soybean proteins: Structure and functionIn W. Y. Aalbersberg, R. J. Hamer, P. Jasperse, H. H. J. de Jongh, C. G. de Kruif, P. Walstra, & F. A. de Wolf (Eds.), *Industrial Proteins in Perspective Progress in Biotechnology* (Vol 23, pp. 55–62). Amsterdam: Elsevier.

Lamarck, J.-B. (1809). Philosophie Zoologique, Vol. 1, 226.

Laskowski, R. A., Watson, J. D., & Thortonton, J. M. (2005). ProFunc: A server for predicting protein function from 3D structure. *Nucleic Acid Research, 33*, W89–W93.

Living Green. (2013). <http://livinggreenmag.com/2013/07/11/people-solutions/sustainability-and-the-world-population-what-is-our-global-limit/>.

Malthus, T.R. (1798). *An essay on the principle of population*. Chapter 1, p. 13 in Oxford World's Classics reprint.

Manceron, S., Ben-Ari, T., & Dumas, P. (2014). Feeding proteins to livestock: Global land use and food vs feed crop competition. *OCL, 21*, D408–D418.

Manjeru, P., Madanzi, T., Makeredza, P., Nciizah, A., & Sithole, M. (2007). Effects of water stress at different growth stages on components and grain yield of common bean (*Phaseolus vulgaris*, L). *African Crop Science Conference Proceedings, 8*, 299–303.

Martiniello, P. (2012). Cereal–forage crop rotations and irrigation treatment effect on water use efficiency and crop sustainability. *Agriculture Science, 3*, 44–57.

Massey, L. K. (2003). Dietary animal and plant protein and human bone health: A whole foods approach. *Journal of Nutrition, 133*, 862S–865S.

McDonald, R. I., Green, P., Balk, D., Fekete, B. M., Revenga, C., Todd, M., & Montgomery, M. (2011). Urban growth, climate change, and freshwater availability. *Proceedings of National Academy of Sciences, 108*(15), 6312–6317.

Myers, S., Zanobetti, A., Kloog, I., Huybers, P., Leakey, A., Bloom, A., ... Usui, Y. (2014). Increasing CO2 threatens human nutrition. *Nature*. Available from http://dx.doi.org/10.1038/nature13179.

Nakai, S. (1983). Structure-function relationships of food proteins with an emphasis on the importance of protein hydrophobicity. *Journal of Agricultural and Food Chemistry, 31*, 676–683.

Nakai, S., & Li-Chan, E. (1993). Recent advances in structure and function of food proteins: QSAR approach. *Critical Reviews in Food Science and Nutrition, 33*, 477–489.

National Geographic. (2014). The next breadbasket. 29-49.

National Research Council (2000). *Nutrient requirements of beef cattle* (p. 232). Washington, DC: National Academy Press.

Neff, R. A., Spiker, M. L., & Truant, P. L. (2015). Wasted food: U.S. consumers' reported awareness, attitudes, and behaviors. *PLoS One, 10*(6), e0127881. Available from http://dx.doi.org/10.1371/journal.pone.0127881.

Orman, S. (2015). Talking top trends from Natural Products Expo West 2015. *Food Drink & Franchise*, March 13. <http://www.fdfworld.com/production/517/Talking-Top-Trends-from-Natural-Products-Expo-West-2015>.

Pimentel, D., & Pimentel, M. (2003). Sustainability of meat-based and plant-based diets and the environment. *American Journal of Clinical Nutrition, 78*(suppl.), 660S–663SS.

Pleijel, H., & Uddling, J. (2011). Yield vs. quality trade-offs for wheat in response to carbon dioxide and ozone. *Global Change Biology, 18*, 596–605.

Prescott-Allen, R., & Prescott-Allen, C. (1990). How many plants feed the world? *Conservation Biology, 4*, 365–374.

Radauer, C., Bublin, M., Wagner, S., Mari, A., & Breiteneder, H. (2008). Allergens are distributed into few protein families and possess a restricted number of biochemical functions. *Allergy and Clinical Immunology, 121*, 847–852.

Ramanathan, V., & Feng, Y. (2008). On avoiding dangerous anthropogenic interference with the climate system: Formidable challenges ahead. *Proceedings of National Academy of Sciences, 105*, 14245–14250.

Richards, M. P. (2002). A brief review of the archeological evidence for Paleolithic and Neolithic subsistence. *European Journal of Clinical Nutrition, 56*, 16. Available from http://dx.doi.org/10.1038/sj.ejcn.1601646.

Rutherfurd-Markwick, K. J. (2012). Food protein as a source of bioactive peptides with diverse functions. *British Journal of Nutrition, 108*, S149–S157.

Segelken, R. (2001). Asians' switch to Western diet might bring Western-type diseases, new China-Taiwan study suggests. *Cornell Chronicle*, June 25. <http://www.news.cornell.edu/stories/2001/06/china-study-ii-western-diet-might-bring-western-disease>.

Sen, M., Kopper, R., Pons, L., Abraham, E. C., Burks, A. W., & Bannon, G. A. (2002). Protein structure plays a critical role in peanut allergen stability and may determine immunodominant IgE-binding epitopes. *Journal of Immunology, 169*, 882–887.

Shewry, P. R., Beaudoin, F., Jenkins, J., Griffiths-Jones, S., & Mills, E. N. C. (2002). Plant protein families and their relationships to food allergy. *Biochemical Society Transactions, 30*, 906–910.

Skirble, R. (2014). Study: Western diet bad for human health, environment. Voice of America. November 14. http://www.voanews.com/content/study-western-diet-bad-human-health-environment/2520952.html.

Terracciano, L., Isoardi, P., Arrigoni, S., Zoja, A., & Martelli, A. (2002). Use of hydrolysates in the treatment of cow's milk allergy. *Annals of Allergy, Asthma and Immunology, 89*, 86−90.

Tilman, D., & Clark, M. (2014). Global diets link environmental sustainability and human health. *Nature, 515*, 518−522.

Trapp, C. B., & Barnard, N. D. (2010). Usefulness of vegetarian and vegan diets for treating type 2 diabetes. *Current Diabetic Reports, 10*, 152−158.

Tuso, P. J., Ismail, M. H., Ha, B. P., & Bartolotto, C. (2013). Nutritional update for physicians: Plant-based diets. *The Permanente Journal, 17*(2), 61−66.

UCAR. (2015). How much has the global temperature risen in the last 100 years? <https://www2.ucar.edu/climate/faq/how-much-has-global-temperature-risen-last-100-years>.

UNEP. (2007). Reactive nitrogen in the environment. Too much or too little of a good thing. <http://www.unep.org/pdf/dtie/Reactive_Nitrogen.pdf>.

UN World Report. (2013). Water cooperation. <http://www.unwater.org/water-cooperation-2013/water-cooperation/facts-and-figures/en/>.

United Nations. (2015). Time for global action. Press release. <http://www.un.org/en/development/desa/population/pdf/events/other/10/World_Population_Projections_Press_Release.pdf>.

USDA. (2015). USDA acreage letter. <http://www.usda.gov/nass/PUBS/TODAYRPT/acrg0615.pdf>.

USDA-ERS. Topics—Corn <http://www.ers.usda.gov/topics/crops/corn/background.aspx>.

Weigel, H. J. (2014). Plant quality declines as CO2 levels increase. *eLife, 3*, e03233. Available from http://dx.doi.org/10.7554/eLife.03233.

WHO. (2010). Communicable diseases and severe food shortage. World Health Organization Technical Note. WHO/HSE/GAR/DC/2010.6.

WHO/FAO/UNU. (2002). Joint WHO/FAO/UNU Expert consultation on protein and amino acid requirement in Human Nutrition WHO Technical Report Series 935. Geneva, Switzerland. <http://whqlibdoc.who.int/trs/who_trs_935_eng.pdf>.

Withana-Gamage, T. S., & Wanasundara, J. P. D. (2012). Molecular modelling for investigating structure-function relationships of soy glycinin. *Trends in Food Science and Technology, 28*, 153−167.

World Commission on Environment and Development. (1987). Our Common Future, Report of the World Commission on Environment and Development, Published as Annex to General Assembly document A/42/427, Development and International Co-operation: Environment August 2, 1987. Accessed 14.11.07.

Part I

Plant Derived Proteins

Chapter 2

Soy Protein: Impacts, Production, and Applications

M. Thrane[1], P.V. Paulsen[2], M.W. Orcutt[2] and T.M. Krieger[3]
[1]DuPont Nutrition Biosciences ApS, Brabrand, Denmark, [2]Solae, LLC, St. Louis, MO, United States, [3]DuPont Engineering Research & Technology, Wilmington, DE, United States

2.1 INTRODUCTION

Soybean (*Glycine max*) is a species of legume rich in both high-quality protein and edible oil. Depending on the context, the plant is classified as either an oilseed (a crop grown primarily for its oil) or a pulse (an annual leguminous crop with seeds in pods), depending on one's perspective. Soybeans contain approximately, 36% protein, 15% soluble carbohydrates, 15% insoluble carbohydrates, and 18% oil (Fig. 2.1).

These values can range depending on variety, geographic location, and weather. Soybean is a rich source of nutritional components due to its unique chemical composition. Between cereal and other legume species, it has the highest protein content. Among legumes, it has the second highest oil content (peanuts are higher). Other valuable components found in soybeans include polysaccharides, phospholipids, vitamins, minerals, oligosaccharides, and isoflavones.

Agronomic practices and seed development have created varieties which can produce high yields in varying climates. These factors should provide for the soybean to be a favorable source of human nutritional ingredients. However, the soybean also contains components, which can prevent successful utilization by humans if not processed appropriately. Raw soybeans cannot be digested and need to be sprouted, or prepared and cooked for human consumption.

Soybean consumption as tofu or other processed soybean foods has been a staple of diets in Asia for several thousand years. This, however, has not been the case for other parts of the world. Introduction of soybean to North America occurred at the beginning of the 20th century for use as an alternative oil source. It was soon realized that the residual meal product from oil processing was a quality protein source as well; this was first proven in animal feeds and later in human foods. Over the past 100 plus years, soybean production and processing have grown globally to become one of the largest sources of plant-derived edible oil and proteins (Berk, 1992; Johnson, White, & Galloway, 2008; WWF, 2014).

The focus of this chapter is a sustainability assessment of soy protein products for human consumption, mainly in the form of isolated soy protein (ISP). ISP is the most concentrated form of commercially available soybean protein and contains a minimum of 90% protein on a dry matter basis (Codex Alimentarius STAN 175-1989). Industrial production of ISP occurred prior to World War II, mainly as adhesives for the paper coating industry. Protein purification technologies have since improved manifold for isolating soy protein for food use. Specific food application examples will be discussed, demonstrating that incorporation of soy protein ingredients can make foods based on traditional animal protein less expensive, and with lower environmental burdens.

2.2 PRODUCTION

Soybeans are grown globally, although the primary producers are in the western hemisphere. The major soybean-producing nations include the United States, Brazil, and Argentina, which grow roughly 90% of the global soybean crop. Total global output of soybeans in 2014 was estimated to be 319 million metric tons, representing a 13% increase over 2013. Thirteen percent (or roughly 41 million metric tons) of these beans go directly into producing foods including soymilk, tofu, miso, and tempeh. Eighty-seven percent (278 million metric tons) of these beans are crushed into

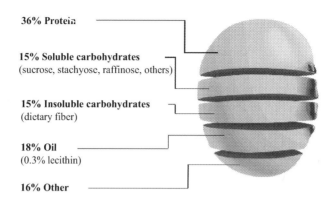

FIGURE 2.1 Composition of typical soybean. *From DuPont Nutrition and Health Internal Data.*

defatted soybean meal and oil. Ninety-five percent of the oil goes into the edible market. Almost 98% of the meal is destined for animal feed, while the remaining 2% serves as raw material for human soy protein products. Global production of soybeans has gradually increased over the past 10 years, totaling 142%. However, the proportion of meal going to soy protein products (2%) has not changed significantly (International Institute for Sustainable Development, 2014; US Department of Agriculture, 2015).

2.3 SOYBEAN PROTEIN RECOVERY: PROTEIN ISOLATION

Soybean pods are harvested from the fields and the seeds separated, dried, and shipped to a soybean processing plant. As a rule, food-grade soy protein products are produced on different lines than those used for feed materials. Soybeans are screened to remove damaged beans and foreign materials. Split and rejected soybeans are diverted to animal feed or industrial extraction operations. Uniform, clean beans pass through serrated rollers to break each bean into several pieces and the outer hulls are removed by aspiration. Typically, hulls are removed prior to crushing, since processors can obtain better value for higher-protein meals, although in some cases, a portion of hulls are retained to assist solvent drainage. The hulls are primarily blended into animal feed, when beans are crushed to prepare defatted flakes for soy protein products. Beans are crushed through smooth rollers to form flakes and the oil extracted using a food-grade solvent (hexane) by a counter-current process. Gums (lecithin) are separated and the oil is refined and deodorized for use as vegetable oil in foods. Fig. 2.2 outlines this process for soybean crushing and extraction to create defatted soy flour.

The defatted soybean flakes are conveyed through a system of steam heating under vacuum to remove the solvent from the materials (flash desolventizing). The industry term for these materials is "white flakes," due to their light-color appearance. Certain defatted soybean flakes alternatively receive a steam heating and cooking (desolventizer toaster) to cause inactivation of enzymes, improve digestibility, and alter functionality. By either desolventizing process, the resulting soybean flakes are typically 52–54% protein. These flakes can be milled into soy flours or grits depending on the end food application and particle size needs. As identified by trading standards, these are sold as soy flour with a minimum protein content of 50% on a dry basis.

Soy protein concentrates can be produced from the defatted flakes by extracting the soluble carbohydrates, either with acidic water (at pH 4.5), with heat denaturation and water leaching, or more traditionally with aqueous ethyl alcohol (60–90%). For each process, the intent is to insolubilize the protein while enabling the soluble carbohydrates to be washed away. These processes are outlined in Fig. 2.3.

Removal of soluble carbohydrates (primarily sucrose, stachyose, and raffinose) increases the protein content to >65%, on a dry basis. This is the trading standard for proteins sold as soy concentrates. The functional properties of concentrates are modified by neutralization (in the case of the acidic process), steam injection, and mechanical shear through homogenization. Soy concentrates, which are modified, will have high water-holding and high emulsifying properties. These modified concentrates have been described as functional concentrates. The soy concentrates are spray dried into a flowable powder as a final process step.

The ISP manufacturing process may deviate slightly depending on the manufacturer, but, in all cases, the objective is to cause separation of the fiber (pectin, cellulose, and hemicellulose) and carbohydrate (sucrose and various oligosaccharides) from the protein. A common approach is to extract the white flakes with alkaline water

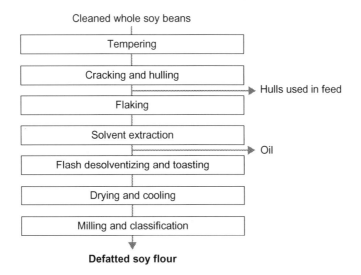

FIGURE 2.2 Flow diagram of typical manufacturing process of defatted soy flour. *Modified from Johnson, L.A., White, P.J., & Galloway, R. 2008. Soybeans—Chemistry, production, processing, and utilization. Urbana, IL: United Soybean Board, AOCS Press.*

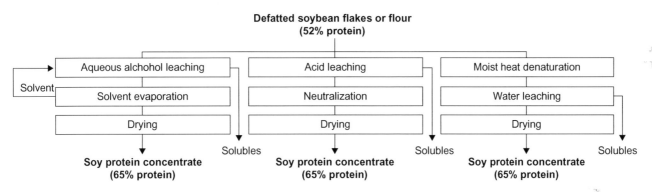

FIGURE 2.3 Flow diagram of typical manufacturing processes of soy protein concentrates. *From Johnson, L.A., White, P.J., & Galloway, R. 2008. Soybeans—Chemistry, production, processing, and utilization. Urbana, IL: United Soybean Board, AOCS Press.*

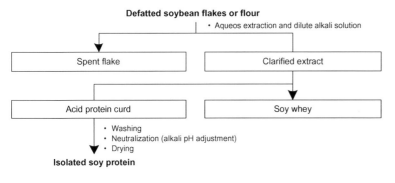

FIGURE 2.4 Flow diagram of the typical manufacturing process of isolated soy protein. *From DuPont Nutrition and Health Internal Data.*

(pH 8–9) and separate the protein and soluble carbohydrate from fibrous materials. The insoluble fiber is called "spent flake." The white flake to water ratio is typically between 1:10 and 1:20 parts. The spent flake materials are cellular wall polysaccharides that can be purified and used as functional dietary fiber ingredients. Fig. 2.4 outlines a process for ISP.

The next step involves the separation of proteins from the carbohydrates by isoelectric precipitation. Soy proteins have minimal solubility at their isoelectric point, which ranges from pH 4.2 to pH 4.5. Food-grade acids, such as hydrochloric or phosphoric, are commonly used to alter protein pH level. The insoluble protein is separated from the soluble carbohydrates by centrifugation. The resulting isolated protein is washed with additional water to continue removal of nonprotein components. Most of the process water is removed via this soluble carbohydrate fraction, also called soy whey. The soy whey fraction also contains dilute levels of albumin proteins. This stream represents a significant disposal issue for the processor today. Innovative handling of soy whey to convert the stream into biogas or collect the sugars and albumins for animal feed use has been implemented to reduce the environmental impacts.

The protein curd will next be adjusted to neutrality (pH 6.8–7.2) with alkaline salts such as sodium or potassium hydroxide. At this point the product should contain >90% protein, dry basis. The protein is processed further to optimize functionality. This could include proteolytic enzyme modification, reduction of disulfide bonds by reducing additives or heat denaturation. The final product is spray-dried (Johnson et al., 2008; Liu, 1999). These steps may be used singly or in combination to achieve the target functional property. Correct drying system operation is critical to retain protein functionality from the previous process steps and impart user-friendliness (nondusting, dispersion, density control) to the ISP powder. The drying systems may include postdrying blending, oil or lecithin spray-on systems, and agglomeration capabilities. The specific treatments for a defined product are closely held trade secrets of manufacturers.

2.4 TYPES OF SOY PROTEINS AND PROTEIN PRODUCTS

The mature soybean contains two main types of storage proteins, in organelles known as protein bodies. These proteins are β-conglycinin and glycinin, which represent 65–89% of the total seed proteins, and are classified as globulin proteins and soluble in a salt solution. These are the primary proteins concentrated and isolated within the previously described processes. In addition, the seed contains other proteins such as lectins, trypsin inhibitors, and lipoxygenases. Purification processes are controlled to either remove or inactivate these latter proteins, which can affect the nutrition and flavor of soy protein ingredients. In addition, minor quantities of other structural and enzymatic proteins are removed in either the spent flake or soy whey stream, respectively.

Glycinin (also called 11S Globulin) is the largest single fraction of total soybean seed protein (25–35%). Glycinin has a high molecular weight (350 kDa) and consists of six acidic and six basic subunits arranged in a hexamer structure. The subunits are held together by disulfide bonding. This protein's properties are low viscosity and high thermal stability. β-Conglycinin (also called 7S Globulin) is a trimer protein with about half the molecular size of glycinin (175 kDa). The three subunits are immunologically distinct, but can vary by bean variety. All three subunit types are glycoproteins with 4–5% carbohydrate. The properties of β-conglycinin are high viscosity and low thermal stability. Due to the differing composition and structures, these soybean globulins have offsetting effects on nutritional and functional properties of soy protein ingredients (Liu, 1999).

The general types of soy protein ingredients are soy flour, soy concentrates, and soy protein isolates, which are primarily differentiated by increasing minimum protein content, respectively. Example proximate composition of these protein products is provided in Section 2.5.2. Most of these ingredients are produced in a dry powder or granular form. The product's characteristics are defined by the targeted food applications. Key properties that may be optimized for a given product are water-holding capacity and gelation, emulsification and fat binding, dispersion and wettability, or low viscosity at high solids.

Soy flour, concentrates, and isolates are also converted into products with defined appearances and textures through the utilization of a single or double screw extruder. Additionally, ISP can be structured by steam injection, jet cooking, or extruding into an acid-salt bath that coagulates protein into fibers. These may be commercially described as textured soy flour, textured soy protein concentrate, structured soy protein products, or soy protein nuggets and crisps, which are valuable and nutritious components of numerous food products.

2.5 SUSTAINABILITY

The environmental profile of ISP produced by DuPont Nutrition & Health (DuPont), has recently been analyzed in a life cycle assessment (LCA) which quantifies the environmental impacts from soy cultivation to final product, referred to as a "cradle-to-gate" perspective. The main scenario represents ISP production during one crop year (CY 2012) from one production site in the United States. Five sites were analyzed as part of a sensitivity analysis, including sites that convert ISP into textured products. The LCA study was independently verified and complies with the ISO 14044 standard for LCA (Muñoz, 2015). It analyzes ISP's contribution to 16 impact categories, but this chapter focuses on the carbon, blue water, and land use footprints.

To provide a context for better understanding the impacts and their magnitude, an additional screening level LCA was completed for the following animal-based protein sources (Muñoz & Schmidt, 2015):

- Beef;
- Pork;
- Chicken;
- Skimmed milk powder (SMP);
- Sodium caseinate;
- Whey protein concentrate (WPC).

Despite applying a less detailed approach, a high level of methodological scrutiny was applied to identify updated and reliable data that match the methodical choices made in the LCA of ISP produced by DuPont. The screening LCAs were based on an initial review of more than 50 existing LCA studies. In several cases, existing data have not been available for certain protein types, footprint types, or modeling approaches. In these cases, new models were developed by modifying and updating existing high-quality LCA studies (Muñoz & Schmidt, 2015).

In terms of geographical scope, the main scenario reflects production of ISP in the United States by DuPont, and is based on soy white flakes produced from average US soybeans (Muñoz, 2015). Except for beef, the analysis of the alternative animal-based protein sources reflects production in European Union and United States (50/50). This scope has been chosen because these regions play an important role in global production of the analyzed protein types, and represent a high-level technology, creating the basis for a fair comparison with ISP produced by DuPont (Muñoz & Schmidt, 2015). Beef is modeled as production from non-dairy cows in Brazil due to its dominating position in the world beef market, and because production from Brazil is expected to represent more than 60% of future expansion of nondairy beef production. Beef produced in the United States and European Union was also analyzed in Muñoz and Schmidt (2015) and showed higher carbon and water use footprints, but somewhat lower land use footprints compared to production in Brazil.

2.5.1 Two Life Cycle Inventory Models

The results presented in this chapter are unique as they represent:

- The first published LCA of ISP that is third-party reviewed and compliant with the ISO 14040/44 standards;
- LCA results based on two different methodologies: consequential modeling and attributional modeling.

The two methods are mainly distinguished by the way they handle calculations of environmental impacts from individual coproducts from multioutput processes, such as a soy mill that produces both soy meal and soy oil, or a cow that produces both milk and meat.

Consequential modeling applies substitution (also known as system expansion). Here, all environmental burdens are allocated to the main product and a credit is given for the products that are being substituted by the by-product(s). In the case of soy, the environmental impacts from soy cultivation and crushing are allocated to the main product soy meal, while a credit is given for vegetable oils substituted by the soy oil byproduct. In the case of milk, the environmental burdens from feed production and cow rearing are allocated to the main product milk, while a credit is given for the meat that substitutes beef from non-dairy cows. Different ways of handling co-product allocation in relation to dairy product are further discussed in Flysjö (2012).

In attributional modeling, different approaches to co-product allocation can be applied, but in the current analysis, economic allocation is applied. This means that the environmental burdens are allocated to the co-products according to their relative contribution to the revenue. Hence, the co-products that represent the highest revenue get the highest share of the environmental impacts. Another term for this method is revenue allocation.

Consequential modeling provides a more accurate description of the market causalities, but can be sensitive to assumptions about displaced products (what they are, where they are produced, and how they are produced). Economic allocation, on the other hand, is widely used in the LCA community and can be easier to comprehend, but is sensitive to assumptions about prices and variations in prices. Furthermore, it can be argued that allocation introduces fictive processes such as a dairy cow that only produces milk. See also Weidema (2014), Sonnemann and Vigon (2011), and Weidema, Ekvall, and Heijungs (2010). In DuPont N&H consequential modeling is generally used as the default LCA methodology.

2.5.2 Cradle-to-Gate Life Cycle Impact Assessment

Greenhouse gas emissions, measured in units of CO_2-equivalents (CO_2e), are assessed by means of the global warming potentials for a time horizon of 100 years, as defined by the fourth assessment report of the Intergovernmental Panel for Climate Change (IPCC) (IPCC, 2007). In the fifth IPCC assessment report, the global warming potential of methane over a time horizon of 100 years was increased from previously 25 CO_2e per kg methane emission, to 28 and even 34 kg CO_2e per kg methane emission if climate carbon feedbacks are included (indirect effects). The result of applying the newer characterization factors would be that beef got an even higher carbon footprint than suggested in this chapter. It would also result in higher impacts for dairy proteins according to the attributional model, but not necessarily according to the consequential model. The reason is that the new characterization factors lead to higher impacts of both the dairy system and the avoided beef from the nondairy beef system (Myhre et al., 2013).

For land use and blue water footprint, the result reflects the inputs of water and land. A conversion of water and land use into more sophisticated impact categories, such as biodiversity loss, would require a more advanced modeling based on detailed geographical information. Table 2.1 provides an overview of life cycle impact assessment results based on consequential and attributional modeling as well as an overview of the maximum and minimum values from a meta-analysis.

The protein sources analyzed in Table 2.1 vary in protein content. When expressed in fresh weight, protein levels are 87% in ISP, 91% in caseinate, 80% in whey protein concentrate, 35% in skim milk powder, and 20% in meat (beef/pork/chicken).

The results show that carbon, blue water, and land use footprints for ISP are among the smallest of all analyzed protein sources. However, it is also clear that different methods provide different results.

2.5.2.1 Carbon Footprint

The carbon footprint of ISP is dependent on the methodology applied: it is 2.4 kg CO_2e per kg protein when consequential modeling (substitution) is applied, and 6.1 kg CO_2e per kg protein when attributional modeling (economic allocation) is applied (Muñoz, 2015). These results do not reflect textured or structured versions of ISP but a sensitivity analysis of other production sites that produce textured and structured versions shows no significant deviations in the carbon footprint. Energy use is the most important driver of the carbon footprint, and DuPont only uses gas as the source of heat energy. But, if the ISP had been produced with coal as the main energy source, the carbon footprint would be more than 3 times higher in the consequential model, and nearly 2 times higher according to the attributional model.

The main reason for the lower footprint when substitution is applied is that a credit is given for the soy oil from soybean milling that substitutes other vegetable oils (notably palm oil) on the world market. The substituted palm oil has a significant carbon footprint for several reasons—the most important factors being carbon emissions associated with cultivation on peat soils, and methane emissions from treatment of palm oil mill effluent in anaerobic ponds (Schmidt, 2015).

Based on the results provided in Table 2.1 for consequential modeling, the carbon footprint of soy protein in ISP is roughly 8–80 times smaller than the alternative animal-based proteins. When attributional modeling is applied soy protein from ISP is roughly 3–30 times smaller than the animal-based proteins. It should be stressed that while the LCA of ISP is highly detailed and third-party reviewed, the LCAs of animal-based proteins are less detailed and represent a higher level of uncertainty. The results, however, are in accordance with a meta review of LCA studies (Nijdam, Rood, & Westhoek, 2012) which concludes "the carbon footprint of the most climate-friendly protein sources is up to 100 times smaller than those of the most climate-unfriendly." The same review identifies the most climate-friendly proteins as soy and pea protein.

Another way to analyze the results is to calculate the amount of CO_2e that is saved by replacing 1 kg animal-based protein with 1 kg proteins from soy (as ISP). In the case of consequential modeling, the savings are 14–176 kg CO_2e per kg replaced animal-based protein, and 12–178 kg CO_2e per kg replaced animal-based protein based on attributional modeling. Quality plant proteins, such as soy protein, perform well for at least three reasons:

- No feed conversion loss;
- No methane emissions from enteric fermentation;
- Legumes, such as soy and peas, have the ability to fix nitrogen from the atmosphere, which reduces (or eliminates) the need for nitrogen fertilizers, that is, less emissions related to the production of fertilizers as well as less field emissions related to N surplus.

TABLE 2.1 Overview of Carbon, Water and Land Use Footprint for Different Protein Sources Based on Consequential and Attributional Modeling.[a] Results From Meta-Analysis Provide an Overview of the Variability in Results in All Included Studies[b] (Muñoz & Schmidt, 2015; Muñoz, 2015)

	Consequential Model (Substitution)			Attributional Model (Economic Allocation)			Range of Results According to Meta-Analysis		
	Carbon Footprint (kg CO_2e/ kg protein)	Blue Water Footprint (L water/kg protein)	Land Use Footprint (m^2 year/ kg protein)	Carbon Footprint (kg CO_2e/ kg protein)	Blue Water Footprint (L water/kg protein)	Land Use Footprint (m^2 year/ kg protein)	Carbon Footprint (kg CO_2e/kg protein)	Blue Water Footprint (L water/kg protein)	Land Use Footprint (m^2 year/kg protein)
Beef, suckler cows	178	1607	1311	184	1607	1310	45–643 (n = 27)	1548–6821 (n = 9)	75–2100 (n = 14)
Beef, dairy cows	n.a.	n.a.	n.a.	125	351	156	45–150 (n = 5)	95–607 (n = 2)	37–210 (n = 3)
Pork	24	1855	59	29	1855	55	22–53 (n = 13)	340–3225 (n = 7)	39–75 (n = 8)
Chicken	17	629	33	18	629	32	10–30 (n = 6)	195–1665 (n = 7)	23–40 (n = 4)
Skim milk powder, SMP	23	n.a.	n.a.	23	153	31	20–26 (n = 3)	0–398 (n = 7)	0–36 (n = 4)
Caseinate	26	n.a.	n.a.	19	170	12	19–30 (n = 3)	0–170 (n = 3)	0–12 (n = 3)
Whey protein, WPC	16	36	19	20	194	14	15–20 (n = 3)	32–203 (n = 4)	12–19 (n = 4)
Isolated soy protein (ISP)	2	38	8	6	205	6	1–7 (n = 10)	38–205 (n = 2)	6–8 (n = 2)

[a]Results for dairy beef have not been separately analyzed based on substitution (noted with n.a. in Table 2.1). The reason is that beef from dairy cows, according to this modeling, is considered to be a byproduct constrained by the demand for product milk (the main product). According to this perspective, an additional demand for beef affects the production of beef from the beef system (suckler cows) instead of beef from the dairy system and the impacts can therefore be seen as identical. This is further elaborated on in Dalgaard et al. (2014).
[b]The number of studies (n) reflects the number of studies published by different authors and times, but also studies of similar products in different geographical contexts or different version of the same study, based on fundamentally different methods, that is, attributional and consequential modeling.

The high footprint for beef is mainly due to methane release from enteric fermentation, which is a characteristic for ruminants. The footprint is significantly lower for monogastric animals, such as pork and chicken, where the carbon footprint measured per kg protein is roughly on the same level as the analyzed dairy-based proteins. As shown in the meta-analysis, results vary significantly and depend on factors such as the exact type of production system, the location, background data as well as the applied LCA methodology, see Table 2.1. However, the meta-analysis shows the same clear tendency toward vegetable proteins having lower environmental burdens, see also Nijdam et al. (2012).

Impacts associated with direct and indirect land use change (ILUC) are not included in the footprint results presented in this chapter. The reason is mainly a lack of methodological consensus in the LCA community of how to include these. ILUC is, however, included in the detailed LCA of ISP in a sensitivity scenario. If included, all carbon footprint results would be higher, but as that would apply to all the analyzed proteins and it would not affect the conclusions.

Energy use is not analyzed separately, but is included in the LCA models. For ISP there is a close relationship between the carbon footprint and energy use, mainly due to the significant energy use related to the separation and drying steps of the process. This is also the case for the dairy proteins. This correlation is less pronounced for chicken and pork—and for beef in particular, the carbon footprint is not a good indicator for energy use, as it is mainly methane and nitrous oxide emissions that drive the carbon footprint.

2.5.2.2 Water Use Footprint (Blue Water)

The blue water footprint of ISP is also dependent on the methodology applied: it is 38 L water per kg protein when consequential modeling (substitution) is applied, and 205 L water per kg protein, based on attributional modeling (Muñoz & Schmidt, 2015). The lower result when substitution is applied is due to the credit obtained for soybean oil (from milling). Soybean oil is a by-product of soybean meal production, and it is substituting other vegetable oils, where palm oil can be identified as the most important marginal source. Furthermore, a by-product from ISP production is carbohydrates, which substitute alternative animal feed, mainly barley. Barley has been identified as the marginal source of feed energy in several studies, for example, Schmidt and Weidema (2008) and Schmidt (2015).

Based on the results provided in Table 2.1 for consequential modeling, the blue water footprint for ISP is about 157–50 times lower than for the analyzed meat proteins. The blue water footprint is, however, on the same level (or slightly higher) that for WPC. For SMP and caseinate, results are not provided for consequential modeling, due to significant uncertainties. Water results for milk proteins are highly site-dependent and very sensitive to assumptions about the location of the avoided beef production. A more detailed level of LCA needs to be applied to provide reliable results in this case. The range for SMP, according to the meta-analysis is 0–398 L water per kg protein. The 398 L water is data for global average SMP according to Mekonnen and Hoekstra (2012) and applies a methodology similar to attributional modeling. The other end of the interval illustrates that the blue water footprint can be very low (and even negative) based on consequential modeling—depending on the assumption about water use for the substituted beef.

According to attributional modeling, the blue water footprint of ISP is 3–9 times lower relative to protein from meat proteins from nondairy beef, pork, and chicken. Beef protein from dairy cows, however, has a relatively low blue water footprint (only 80% higher than for ISP) and the blue water footprints for WPC, SMP, and caseinate are all slightly lower than for ISP.

The meta-analysis in Muñoz and Schmidt (2015) suggests a wide range of results for the blue water footprint and the uncertainty is greater than for carbon footprint. The reason is that water use is highly site-dependent and that water use data historically have been prioritized lower in LCA studies (and databases).

2.5.2.3 Land Use Footprint

The land use footprint of ISP amounts to 8 m^2 year per kg protein when substitution is applied and 6 m^2 year per kg protein, when economic allocation is applied (Muñoz & Schmidt, 2015). Here, consequential modeling represents the highest results, which is mainly because the substituted palm oil uses little land, thus providing only a small credit to ISP.

According to Table 2.1, the land use footprint of ISP is nearly 160 times smaller than for beef—a difference that is particularly large because the analyzed beef is from pasture-based production systems in Brazil. The land use for ISP is 2–7 times smaller than for pork, chicken, and whey protein, based on consequential modeling. For similar reasons as for water, consequential results for land use are not provided for SMP and caseinate.

Based on attributional modeling, the land use footprint of ISP is nearly 30–220 times smaller compared to protein from beef (from dairy and nondairy cows), and 2–9 times lower compared to pork, chicken, and dairy proteins. The reason for the relatively low land use of ISP is mainly the high yield of soy. According to WWF (2014), soy produces

TABLE 2.2 Energetic Efficiencies Presented in Kcal and Grams of Protein Based on Eshel and Martin (2006) and LMC International (2011)

	Energetic Efficiencies	
	100* g kcal Output/kcal Input	100* g Protein Output/kcal Input
Livestock		
Milk	20.6	1.3
Chicken	18.1	1.6
Eggs	11.2	0.9
Beef (grain fed)	6.4	0.7
Pork	3.7	0.4
Lamb	1.2	0.1
Fish		
Herring	110	12.5
Tuna	5.8	1.2
Farmed salmon	5.7	0.6
Shrimp	0.9	0.2
Plants		
Soybeans (farm gate)	415	34.0
Corn	250	6.5
Apple	110	0.6
Potatoes	123	3.2

more protein per hectare than any other major crop. The meta-analysis in Muñoz and Schmidt (2015) suggests a wide range of results for land use, and especially for nondairy beef that range from 75 to 2100 m^2 year per kg protein. These extremes represent intensive production in the Netherlands and extensive production in Brazil (Nijdam et al., 2012).

2.5.3 Other Perspectives on Sustainability of Soy

The previous sections focused on LCAs of different protein sources. They represent a sophisticated life cycle-oriented approach to assess the sustainability profile of products. However, simpler approaches that only focus on one specific life cycle stage (or issue) are also relevant as they provide another perspective. The following focus on the farm level inputs in terms of energy, water, and land use associated with soybean production.

2.5.3.1 Energy Use at Farm Level

Muñoz (2015) and Muñoz and Schmidt (2015) do not separately address energy use at the farm level. However, Eshel and Martin (2006) provide an interesting comparison between the energetic efficiencies of soybeans at farm level compared to other foods based on livestock, fish, and plants. The energy efficiency is defined as 100 * kcal output/kcal of input. LMC International (2011) extended the calculations to include the energetic efficiency measured in terms of gram protein output per kcal input. The results are provided in Table 2.2.

The comparison shows that soybeans have the highest energetic efficiency among the analyzed foods—both measured as kcal output per kcal input, and as gram protein output per kcal input. It is, however, important to understand that the results represent soybeans at farm gate, and hence do not include energy use related to downstream processing and transport. The comparison is also based on older and arguably less sophisticated studies than the LCA studies in this chapter.

TABLE 2.3 The Green, Blue, and Gray Water Footprint of Selected Crops and Animal-Based Products (Mekonnen and Hoekstra, 2011, 2012)

	Global Average Water Footprints			
	Blue Water (Focus in LCA) (m^3/ton)	Green Water (m^3/ton)	Gray Water (m^3/ton)	Total Water (m^3/ton)
Livestock				
Milk	86	863	72	1020
Eggs	244	2592	429	3265
Chicken	313	3545	467	4325
Pork	459	4907	622	5988
Lamb/sheep	522	9813	76	10,415
Beef	550	14,414	451	15,415
Plants				
Potatoes	33	191	63	287
Soybean (farm gate)	70	2037	37	2145
Corn	81	947	194	1222
Apple	133	561	127	822

2.5.3.2 Water Use at Farm Level

The LCA study included use of blue water from cradle-to-gate. Water use at farm level was not separately analyzed, but an overview of farm level blue, green,[1] and gray[2] water is provided by Mekonnen and Hoekstra (2011, 2012) (see Table 2.3).

The water footprint results for soybeans are among the lowest of the analyzed foods. But it is also varied by different products with different protein-, energy-, and dry matter content. Even though the data from Mekonnen and Hoekstra (2011, 2012) have been used as background references for the LCA, the results cannot be compared directly. For instance, the LCA includes post farm-gate processes and results are expressed per kg protein and not per kg product. The general conclusion, however, points in the same direction.

According to WWF (2014), the water use in soy production varies greatly between countries and regions. Soybean used 4% of global irrigation water in 1997–2000, but is not evenly spread. As an example, soy is generally rainfed in South America, while it is more frequently irrigated elsewhere (blue water footprint results for ISP in the LCA, are based on soy grown in North America).

2.5.3.3 Land Use at Farm Level and Deforestation

Based on modification of the LCA of ISP, it can be calculated that the land use at farm level amounts to an annual output of 1000 kg protein per hectare. The protein yields for chicken, pork, and beef at farm level correspond to an annual output of 300, 182, and 8 kg protein per hectare (Muñoz & Schmidt, 2015).

The following numbers clearly show that it is important to reduce land use. Globally, croplands cover 1.53 billion hectares (12% of the earth's ice-free land), while pastures cover another 3.38 billion hectares (about 26% of the earth's

---

1. The green water footprint is the volume of rainwater consumed during the production process. It refers to the total rainwater evapotranspiration (from fields and plantations) plus the water incorporated into the harvested crop or wood (Hoekstra et al., 2011).
2. The gray water footprint of a product is an indicator of freshwater pollution that can be associated with the production of a product over its full supply chain. It is calculated as the volume of water that is required to dilute pollutants to such an extent that the quality of the water remains above agreed water quality standards (Hoekstra et al., 2011).

ice-free land). In total, agriculture occupies 38% of the earth's terrestrial surface. Adding croplands devoted to animal feed to pasture and grazing lands gives the total land devoted to raising animals as 3.73 billion hectares, an astonishing 75% of the world's agricultural land (Foley et al., 2011).

According to Boucher et al. (2011), cattle pasture is the main driver of deforestation in Latin America, but rainforest depletion is also associated with soybeans, notably in South America. Schmidt et al. (2015) points more broadly on all land uses as drivers of deforestation, namely that all land uses contribute to a common pressure on the frontiers between nature and utilized land. There exist various ways to reduce undesirable effects on deforestation, such as maximizing yields, supporting nature conservation, and avoiding sourcing crops from suppliers who are associated with transformation of high-value conservation land. The latter can be addressed by sourcing from certified sustainable soy, for example, based on RTRS (round table on responsible soy). Other actions and engagements that can be taken by various stakeholders are discussed in WWF (2014). Ideally, considerations about ILUC also need to be taken, and research is needed about the effectiveness of different means of action including different certification schemes.

In 2006, the Brazilian Association of Vegetable Oil Industries and the National Association of Cereal Exporters, announced a moratorium on deforestation, implying that members would not buy soybeans produced on Amazon farmland deforested after Jun. 24, 2006. According to Boucher et al. (2011) and WWF (2014), this has significantly reduced soy cultivation as a driver of rain forest depletion. As mentioned in Section 2.2, it should also be considered that almost 98% of the soy meal becomes animal feed, while only 2% is used as raw material for human soy protein products.

2.5.3.4 Use of Hexane in Soy Milling

Another issue that sometimes gets attention among customers and the public is the use of hexane during the separation of soy oil and soy meal in the crushing stage. Hexane is a solvent used to extract and separate vegetable oil from almost all oilseeds, including soybean oil, canola oil, sunflower oil, olive oil, and many others. Impacts associated with the production of hexane, as well as the emissions of hexane during the milling stage, are included in the LCA. The hexane emissions do not contribute to global warming, and do not have a significant contribution to any impact categories beyond photochemical ozone formation. The contribution to the latter by hexane is 16%, whereas the remaining 84% is associated with energy use by different activities in the ISP life cycle (heat, electricity, and transport-related). The residual level of hexane found in soy products including ISP produced by DuPont are typically less than 1 ppm. There is no specific regulation for hexane residues for production of soy products in the United States. In the EU hexane is permitted (Directive 2009/32/EC) for use in "preparation of defatted protein products and flours" with a 10 ppm residue limit for the finished food that contains the protein ingredient, and a 30 ppm limit for the protein product sold by itself to the final consumer. Residual solvents are reviewed annually as part of DuPont's ongoing Product Stewardship Program.

2.5.3.5 ISP Manufacturing

From a manufacturing point of view, it is important to understand that despite the excellent environmental profile of ISP, as expected, there are continual challenges and steps that need to be taken to make the ISP production even more sustainable. This includes:

- Improvement of protein recovery from soy white flakes;
- Recovery and utilization of ISP manufacturing waste streams contributing to biological and chemical oxygen demand;
- Value creation for ingredients derived from ISP processing waste streams, such as soy hull and soy cotyledon fiber;
- Reduction of water use in manufacturing.

This chapter has not dealt with all impact categories analyzed in the LCA of ISP, nor have social or economic aspects such as affordable food, been addressed. However, there is plenty of evidence that soy protein represents a more affordable alternative to animal proteins and there are no indications that an inclusion of social aspects would change the conclusions.

2.6 NUTRITIVE VALUE

2.6.1 Protein Nutrition

Protein needs vary throughout the human life cycle, as it is the primary tissue-repair and growth nutrient in the body. Adequate protein is especially important during times of rapid growth, such as infancy, childhood, and adolescence.

TABLE 2.4 Amino Acid Composition of Soy Protein Products[a]

Analysis	ISP[b]	SPC[c]	Soy Flour[d]	FAO/WHO Amino Acid Ref Pattern[e]
Alanine	4.3	4.4	4.4	–
Arginine	8.5	7.8	7.3	–
Aspartic acid	12.4	11.6	11.9	–
Cysteine	1.3	1.5	1.5	–
Glutamic acid	19.6	18.9	18.3	–
Glycine	4.2	4.3	4.4	–
Histidine	2.6	2.5	2.5	1.9
Isoleucine	4.9	4.6	4.6	2.8
Leucine	8.2	7.9	7.7	6.6
Lysine	6.4	6.5	6.3	5.8
Methionine	1.3	1.4	1.3	–
Phenylalanine	5.2	5.0	4.9	–
Proline	5.2	5.3	5.5	–
Serine	5.1	5.2	5.5	–
Threonine	3.7	4.0	4.1	3.4
Tryptophan	1.4	1.3	1.4	1.1
Tyrosine	3.9	3.7	3.6	–
Valine	5.1	5.0	4.7	3.5
Methionine + cysteine	2.6	3.0	2.8	2.5
Phenylalanine + tyrosine	9.2	8.8	8.5	6.3
True digestibility[f]	97%	95%	84%	n.a.
PDCAAS, truncated[g]	1.00	1.00	0.94	n.a.

[a]Amino acids are g per 100 g protein (16 g N).
[b]Isolated soy protein (Hughes, Ryan, Mukherjea, & Schasteen, 2011).
[c]Soy protein concentrate (DuPont Nutrition & Health internal data).
[d]Soy flour, defatted (USDA, National Nutrient Database, 2011).
[e]Recommended essential amino acid pattern for preschool child (2–5 years) (FAO/WHO, 1991).
[f]By rat fecal digestibility method. ISP (Hughes et al., 2011); SPC (FAO/WHO, 1991); Soy flour, defatted (Food and Drug Administration, HHS, 1993).
[g]Calculated using PDCAAS method (FAO/WHO, 1991).

Soy is a high-quality source of protein that provides adequate amounts of essential amino acids to meet the needs for growth and repair of both children and adults. Table 2.4 contains amino acid compositions for soybean protein from flour, concentrate, and isolate products. The amino acid data are provided on a protein basis and are compared to FAO/WHO guidelines for amino acid requirements of the 2–5-year-old. All of these soy protein products meet the requirements for 2-year-old or older individuals. For infants, methionine fortification is recommended to match breast milk. After correcting the amino acid contents for digestibility, all soybean protein products would be considered high-quality according to protein digestibility corrected amino acid scores (PDCAAS). These soy protein products provide PDCAAS values similar to milk or egg, and higher than other plant proteins (see Fig. 2.5).

2.6.2 Muscle Health

Protein is a key nutritional component needed to promote muscle growth and strength. A large body of clinical evidence has shown that soy protein can help resistance-trained people achieve significant muscle growth (Brown, DiSilvestro,

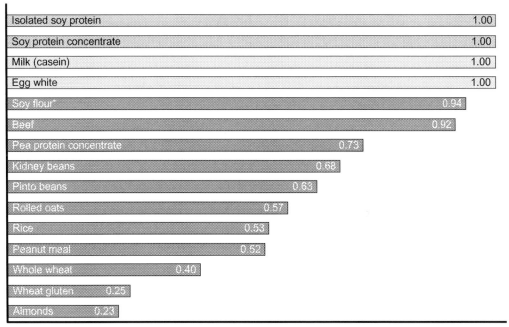

FIGURE 2.5 Protein quality (PDCAAS values) of common sources of protein. *From Hughes, G.J., Ryan, D.J., Mukherjea, R., & Schasteen, C.S. (2011). Protein digestibility-corrected amino acid scores (PDCAAS) for soy protein isolates and concentrate: Criteria for evaluation.* Journal of Agricultural and Food Chemistry, 59*(23), 12707–12712.*

Babaknia, & Devor, 2004; Candow, Burke, Smith-Palmer, & Burke, 2006; Deibert et al., 2011; Dragan, Stroescu, Stoian, Georgescu, & Baloescu, 1992; Hartman et al., 2007; Haub, Wells, Tarnopolsky, & Campbell, 2002; Maesta et al., 2007). Soy protein is a high-quality, complete protein that provides the indispensable amino acids necessary for protein synthesis in muscle and other tissues. Therefore, soy protein can be effectively used for the maintenance, repair, and synthesis of skeletal muscle proteins in response to training (Rodriguez, Di Marco, & Langley, 2009).

Soy protein, alone or as part of a blend, supports muscle health and muscle protein synthesis (MPS), as part of an exercise program. New research suggests that combining animal and plant proteins that have different absorption rates, such as soy protein, whey, and casein, can prolong delivery of amino acids to the muscle. These three proteins have unique characteristics and thus combining them creates an opportunity to optimize muscle growth. A recent animal study compared soy–dairy blends versus isolated protein sources on their ability to stimulate MPS as measured by muscle protein fractional synthetic rates. Single-source proteins and soy–dairy blends all enhanced MPS; however, the soy–dairy blend extended the amount of time that MPS was activated (Butteiger et al., 2013). Reidy et al. (2013) subsequently conducted a randomized controlled trial in healthy young adults and found that consuming a soy–dairy blend after resistance training extended MPS as well as amino acid delivery compared to whey protein isolate (Reidy et al., 2013). Further analyses also determined that the soy–dairy blend prolonged skeletal muscle net protein balance following resistance exercise using an established isotope tracer infusion method (Reidy et al., 2014). Fig. 2.6 presents the net protein synthesis time charting for the soy–dairy blend. Collectively, these studies demonstrate that soy–dairy blends extend the anabolic window following resistance exercise. Individuals seeking to optimize muscle growth would benefit from consuming soy–dairy blends after exercise training.

2.6.3 Weight Management and Satiety

Soy protein, like other high-quality proteins, is satiating, an attribute that allows foods to be more satisfying and supports reduction of daily energy intake, assisting weight management. Dietary protein influences satiety and plays a key

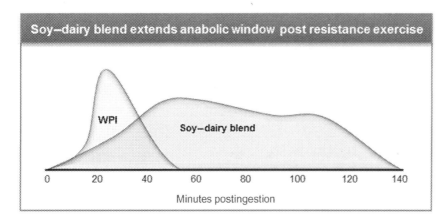

FIGURE 2.6 Plot of net protein synthesis rates post exercise for consumed whey protein isolate versus blend of whey protein isolate, soy protein isolate, and casein. *From Reidy, P. T., Walker D.K., Dickinson, J.M., Gundermann, D.M., Drummond, M.J., Timmerman, K.L., ... Rasmussen, B.B. (2014). Soy-dairy protein blend and whey protein ingestion after resistance exercise increases amino acid transport and transporter expression in human skeletal muscle. Journal of Applied Physiology, 116(11), 1353—1364.*

role in supporting weight management strategies, and, in fact, protein is viewed as the most satiating macronutrient (Astrup, 2005). Diets high in protein increase satiety more than high-carbohydrate diets and can help reduce food intake (Astrup, 2005; Bensaid et al., 2002; Halton & Hu, 2004). High-quality proteins, such as soy, have been shown to suppress appetite in part by stimulating the release of cholecystokinin, which regulates satiety and gastric emptying (Anderson & Moore, 2004; Nishi, Hara, & Tomita, 2003).

High-protein diets (>0.8 g protein per kg body weight per day) help preserve lean body mass (ie, muscle) during weight loss, which in turn, improves the metabolic profile of dieters (Layman, 2004; Paddon-Jones et al., 2008). Several studies have demonstrated the efficacy of soy protein for promoting fat loss, including abdominal fat, while preserving muscle mass (Christie et al., 2010; Deibert et al., 2004; Neacsu, Fyfe, Horgan, & Johnstone, 2014; Sites et al., 2007; Van Nielen, Feskens, Rietman, Siebelink, & Mensink, 2014). Soy protein and animal-based proteins both support weight loss and weight maintenance equally as part of energy-restricted diet; however, soy protein offers additional cardiometabolic advantages, such as maintenance of blood glucose and reduced risk for cardiovascular disease (Neacsu et al., 2014; Van Nielen et al., 2014).

In a recent randomized controlled crossover study, high-soy protein diets were as effective as high-meat protein diets for appetite control and weight loss in obese men; however, the soy protein diet led to greater improvements in blood lipid levels (Neacsu et al., 2014). Similarly, another recent randomized controlled crossover study found that both high-meat protein and high-soy protein diets lowered body weight and improved body composition of postmenopausal women, yet, partly replacing meat with soy protein further improved blood lipid levels and insulin sensitivity independent of changes in body weight (Van Nielen et al., 2014). Collectively, these recent findings indicate the benefits of incorporating soy protein in the diet for healthy weight management go beyond improvements in body composition.

2.6.4 Cardiovascular Health

Cardiovascular fitness and heart health are important for active individuals, as well as to support an improved quality of life. Nutritional interventions can help improve cardiovascular fitness through arterial health and may support blood flow. Another aspect of blood vessel health is blood pressure, and when elevated can lead to endothelial dysfunction. Oftentimes this limits participation in vigorous physical activities (Leddy & Izzo, 2009). A meta-analysis of 27 randomized controlled trials concluded that soy protein intake, compared with a control diet, reduced both systolic and diastolic blood pressure by 2.2 and 1.4 mmHg, respectively. It has been estimated that a 2-mmHg reduction in population systolic blood pressure could lead to a 6% reduction in stroke mortality, 4% reduction in coronary heart disease, and 3% reduction in all-cause mortality (Whelton et al., 2002).

Soy protein has well-tested effects on circulating cholesterol concentrations, as well as blood pressure and blood vessels. A significant number of clinical studies have examined the cholesterol-lowering effects of soy protein, which formed the basis of the FDA-approved health claim that soy protein, as part of a diet low in saturated fat and cholesterol, may reduce the risk of heart disease (US-FDA, 1999). In fact, a total of 13 countries have an approved health claim for soy protein based on its ability to lower plasma cholesterol, these countries include Canada, the United States, Japan, South Africa, The Philippines, Brazil, Indonesia, Korea, Turkey, Malaysia, Chile, Colombia, and India.

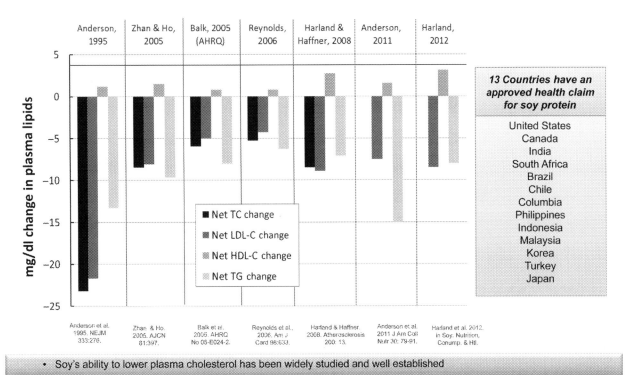

FIGURE 2.7 The cholesterol-lowering effect of soy protein is well established.

Jenkins et al. (2010) conducted a meta-analysis of clinical studies that controlled diets so that the only difference between groups was the source of protein. Soy protein consumption resulted in an average intrinsic reduction in low-density lipoprotein (LDL) cholesterol of 4.3%. This LDL cholesterol-lowering effect was observed with both solid and liquid food forms. The authors also found that replacement of meat or dairy protein with 13 g of soy protein per day resulted in an LDL cholesterol reduction of 3.6% and a maximum lowering of 6.0% was observed at 50 g of soy protein per day (Jenkins et al., 2010). Every 1% reduction in LDL cholesterol equates to a reduction in risk of heart disease from 1 to 3% depending on age, gender, etc. (Law, Wald, & Thompson, 1994). Collectively, this meta-analysis demonstrated that soy protein can reduce LDL cholesterol by 10.3%, with a 4.3% reduction coming from an intrinsic effect of soy protein and then an additional 6.0% lowering when soy protein replaces saturated fat and cholesterol. Multiple metastudies have reached similar conclusions regarding the connection between soy protein consumption and blood lipids (see Fig. 2.7).

2.6.5 Nutritional Relevance of Other Seed Constituents

Soy, like other plant proteins, contains minor constituents associated with the protein fraction, some of which have been reported to have bioactive or antinutritional effects (Macready et al., 2014). These compounds have been the subject of research to better understand how they may interfere with the digestion or absorption of other nutrients but also exert beneficial effects on health outcomes.

2.6.5.1 Trypsin Inhibitors

Trypsin inhibitors are present in a variety of foods including soybeans, potatoes, peas, beans, peanuts, sweet corn, and other vegetables and cereals. Studies have shown trypsin inhibitors can interfere with protein digestion and lead to pancreatic hypertrophy in rats (Folsch, Winckler, & Wormsley, 1974; Neiss, Ivey, & Nesheim, 1972). They evoke increased pancreatic trypsin secretion by forming inactive trypsin—trypsin complexes, which thereby decrease the feedback suppression exerted by free trypsin (Ishe, Lilja, & Lundquist, 1977). Long-term studies in other animals, including primates and swine, however, have not shown negative effects on the pancreas with soy food intake (Ausman et al., 1985; Garthoff et al., 2002).

Heat processing can effectively reduce levels of trypsin inhibitor activity in soy products. Therefore, products that are less heat-processed, such as soymilk or tofu, have higher trypsin inhibitors than SPC and ISP. ISPs are carefully processed to decrease the trypsin inhibitor activity level and thus maintain digestibility and protein quality.

2.6.5.2 Phytates

Phytates are naturally occurring compounds found in many cereals and legumes, including soy. Though phytates are associated with protein, phytate levels do not increase as protein content increases in soy protein products. Phytates are the main storage form of phosphorus in legumes, nuts, seeds, and grains and pass through the digestive tract unabsorbed, as humans lack the enzyme phytase. These compounds can bind to specific minerals and reduce absorption in the digestive tract, however, mineral deficiencies due to phytate consumption are uncommon in developed countries and other food compounds, such as vitamin C, help enhance micronutrient absorption (Mega, 1982).

2.6.5.3 Oxalates

Oxalates are another common constituent of plants that can bind calcium and reduce its absorption (Schlemmer, Frølich, Prieto, & Grases, 2009). Spinach is one of the highest sources of oxalates, rendering the calcium found in spinach much less readily available (Heaney, Weaver, & Recker, 1988). However, when absorbability of calcium from soy-based sources was compared with oxalate-free sources, such as cow's milk, calcium from soymilk and tofu was comparable (Weaver et al., 2002; Zhao, Martin, & Weaver, 2005).

2.6.5.4 Isoflavones

Isoflavones are a type of polyphenol found in legumes, including soybeans, chickpeas, fava beans, pistachios, peanuts, and other fruits and nuts (USDA, 2008). Soybeans are the richest source of isoflavones, and soy foods and ingredients contain varying concentrations of isoflavones. Isoflavone content is affected to some extent by processing, with the highest levels in whole-bean products, such as tofu and cooked soybeans (3−4 mg isoflavones, expressed as aglycones, per gram of protein). That level is reduced during processing to produce ISP (1 mg per g protein) and is further reduced in alcohol-extracted soy protein concentrate (0.2 mg per g protein). Soy isoflavones are only a small constituent of soybeans and thus soy protein ingredients. Therefore, soy-containing foods should not be equated with isoflavones.

Isoflavones have been associated with a number of health benefits. Isoflavones, consumed at levels found in soy foods can help maintain blood vessel health (Messina, 2010). Consumption of foods containing isoflavones may increase the body's level of antioxidants and help support cellular health (Brown et al., 2004; DiSilvestro, Mattern, Wood, & Devor, 2006).

2.6.6 Protein Allergies

According to WHO/IUIS there are eight registered proteins within the soybean which can elicit an allergic response (www.allergen.org). Two of these, β-conglycinin and glycinin, represent 70% of the soybean protein and will be the predominant proteins in commercial soy protein products (Helm et al., 2000; Verhoeckx et al., 2015). FAO includes soy proteins in its list of significant food allergens (FAO/WHO Food Standards, 1991) and the US-FDA and USDA Food Safety and Inspection Service require that these proteins must be declared on all food packages and a warning made separate from the ingredient statement on food labels declaring contained allergens (USDA FSIS, 2015; US-FDA, 2004).

Further processing can reduce soybean allergenicity (Verhoeckx et al., 2015). Thermal processing has been demonstrated to reduce IgE and IgG binding by soy 7S and 11S proteins; moreover, subjecting soybean meal to thermal plastic extrusion with extrudate temperatures greater than 66°C reduced IgG-specific binding to the extrudate soybean meal proteins significantly (Ohishi et al., 1994). Protease enzymatic hydrolysis can be very effective in reducing but not eliminating soybean protein allergenicity (Verhoeckx et al., 2015). Currently, no processes are available that would provide 100% assurance for soybean protein antigen inactivation.

According to Sicherer, Morrow, and Sampson (2000), the incidence of soy protein allergy is much lower (0.4%) than other food allergens, such as milk proteins (2.5%) or peanut proteins (0.8%). In fact, in vitro and blinded food challenge studies with susceptible subjects "show lower allergenic reactivity for soy protein verses other food allergens." Investigations in animal models confirm these clinical studies of diminished immunological reactivity for soy

FIGURE 2.8 Existing clinical research of protein sources for health outcomes. *Internal data from DuPont Nutrition and Health, 2015.*

Protein sources	Quality	Muscle health	Weight management/satiety	Body composition	Heart health
Pea	Digestibility lower, limited in sulfur amino acids, Met & Cys	−	−	−	−
Rice	Digestibility lower, limited in Lys	−	−	−	−
Soy	•••	••	••	••	•••
Casein	•••	••	••	•	•
Whey	•••	•••	••	••	•

Number of symbols reflects strength/depth of the body of evidence to support

proteins (Cordle, 2004). Food allergy reactions to soy proteins do occur and hence enforcement of proper labeling is vital to assure susceptible consumers avoid ingestion.

2.6.7 A Good Source of Protein Across the Lifespan

Soy protein has been shown to support health needs across the lifespan as a source of lean, cholesterol-free and lactose-free protein. The field of nutrition science and exercise physiology supports the need for physical activity in combination with more nutritious choices—such as consuming sources of soy protein, to maintain a healthy quality of life. DuPont Nutrition and Health scientists have assessed the human clinical research supporting source protein impact on different health outcomes; the report summary is provided in Fig. 2.8. From a standpoint of nutritional efficacy and health benefits, soy protein has been one of the most studied ingredients, offering multiple benefits to the consumer.

2.7 USES AND FUNCTIONALITY

ISP is an economic and reliable protein source, which can be used as an alternative to meat and dairy proteins to control costs and improve the nutritional value of various food products. Moreover, soy protein provides both nutritional and functional advantages over animal-based proteins. It is a high-quality and complete protein that contains all of the essential amino acids required to support human nutrition and is supported by an FDA-approved health claim describing its positive effect on heart health. Functionally, soy protein ingredients can replace animal-derived protein (meat, dairy, and egg) and reduce costs without changing taste and quality.

As an ingredient, soy has several functions when used with food products. The versatile nature of the various soy proteins allow it to deliver the following functions within foods:

- Solubility;
- Emulsification;
- Gelation;
- Water binding;
- Whipping/foaming;
- Viscosity;
- Flavor/aroma.

Soy protein products are used in a variety of foods, such as salad dressings, soups, nutrition bars, meat analogs, beverage powders, cheeses, nondairy creamers, frozen desserts, whipped toppings, infant formulas, breads, breakfast cereals, pastas, and pet foods. As described earlier, any given ISP ingredient cannot offer all the functions listed above for use in a given food product. The appropriately processed or modified ISP must be matched to specific functional requirements. For example, a strong gelling ISP would be selected to improve texture and replace meat in a finely comminuted sausage formulation. This same ISP likely would not function well when used to augment an intact muscle meat product such as tumble-marinated chicken breast or marinade-injected cooked roast beef. Such products would require a partially hydrolyzed ISP product possessing lower viscosities and lower gel strengths than used for finely comminuted sausage. Both dairy and soy beverages require different modified ISP ingredients than used for meat. Furthermore, whipped or air-entrained foods require ISP functional characteristics different from those needed for meat and dairy foods; moreover, physical properties required of ISP would be different for extrusion.

2.8 APPLICATION AND CURRENT PRODUCTS

Using soy protein ingredients to replace poultry, meat, fish, egg, and dairy proteins, can enhance quality of food products, reduce costs of various food formulations, and improve environmental sustainability associated with supply of quality protein. Examples of soy applications include:

- Meat extension (beef, pork, poultry, and fish);
- Meat analogs (100% replacement meat);
- Infant formula (replacement of dairy proteins);
- Clinical nutrition (replacement of dairy proteins);
- Dairy (replacement of dairy proteins in, eg, yogurt, cheese, and milk);
- Sports nutrition (replacement of dairy proteins in bars and protein beverages);
- Bread, pasta, etc. (protein fortification);
- Affordable food, such as milk drinks for low-income segments.

Often, soy protein is combined with other protein sources to achieve certain functionalities of nutritional attributes—and in many cases, only partial replacements are possible. It will not be possible to go through each application area and, thus, the following only addresses meat applications as an example.

Textured soy proteins (based on ISP, soy protein concentrates, and soy flours) are common, yet important ingredients of many meat and meat analog products. It is common to replace 30–40% of the meat in foods such as beef patties and chicken nuggets. After hydration, texturized soy protein of the various sizes and densities contributes both meat-like appearance and texture to meat and meat-like food products, while providing an excellent source of high-quality protein similar to that of lean meat. Though inherently bland regarding flavor, textured soy proteins are excellent absorbers of artificial and natural flavors. Additionally, textured soy protein ingredients can be colored using caramel colors, malt extracts, synthetic colors, spice extractives, and seasoning ingredients.

Textured soy proteins are used throughout the world primarily to replace meat for the purpose of formulation cost reduction and processing yield improvements, as well as to improve nutrition. However, these textured ingredients contribute other important attributes to the foods into which they have been formulated. Both ISP powders and textured soy proteins hold water very tenaciously. This attribute allows meat products made with textured soy ingredients and ISP to have greater moisture retention during cooking, reheating, through freezing and thawing, and retaining under heat lamps or steam tables in readiness for serving compared to similar meat products made without such ingredients. Thus, use of both textured soy protein ingredients and functional soy protein ingredients, such as ISP, allows the manufacture of improved meat products.

Meat products formulated with ISP or related soy ingredients provide significant cost savings to processors by replacing expensive lean meats with soy ingredients and water. Meat replacement usually involves maintaining similar fat content as an all-meat product. Since the soy ingredients have extremely low lipid composition, additional meat fat must be added to formulations compensating for the fat removed by the lean substitution with ISP or related soy ingredients. This offers additional formulation cost as fatter meats are valued at lower values than leaner meats. Cost savings and product characterization associated with replacing lean meat with a textured soy protein ingredient and water are described in Table 2.5.

As appears from the formulation examples, the footprint reductions are rather significant for 20–40% meat replacements. More interestingly, this is achieved while reducing costs, and without diluting the nutritional quality (all recipes reflect a protein content of 20%).

2.9 POTENTIAL NEW USES, ISSUES, AND CHALLENGES

A growing international food consumption phenomenon is the flexitarian movement. Technically, the term flexitarian refers to individuals who are primarily vegetarians but indulge in animal foods occasionally. More recently, the term flexitarian has been used to describe consumers structuring their diets to intentionally eat less meat for any given

TABLE 2.5 Example Cost, Yield, and Footprint Impacts of Replacing Meat With Hydrated Textured Soy Protein

	Meat Replacements			
	0%	20%	30%	40%
Ingredients				
90% Lean beef. USD 6.31/kg (%)	75	49.48	36.5	25
50% Lean beef. USD 2.84/kg (%)	24.5	30	33	34.5
Soy protein as ISP or TSPC (%)	0	5.56	8.33	11.11
Water (%)	0	14.46	21.66	28.89
Salt (%)	0.5	0.5	0.5	0.5
Total (%)	100	100	100	100
Costs and Yields of Formulations				
Ingredients cost. Raw (USD/kg beef patty)	5.04	3.81	3.19	2.62
Cooking yield (%)	70	76	77	78
Ingredients cost. Cooked (USD/kg beef patty)	7.2	5.01	4.14	3.36
Footprint of Formulations[a]				
Carbon footprint (kg CO_2e/kg beef patty)	35.6	28.5	25	21.5
Blue water footprint (L/kg beef patty)	321	259	228	197
Land use footprint (m^2 year/kg beef patty)	262	210	184	159

[a]The footprints associated with the creation of the various beef patty formulations were determined using the carbon, blue water, and land use footprint results provided for beef meat based on consequential modeling, and adjusted for protein content, which is assumed be to 20%. The footprints for soy protein are conservatively estimated to be the same as for ISP (90% protein) despite a protein content around 72% in the actual formulations. The footprints for salt and water are assumed to be zero for the sake of simplification.
TSPC, Textured soy protein concentrate

number of reasons regardless of their meat consumption habits. The rationale offered for individuals wishing to consume less meat includes reduced reliance on animal harvesting, improved agricultural sustainability, and personal health improvement. Meat analogs and nonmeat protein meals comprised of any number of vegetable proteins are significant components of flexitarian, vegetarian, and vegan diets. Additionally, soy beverages, nutrition snack bars, snack chips, etc., containing significant quantities of ISP can fully or partially replace animal protein portions of meals. These soy-containing foods are recent developments. Numerous more traditional soy foods such as soymilk, tofu, tempeh, roasted soy nuts, yuba, and miso continue to offer alternatives to animal proteins.

This movement appears to have generated business development opportunities, as recently several new companies have emerged to take advantage of this food trend. The common goal of these companies is to create great vegetarian foods such as salad dressings, snacks, beverages, and meat analog products possessing all the eating quality characteristics of animal protein-based foods. The business model of each of these companies includes a "no compromise" strategy to food product design such that the engineered foods precisely mimic those of animal protein foods. Moreover, the emergence of these new companies has pressured existing companies to improve their current products and expand product offerings.

In addition, consumers are interested in where and how their foods are made. There is a clear trend toward foods made with simpler ingredients; ingredients considered "natural" and "organic" and ingredients (and foods) considered "good-for-you."

2.9.1 Generational Flavor Improvements

Characteristic "beany and grassy" flavor limited early market growth of soybean protein products in Western-culture foods. The flavors, which are generally desired in Eastern culture foods, were put-offs for consumers without familiarity.

Considerable research was done in the early 1960–70s that identified lipoxygenase enzyme (Lox) oxidation of lipids as a key factor. Over the years, several steps have been taken to significantly reduce this defect. These include breeding of seeds with low or no Lox, and reducing the content of oxidation-susceptible fatty acids, linoleic, and linolenic acids. Processors also adopted methods to maintain seeds at low enough water activity to inhibit Lox and then heat-inactivate Lox quickly during aqueous extraction processing. Unfortunately, since soybean oil is polyunsaturated oil, autoxidation can occur without enzymatic catalysis. For this reason, protein product processors also focused efforts on removing as much oil as possible during extraction, which resulted in better flavor and long-term flavor stability. Finally, soybean protein processors have borrowed separation and heat-processing techniques from other analogous industries (such as dairy) to move beyond the previous flavor limitations for Western-culture foods (Johnson et al., 2008).

2.9.2 Genetic Modified and Identity Preserved

Over the past 20 years, there has been a tidal wave of farmer conversion from growing traditionally crossbred soybeans to genetically engineered modified (GE M) soybeans (Genetic engineering (GE) is the term recommended by the US-FDA, however it is important to note that in some media, publications, and discussions the terms used to refer to the same material could be genetically modified (GM), genetically modified organism (GMO). Today, there are a number of traits (primarily HT (herbicide-tolerant) and IR (insect-resistant) traits) relevant to the farmer and processor, which have been enabled by genetic modification techniques. The GE M HT technology in soybeans has boosted farm incomes by $5.3 billion in 2013 over 2012, and since 1996 has delivered an estimated $41.4 billion of extra farm income (Brookes & Barfoot, 2015).

However, public concern over GE M foods since 1996 has created demand for product lines with controlled soybean (non-GE M) sources. These needs have been met through the creation of supply chains that enable delivery of identity preserved (IP) non-GE M beans. So today, food processors and consumers have GE M or IP choices regarding soybean protein products as well.

Identity preservation is a standardized and controlled process designed to minimize adventitious comingling of diverse product streams. An IP program requires use of best practices for agricultural management—starting with certified non-GE M soybean seeds, enabling controlled soybean delivery and processing throughout the supply chain. These practices are managed under defined terms and procedures with documentation of conformance with IP procedures. Even though the United States does not require labeling of GE M products that meet the substantial equivalence criteria, other countries have labeling standards that require conformance to maximum levels for labeling purposes (such as EU labeling laws and regulations $\leq 0.9\%$ threshold of GE M DNA; EU 1829/2003 and EU 1830/2003). Typically, there will be third-party audits of conformance to IP procedures. Finally, periodic testing to validate effectiveness of the IP system will be conducted using methods such as ELISA and PCR at qualified laboratories.

Soybean seed certification programs are going beyond IP though. No matter how the seed genetics are derived, the industry, regulators, financiers, buyers, and other stakeholders must work collectively to develop and promote environmentally appropriate, socially beneficial, and economically viable practices to minimize the potential negative effects of increased soybean production and trade. Working groups such as RTRS provide guidelines which move soybean producers and traders toward soy production that is socially equitable, economically feasible, and environmentally sound (RTRS, 2013). The Soybean Sustainability Assurance Protocol (SSAP) is another program established in the United States by the US Soybean Export Council and American Soybean Association (USB, 2014).

2.10 CONCLUDING REMARKS

It is estimated that demand for protein will grow 110% between 2005 and 2050 (Tilman, Balzer, Hill, & Befort, 2011). Both global population and improved standards of living in the developing nations serve as drivers for the additional protein required to feed the world in 2050. Per capita meat consumption tied to anticipated improved per capita incomes in many of the developing countries will constitute, in no small way, the increased global protein demand through 2050. Meeting future world requirements for protein will require significant expansion of plant and animal production through advances in agricultural technologies, increased acreage devoted to intensified agriculture, finding additional water that can be used for agriculture and probable global reallocation of land and water resources for animal and crop production (Tilman et al., 2011). This necessary change in agricultural production will not be trivial nor without some degree of risk, requiring considerable international cooperation. Increasing human soybean protein ingredient consumption, as demonstrated in this chapter, would allow water and land use conservation for the purpose of protein production while significantly reducing the carbon emissions required to produce each kg of protein of high nutritive value.

REFERENCES

Anderson, G., & Moore, S. (2004). Dietary proteins in the regulation of food intake and body weight in humans. *The Journal of Nutrition, 134*, 974S–979S.

Astrup, A. (2005). The satiating power of protein—A key to obesity prevention? *American Journal of Clinical Nutrition, 82*, 1–2.

Ausman, L. M., Harwood, J. P., King, N. W., Sehgal, P. K., Nicolosi, R. J., Hegsted, D. M., . . . Tarcza, J. (1985). The effects of long term soy protein and milk protein feeding on the pancreas of *Cebus albifrons* monkeys. *Journal of Nutrition, 115*(12), 1691–1701.

Bensaid, A., Tome, D., Gietzen, D., Even, P., Morens, C., Gausseres, N., & Fromentin, G. (2002). Protein is more potent than carbohydrate for reducing appetite in rats. *Physiological Behavior, 75*, 577–582.

Berk, Z. (1992). Isolated soybean protein. In: *Technology of production of edible flours and protein products from soybeans*. FAO Agricultural Services Bulletin no. 97.

Boucher, D., Elias, P., Lininger, K., May-Tobin, C., Roquemore, S., & Saxon, E. (2011). *The root of the problem—What's driving tropical deforestation today? Union of concerned scientist*. Cambridge, MA: UCS Publications.

Brookes, G., & Barfoot, P. (2015). *GM crops: Global socio-economic and environmental impacts 1996–2013*. Dorchester: PG Economics Ltd.

Brown, E., DiSilvestro, R., Babaknia, A., & Devor, S. (2004). Soy versus whey protein bars: Effects on exercise training impact on lean body mass and antioxidant status. *Nutrition Journal, 3*, 22–26.

Butteiger, D., Cope, M., Liu, P., Mukherjea, R., Volpi, E., Rasmussen, B. B., & Krule, E. S. (2013). A soy, whey and caseinate blend extends postprandial skeletal muscle protein synthesis in rats. *Clinical Nutrition, 32*, 585–591.

Candow, D. G., Burke, N. C., Smith-Palmer, T., & Burke, D. G. (2006). Effect of whey and soy protein supplementation combined with resistance training in young adults. *International Journal of Sport Nutrition and Exercise Metabolism, 6*, 233–244.

Christie, D. R., Grant, J., Darnell, B. E., Chapman, V. R., Gastaldelli, A., & Sites, C. K. (2010). Metabolic effects of soy supplementation in postmenopausal Caucasian and African American women: A randomized, placebo-controlled trial. *American Journal of Obstetrics and Gynecology, 203* (153), e1–e9.

Cordle, C. (2004). Soy protein allergy: Incidence and relative severity. *Journal of Nutrition, 134*, 1213S–1219S.

Dalgaard, R., Schmidt, J. H., & Flysjö, A. (2014). Generic model for calculating carbon footprint of milk using four different LCA modelling approaches. *Journal of Cleaner Production, 73*, 146–153.

Deibert, P., Konig, D., Schmidt-Trucksaess, A., Zaenker, K. S., Frei, I., Landmann, U., & Berg, A. (2004). Weight loss without losing muscle mass in pre-obese and obese subjects induced by a high-soy-protein diet. *International Journal of Obesity and Related Metabolic Disorders, 28*, 1349–1352.

Deibert, P., Solleder, F., Konig, D., Vitolins, M. Z., Dickhuth, H. H., Gollhofer, A., & Berg, A. (2011). Soy protein based supplementation supports metabolic effects of resistance training in previously untrained middle aged males. *Aging Male, 14*, 273–279.

DiSilvestro, R. A., Mattern, C., Wood, N., & Devor, S. T. (2006). Soy protein intake by active young adult men raises plasma antioxidant capacity without altering plasma testosterone. *Nutrition Research, 26*, 92–95.

Dragan, I., Stroescu, V., Stoian, I., Georgescu, E., & Baloescu, R. (1992). Studies regarding the efficiency of Supro isolated soy protein in Olympic athletes. *Revue Roumaine de Physiologie, 29*, 63–70.

Eshel, G., & Martin, P.A. (2006). Diet, energy, and global warming. *Earth Interactions, 10*, paper no. 9. <http://www.fao.org/fileadmin/templates/wsfs/docs/expert_paper/How_to_Feed_the_World_in_2050>.

FAO/WHO. (1991). *Protein quality evaluation, Report of Joint FAO/WHO Expert Consultation*. Rome: Food and Agriculture Organization of the United Nations.

FAO/WHO Food Standards. (1991). Codex Alimentarius. The Codex General Standard for the Labelling of Prepackaged Foods. CODEX STAN 1-1985 (Rev. 1-1991).

Flysjö, A. (2012). *Greenhouse gas emissions in milk and dairy product chains—Improving the carbon footprint of dairy products (PhD thesis)*. Denmark: Science and Technology, Aarhus University.

Foley, J. A. (2011). Solutions for a cultivated planet. *Nature, 478*, 337–342.

Folsch, U. R., Winckler, K., & Wormsley, K. A. (1974). Effect of soybean diet on enzyme content and ultra-structure of the rat exocrine pancreas. *Digestion, 11*, 161–171.

Garthoff, L. H., Henderson, G. R., Sager, A., Sobotka, T., Gaines, D., O'Donnell, M., & Khan, M. (2002). Pathological evaluation, clinical chemistry and plasma cholecystokinin in neonatal and young miniature swine fed soy trypsin inhibitor from 1 to 39 weeks of age. *Food and Chemical Toxicology, 40*(4), 501–516.

Halton, T. L., & Hu, F. B. (2004). The effects of high protein diets on thermogenesis, satiety and weight loss: A critical review. *Journal of the American College of Nutrition, 23*, 373–385.

Hartman, J. W., Tang, J. E., Wilkinson, S. B., Tarnopolsky, M. A., Lawrence, R. L., Fullerton, A. V., & Phillips, S. M. (2007). Consumption of fat-free fluid milk after resistance exercise promotes greater lean mass accretion than does consumption of soy or carbohydrate in young, novice, male weightlifters. *American Journal of Clinical Nutrition, 86*, 373–381.

Haub, M. D., Wells, A. M., Tarnopolsky, M. A., & Campbell, W. W. (2002). Effect of protein source on resistive-training-induced changes in body composition and muscle size in older men. *American Journal of Clinical Nutrition, 76*, 511–517.

Heaney, R. P., Weaver, C. M., & Recker, R. R. (1988). Calcium absorbability from spinach. *American Journal of Clinical Nutrition, 47*(4), 707–709.

Helm, R. M., Cockwell, G., Connaughton, C., Sampson, H. A., Bannon, G. A., Beilinson, V., & Burks, A. W. (2000). A soybean G2 glycinin allergen. 1. Identification and characterization. *International Archive of Allergy and Immunology, 123*, 205–212.

Hoekstra, A. Y., Chapagain, A. K., Aldaya, M. M., & Mekonnen, M. M. (2011). *The Water Footprint Assessment Manual: Setting the Global Standard*. London, UK: Earthscan.

Hughes, G. J., Ryan, D. J., Mukherjea, R., & Schasteen, C. S. (2011). Protein digestibility-corrected amino acid scores (PDCAAS) for soy protein isolates and concentrate: Criteria for evaluation. *Journal of Agricultural and Food Chemistry, 59*(23), 12707–12712.

International Institute for Sustainable Development. (2014). *The state of sustainability issues review* (pp. 253–273). Manitoba: International Institute for Sustainable Development, Chapter 12.

IPCC. 2007. Climate change 2007: Synthesis report. In Core Writing Team, R. K. Pachauri, & A. Reisinger (Eds.), *Contribution of working groups I, II and III to the fourth assessment report of the intergovernmental panel on climate change* (104 pp.). Geneva, Switzerland: IPCC.

Ishe, I., Lilja, P., & Lundquist, I. (1977). Feedback regulation of pancreatic enzyme secretion by intestinal trypsin in man. *Digestion, 15*, 303–308.

Jenkins, D. J., Mirrahimi, A., Srichaikul, K., Berryman, C. E., Wang, L., Carleton, A., & Kris-Etherton, P. M. (2010). Soy protein reduces serum cholesterol by both intrinsic and food displacement mechanisms. *The Journal of Nutrition, 140*(12), 2302S–2311S.

Johnson, L. A., White, P. J., & Galloway, R. (2008). *Soybeans—Chemistry, production, processing, and utilization*. Urbana, IL: United Soybean Board, AOCS Press.

Law, M. R., Wald, N. J., & Thompson, S. G. (1994). By how much and how quickly does reduction in serum cholesterol concentration lower risk of ischaemic heart disease? *British Medical Journal, 308*, 367–372.

Layman, D. K. (2004). Protein quantity and quality at levels above the RDA improves adult weight loss. *Journal of the American College of Nutrition, 23*, 631S–636S.

Leddy, J. J., & Izzo, J. (2009). Hypertension in athletes. *The Journal of Clinical Hypertension, 11*, 226–233.

Liu, K. (1999). *Soybeans chemistry, technology, and utilization*. Gaithersburg, MD: Aspen Publication.

LMC International. (2011). Soyfoods and soy protein in the human diet: A tool in the quest for food sustainability—Review and interpretation of the literature. Report for: Soyfoods Association of North America (SANA), Washington, DC.

Macready, A., George, T., Chong, M., Alimbeov, D., Jin, Y., Vidal, A., & Gordon, J. (2014). Flavonoid-rich fruit and vegetables improve microvascular reactivity and inflammatory status in men at risk of cardiovascular disease—FLAVURS: A randomized controlled trial. *American Journal of Clinical Nutrition, 99*(3), 479–489.

Maesta, N., Nahas, E. A., Nahas-Neto, J., Orsatti, F. L., Fernandes, C. E., Traiman, P., & Burini, R. C. (2007). Effects of soy protein and resistance exercise on body composition and blood lipids in postmenopausal women. *Maturitas, 56*, 350–358.

Mega, J. A. (1982). Phytate: Its chemistry, occurrence, food interactions, nutritional significance, and methods of analysis. *Journal of Agricultural and Food Chemistry, 30*, 1–9.

Mekonnen, M. M., & Hoekstra, A. Y. (2011). The green, blue and grey water footprint of crops and derived crop products. *Hydrology and Earth System Sciences, 15*, 1577–1600.

Mekonnen, M. M., & Hoekstra, A. Y. (2012). A global assessment of the water footprint of farm animal products. *Ecosystems, 15*, 401–415.

Messina, M. (2010). A brief historical overview of the past two decades of soy and isoflavone research. *Journal of Nutrition, 140*, 1350S–1354S.

Muñoz, I. (2015). Life cycle assessment of isolated soy protein produced by DuPont Nutrition and Health. In Prepared by Ivan Muñoz, 2-0 LCA Consultants for DuPont Nutrition and Health. Made in accordance with the ISO 14044 standard 3rd party reviewed by SP Food and Bioscience in Gothenburg, Sweden. Confidential.

Muñoz, I., & Schmidt J. (2015). Life cycle screening of animal and vegetable derived protein sources. In Prepared by Ivan Muñoz and Jannick Schmidt, 2-0 LCA Consultants for DuPont Industrial Biosciences ApS.

Myhre, G., Shindell, D., Bréon, F.-M., Collins, W., Fuglestvedt, J., Huang, J., & Zhang, H. (2013). Anthropogenic and natural radiative forcing. In T. F. Stocker, D. Qin, G.-K. Plattner, M. Tignor, S. K. Allen, J. Boschung, A. Nauels, Y. Xia, V. Bex, & P. M. Midgles (Eds.), *Climate change 2013: The physical science basis. Contribution of Working Group I to the Fifth Assessment Report of the Intergovernmental Panel on Climate Change*. New York, NY: Cambridge University Press.

Neacsu, M., Fyfe, C., Horgan, G., & Johnstone, A. M. (2014). Appetite control and biomarkers of satiety with vegetarian (soy) and meat-based high-protein diets for weight loss in obese men: A randomized crossover trial. *American Journal of Clinical Nutrition, 100*, 548–558.

Neiss, I., Ivey, C. A., & Nesheim, M. C. (1972). Stimulation of gall bladder emptying and pancreatic secretion in chicks by soybean whey protein. *Proceedings of the Society for Experimental Biology and Medicine, 140*, 291–296.

Nijdam, D., Rood, T., & Westhoek, H. (2012). The price of protein: Review of land use and carbon footprints from lie cycle assessments of animal food products and their substitutes. *Food Policy, 37*, 760–770.

Nishi, T., Hara, H., & Tomita, F. (2003). Soybean beta-conglycinin peptone suppresses food intake and gastric emptying by increasing plasma cholecystokinin levels in rats. *The Journal of Nutrition, 133*, 352–357.

Ohishi, A., Watanabe, K., Urushibata, M., Utsuno, K., Ikuta, K., Sugimoto, K., & Harada, H. (1994). Detection of soybean antigenicity and reduction by twin screw extrusion. *Journal American Oil Chemists Society, 71*, 1391–1396.

Paddon-Jones, D., Westman, E., Mattes, R. D., Wolfe, R. R., Astrup, A., & Westerterp-Plantenga, M. (2008). Protein, weight management, and satiety. *American Journal of Clinical Nutrition, 87*, 1558S–1561S.

Reidy, P. T., Walker, D. K., Dickinson, J. M., Gundermann, D. M., Drummond, M. J., Timmerman, K. L., & Rasmussen, B. B. (2013). Protein blend ingestion following resistance exercise promotes human muscle protein synthesis. *The Journal of Nutrition, 143*, 410–416.

Reidy, P. T., Walker, D. K., Dickinson, J. M., Gundermann, D. M., Drummond, M. J., Timmerman, K. L., & Rasmussen, B. B. (2014). Soy-dairy protein blend and whey protein ingestion after resistance exercise increases amino acid transport and transporter expression in human skeletal muscle. *Journal of Applied Physiology, 116*(11), 1353–1364.

Rodriguez, N. R., Di Marco, N. M., & Langley, S. (2009). American College of Sports Medicine position stand. Nutrition and athletic performance. *Medicine & Science in Sports & Exercise, 41*, 709–731.

RTRS. (2013). RTRS standard for responsible soy production version 2.0_ENG. Round Table on Responsible Soy Association (RTRS). <http://www.responsiblesoy.org/documentos/rtrs-standard-for-responsible-soy-production/?lang=en>. Accessed September 2015.

Schlemmer, U., Frølich, W., Prieto, R. M., & Grases, F. (2009). Phytate in foods and significance for humans: Food sources, intake, processing, bioavailability, protective role and analysis. *Molecular Nutrition and Food Research, 53*, 330–375.

Schmidt, J. H. (2015). Life cycle assessment of five vegetable oils. *Journal of Cleaner Production, 87*, 130–138.

Schmidt, J. H., & Weidema, B. P. (2008). Shift in the marginal supply of vegetable oil. *International Journal of Life Cycle Assessment, 13*(3), 235–239. <http://lca-net.com/p/995>.

Sicherer, S., Morrow, E., & Sampson, H. (2000). Dose-response in double-blind, placebo-controlled oral food challenges in children with atopic dermatitis. *Journal of Allergy and Clinical Immunology, 105*, 582–586.

Sites, C. K., Cooper, B. C., Toth, M. J., Gastaldelli, A., Arabshahi, A., & Barnes, S. (2007). Effect of a daily supplement of soy protein on body composition and insulin secretion in postmenopausal women. *Fertility and Sterility, 88*(6), 1609–1617.

Sonnemann, G., & Vigon, B. (2011). *UNEP/SETAC Life Cycle Initiative workshop report: Global Guidance Principles for Life Cycle Assessment Databases*. France: United Nations Environmental Programme (UNEP).

Tilman, D., Balzer, C., Hill, J., & Befort, B. (2011). Global food demand and the sustainable intensification of agriculture. *Proceedings of the National Academy of Sciences, 108*, 20260–20264.

United States Department of Agriculture. (2008). A Database for the Isoflavone Content of Selected Foods, Release 2.0. September.

United States Department of Agriculture. (2011). Soy Flour, Defatted. National Nutrient Database for Standard Reference Release 27, NDB 16417, Accessed September 25, 2015.

United States Department of Agriculture. (2015). World Agriculture Supply and Demand Estimates, WASDE—543, July 10, p. 28.

USB. (2014). Certified Sustainable, Chesterfield, MO, Nov. 10. United Soybean Board (USB), US. <http://unitedsoybean.org/article/certified-sustainable/>.

USDA FSIS. (2015). FSIS Directive 7230.1 Ongoing Verification of Product Formulation and Labeling Targeting the Eight Most Common ("Big Eight") Food Allergens. Issue Date March 10, 2015. Food Safety and Inspection Service (FSIS), US.

US-FDA. (1999). Food labelling: Health claims; soy protein and coronary heart disease. Final rule. Federal Register 64:57700-33. United States Food and Drug Administration (US-FDA), HHS.

US-FDA. (2004). Food Allergen Labeling and Consumer Protection Act of 2004 (Public Law 108-282, Title II). Food and Drug Administration (FDA).

Van Nielen, M., Feskens, E. J., Rietman, A., Siebelink, E., & Mensink, M. (2014). Partly replacing meat protein with soy protein alters insulin resistance and blood lipids in postmenopausal women with abdominal obesity. *The Journal of Nutrition, 144*, 1423–1429.

Verhoeckx, K. C., et al. (2015). Food processing and allergenicity. *Food and Chemical Toxicology, 80*(2015), 223–240.

Weaver, C., Heaney, R. P., Connor, L., Martin, B. R., Smith, D. L., & Nielsen, S. (2002). Bioavailability of calcium from tofu as compared with milk in premenopausal women. *Journal of Food Science, 67*(8), 3144–3147.

Weidema, B. (2014). Has ISO 14040/44 failed its role as a standard for life cycle assessment? *Journal of Industrial Ecology, 18*, 324–326. Available from http://dx.doi.org/10.1111/jiec.12139.

Weidema, B.P., Ekvall, T., & Heijungs, R. (2010). Guidelines for application of deepened and broadened LCA. Deliverable D18 of work package 5 of the CALCAS project (Co-ordination Action for innovation in Life-Cycle Analysis for Sustainability). July 2009.

Whelton, P. K., He, J., Appel, L. J., Cutler, J. A., Havas, S., Kotchen, T. A., & Karimbakas, J. (2002). Primary prevention of hypertension: Clinical and public health advisory from The National High Blood Pressure Education Program. *Journal of American Medical Association, 288*, 1882–1888.

WWF. (2014). *The growth of soy: Impacts and solutions*. Gland: WWF International.

Zhao, Y., Martin, B., & Weaver, C. (2005). Calcium bioavailability of calcium carbonate fortified soymilk is equivalent to cow's milk in young women. *Journal of Nutrition, 135*(10), 2379–2382.

Chapter 3

Rice Protein and Rice Protein Products

H. Hoogenkamp[1], H. Kumagai[2] and J.P.D. Wanasundara[3]

[1]*RiceBran Technologies Inc., Scottsdale, AZ, United States,* [2]*Nihon University, Fujisawa-shi, Japan,* [3]*Agriculture and Agri-Food Canada, Saskatoon SK, Canada*

3.1 INTRODUCTION

Rice (*Oryza sativa* L.) is often referred to as the "gold of the Orient" and is the most universally eaten daily staple for nearly half of the global population; more than 3.5 billion people mostly from Asia, Africa, parts of Latin America, and the Caribbean. Rice plays a critical role in food security of developing countries of the world. It is estimated that China and India together account for ∼50% of the global rice consumption. Daily consumption of rice is highest among Asian countries. In 2011, average global per capita rice consumption reached close to 60 kg/year, while it reached ∼100 kg/year for Asian countries.[1] Rice provides nearly 20% of human calorie intake worldwide, making it the most important crop in the global human nutrition (Zeigler & Barclay, 2008). It is also estimated that rice provides up to 50% of the daily caloric supply and a substantial amount of the dietary protein requirement for about 520 million people living in poverty in Asian region (Muthayya, Sugimoto, Montgomery, & Maberly, 2014). Rice has been one of the major sources of protein in Asian countries (Grigg, 1995; Wang et al., 2015), and the most abundant vegetable protein source in Japan (Kubota et al., 2013). Rice production in Asia has deep sociopolitical and sociocultural roots and accounts for about 90% of global production.

A major fraction of global rice consumption is in the form of whole or broken kernel. Increase in the consumption of rice-based noodles, and value-added products such as breakfast cereals, baked product paste, rice flakes, crackers, snacks is evident in addition to whole grain. Rice is a fast-growing healthy grain option in Canada and the US.[2] Rice and rice products provide gluten-free product development options and are therefore available in a wide range of food products.

As a food crop, rice was late in domestication compared to barley and wheat and may have happened about 8000–10,000 years ago. Since then this grass species has been constantly selected for improved traits and has become an economic giant providing the world's staple (Bhattachrya, 2011). Rice is a semiaquatic annual grass and belongs to the genus *Oryza*. Among the 22 species found in this genus, only *O. glaberrina* (confined to the African continent) and *O. sativa* (widely cultivated globally) are important for human consumption. *Japonica* and *indica* rice are two major subspecies of *O. sativa*: the former is a short and sticky type with amylose content of 15–26% (Biselli et al., 2014), and the latter is a long and nonsticky type with amylose content of 23–31%. Subspecies *japonica* is usually cultivated in temperate areas such as East Asia, while *indica* is grown in tropical areas such as South Asia. Among more than 13,000 varieties of rice that have been reported, three groups of widely cultivated ecological varieties can be identified: (1) long-grain *indica* varieties grown in tropical and subtropical Asia, (2) short/medium-grained *japonica* rice cultivated in temperate regions such as Japan and Northern China, and (3) medium-grain *javonica* rice grown in the Philippines and the mountainous areas of Madagascar and Indonesia.[3] According to the book "Rice quality − A guide to rice properties and analysis" by Kshirod R. Bhattacharya (2011), it is difficult to find a set of rules to describe the variation found in rice for all the aspects; contradictions and paradoxes are part of the nature of rice. This book provides information on rice in a wider scope than what is condensed in this chapter.

---

1. <http://irri.org/rice-today/trends-in-global-rice-consumption/> Accessed November 2, 2015.
2. <http://www5.agr.gc.ca/resources/prod/Internet-Internet/MISB-DGSIM/ATS-SEA/PDF/6216-eng.pdf> Accessed November 2, 2015.
3. <http://ricepedia.org/rice-as-a-plant/rice-species/>.

3.2 PRODUCTION OF RICE

According to FAOSTAT data, nearly 115 countries contribute to global rice production in which >90% is from 13 rice-producing countries. Global paddy rice (before processing to rice grains) production in 2013 was estimated 740.9 million metric tons (MT).[4] Rice occupies second place after corn in the world's food grain production. Global milled rice production has increased from 484 million MT in 2011/12 to 494.9 million MT in 2014/15.[5] Rice is grown on ~160 million ha and 90% of that land is in Asia. In large part, ~200 million smallholders contribute to world rice production and also about 20% of the world's population depends on rice cultivation for their livelihood. China is not only the world's largest consumer of rice; it is also the largest producer, accounting for a quarter of the global input.

Rice is thinly traded for two main reasons. One is that many countries subsidize their rice production and impose trade restrictions or tariffs on imported rice. The other is the wide range of rice types in the market. Rice is classified by grain length (long, medium, short), by form (*japonica, indica*, aromatic, wild), by the type of processing (white, brown, parboiled), and by any combination thereof (Hoogenkamp, 2015). Although long-grain white rice is the most common, specific varieties of rice are traded in small volumes. Most of the rice produced around the world is consumed domestically. China, Thailand, India, and Vietnam constitute 66% of world rice trade. The United States produces on average ~9 million tons of rice and occupies fifth place among global rice-exporting countries (USA Rice[6]). In the 2013–14 trade years, only 9% of the world's rough rice (43.4 million MT of 478.2 million MT) was exported.

3.2.1 Land Use

Rice farming is the largest single use of land for food production, the most important economic activity on earth, and the single most important employment and income source for rural communities (Bhattacharya, 2011). Rice crop is grown in different parts of the world under a range of climates including temperate, subtropical, and tropical. Within these climatic regions, the weather varies from arid, semiarid to subhumid and humid. Rice is produced in different ecosystems under these climatic regions and weather conditions. Based on soil–water conditions these ecosystems include irrigated lowland, irrigated upland, rain-fed lowland, rain-fed upland, and deep water/floating. Rice is cultivated in saline, alkaline, and acid-sulfur soils.

In South Asia, Southeast Asia, East Asia, and Africa, farm size for rice cultivating is generally small, less than one or few hectares. In most of these countries, except Japan and the Korean Republic, rice cultivation still uses human labor to a great extent. Rice cultivation in Australia, Europe, and the USA is on large farms and is highly mechanized (Muthayya et al., 2014). It is estimated that the global rice-producing area is declining due to land conversion and urbanization, salinization, and increased water scarcity.

Although global rice production shows a continuous increase from 1961, fluctuations in the volume of rice produced/year are mainly due to declining rice harvest area around the world.[5] Rice production is known for low N-use efficiency compared to other cereals. Although the yield potential of modern rice varieties is 10 tons/ha, on average farmers harvest 5 tons/ha (Khush and Virk, 2010). According to FAO reporting, global average for annual yield of rice is 4.49 tons/ha.[7] The rice-yield has reached a plateau and technological innovation on rice grain is needed to break through the current yield limits to provide adequate nutrition and food security for the growing world populations (Hoogenkamp, 2015).

3.2.2 Water Use

Approximately, world rice production areas are divided as 85% under wetland and 15% under upland systems. Wetland cultivation is either irrigated or rain-fed. Soil is kept saturated with water during the entire period of rice cultivation except for the last 15 days to have dry fields for easy harvesting. Rain-fed lowland wet cultivation occurs in bunded fields that are flooded with rainwater. About 20% of world rice production is from rain-fed lowland cultivation. Irrigated lowland cultivation is on bunded fields with assured water supply and produces two to three crops per year. This irrigated wetland production system contributes ~75% of world rice production. The work of Chapagain and Hoekstra (2010) extensively describes the water footprint of rice production for individual rice-producing countries and also in global terms. It is estimated that the global water footprint of rice production is 784 billion m^3/year that can be

---

4. <http://www.statista.com/statistics/263977/world-grain-production-by-type/> Accessed November 2, 2015.
5. <http://www.fao.org/worldfoodsituation/csdb/en/> Accessed November 2, 2015.
6. <http://usarice.com/news-resources/archive> Accessed November 2, 2015.
7. <http://www.fao.org/fileadmin/templates/agphome/documents/Rice/sustintriceprod.pdf>.

broken down as 48% green, 44% blue, and 8% gray water. In South Asian countries, although the water footprint is quite significant for rice production, the contribution to water scarcity is relatively low because rice growing occurs in the wet monsoon season. It is clear that water cost for rice production varies in a wide range from place to place, and the production system whether wet or dry (Chapagain & Hoekstra, 2010).

3.2.3 Energy Use

Energy involved in producing rice varies with production system and country because of the involvement of irrigation and labor (human and animal) depending on the practices of the region. According to Pimentel and Pimentel (2003), kcal energy output/kcal energy input for rice production varies among the countries and localities. In Borneo, the Iban tribe uses only human labor and no fossil fuel for rice cultivation, and has a relatively high return for energy investment with the kcal output to input ratio of 7.1:1. In Japan, employing human power, high-yielding varieties, fertilizers, and other technologies results in a kcal output/kcal input ratio of 2.80:1. Both human and animal power are used in rice production in the Philippines which has an estimated energy output/input ratio of 3.29:1. Rice production in the United States uses considerable input of fossil fuel energy and receives significantly higher yields (similar to Japan) than some other production systems discussed above and results in 2.2:1 energy output/input ratio.

3.3 PROCESSING OF RICE AND RICE PROTEINS

Paddy is the end product that is obtained from harvesting and threshing of the mature rice plant. The edible rice kernel (true fruit or caryopsis) is encased in the protective husk or hull that is inedible. Removal of hull produces brown rice coated with several coatings or "bran" (Fig. 3.1). Multistage milling, involving dehusking, milling, and polishing, produces white rice.

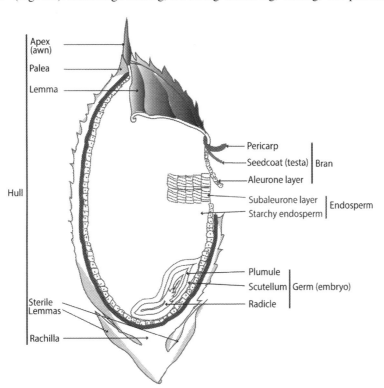

FIGURE 3.1 A schematic depicting rice grain and associated structural components. Rice grain with husk makes paddy. Bran, germ, and endosperm together make brown rice. White rice is made up of endosperm only. The husk of *japonica* rice includes rudimentary glumes and a portion of the pedicel.[8] *Redrawn from figures in Rice Almanac.*

---

8. <http://ricepedia.org/rice-as-a-plant/parts-of-the-rice-plant>.

TABLE 3.1 Basic Composition, Mineral, and Vitamin Levels of Uncooked Brown and White Rice From Japan

Type	Water (%)	Protein (%)	Fat (%)	Carbohydrates (%)	Ash (%)	Minerals (mg%)			Vitamins (mg%)		
						K	Mg	Fe	B1	B2	B6
Brown	15.5	6.8	2.7	73.8	1.2	230	110	2.1	0.41	0.04	0.45
White	15.5	6.1	0.9	77.1	0.4	88	23	0.8	0.08	0.02	0.12

Source: Food Composition Database, Ministry of Education, Culture, Sports, Science and Technology in Japan.

White rice is produced from further milling and whitening (polishing) of brown rice that results in removal of bran and germ. On average, paddy rice produces 25% husk, 10% bran and germ, and 65% white rice (Chen, Siebenmorgen, & Griffin, 1998).

Anatomical details of the rice seed are depicted in Fig. 3.1. Interlocked lemma and palea constitute the husk. The husk is composed mostly of cellulosic and fibrous tissue (38–48% cellulose; 23–28% hemicellulose; 12–16% lignin; 1.9–3.7% protein; and 0.3–0.8% fat; Klyosov, 2007) and is covered with hard glass-like spines or trichomes providing abrasive characteristics that are helpful in protecting seed. Rice hull contains about 18–20% amorphous silica by weight (Luh, 1991). Silica is bound by cellulose and lignin, making the stalks and hulls resistant to water and fungal decomposition. The high calorific value of rice hull, ranging from 3000 to 3500 kcal/kg, makes it an important source of energy for various uses.

The pericarp is the thin fibrous layer remaining on the grain after removing hull. The epicarp, mesocarp, and cross layer compose the pericarp and protect the seed from oxidative, enzymatic, and moisture damage. Usually the pericarp is translucent, grayish, and silvery; when not translucent, it could be pigmented (red, purple, and black) and an integral part of the brown rice kernel that is lost in the whitening process. Anthocyanin pigments, cyanidin 3-glucoside, cyanidin 3-galactoside, cyanidin 3-rutinoside, cyanidin 3,5-di glucoside, malvidin 3-galactoside, peonidin 3-glucoside, and pelargonidin 3,5-diglucoside are found in the pigmented rice (Abdel-Aal, Young, & Rabalski, 2006; Deng et al., 2013). The less fibrous seed coat (testa, tegument layer) is found immediately below the pericarp (Fig. 3.1). Testa is rich in oil and protein, and very low in starch. The aleurone layer is found between testa and starch-filled endosperm. The embryo (germ) of rice grain is more close to where the grain is attached to the panicle of the plant and is at central bottom portion of the grain.

Once the hull is removed, the rice grain contains bran, germ, and endosperm, which is brown rice. When the hull, pericarp, bran, and the embryo are removed, endosperm rich in starch or white rice can be obtained. On average, bran and germ together constitute 6–8% of the rice grain by weight. Rice endosperm has only a small concentration of protein and very low levels of minerals, vitamins, or oil. White rice has high energy value because of its high percentage of carbohydrates. The bran has very low starch content but a high percentage of oil, protein, vitamins, and minerals. Bran is known to be rich in B-complex vitamins and minerals (Table 3.1), the approximate composition being 13% protein, 25% fat, 6% fiber, 44% carbohydrate, 11 mg% ion, 670 mg% magnesium, 5 mg% zinc, 49 mg% calcium, 19 ppm vitamin B_1, 350 ppm vitamin B_3, and 34 ppm vitamin B_6 (Satter et al., 2014). Therefore, white rice has a lower content of B-complex vitamins and minerals than brown rice (Table 3.1). The high oil content of the bran is one of the factors that make rice bran highly prone to oxidation.

Various rice milling systems are in use: simple, one- or two-stage, and multiple-stage processes. Use of motor and pestle to handpound paddy to remove husk is done by remote, village communities to process rice for personal use. Commercial rice milling is done in multiple stages to ensure rice that is sufficiently milled for customer appeal while maximizing total milled rice recovery from paddy with minimum grain breakage. During milling, the bran layer and embryo are removed, resulting in an indented shape at one end of the milled rice grain. Degree of milling (DM) is the extent that the bran layer is removed during milling. Rice bran is a byproduct of rice milling. Edible rice grain can be in various forms, for example, different sizes (small, large), shapes (round, elongated, long), colors (white, red, purple), process forms (brown, white, parboiled), and aroma characteristics (basmati, jasmine), and cooking characteristics (waxy, sticky, low-amylose).

Table 3.2 provides different systems of rice milling processes and their products. Table 3.3 provides crude protein content of different fractions results in from rice milling. Upon milling, different varieties of rice produce 20–25% husk fraction, 10–11% bran and germ fraction, and 65–69% starchy endosperm or total milled rice fractions. Brown rice has intact bran layers that give the characteristic tan color and nutty flavor. Boiled brown rice is edible, high in fiber, and chewier than white rice. Milled rice contains whole grains or head rice, and broken kernels. Rice milling in small-scale processing produces a high proportion of broken kernels: 53–55% white rice and ∼30% head rice (whole

TABLE 3.2 Products of Various Systems of Rice Milling and the Protein Levels of the Products

Processing System	Products	Product Protein Levels (%N × 5.95)
One-step milling	Milled or partially polished brown rice	
Husk and bran removal in one pass	Husk	
Two-step milling	Brown rice (intermediate product)	Rough rice: 5.6–7.7%
Removing husk and removing bran is done separately	White rice	Brown rice: 7.1–8.3%
	Rice bran	Milled rice: 6.3–7.1
	Husk	Rice bran: 11.3–14.9
Multistage milling:	Head rice (whole grain)	Rice hull: 2.0–2.8
Various stages:	Broken rice	
	Rice germ and bran	
	Husk	

Source: Shih, F. F. (2003). An update on the processing of high-protein rice products. Review. *Nahrung/Food, 6,* 420–424.

TABLE 3.3 Composition of Rice Bran in Comparison With Brown and White Rice (Park et al., 2009)

Component (%)	Rice Bran, Untreated	Rice Bran, Defatted	Brown Rice	White Rice
Moisture	10.6	12.3	12.4	13.1
Fat	19.2	0.9	2.4	0.47
Protein	14.0	18.0	8.1	5.9
Ash	7.1	11.9	1.2	0.43
Crude fiber	9.3	8.1	1.3	0.5

kernels). Medium- to large-scale processing (60–220 tons paddy/d) mills produces 50–60% head rice, 5–10% large broken kernels, and 10–15% small broken kernels (Chapagain & Hoekstra, 2010; Chen et al., 1998; IRRI, 2015[9]). Milled rice, depending on DM, has a low content of protein, oil, vitamins (B complex), and minerals. In rice processing, the vitamins in the grain can be retained by parboiling before milling. The process of parboiling involves steam in a large industrial setting, and ensures movement of nutrients from the bran layers to the inner parts of the rice grain (endosperm) making these micronutrients available after milling.

3.3.1 Proteins in Rice

3.3.1.1 Protein Localization

Storage proteins of rice are sequestrated in the cells as dense deposits or protein bodies (PB). Two morphologically distinct PB are found in rice, spherical with concentric strata (PB-I, 1–2 μm) and irregularly shaped electron dense

---
9. *International Rice Research Institute (IRRI) Rice knowledge bank.* <http://www.knowledgebank.irri.org/step-by-step-production/postharvest/milling> Accessed November 10, 2015.

strata (PB-II, 2–3 μm). PB with concentric strata PB-I are described as cytoplasmic, bounded by a double membrane, and rich in prolamin (10, 13, and 16 kDa, that of 13 kDa being the major one) (Kawagoe, et al., 2005). Prolamin accounts for 20–30% of total seed protein. The irregularly shaped PB-II secretes into the vacuole and is called crystalline PB containing more glutelin (34–37 kDa acidic, α-subunit, and 21–23 kDa basic β-subunit) than globulin (α-globulin, 21 kDa precursor). Glutelin accounts for 60–80% and α-globulin 2–8% of total seed protein (de Lumen & Chow, 1991; Fabian & Ju, 2011; Kim et al., 2013; Mitsukawa, Konishi, Uchiki, Masumura, & Tanaka, 1999; Ogawa et al., 1987, 1989; Shyur, Wen, & Chen, 1992; Tanaka, Sugimoto, Ogawa, & Kasai, 1980; Yamagata, Sugimoto, Tanaka, & Kasai, 1982; Zhou, Robards, Helliwell, & Blanchard, 2002). The aleurone and subaleurone layers of rice are rich in storage protein and more PBs are found in the subaleurone layer (Takaiwa et al., 1999). Starchy endosperm also contains both types of PBs. PB-I is known to be less digestible than PB-II (Resurreccion, Li, Okita, & Juliano, 1993; Tanaka, Resurreccion, Juliano, & Bechtel, 1978).

Since the milling operation is done to various degrees of milling, a variable quantity of subaleurone layer partitions into bran fraction and endosperm (white rice). Rohrer and Siebenmorgen (2005) showed that longer milling times remove more of the bran layers that contain most of the rice grain proteins and result in a decreased level of protein in milled rice. Rice bran that contains the aleurone layer and the germ together has more protein than the endosperm (white rice) and can be up to 15% (full fat) and 18% (oil-free) (Kahlon, 2009; Fabian & Ju, 2011). Besides storage proteins, rice bran contains various biologically active proteins, mainly enzymes, several types of lipases, those specific to 1,3-triacylglycerol (Prabhu, Tambe, Gandhi, Sawant, & Joshi, 1999; Ramezanzadeh et al., 1999), amylases, catalase, ascorbic acid oxidase, cytochrome oxidase, lipoxygenases, polyphenol oxidase, dehydrogenase, and esterases.

3.3.1.2 Protein Types

Estimation of protein types of rice grain according to Osborne solubility classification shows varietal differences. Rice grain contains albumin (4–22%), globulin (5–13%), and prolamin (1–5%), and the majority consists of glutelin (60–80% of total protein) (Chavan & Duggal, 1978; Ju & Rath, 2001; Kim et al., 2013). On average, rice bran contains 24–37% albumin, 15–36% globulin, 11–38% glutelin, and 2–6% prolamin (Fabian & Ju, 2011; Hamada, 1997; Wang, Li, Xu, Hao, & Zhang, 2014). Proteins in rice are mostly water-insoluble, however rice bran contains a rather high amount of water- and salt-soluble proteins. Albumin and globulin content are higher in brown rice than in white rice (Kim & Jeong, 2002).

3.3.1.2.1 Albumins

Rice albumins are water-soluble, coagulated by heat, and possess a lower amount of disulfide crosslinking and comprise about 2–6% of total seed protein and 24–37% of bran proteins (Hamada, 1997; Shewry & Casey, 1999). Rice albumin is readily digestible and absorbable. Albumin fraction contains protein with molecular weight in the range of 10–200 kDa, and the 16 kDa protein and 60 kDa glycoprotein are predominant (Fabian & Ju, 2011; Mawal, Mawal, & Ranjekar, 1987; Wei, Nguyen, Kim, & Sok, 2007). The albumin fraction of rice bran contains proteins less than 100 kDa molecular weight (Hamada, 1997). The isoelectric point of albumin is pH 4.1 and 6.4 (Ju & Rath, 2001; Padhye & Salunkhe, 1979).

3.3.1.2.2 Globulins

The salt-soluble globulin fraction of rice contains proteins rich in cysteine and methionine but very low in lysine and constitutes about 15–36% of storage proteins of the bran. Reduction of disulfide bonds in globular fraction proteins results in polypeptides of 16 kDa γ-globulin and 21 kDa α-globulin. These can be traced back to the localized discrete zones of irregular shaped (PB-II) PB (Houston & Mohammad, 1970; Krishnan, White, & Pueppke, 1992; Morita & Yoshida, 1968; Pan & Reeck, 1988). The isoelectric point of globulin is pH 4.3, 5.85–7.27, and 7.9 (Ju & Rath, 2001; Padhye & Salunkhe, 1979).

3.3.1.2.3 Prolamins

Rice prolamins that are soluble in aqueous (60–70%) ethanol are about 4% of the bran. Polypeptides of prolamin fraction are between 12 and 17 kDa that are rich in glutamine/glutamic acid, alanine, glycine, and arginine but low in lysine (Shyur & Chen, 1994). Prolamin fraction contains proteins in the molecular weight range of 10–17 kDa (Kim & Okita, 1988). The 13-kDa prolamin is rich in hydrophobic amino acids such as leucine, valine, and glutamine, but lacks lysine (Masumura et al., 1990). On the other hand, prolamins of 16 kDa and 10 kDa are rich sulfur-containing amino acids, such as cysteine and methionine (Hibino et al., 1989; Mitsukawa et al., 1999; Masumura et al. 1989a,b). Among all the protein fractions of rice grain, prolamin contains the highest amount of glutamine/glutamic acid (19.9 mol%) and isoleucine (12.3 mol%) and the lowest amount of threonine (1.3 mol%), cysteine (0.0 mol%), glycine (6.2 mol%), histidine (1.7 mol%), arginine (4.6 mol%), lysine (1.0 mol%), and methionine (0.8 mol%) (Hibino et al., 1989; Padhye & Salunkhe, 1979). The high content of acid amides and low content of polar amino acids would be one of the reasons for the low solubility of prolamin in water. The isoelectric point of prolamin is pH 6.0–6.5 (Ju & Rath, 2001; Padhye & Salunkhe, 1979).

3.3.1.2.4 Glutelins

The majority of rice grain proteins are in the glutelin fraction. Proteins in the glutelin fraction are extensively aggregated, disulfide bonded, and glycosylated and difficult to solubilize (Fabian & Ju, 2011). Rice glutelins are composed of high-molecular-weight proteins ranging from 45 to 150 kDa. The amino-acid composition of glutelin is not so distinct from that of total rice protein because it is the most abundant protein. The glutelin fraction in rice endosperm contains several polypeptides of 57 kDa, 34–37 kDa, 25 kDa, 21–23 kDa, 16 kDa, and 14 kDa, and the 57-kDa protein consists of two subunits of 34–37 kDa (acidic α-subunit) and 21–23 kDa (basic β-subunit) linked by disulfide bonds (Krishnan et al., 1992; Takaiwa, Kikuchi, & Oono, 1986, 1987). Rice glutelins are considered similar to legumins in soy and pulses and are of types A and B. Glutelin type B is rich in lysine and considered a good genetic resource to increase the lysine content in rice. The isoelectric point of glutelin is reported as pH 4.8 , 5.7–6.8 and 8.0–8.7 (Ju & Rath, 2001; Padhye & Salunkhe, 1979; Shyur, Zia & Chen, 1988).

3.3.2 Production of Rice Protein

Rice-based protein-rich products (eg, protein concentrates, protein isolates, milk) have become available recently, especially in the geographical regions where traditional rice consumption is low, for example, North America. Recognized health benefits and hypoallergenic properties are the main reasons for this recent popularity of rice protein products. Soluble rice protein products can improve formulations of rice-based infant formula. Rice is not a seed rich in protein (Tables 3.1 and 3.2) compared to soy or pulses that are used for protein product preparation (Shih, 2003). Brown or white rice is an expensive starting material for protein product preparation besides its inherently low protein content. Rice bran, broken rice kernels, and also the residue of rice starch extraction, which has lesser economic value than rice endosperm, are the sources to obtain rice protein. Obtaining high-protein rice flour, while producing rice syrup sweeteners has been described by Chen and Chang (1984), Chang, Lee, and Brown (1986) and the patent by Mitchell, Mitchell, and Mitchell (1988). In addition, sprouted rice-based products are also available in the market.

3.3.2.1 Rice Bran Protein Products

Rice bran is usually contaminated with hull particles and to some extent with broken rice. Traditional use of rice bran in animal feed formulation in the heavy-rice-consuming countries ensures this energy, protein, and micronutrient-rich rice milling coproduct is diverted to animal protein production including premium equine nutrition (Hoogenkamp, 2015). This is the most economical and sustainable use of rice bran in the socioeconomic environment in which rice cultivation and production occur. Further scientific investigations and technological developments, particularly in the same rice-growing countries, have been able to obtain high-value products from rice bran that are suitable for human nutrition. Rice bran oil that is rich in phytosterols, such as γ-oryzanol and tocopherols, are obtained through hexane or supercritical carbon dioxide extraction and used in a variety of high-value applications.

The proteins of rice bran are less soluble in water. The bran lipids are highly prone to lipolysis and oxidation due to the enzymes present, as well as the polyunsaturated nature of fats. Stabilization of bran using heat treatment to inactivate these enzymes renders proteins further insoluble due to heat denaturation and aggregation. In a patent, Park et al. (2009) describe pelletizing of rice bran that can stabilize bran oil as well as making suitable physical forms for efficient oil extraction with hexane. Besides that, the phytates in the bran (∼1.6%; Juliano, 1985) may also complex with protein depending on the pH.

Two methods have been described to obtain protein from stabilized rice bran. Products with high protein levels can be obtained by alkali extraction of rice bran followed by acid precipitation of solubilized protein. Manipulation of temperature and extraction time can bring higher protein yields during extraction at low-alkaline pH than using high-alkaline pH that is detrimental to lysine, serine, and cysteine. Although most of the proteins found in other seed sources (eg, oilseeds) can be extracted under alkaline conditions, only about 48% of rice bran proteins can be extracted

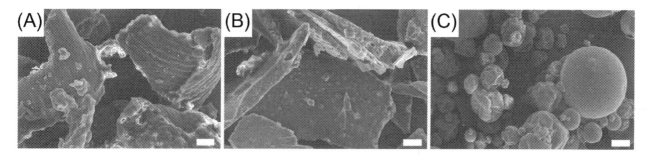

FIGURE 3.2 Scanning electron micrographs of rice-bran derived products: (A) stabilized rice bran; (B) defatted and stabilized rice bran; and (C) spray dried rice protein 80% (w/w). Bar = 20 μm. *Copyright Henk Hoogenkamp, Radboud University Nijmegen Netherlands.*

(Fabian & Ju, 2011). Extraction of oil-free rice bran in a sequential manner with water, NaCl solution, 60% ethanol, and 0.1 M NaOH, respectively, resulted in >90% protein extraction yield (Adebiyi, Adebiyi, Hasegawa, Ogawa, & Muramoto, 2009; Hamada, 1997). Several studies have indicated that a reduction of disulfide bonds of rice proteins may enhance protein extractability. Fig. 3.2 provides scanning electron micrographs of rice-bran-derived protein products.

Enzyme-assisted aqueous extraction has been successful in obtaining high protein yield from rice bran. Carbohydrates found in rice bran are mostly cellulose and hemicellulose (Ansharullah, Hourigan, & Chesterman, 1997; Shih et al., 1999). Use of food-grade cellulase or hemicellulase (65°C, pH 4.0) for rice bran protein extraction resulted in 35% and 46% protein yield, respectively (Ansharullah et al., 1997), and ~55% protein yield when xylanase was used (Wang, Hettiarachchy, Qi, Burks, & Siebenmorgen, 1999). Use of commercial enzyme Viscozyme L (50°C, pH 3.8) that has mixed activities (arabinase, cellulase, hemicellulase, and xylanase) effectively cleaves linkages within the polysaccharide matrix releasing more intercellular proteins, providing higher protein yield (57%) than using carbohydrases with single activity (Guan & Yao, 2008). Although starch is not a component of true bran, depending on milling conditions broken starch-rich endosperm particles may contaminate, therefore use of α-amylase improves the yield of unbound protein (Fabian & Ju, 2011). Phytases that cleave bonds between protein and phytate when in combination with xylanase can provide higher protein yield up to 74.6% (Wang et al., 1999). Proteolytic enzymes such as Flavourzyme, having both endoproteolytic and exopeptidasic activity, can release partially hydrolyzed proteins from the bran cellular matrix. Use of these proteases helps in recovering more protein nitrogen (81.4%, 50°C, pH 8.0) from rice bran (Hamada, 1999) than other combinations.

Physical processes can also be used to release and concentrate rice bran proteins without forming chemical artifacts. These include colloidal milling, homogenization, and high-speed blending that provide shear forces to disrupt cells walls, freeze–thaw process that causes cell lysis, and intercellular membrane structure rupture due to ice crystal formation, cell wall breakage, and molecular bond breakage by high pressure, high temperature, and shock waves (sonication). Combination of sonication (5 min) with amylase and protease treatment resulted in ~56.2% protein recovery (Tang, Hettiararchy, & Shellhammer, 2002). Use of subcritical water as the extraction medium resulted in 84% protein recovery yield from rice bran (Watchararuji, Goto, Sasaki, & Shotipruk, 2008).

3.3.2.2 Endosperm Protein

When broken rice (endosperm, ~7–8% protein) is the substrate for rice protein extraction, use of α-amylase, glucoamylase, and pullulanase helps in degrading and removing starch and generating protein concentrates (25% protein) and isolates (>90% protein). Since the majority of rice proteins are glutelins that require high-alkaline pHs to be soluble, most of the processes (Euber, Puski, & Hartman, 1991; Mitchell et al., 1988; Park et al., 2009; Tokuba, 1997) tend to use alternative approaches to remove nonprotein components from the substrate in order to increase the protein content of the resulting product. In rice syrup generation, heat stable α-amylases to liquefy starch and proteases to release protein embedded in fiber and starch granules are used. This process gives rice syrup, insoluble rice residue, and soluble rice protein concentrates with varying levels of protein content. Using protein-rich coproduct (50% protein-containing residue) of rice-syrup manufacturing, Shih and Daigle (2000) were able to obtain a protein product with 85% protein. It is noted that tightly associated proteins (PB) on the rice starch granule surface are difficult to remove, therefore high-alkaline conditions or protease treatments are needed (Puchongkavarian, Varavinit, & Bergthaller, 2005).

Digestibility of rice protein obtained from alkaline treatment and α-amylase degradation (two major industrial processes for rice protein extraction) is different (Yang et al., 2011). Prolamin of 13 kDa extracted by starch degradation is indigestible, but that extracted by alkaline is digested and absorbed in the intestine (Kubota et al., 2010). As the digestibility of rice protein extracted under alkaline conditions is higher than that extracted by starch degradation, their polypeptide compositions do not differ from one another (Yang et al., 2011). The bioavailability of protein extracted by alkaline is also higher than that of protein extracted by removing starch by enzymatic degradation (Kumagai et al., 2009).

3.4 FUNCTIONAL PROPERTIES AND APPLICATIONS

Most of the proteins found in rice exhibit poor solubility properties because of a high degree of intermolecular S—S bonds and comparatively high molecular weights. Particularly, rice bran goes through heat treatment for stabilization making bran proteins more insoluble (Shih, 2003). Freeze-dried protein concentrate obtained from both heat-stabilized and parboiled rice bran showed low water absorption capacity and high fat absorption capacity. Rice protein products are available in the market and used in several product formulations. Solubility is the major concern with rice protein that is discussed in literature; however depending on the process used, partial hydrolysis (due to use of proteases) may occur during protein processing to overcome this. Rice bran proteins show comparable foaming capacity and stability as egg albumin (Wang et al., 1999) and emulsifying properties comparable with casein (Fabian & Ju, 2011). The denaturation temperatures of rice albumin, globulin, and glutelin are 73.3°C, 78.9°C, and 82.2°C, respectively (Ju & Rath, 2001). Rice prolamin does not show any thermal transition as observed in differential scanning calorimetry (DSC).

Sagum and Arcot (2000) showed boiling, parboiling, and extrusion process to increase in vitro digestibility of rice proteins. According to Eggum, Resurreccion, & Juliano (1977) heat treatment reduces in vivo digestibility of rice protein, resulting in low biological value (BV) and net protein utilization (NPU). Tanaka et al. (1978) and Resurreccion et al. (1993) showed that poorly digested proteins represent lipid-rich core proteins that are poor in lysine and rich in cysteine, which may be prolamins. According to FAO data,[10] true digestibility value of protein of milled rice compared to reference egg protein is 93% while both whole wheat and oat are at 90%. Kalman (2014) has studied the amino acid composition of commercial rice protein products and compared that with cooked rice and soy protein products in the market (Table 3.4) and it is noted that high arginine levels and considerably high branched chain amino acid levels are present in rice protein products.

Rice bran is an approved functional ingredient in processed meat products in the US and labeled as "isolated rice product." Fiber and protein components in the bran help to bind and immobilize moisture and oil of the products, thus inhibiting purge and moisture migration during freezing and thawing besides providing good emulsifying and gelling ability in meat batters (Hoogenkamp, 2015; Fig. 3.3).

Several commercial entities produce rice protein products derived from rice bran, rice syrup coproduct, broken rice, or germinated rice.[11] Rice bran protein hydrolysates are used in nutritional supplements, functional ingredients, and flavor ingredients in foods. Rice proteins are used in confectionary, soft drinks and juices, soups, sauces, gravies, meat products, and other savory applications, besides cosmetic and personal care products (Fabian & Ju, 2011). Brown-rice-derived protein product has GRAS status and also parallel properties, such as building and repairing muscles, similar to whey is also available.[12] Protein products derived from germinated brown rice (eg, Oryzatein[11]) with increased GABA content, improved mineral availablity, and reduced phytate levels, are also available. Rice protein is considered as hypoallergenic and suitable for infant food formulations. Hypoallergenicity and the health benefits of rice protein products outweigh any shortcomings of the functional properties.

3.5 ALLERGENICITY, OFF TASTES, AND ANTINUTRITIONAL FACTORS

3.5.1 Allergenicity

As mentioned earlier, rice protein is considered hypoallergenic. Rice is the cereal that is fed to infants as the first introduction to solid foods in their life. Rice protein products are commonly used in formulating infant food. In the communities where rice is the staple food, allergic reactions to rice prevail. Symptoms related to rice allergy are reported

---

10. <http://www.fao.org/docrep/t0567e/t0567e0d.htm>.
11. <http://www.hillpharma.com/ortiva-whole-grain-brown-rice-protein/>.
12. <http://axiomfoods.com/product_details.php?main_cat=3&sub_cat=19&prod_id=28/>.

TABLE 3.4 Amino Acid Composition (g/100 g) of Commercial Rice Products in Comparison With Brown Cooked Rice

Amino Acid	Oryzatein 90 Silk Protein Isolate[a]	Oryzatein 80 Silk Protein Concentrate[a]	Oryza sativa L. (Brown, Cooked)
Alanine	4.38–4.47	4.32	0.151
Arginine	6.32–6.35	6.11	0.196
Aspartic acid	6.94–6.79	6.76	0.242
Cysteine	1.70–1.80	1.63	0.031
Glutamic acid	13.9–13.7	13.49	0.526
Glycine	3.53–3.41	3.41	0.127
Histidine	1.82–1.67	1.67	0.066
Isoleucine	3.45–3.23	3.38	0.109
Leucine	6.41–6.32	6.20	0.214
Lysine	2.42–2.19	2.12	0.099
Methionine	2.27–2.26	2.29	0.058
Phenylalanine	4.41–4.29	4.11	0.133
Proline	2.88–3.67	3.56	0.121
Serine	3.91–3.88	3.79	0.134
Threonine	2.92–2.86	2.80	0.095
Tryptophan	1.17–1.15	1.12	0.033
Tyrosine	4.26–4.26	6.20	0.097
Valine	4.56–4.26	4.47	0.151
Total amino acids	76.5–77.4	77.5	2.58
EAA,[b] total (%)	29.4–66.9	28.19	0.958
BCAA,[c] total (%)	14.4–13.8	14.05	0.474

[a]Products of Axiom Foods, Los Angeles, CA, USA.
[b]Essential amino acids and include histidine, isoleucine, leucine, lysine, methionine, phenylalanine, threonine, tryptophan, and valine.
[c]Branched chain amino acids and include leucine, isoleucine, and valine.
Source: Kalman, D. S. (2014). Amino acid composition of an organic brown rice protein concentrate and isolate compared to soy and whey concentrates and isolates. *Foods, 3,* 394–402.

as abdominal cramping, nausea, vomiting, rhinitis, rhinoconjunctivitis, asthma, contact urticaria, atopic dermatitis, dermatitis, and angioedema.[13] Increasing rice consumption in the West may show some prevalence of allergy to rice.

There are four allergens reported for *Oryza sativa* unpolished rice. A lipid transfer protein (LTP) of 14 kDa (Ory s LTP) (Asero, Amato, Alfieri, Folloni & Mistrello, 2006; Asero et al., 2002; Asero, Mistrello, Roncarolo, Amato, & van Ree, 2001; Enrique et al., 2005; Poznanski et al., 1999), a 16 kDa α-amylase/trypsin inhibitor Ory s aA/TI (Adachi, Izumi, & Yamada, 1993; Alvarez et al., 1995; Izumi, Sugiyama, Matsuda, & Nakamura, 1999; Nakase et al., 1998; Yamada et al., 2006), a glyoxalase (Ory s Glyoxalase I) (Kato, Katayama, Matsubara, Omi, & Matsuda, 2000; Urisu et al., 1991; Usui et al., 2001), and a profilin (Ory s 12) (van Ree et al., 1992). The majority of rice allergens are in the albumin protein fraction having a molecular weight between 14 and 16 kDa, however proteins with molecular masses of 26, 33, and 56 kDa have also exhibited potential allergenicity (Nakamura & Matsuda, 1996; Usui et al., 2001). The 33-kDa allergen is a novel type of plant glyoxalase I found in various plant tissues, including maturing seeds. The 16-kDa protein in rice is reported to be a major allergen and responsible for cross-allergenicity between cereal grains in

---

13. <http://www.phadia.com/en/Products/Allergy-testing-products/ImmunoCAP-Allergen-Information/Food-of-Plant-Origin/Grains/Rice/>.

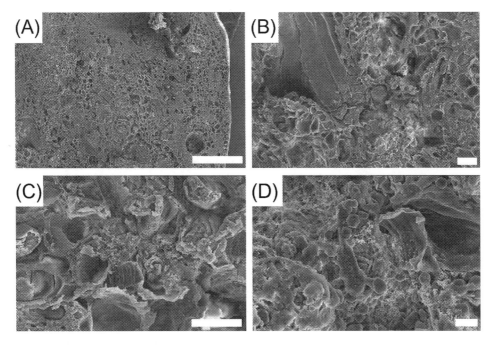

FIGURE 3.3 Scanning electron micrograph of stabilized rice bran used in emulsion-type products. (A) All beef frankfurter with 2% (w/w) stabilized rice bran, bar = 1 mm; (B) enlarged (A), bar = 100 μm; (C) and (D) Close-up image of defatted stabilized rice bran particles in emulsion, bars are 100 and 10 μm, respectively. *Copyright Henk Hoogenkamp, Radboud University Nijmegen Netherlands.*

the Poaceae family (Urisu et al., 1991) and a member of the α-amylase/trypsin inhibitor protein family (Adachi et al., 1993; Izumi et al., 1999). Raw rice is reported to be more allergenic than cooked, however some of the allergens may be heat-stable and resist proteolysis (Shibasaki, Suzuki, Nemoto, & Kuroume, 1979). Evaluation of rice-allergic patient sera has revealed that 14–16-, 33-, 56-, and 60-kDa proteins of rice are the major IgE-binding components and the boiled rice retained IgE-reactivity of 16-, 23-, 33-, and 53-kDa proteins (Kumar et al., 2007). Rice pollen also contributes to allergic rhinitis and allergic conjuctivitis, and Ory s 12 profilin is found in both rice seed and rice pollen (van Ree et al., 1992).[13] LTPs are heat-stable proteins and may play a role in allergy to cooked rice, however there is evidence that rice LTP may modify during cooking (Enrique et al., 2005). Hydrolyzed (enzymatically or alkali-induced) and high-pressure-treated rice protein products are reported as hypoallergenic.[14]

3.5.2 Flavor Compounds and Off Tastes

Flavor is one of the attributes that determine eating quality of rice; it is an especially strong consideration among rice eaters of the Indian subcontinent. Among the more than 320 compounds identified from cooked rice aroma, only a small subset of compounds is odor-active. The origin of these volatile compounds is by lipid oxidation/degradation reactions, Maillard-type reactions, and thermal-induced volatile formation. In scented rice (basmati and jasmine), N-containing 2-acetyl-1-pyrroline (2-AP) is considered as important for the butter-like or popcorn like aroma (Buttery, Ling, Juliano, & Turnbaugh, 1983). This compound is found in nonscented rice in negligible amounts (Buttery, Turnbaugh, & Ling, 1988; Grosch & Schieberle, 1997). In the scented rice varieties 2-AP is synthesized in the plants using L-proline and L-ornithine (Yoshihashi, Huong, & Inatomi, 2002), and the genetic and environmental factors affect the level of accumulation in the seed (Itani, Tamaki, Hayata, Fushimi, & Hashizume, 2004). Although 2-AP has a very low threshold value, the work of Yang (2007) showed that the balance of several odor-active volatiles is responsible for the typical aroma of scented rice not only 2-AP. Among the Maillard reaction products found in cooked rice volatiles, the compounds 2-phenylethanol (rose-like) and phenylacetic acid (rose-like) are Strecker degradation products of L-phenylalanine. The Strecker degradation product of tryptophan, 2-aminoacetophenone, has a naptheline-like, nail polish-like aroma note (Rapp, Versini, & Ullemeyer, 1993) and considered responsible for the floor-polish like off-odor

---

14. <http://www.food-allergens.de/symposium-3-1/rice/rice-allergens.htm>.

in brown rice (Yang, 2007). Lipid oxidation products found in cooked rice are from degradation of major unsaturated fatty acids (oleic, linoleic, and linolenic acids) found in rice. These compounds include octanal, heptanal, nonanal, (*E*)-2-nonenal, decanal, and 2-heptanone derived from oleic acid, and hexanal, pentanol, pentanal, (*E*)-2-octenal, (*E*,*E*)-2,4-decadienal, and 2-pentylfuran formed from linoleic acid (Monsoor & Proctor, 2004). Vanillin found in cooked brown rice (Jezussek, Juliano, & Schieberle, 2002) contributes to positive flavor attributes of rice, while hexanal contributes to rancid odor. According to Lam and Proctor (2003), more hexanal is formed in partially milled rice than fully milled rice and with storage time (*E*)-2-nonenal (rancid), octanal (fatty), and hexanal (green) significantly increase while contributing to off-flavors. Among thermally induced volatile compounds, 3-hydroxy-4, 5-dimethyl-2(5H)-furanone and *bis*-(2-methyl-3-furyl)-disulfide formed in cooked rice possess seasoning-like and meaty-like aromas, respectively (Jezussek et al., 2002). 2-Methoxy-4-vinylphenol, 4-vinylguaiacol, and 4-vinylphenol are formed in cooked rice due to thermal and enzymatic reaction that confer decarboxylation of ferulic acid and cause undesirable pharmaceutical odors (Coghe, Benoot, Delvaux, Vanderhaegen, & Delvaux, 2004). Working with scented and unscented rice of both *indica* and *japonica* eco-types, Yang, Shewfelt, Lee, and Kays (2008) showed that 2-AP, hexanal, (*E*)-2-nonenal, octanal, hepatanal, and nonanal constituted >97% of the relative proportion of odor activity values of cooked rice volatiles which are found in different proportions. Among the six flavor types of rice in their study (basmati, jasmine, two *japonica* varieties of Korea, black, and nonaromatic), 13 odor-active compounds; 2-AP, hexanal, (*E*)-2-nonenal, octanal, hepatanal and nonanal, 1-octen-3-ol, (*E*)-2-octenal, (*E*,*E*)-2,4-nonadienal, 2-heptanone, (*E*,*E*)-2,4-decadienal, decanal, and guaiacol are found to contribute to odor differences.

3.5.3 Antinutritional Factors

Antinutritional factors of rice are not discussed in the literature. Only phytates in rice bran is mentioned. Some details about enzymes and enzyme inhibitors of rice grain have been described.

3.5.3.1 Enzymes

Among the enzymes reported in rice, α-amylase is a glycoprotein of 44 kDa, that is synthesized de novo in the scutellar epithelium in the initial stage of germination (Miyata, Okamoto, Watanabe, & Akazawa, 1981), while biosynthesis spreads into the aleurone layer of the seed in the later stage (O'Neill et al., 1990). Then, α-amylase is subsequently secreted into the endosperm to hydrolyze the stored starch (Kashem, Itoh, Iwabuchi, Hori, & Mitsui, 2000) Mitsui, Christeller, Hara-Nishimura & Akazawa (1984). Cysteine proteinases found in rice are oryzains α, β, and γ, that have a molecular mass around 23 kDa and an isoelectric point at pH 5.15 (Abe, Kondo, & Arai, 1987b; Watanabe, Abe, Emori, Hosoyama, & Arai, 1991). Oryzains α and β are similar to each other and also to actinidin and papain, while oryzain γ is similar to aleurain and cathepsin H. Oryzains α and γ are expressed continuously during germination with a maximum expression of 5 days from germination. On the other hand, oryzain β is expressed not only during germination but also in ripened seeds before germination. Expression of oryzain α increases with stress conditions such as pathogen attack. Oryzasin is an aspartic proteinase found in rice seeds (Asakura, Watanabe, Abe, & Arai, 1997). The molecular mass of oryzasin is 57 kDa and optimum pH for hydrolysis is 3.0. It is completely inhibited by pepstatin but not affected by other proteinase inhibitors such as EDTA, leupeptin, PMSF, and E-64. Carboxypeptidases exist in germinating rice seeds (Doi, Komori, Matoba, & Morita, 1980). Carboxypeptidases-4, -5, and -7 optimally hydrolyze carbobenzoxy-L-phenylalanyl-L-alanine at pH 4, 5–5.5, and 7, respectively. The activity of carboxypeptidase-4 is at the maximum in resting seeds and gradually decreases during germination. Carboxypeptidase-5 is absent in resting seeds, and appears in endosperms and seedlings in the later stages after germination. Carboxypeptidase-7 is detected in the young shoots and young roots during a limited period of germination.

3.5.3.2 Enzyme Inhibitors

α-Amylase inhibitor, a rice albumin of 14 kDa contains several α-amylase inhibitors of different pIs, mostly between pH 8 and 9 (Feng, Chen, Kramer, & Reeck, 1991). Some of these albumin fractions inhibit only one of the four insect α-amylases tested, whereas others inhibit both insect and mammalian α-amylases. But none of them inhibit bacterial α-amylase. α-Amylase inhibitor of 25 kDa and isoelectric point at pH 4.7 inhibits insect α-amylase, and the inhibitory activity is the highest at pH 6.9 and 37°C (Katoch & Jamwal, 2013).

Bifunctional α-amylase/subtilisin inhibitor, a member of the soybean Kunitz trypsin-inhibitor family with a molecular mass of 20–21 kDa, only weakly inhibits α-amylase from germinating rice seeds, but strongly inhibits serine proteases of the bacterial subtilisin family (Yamasaki et al., 2006). Different from cereal α-amylase/trypsin inhibitor with a molecular mass of 14–16 kDa, α-amylase/subtilisin inhibitor does not inhibit insect α-amylase nor serine protease of the mammalian trypsin-chymotrypsin family. α-Amylase/subtilisin inhibitor contains two intramolecular disulfide bridges, and its isoelectric point is pH 9.05. It exists in the outermost part of the rice grain, synthesized in the late milky stage in developing seeds and retained constantly during the first 7 days of germination.

Oryzacystatin-I, -II, and -III are cysteine proteinase inhibitors found in rice and are 12 kDa in molecular weight without disulfide bonding. They inactivate cysteine proteases, oryzain-α, -β, and -γ that are found in rice (Udenigwe, 2016). An isoelectric point of oryzacycstatin-I is at pH 5.3, and the inhibitory activity is stable between pH 2 and 9, and is retained even after heating at 100°C (Abe, Kondo & Arai, 1987a; Ohtsubo, Kobayashi, Noro, Taniguchi, & Saitoh, 2005). Oryzacystatin-I, -II, and -III inhibit papain and ficin (Ohtsubo et al., 2005). Oryzacystatin-I inhibits papain more effectively than cathepsin H, whereas oryzacystatin-II inhibits cathepsin H better than papain (Kondo et al., 1990). Oryzacystatin-I and oryzacystatin-II do not inhibit cathepsin B that is effectively inhibited by oryzacystatin-III (Ohtsubo et al., 2005). The mRNA for oryzacystatin-I is expressed predominantly 2 weeks after flowering and is not detected in mature seeds, while that for oryzacystatin-II is constantly expressed throughout the seed maturation and is detected even in mature seeds.

3.6 POTENTIAL NEW USES AND EMERGING HEALTH BENEFITS

Rice protein is widely used in several applications, including sports nutrition, and is reported to have several other health benefits. Germinated brown rice obtained by soaking for 24–48 h at 30–40°C has good digestion and absorption properties, containing ferulic acid in a more accessible form and also containing gamma-aminobutyric acid (GABA, 0.01–0.1 mg/g). A significant correlation has been observed between the glutamic acid level of rice grain and the GABA content when germinated (Roohinejad et al., 2009). Intake of germinated brown rice can reduce hyperglycemia, boost immune responses, lower blood pressure, and assist in anxiety disorders compared to consuming white rice (Patil & Khan, 2011). Increasingly, rice protein is extruded into small (~3 mm) particles to provide crunchy texture to cereals and nutrition bars in which they are included (Hoogenkamp, 2015).

3.6.1 Reduction of Cholesterol and Triacylglycerol Levels

Rice protein extracted by alkaline with different composition of 23 kDa glutelin and 13 kDa prolamin both reduces the cholesterol level in plasma and liver and the triacylglycerol level in liver, one of the reasons for this effect being attributed to the enhancement of fecal steroid excretion (Yang et al., 2007).

Rice protein extracted by alkaline or α-amylase reduces both cholesterol and triacylglycerol levels in the liver, suppressing activities of fatty acid synthase, glucose 6-phosphate dehydrogenase and malate dehydrogenase in liver and enhancing those of lipoprotein lipase and hepatic lipase (Yang et al., 2012). However, rice protein extracted by α-amylase is more effective to reduce the cholesterol level in liver than that extracted under alkaline conditions, probably because the former is more indigestible than the latter and promotes fecal excretion of bile acids (Yang et al., 2011). Rice protein extracted by alkaline or α-amylase suppresses activities of fatty acid synthase, glucose 6-phosphate dehydrogenase, and malate dehydrogenase in liver, and enhances those of lipoprotein lipase and hepatic lipase (Yang et al., 2012).

3.6.2 Suppression of Hyperglycemia

Albumin of 14–16 kDa suppresses postprandial hyperglycemia after starch or glucose intake. As the albumin fraction does not inhibit mammalian α-amylase, one of the reasons for this effect is attributed to the indigestibility of rice albumins by pepsin, trypsin, and chymotrypsin. Rice glutelin and prolamin extracted by alkaline suppress excretion of albumin in urine and diabetic nephropathy fed a high-sucrose diet (Kubota et al., 2013).

3.6.3 Antioxidative Activity

Rice albumin fraction has higher antioxidative activity than other fractions. Albumin of 16 kDa with N-terminal sequence of Asp-His-His-Gln is the responsible protein to prevent the oxidation of low-density lipoprotein (LDL) induced by Cu^{2+} as the sequence is homologous to that of human serum albumin having Asp-Ala-His-Lys, high-affinity binding site for cations (Wei et al., 2007). This rice albumin maintained its effect to inhibit Cu^{2+}-induced oxidation of LDL even after hydrolysis with trypsin or chymotrypsin.

Globulin in rice bran does not have remarkable antioxidative activity, but peptides of 670–3611 Da produced by peptic hydrolysis show high antioxidative activity, Tyr-Leu-Ala-Gly-Met-Asn having the highest activity (Adebiyi, Adebiyi, Yamashita, Ogawa, & Muramoto, 2008).

Intake of rice glutelin and prolamin extracted by alkaline with and without cholesterol enhances total antioxidative capacity, reduces glutathione level in plasma, activities of antioxidant enzymes (total superoxide dismutase and catalase) and glutathione-metabolizing enzymes (γ-glutamylcysteine synthetase, glutathione reductase, and glutathione peroxidase) and reduces accumulations of malondialdehyde, protein carbonyl, and oxidized glutathione in liver and plasma, indicating that the hypocholesterolemic effect of rice protein is attributed to its antioxidative activity (Cai et al., 2014).

3.6.4 Reduction in Hypertension

Rice protein extracted under alkaline conditions and hydrolyzed by Alcalase enzyme inhibited the activity of angiotensin I-converting enzyme (ACE), an enzyme to convert angiotensin I to vasoconstrictor angiotensin II and to inactivate the antihypertensive vasodilator bradykinin (Li, Qu, Wan, & You, 2007). Peptide with the amino-acid sequence of Thr-Gln-Val-Tyr produced from rice protein potently inhibits ACE activity. Protein hydrolysates produced from albumin and glutelin of rice-bran with Alcalase and/or Protamax as the enzyme catalysts inhibited ACE, α-amylase, and β-glucosidase activities more strongly than those obtained from globulin and prolamin hydrolysis (Uraipong & Zhao, 2016).

3.6.5 Ileum-Contracting, Antiopioid, and Phagocytosis-Promoting Activities

Oryzatensin, a peptide of Gly-Tyr-Pro-Met-Tyr-Pro-Leu-Pro-Arg, produced from rice albumin by trypsin has ileum-contracting, antiopioid, and phagocytosis-promoting activities (Takahashi, Moriguchi, Yoshikawa, & Sasaki, 1994). The rapid contraction of ilium is mediated by histamine release and the slow contraction of ileum is mediated by a prostaglandin E_2-like substance through the cholinergic nervous system, which is associated with antiopioid activity (Takahashi et al., 1996). The contraction profile of oryzatensin is similar to that of human complement C3a (70–77; ASHLGLAR, has partial activity of anaphylatoxin), the COOH-terminal octapeptide of C3a and oryzatensin has affinity for C3a receptors. Complement C3a is a 77-amino-acid peptide found in serum, produced by the cleavage of complement C3 protein, and mediates chemotaxis of mast cells and eosinophils, degranulation of mast cells and basophils, smooth muscle contraction, induction of lysosomal release from leukocytes, and increases vascular permeability (Jinsmaa, Takenaka, & Yoshikawa, 2001). C3a receptors are expressed throughout the body, including brain, lung, spleen, placenta, and small intestine in the cells of myeloid lineage such as neutrophils, macrophages, eosinophils, basophils, and mast cells. Although neither C3a nor C3a agonists have the central effects after oral administration, a pentapeptide at the carboxyl terminus of oryzatensin, Tyr-Pro-Leu-Pro-Arg, shows C3a activity antagonizing morphine-induced analgesia and improving scopolamine- and ischemia-induced amnesia even after oral administration. In addition, this pentapeptide of Tyr-Pro-Leu-Pro-Arg after intracerebroventricular or intraperitoneal administration suppresses food intake decreasing gastric emptying through prostaglandin E_2 production followed by the activation of EP_4 receptor, one of the subtypes (EP_1–EP_4) for prostaglandin E_2 (Ohinata, Suetsugu, Fujiwara, & Yoshikawa, 2007).

3.7 CONCLUDING REMARKS

As the major cereal consumed by nearly half of the world population, rice is an important protein source. Rice production, processing, and trade are an integral component of the sociocultural fabric of the major rice-producing and -consuming countries and provide sustainability of the rural economies of several countries in the Asian continent. In the American continent, rice production is for trading. Although rice is not a protein crop, coproducts of rice processing, the bran and the broken rice, can be sources for obtaining high-protein rice products without interfering with the rice grain that is used as a food staple. Current uses of rice protein products are mostly in sports nutrition, hypoallergenic formulas, and beverage-type products. More beneficial biochemical advantages are found in rice protein-derived peptides which help to enrich the overall value of rice protein products.

REFERENCES

Abdel-Aal, E. S. M., Young, J. C., & Rabalski, I. (2006). Anthocyanin composition in black, blue, pink, purple, and red cereal grains. *Journal of Agricultural and Food Chemistry, 54*, 4696–4704.

Abe, K., Kondo, H., & Arai, S. (1987a). Purification and characterization of a rice cysteine proteinase inhibitor. *Agricultural and Biological Chemistry, 51*(10), 2763–2768.

Abe, K., Kondo, H., & Arai, S. (1987b). Purification and properties of a cysteine proteinase from germinating rice seeds. *Agricultural and Biological Chemistry, 51*(6), 1509–1514.

Adachi, T., Izumi, H., Yamada, T., et al. (1993). Gene structure and expression of rice seed allergenic proteins belonging to the alpha-amylase/trypsin inhibitor family. *Plant Molecular Biology, 21*, 239–248.

Adebiyi, A. P., Adebiyi, A. O., Hasegawa, Y., Ogawa, T., & Muramoto, K. (2009). Isolation and characterization of protein fractions from deoiled rice bran. *European Food Research and Technology, 288*, 391–401.

Adebiyi, A. P., Adebiyi, A. O., Yamashita, J., Ogawa, T., & Muramoto, K. (2008). Purification and characterization of antioxidative peptides derived from rice bran protein hydrolysates. *International Journal of Food Science and Technology, 43*(1), 35–43.

Alvarez, A. M., Adachi, T., Nakase, M., Aoki, N., Nakamura, R., & Matsuda, T. (1995). Classification of rice allergenic protein cDNAs belonging to the alpha-amylase/trypsin inhibitor gene family. *Biochimica Biophysica Acta, 1251*, 201–204.

Ansharullah, Hourigan, J. A., & Chesterman, C. F. (1997). Application of carbohydrases in extracting protein from rice bran. *Journal of the Science Food and Agriculture, 74*, 141–146.

Asakura, T., Watanabe, H., Abe, K., & Arai, S. (1997). Oryzasin as an aspartic proteinase occurring in rice seeds: Purification, characterization, and application to milk clotting. *Journal of Agricultural and Food Chemistry, 45*(4), 1070–1075.

Asero, R., Amato, S., Alfieri, B., Folloni, S., & Mistrello, G. (2006). Rice: Another potential cause of food allergy in patients sensitized to lipid transfer protein. *International Archives of Allergy and Immunology, 143*(1), 69–74.

Asero, R., Mistrello, G., Roncarolo, D., Amato, S., Caldironi, G., Barocci, F., & van Ree, R. (2002). Immunological cross-reactivity between lipid transfer proteins from botanically unrelated plant-derived foods: A clinical study. *Allergy, 57*(10), 900–906.

Asero, R., Mistrello, G., Roncarolo, D., Amato, S., & van Ree, R. (2001). A case of allergy to beer showing cross-reactivity between lipid transfer proteins. *Annals of Allergy, Asthma and Immunology, 87*(1), 65–67.

Bhattachrya, K. R. (2011). *A guide to rice properties and analysis*. Cambridge, UK: Woodhead Publishing Ltd.

Biselli, C., Cavalluzzo, D., Perrini, R., Gianinetti, A., Bagnaresi, P., Urso, S., ... Valè, G. (2014). Improvement of marker-based predicability of apparent amylose content in japonica rice through GBSSI allele mining. *Rice, 7*(1), 1–18.

Buttery, R. G., Ling, L. C., Juliano, B. O., & Turnbaugh, J. G. (1983). Cooked rice aroma and 2-acetyl-1-pyrroline. *Journal of Agricultural and Food Chemistry, 31*, 823–826.

Buttery, R. G., Turnbaugh, J. G., & Ling, L. C. (1988). Contribution of volatiles to rice aroma. *Journal of Agricultural and Food Chemistry, 36*, 1006–1009.

Cai, J., Yang, L., He, H.-J., Xu, T., Liu, H.-B., Wu, Q., ... Nie, M.-H. (2014). Antioxidant capacity responsible for a hypocholesterolemia is independent of dietary cholesterol in adult rats fed rice protein. *Gene, 533*(1), 57–66.

Chang, K. C., Lee, C. C., & Brown, G. (1986). Production and nutritional evaluation of high protein rice flour. *Journal of Food Science, 51*, 464–467.

Chapagain, A. K., & Hoekstra, A. Y. (2010). The green, blue and grey water footprint of rice from both a production and consumption perspective. *Value of water research report series no 40. UNESCO-IHE*. Institute for Water Education.

Chavan, J., & Duggal, S. (1978). Studies on the essential amino acid composition, protein fractions and biological value (BV) of some new varieties of rice. *Journal of Science Food Agriculture, 29*(3), 225–229.

Chen, H., Siebenmorgen, T., & Griffin, K. (1998). Quality characteristics of long grain rice milled in two commercial systems. *Cereal Chemistry, 75*, 560–565.

Chen, W.-P., & Chang, Y.-C. (1984). Production of high-fructose rice syrup and high-protein rice flour from broken rice. *Journal of Science Food and Agriculture, 35*, 1128–1135.

Coghe, S., Benoot, K., Delvaux, F., Vanderhaegen, B., & Delvaux, F. R. (2004). Ferulic acid release and 4-vinylguaiacol formation during brewing and fermentation: Indications for feruloyl esterase activity in *Saccharomyces cerevisiae*. *Journal of Agricultural and Food Chemistry, 52*, 602–608.

de Lumen, B. O., & Chow, H. (1991). Endosperm: Nutritional quality. In B. S. Luh (Ed.), *Rice, volume 2: Utilization* (p. 367). New York: Springer Science & Business Media.

Deng, G. F., Fu, Y.-R., Zhang, Y., Li, D., Gan, R.-Y., & Li, H.-B. (2013). Phenolic compounds and bioactivities of pigmented rice. *Critical Reviews in Food Science and Nutrition, 53*, 296–306.

Doi, E., Komori, N., Matoba, T., & Morita, Y. (1980). Some properties of carboxypeptidases in germinating rice seeds and rice leaves. *Agricultural and Biological Chemistry, 44*(1), 77–83.

Eggum, B. O., Resurreccion, A. P., & Juliano, B. O. (1977). Effects of cooking on nutritional value of milled rice in rats. *Nutrition Reports International, 16*, 649–655.

Enrique, E., Ahrazem, O., Bartra, J., Latorre, M. D., Castello, J. V., de Mateo, J. A., ... Salcedo, G. (2005). Lipid transfer protein is involved in rhinoconjunctivitis and asthma produced by rice inhalation. *Journal of Allergy and Clinical Immunology, 116*, 4–928.

Euber, J. R., Puski, G., & Hartman, G. H. (1991). *Method for making soluble rice protein concentrate and the product produced therefrom*. US Patent 4,990,344.

Fabian, C., & Ju, Y.-H. (2011). A review on rice bran protein: Its properties and extraction methods. *Critical Reviews in Food Science and Nutrition, 51*(9), 816–827.

Feng, G.-H., Chen, M., Kramer, K. J., & Reeck, G. R. (1991). α-Amylase inhibitors from rice: Fractionation and selectivity toward insect, mammalian, and bacterial α-amyases. *Cereal Chemistry, 68*(5), 516–521.

Grigg, D. (1995). The pattern of world protein consumption. *Geoforum, 26*(1), 1–17.

Grosch, W., & Schieberle, P. (1997). Flavor of cereal products – A review. *Cereal Chemistry, 74*, 91–97.

Guan, X., & Yao, H. (2008). Optimization of Viscozyme L-assisted extraction of oat bran protein using response surface methodology. *Food Chemistry, 106*, 345–351.

Hamada, J. S. (1997). Characterization of protein fractions of rice bran to devise effective methods of protein solubilization. *Cereal Chemistry, 74*(5), 662–668.

Hamada, J. S. (1999). Use of protease to enhance stabilization of rice bran proteins. *Journal of Food Biochemistry, 23*, 307–321.

Hibino, T., Kidzu, K., Masumura, T., Ohtsuki, K., Tanaka, K., & Kawabata, M. (1989). Amino acid composition of rice prolamin polypeptides. *Agricultural and Biological Chemistry, 53*(2), 513–518.

Hoogenkamp, H. (2015). *Plant protein vision. Chapter 6. Rice bran: The complete super food* (pp. 91–130). E-Book, ISBN-10:1511910291/13:978-1511910293, CreativeSpace, San Bernadino, CA.

Houston, D. F., & Mohammad, A. (1970). Purification and partial characterization of a major globulin from rice endosperm. *Cereal Chemistry, 47*(1), 5–9.

Itani, T., Tamaki, M., Hayata, Y., Fushimi, T., & Hashizume, K. (2004). Variation of 2-acetyl-1-pyrroline concentration in aromatic rice grains collected in the same region in Japan and factors affecting its concentration. *Plant Production Science, 7*, 178–183.

Izumi, H., Sugiyama, M., Matsuda, T., & Nakamura, R. (1999). Structural characterization of the 16-kDa allergen, RA17, in rice seeds. Prediction of the secondary structure and identification of intramolecular disulfide bridges. *Bioscience, Biotechnology and Biochemistry, 63*, 2059–2063.

Jezussek, M., Juliano, B. O., & Schieberle, P. (2002). Comparison of key aroma compounds in cooked brown rice varieties based on aroma extract dilution analysis. *Journal of Agricultural and Food Chemistry, 50*, 1101–1105.

Jinsmaa, Y., Takenaka, Y., & Yoshikawa, M. (2001). Designing of an orally active complement C3a agonist peptide with anti-analgesic and anti-amnesic activity. *Peptides, 22*(1), 25–32.

Ju, Z. Y., & Rath, H. N. (2001). Extraction, denaturation and hydrophobic properties of rice flour proteins. *Journal of Food Science, 66*(2), 229–232.

Juliano, B. O. (Ed.), (1985). Rice bran. *Rice chemistry and technology* St. Paul, MN: American Association of Cereal Chemists.

Kahlon, T. S. (2009). Rice bran: Production, composition, functionality and food applications, physiological benefits. In S. S. Cho, & P. Samuel (Eds.), *Fiber ingredients: Food applications and health benefits* (p. 306). Parkway: CRC Press, Taylor & Francis Group.

Kalman, D. S. (2014). Amino acid composition of an organic brown rice protein concentrate and isolate compared to soy and whey concentrates and isolates. *Foods, 3*, 394–402.

Kashem, M. A., Itoh, K., Iwabuchi, S., Hori, H., & Mitsui, T. (2000). Possible involvement of phosphoinositide-Ca^{2+} signaling in the regulation of α-amylase expression and germination of rice seed (*Oryza sativa* L.). *Plant and Cell Physiology, 41*(4), 399–407.

Kato, T., Katayama, E., Matsubara, S., Omi, Y., & Matsuda, T. (2000). Release of allergenic proteins from rice grains induced by high hydrostatic pressure. *Jouranl of Agricultural and Food Chemistry, 48*(8), 3124–3129.

Katoch, R., & Jamwal, A. (2013). Characterization of α-amylase inhibitor from rice bean with inhibitory activity against midgut α-amylases from *Spodoptera litura*. *Applied Biochemistry and Microbiology, 49*(4), 419–425.

Kawagoe, Y., Suzuki, K., Tasaki, M., Yasuda, H., Akagi, K., Katoh, E., … Takaiwa, F. (2005). The critical role of disulfide bond formation in protein sorting in the endosperm of rice. *The Plant Cell, 17*(4), 1141–1153.

Khush, G. S., & Virk, P. S. (2010). A century of rice breeding, its impact and challenges ahead. In S. D. Sharma (Ed.), *Rice, origin, antiquity and history* (pp. 486–512). British Channel, Islands: Science Publishers.

Kim, M., & Jeong, Y. (2002). Extraction and electrophoretic characterization of rice proteins. *Nutraceuticals and Food, 7*(4), 437–441.

Kim, J.-W., Kim, B.-C., Lee, J.-H., Lee, D.-R., Rehman, S., & Yun, S. J. (2013). Protein content and composition of waxy rice grains. *Pakistan Journal of Botany, 45*(1), 151–156.

Kim, W. T., & Okita, T. W. (1988). Structure, expression, and heterogeneity of the rice seed prolamins. *Plant Physiology, 88*(3), 649–655.

Klyosov, A. A. (2007). *Wood-plastic composites* (p. 106). New York: John Wiley & Sons.

Kondo, H., Abe, K., Nishimura, I., Watanabe, H., Emori, Y., & Arai, S. (1990). Two distinct cystatin species in rice seeds with different specificities against cysteine proteinases. *The Journal of Biological Chemistry, 265*(26), 15832–15837.

Krishnan, H. B., White, J. A., & Pueppke, S. G. (1992). Characterization and localization of rice (*Oryza sativa* L.) seed globulins. *Plant Science, 81*(1), 1–11.

Kubota, M., Saito, Y., Masumura, T., Kumagai, T., Watanabe, R., Fujimura, S., & Kadowaki, M. (2010). Improvement in the in vivo digestibility of rice protein by alkali extraction is due to structural changes in prolamin/protein body-I particle. *Bioscience, Biotechnology, and Biochemistry, 74*(3), 614–619.

Kubota, M., Watanabe, R., Kabasawa, H., Iino, N., Saito, A., Kumagai, T., & Kadowaki, M. (2013). Rice protein ameliorates the progression of diabetic nephropathy in Goto-Kakizaki rats with high-sucrose feeding. *British Journal of Nutrition, 110*(7), 1211–1219.

Kumagai, T., Watanabe, R., Saito, M., Watanabe, T., Kubota, M., & Kadowaki, M. (2009). Superiority of alkali-extracted rice protein in bioavailability to starch degraded rice protein comes from digestion of prolamin in growing rats. *Journal of Nutritional Science and Vitaminology, 55*(2), 170–177.

Kumar, R., Srivastava, P., Kumari, D., Fakhr, H., Sridhara, S., Arora, N., ... Singh, B. P. (2007). Rice (*Oryza sativa*) allergy in rhinitis and asthma patients: A clinico-immunological study. *Immunobiology, 212*(2), 141−147.

Lam, H. S., & Proctor, A. (2003). Milled rice oxidation volatiles and odor development. *Journal of Food Science, 68*, 2676−2681.

Li, G.-H., Qu, M.-R., Wan, J.-Z., & You, J.-M. (2007). Antihypertensive effect of rice protein hydrolysate with in vitro angiotensin I-converting enzyme inhibitory activity in spontaneously hypertensive rats. *Asia Pacific Journal of Clinical Nutrition, 16*(1), 275−280.

Luh, B. S. (1991). Rice hulls. In B. S. Luh (Ed.), *Rice, volume 2: Utilization* (p. 271). New York: Springer Science & Business Media.

Masumura, T., Hibino, T., Kidzu, K., Mitsukawa, N., Tanaka, K., & Fujii, S. (1990). Cloning and characterization of a cDNA encoding a rice 13 kDa prolamin. *Molecular and General Genetics, 221*(1), 1−7.

Masumura, T., Kidzu, K., Sugiyama, Y., Mitsukawa, N., Hibino, T., Tanaka, K., & Fujii, S. (1989a). Nucleotide sequence of a cDNA encoding a major rice glutelin. *Plant Molecular Biology, 12*(6), 723−725.

Masumura, T., Shibata, D., Hibion, T., Kato, T., Kawabe, K., Takeba, G., & Fujii, S. (1989b). cDNA cloning of an mRNA encoding a sulfur-rich 10 kDa prolamin polypeptide in rice seeds. *Plant Molecular Biology, 12*(2), 123−130.

Mawal, Y. R., Mawal, J. R., & Ranjekar, P. K. (1987). Biochemical and immunological characterization of rice albumin. *Bioscience Reports, 7*(1), 1−9.

Mitchell, C. R., Mitchell, P. R., & Mitchell, W. A. (1988). *Rice syrup sweetner production.* US Patent 4,756,912.

Mitsui, T., Christeller, J. T., Hara-Nishimura, I., & Akazawa, T. (1984). Possible roles of calcium and calmodulin in the biosynthesis and secretion of α-amylase in rice seed scutellar epithelium. *Plant Physiology, 75*(1), 21−25.

Mitsukawa, N., Konishi, R., Uchiki, M., Masumura, T., & Tanaka, K. (1999). Molecular cloning and characterization of a cysteine-rich 16.6-kDa prolamin in rice seeds. *Bioscience Biotechnology and Biochemistry, 63*(11), 1851−1858.

Miyata, S., Okamoto, K., Watanabe, A., & Akazawa, T. (1981). Enzymic mechanism of starch breakdown in germinating rice seeds. 10. The in vivo and in vitro synthesis of α-amylase in rice seed scutellium. *Plant Physiology, 68*(10), 1314−1318.

Monsoor, M. A., & Proctor, A. (2004). Volatile component analysis of commercially milled head and broken rice. *Journal of Food Science, 69*, C632−C636.

Morita, Y., & Yoshida, C. (1968). Studies on γ-globulin of rice embryo. Part I. Isolation and purification of γ-globulin from rice embryo. *Agricultural and Biological Chemistry, 32*(5), 664−670.

Muthayya, S., Sugimoto, J. D., Montgomery, S., & Maberly, G. F. (2014). An overview of global rice production, supply, trade, and consumption. *Annals of the New York Academy of Sciences, 1324*, 7−14.

Nakamura, R., & Matsuda, T. (1996). Rice allergenic protein and molecular-genetic approach for hypoallergenic rice. *Bioscience, Biotechnology and Biochemistry, 60*(8), 1215−1221.

Nakase, M., Usui, Y., Alvarez-Nakase, A. M., Adachi, T., Urisu, A., Nakamura, R., ... Matsuda, T. (1998). Cereal allergens: Rice-seed allergens with structural similarity to wheat and barley allergens. *Allergy, 53*(46 Suppl.), 55−57.

O'Neill, et al. (1990). The α-amylase genes in *Oryza sativa*: Characterization of cDNA clones and mRNA expression during seed germination. *Molecular and General Genetics, 221*(2), 235−244.

Ogawa, M., Kumamaru, T., Satoh, H., Iwata, N., Omura, T., Kasai, Z., & Tanaka, K. (1987). Purification of protein body-I of rice seed and its polypeptide composition. *Plant Cell Physiology, 28*(8), 1517−1527.

Ogawa, W., Kumamaru, T., Satoh, H., Omura, T., Park, T., Shintaku, K., & Baba, K. (1989). Mutants of rice storage proteins: 2. Isolation and characterization of protein bodies from rice mutants. *Theoretical and Applied Genetics, 78*(3), 306−309.

Ohinata, K., Suetsugu, K., Fujiwara, Y., & Yoshikawa, M. (2007). Suppression of food intake by a complement C3a agonist [Trp^5]-oryzatensin(5-9). *Peptides, 28*(3), 602−606.

Ohtsubo, S., Kobayashi, H., Noro, W., Taniguchi, M., & Saitoh, E. (2005). Molecular cloning and characterization of oryzacystatin-III, a nove. Member of phytocystatin in rice (*Oryza sativa* L. japonica). *Journal of Agricultural and Food Chemistry, 53*(13), 5218−5224.

Padhye, V. W., & Salunkhe, D. K. (1979). Extraction and characterization of rice proteins. *Cereal Chemistry, 56*(5), 389−393.

Pan, S.-J., & Reeck, G. R. (1988). Isolation and characterization of rice α-globulin. *Cereal Chemistry, 65*(4), 316−319.

Park, H.-J., Han, S.-W., Lee, D.-Y., Kim, H. K., Jeong, H.-C., Park, H. H., & Song, H.-S. (2009). *A method for preparing protein concentrate from rice bran.* WO 2009035186 A1.

Patil, S. B., & Khan, M. K. (2011). Germinated brown rice as a value added rice product: A review. *Journal of Food Science and Technology, 48*, 661−667.

Pimentel, D., & Pimentel, M. (2003). Sustainability of meat-based and plant diets and the environment. *American Journal of Clinical Nutrition, 78* (Suppl), 660S−663S.

Poznanski, J., Sodano, P., Suh, S. W., Lee, J. Y., Ptak, M., & Vovelle, F. (1999). Solution structure of a lipid transfer protein extracted from rice seeds. Comparison with homologous proteins. *European Journal of Biochemistry, 259*(3), 692−708.

Prabhu, A. V., Tambe, S. P., Gandhi, N. N., Sawant, S. B., & Joshi, J. B. (1999). Rice bran lipase: Extraction, activity and stability. *BiotechnologyProgress, 15*, 1083−1089.

Puchongkavarian, H., Varavinit, S., & Bergthaller, W. (2005). Comparative study of pilot scale rice starch production by alkaline and enzymatic process. *Starch, 57*, 134−144.

Ramezanzadeh, F. M., Rao, R. M., Windhauser, M., Prinyawiwatkul, W., Tulley, R., & Marshall, W. E. (1999). Prevention of hydrolytic rancidity in rice bran during storage. *Journal of Agricultural and Food Chemistry, 47*, 3050−3952.

Rapp, A., Versini, G., & Ullemeyer, H. (1993). 2-Aminoacetophenone — Acusal component of untypical aging flavor (naphthalene note, hybrid note) of wine. *VITIS, 32*, 61−62.

Resurreccion, A. P., Li, X., Okita, T. W., & Juliano, B. O. (1993). Characterization of poorly digested protein of cooked rice protein bodies. *Cereal Chemistry, 70*, 101–104.

Rohrer, C., & Siebenmorgen, T. (2005). Nutraceutical concentrations within the bran of various rice kernel thickness fractions. *Biosystem Engineering, 88*, 453–460.

Roohinejad, S., Mirhosseini, H., Saari, N., Mustafa, S., Alias, I., Husin, A. S. M., … Manap, M. Y. (2009). Evaluation of GABA, crude protein and amino acid composition from different varieties of Malaysian brown rice. *Australian Journal of Crop Science, 3*, 184–190.

Sagum, R., & Arcot, J. (2000). Effect of domestic processing methods on the starch, non-starch polysaccharides and in vitro starch and protein digestibility of three varieties of rice with varying levels of amylose. *Food Chemistry, 70*, 107–111.

Satter, M. A., Ara, H., Jabin, S. A., Abedin, N., Azad, A. K., Houssain, A., & Ara, U. (2014). Nutritional composition and stabilization of local variety rice bran BRRI-28. *The International Journal of Science and Technology, 3*(5), 306–313.

Shewry, P. R., & Casey, R. (1999). *Seed proteins*. The Netherlands: Kluwer Academic Publishers.

Shibasaki, M., Suzuki, S., Nemoto, H., & Kuroume, T. (1979). Allergenicity and lymphocyte-stimulating property of rice protein. *Journal of Allergy and Clinical Immunology, 64*(4), 259–265.

Shih, F. F. (2003). An update on the processing of high-protein rice products. Review. *Nahrung/Food, 6*, 420–424.

Shih, F. F., Champagne, E. T., Daigle, K., & Zarins, Z. (1999). Use of enzymes in the processing of protein products from rice bran and rice flour. *Die Nahrung, 43*, 14–18.

Shih, F. F., & Daigle, K. W. (2000). *Use of enzymes for the separation of protein from rice flour Cereal Chemistry, 77*, 885–889.

Shyur, L. F., & Chen, C. S. (1994). Purification and characterization of rice prolamins. *Botanical Studies, 35*, 65–71.

Shyur, L.-F., Wen, T.-N., & Chen, C.-S. (1992). cDNA cloning and gene expression of the major prolamins of rice. *Plant Molecular Biology, 20*(2), 323–326.

Shyur, L.-F., Zia, K. K., & Chen, C.-S. (1988). Purification and some properties of storage proteins in *japonica* rice. *Botanical Bulletin of Academia Sinica, 29*(2), 113–122.

Takahashi, M., Moriguchi, S., Ikeno, M., Kono, S., Ohata, K., Usui, H., … Yoshikawa, M. (1996). Studies on the ilium-contracting mechanisms and identification as a complement C3a receptor agonist of oryzatensin, a bioactive peptide derived from rice albuin. *Peptides, 17*(1), 5–12.

Takahashi, M., Moriguchi, S., Yoshikawa, M., & Sasaki, R. (1994). Isolation and characterization of oryzatensin: A novel bioactive peptide with ileum-contracting and immunomodulating activities derived from rice albumin. *Biochemistry and Molecular Biology International, 33*(6), 1151–1158.

Takaiwa, F., Kikuchi, S., & Oono, K. (1986). The structure of rice storage protein glutelin precursor deduced from cDNA. *FEBS Letters, 206*(1), 33–35.

Takaiwa, F., Kikuchi, S., & Oono, K. (1987). A rice glutelin gene family — A major type of glutelin mRNAs can be divided into two classes. *Molecular and General Genetics, 208*(1), 15–22.

Takaiwa, F., Ogawa, M., & Okita, T. W. (1999). Rice glutellins. In P. R. Shewry, & R. Casey (Eds.), *Seed Proteins* (pp. 401–425). The Netherlands: Kluwer Academics Publishers.

Takubo, Y. (1997). *Method for producing halk-hulled rice milk*. US patent 5,609,895.

Tanaka, K., Sugimoto, T., Ogawa, M., & Kasai, Z. (1980). Isolation and characterization of two types of protein bodies in the rice endosperm. *Agricultural and Biological Chemistry, 44*(7), 1633–1639.

Tanaka, Y., Resurreccion, A. P., Juliano, B. O., & Bechtel, D. B. (1978). Properties of whole and undigested fraction of protein bodies of milled rice. *Agricultural and Biological Chemistry, 42*, 2015–2023.

Tang, S., Hettiararchy, N. S., & Shellhammer, T. H. (2002). Protein extraction from heat-stabilized defatted rice bran. 1. Physical processing and enzyme treatments. *Journal of Agricultural and Food Chemistry, 50*, 7444–7448.

Udenigwe, C. C. (2016). Towards rice bran protein utilization: In silico insight on the role of oryzacystatins in biologically-active peptide production. *Food Chemistry, 191*, 135–138.

Uraipong, C., & Zhao, J. (2016). Rice bran protein hydrolysates exhibit strong in vitro α-amylase, β-glucosidase and ACE-inhibition activities. *Journal of the Science of Food and Agriculture, 96*(4), 1101–1110.

Urisu, A., Yamada, K., Masuda, S., Komada, H., Wada, E., Kondo, Y., … Yamada, M., et al. (1991). 16-kilodalton rice protein is one of the major allergens in rice grain extract and responsible for cross-allergenicity between cereal grains in the Poaceae family. *International Archives of Allergy and Applied Immunology, 96*(3), 244–252.

Usui, Y., Nakase, M., Hotta, H., Urisu, A., Aoki, N., Kitajima, K., & Matsuda, T. (2001). A 33-kDa allergen from rice (*Oryza sativa* L. *japonica*). cDNA cloning, expression, and identification as a novel glyoxalase I. *Journal of Biological Chemistry, 276*(14), 11376–11381.

van Ree, R., Voitenko, V., et al. (1992). Profilin is a cross-reactive allergen in pollen and vegetable foods. *International Archives of Allergy and Immunology, 98*, 97–104.

Wang, C., Li, D., Xu, F., Hao, T., & Zhang, M. (2014). Comparison of two methods for the extraction of fractionated rice bran protein. *Journal of Chemistry*, , 546345/1–546345/11.

Wang, H., Denney, L., Zheng, Y., Vinyes-Pares, G., Reldy, K., Wang, P., & Zhang, Y. (2015). Food sources of energy and nutrients in the diets of infants and toddlers in urban areas of China, based on one 24-hour dietary recall. *BMC Nutrition, 1*, 19.

Wang, M., Hettiarachchy, N. S., Qi, M., Burks, W., & Siebenmorgen, T. (1999). Preparation and functional properties of rice bran protein isolate. *Journal of Agricultural and Food Chemistry, 47*, 411–416.

Watanabe, H., Abe, K., Emori, Y., Hosoyama, H., & Arai, S. (1991). Molecular cloning and gibberellin-induced expression of multiple cysteine proteinases of rice seeds (oryzains). *The Journal of Biological Chemistry, 266*(25), 16897–16902.

Watchararuji, K., Goto, M., Sasaki, M., & Shotipruk, A. (2008). Value-added subcritical water hydrolysate from rice bran and soybean meal. *Bioresources Technology, 99*, 6207–6213.

Wei, C., Nguyen, S. D., Kim, M. R., & Sok, D.-E. (2007). Rice albumin N-terminal (Asp-His-His-Gln) prevents against copper ion-catalyzed oxidations. *Journal of Agricultural and Food Chemistry, 55*(6), 2149–2154.

Yamada, C., Yamashita, Y., Seki, R., Izumi, H., Matsuda, T., & Kato, Y. (2006). Digestion and gastrointestinal absorption of the 14-16-kDa rice allergens. *Bioscience Biotechnology and Biochemistry, 70*(8), 1890–1897.

Yamagata, H., Sugimoto, T., Tanaka, K., & Kasai, Z. (1982). Biosynthesis of storage proteins in developing rice seeds. *Plant Physiology, 70*(4), 1094–1100.

Yamasaki, T., Deguchi, M., Fujimoto, T., Masumura, T., Uno, T., Kanamaru, K., & Yamagata, H. (2006). Rice bifunctional α-amylase/subtilisin inhibitor: Cloning and characterization of the recombinant inhibitor expressed in *Escherichia coli*. *Bioscience Biotechnology and Biochemistry, 70*(5), 1200–1209.

Yang, D. S., Shewfelt, R. J., Lee, K.-S., & Kays, S. J. (2008). Comparison of odor-active compounds from distinctly different rice flavor types. *Journal of Agricultural and Food Chemistry, 56*, 2780–2787.

Yang, L., Chen, J., Xu, T., Qiu, W., Zhang, Y., Zhang, L., et al. (2011). Rice protein extracted by different methods affects cholesterol metabolism in rats due to its lower digestibility. *International Journal of Molecular Sciences, 12*(11), 7594–7608.

Yang, L., Chen, J.-H., Lv, J., Wu, Q., Xu, T., Zhang, H., et al. (2012). Rice protein improves adiposity, body weight and reduces lipid level in rats through modification of triglyceride metabolism. *Lipids in Health and Disease, 11*, 24.

Yang, L., Kumagai, T., Kawamura, H., Watanabe, T., Kubota, M., Fujimura, S., ... Kadowaki, M. (2007). Effects of rice proteins from two cultivars, *Koshihikari* and *Shunyo*, on cholesterol and triglyceride metabolism in growing and adult rats. *Bioscience, Biotechnology, and Biochemistry, 71*(3), 694–703.

Yang, T. S. (2007). *Flavor chemistry of rice*. Doctoral Dissertation. Athens, USA: University of Georgia.

Yoshihashi, T., Huong, N. T. T., & Inatomi, H. (2002). Precursors of 2-acetyl-1-pyrroline, a potent flavor compound of an aromatic rice variety. *Journal of Agricultural and Food Chemistry., 50*, 2001–2004.

Zeigler, R. S., & Barclay, A. (2008). The relevance of rice. *RICE, 1*, 3–10.

Zhou, Z., Robards, K., Helliwell, S., & Blanchard, C. (2002). Composition and functional properties of rice. *International Journal of Food Science and Technology, 37*(8), 849–868.

Chapter 4

Proteins From Wheat: Sustainable Production and New Developments in Nutrition-Based and Functional Applications

M. Flambeau, A. Redl and F. Respondek
Tereos, Marckolsheim, France

4.1 INTRODUCTION

4.1.1 Agricultural Production

Wheat is an important cereal grain originating from the Near East and is currently cultivated worldwide. Wheat and wheat products are ubiquitous in a variety of the foods we consume, including bread and pasta. Annual production of wheat is 715 million tonnes based on FAO data 2013.[1] It is the third most produced cereal after corn and rice. Wheat is cultivated on 224 million hectares worldwide. India represents 31 million hectares, EU27 has 27 million hectares, and the US 18 million hectares. Worldwide wheat production was 715 million tonnes in 2014 (out of a worldwide cereal production of 2522 million tonnes). The top wheat-producing countries include the EU27 (156 million tonnes), China (126 million tonnes), India (96 million tonnes), Russia (59 million tonnes), the US (55 million tonnes), and Canada (29 million tonnes).[2] The volatility of wheat prices is quite high and this impacts the cost of the wheat proteins (Fig. 4.1).

Most of the wheat produced is transformed into flour for food consumption, while a portion goes toward animal feed. A significant proportion of European wheat (approximately 8 million tons) is transformed into starch and wheat protein with the production of wheat gluten representing approximately 560,000 tonnes.

4.1.2 Land Use

Wheat crop is cultivated in spring and winter, with the winter crop being more resistant to frost.[3] However, it is the early-stage crop that is resistant to cold temperatures. Once the plants are growing, both the spring and winter crops are more susceptible to the onset of cold weather. Spring wheat is harvested in 3–4 months, while winter wheat requires about 7–8 months for harvest.[4]

Wheat plants can grow in a wide range of soils as shown by the diverse cultivation spread all over the world, however, medium-texture soils with a pH range from 6 to 8 are more adapted. Yields vary largely depending on soil, fertilization, irrigation, and variety. For example, wheat yield is as low as 1 tonne/ha in Kazakhstan, but reaches a high of 9 tonnes/ha in New Zealand. Typical yields are about 3 tonnes/ha in the US and range from 5 to 6 tonnes/ha in EU27.

---

1. <http://www.fao.org/worldfoodsituation/csdb/en/>.
2. <http://www.indexmundi.com/agriculture/?commodity=wheat>.
3. <http://www.fao.org/nr/water/cropinfo_wheat.html>.
4. <http://homeguides.sfgate.com/long-wheat-plants-before-harvest-69823.html>.

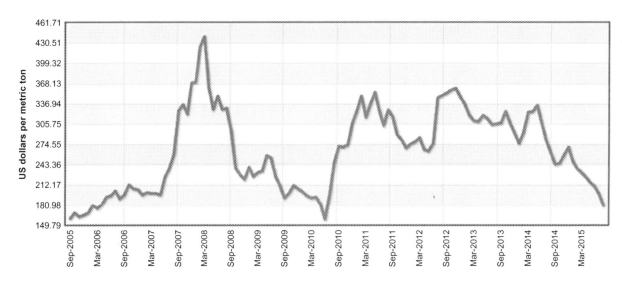

FIGURE 4.1 Monthly prices of wheat in US dollars per metric ton from Sep. 2005 to Sep. 2015 (Wheat N°1 hard red winter). *From Index Mundi, World Bank.*

4.1.3 Water Use

Wheat plants grow best in regions away from the tropical regions and typically thrive in temperate climates. Rainfall and irrigation are required for good yields. Suitable temperatures for optimum plant growth range from 7°C to 21°C[5] with water requirements of at least 60 cm/year to about 150 cm/year.[6] Water is essential for proper germination and early-stage plant development.[7] If rainfall is sparse, then farmers have to depend on irrigation, although irrigation is reduced during the flowering stage and should stop when the seeds have ripened. Water requirements are higher for the grain-filling stage of the wheat ears. Excess moisture via rainfall during the early stages of wheat plant growth can cause blight. Diseases such as *Fusarium* head blight caused by *Fusarium graminearum*, can greatly reduce yields.[8]

4.1.4 Energy Use

Wheat crop requires the addition of various nutrients for yielding a good harvest. Nitrogen is very important for good crop yields and is transformed into protein by the plant. Thus, plants provided sufficient nitrogen develop dark green shoots and grow rapidly.[9] Sulfur is a limiting component and is typically added at a tenth of the amount of nitrogen. Sulfur is essential for producing flour for baking needs.[10] Potassium helps maintain the balance between carbohydrates and protein, while providing strength to wheat straws.[11] Finally, phosphorus is critical for cellular processes, such as energy transfer and photosynthesis. Thus, potassium should be added, especially early in the growing cycle.[12]

4.1.5 Sustainability of Wheat

While worldwide production of cereals has nearly tripled in the last 40 years (Tilman et al., 2002) from 800 million tonnes in 1960 to 2000 million tonnes in 2000, the worldwide use of fertilizer (nitrogen (N) and phosphorous (P)) has increased from 10 million tonnes to 80 or 60 million tonnes/year, respectively, for nitrogen and phosphorous fertilizers. When dividing the annual global cereal production by the annual global application of nitrogen fertilizers it appears that nitrogen efficiency of cereal production has decreased from 80 tonnes of cereal produced per tonne of nitrogen

---

5. <http://www.agriinfo.in/default.aspx?page=topic&superid=1&topicid=1172>.
6. <http://www.nda.agric.za/docs/brochures/wheat.pdf>.
7. <http://www1.agric.gov.ab.ca/$Department/deptdocs.nsf/all/agdex13535>.
8. <https://www.extension.purdue.edu/extmedia/BP/BP-33-W.pdf>.
9. <http://www1.agric.gov.ab.ca/$department/deptdocs.nsf/all/crop1273>.
10. <http://extension.oregonstate.edu/umatilla/sites/default/files/cereals/Publications/fg81-e.pdf>.
11. <http://www1.agric.gov.ab.ca/$department/deptdocs.nsf/all/crop1296>.
12. <http://www.ipni.net/ppiweb/ppinews.nsf/0/fad7efc77845297585256db4004f8670/$FILE/P%20on%20Wheat.pdf>.

fertilizer in the 1960s down to 25 tonnes of cereals produced per tonne of nitrogen fertilizer used in 2000 (data from FAO statistical database 2001, cited in Tilman et al., 2002). One of the main issues of intensive cereal production is the leaching of fertilizers, while a corresponding main challenge of sustainable cereal production is to increase the fertilizer efficiency ratio again. Applying fertilizers during periods of highest crop demand and in smaller and more frequent applications has great potential in improving fertilizer efficiency and reducing leakages.

Farmer incentives are also a central issue facing sustainable agriculture. A number of countries, including Australia, Canada, the European Union, and the United States have implemented various forms of green payments to farmers who adopt sustainable or environmentally benign farming practices. In Europe, for example, the new revision of the common agricultural policy introduced the conditioning of up to 30% of the EU payments to mandatory additional practices beneficial to the environment and climate. These translate to a number of benefits to the environment such as:

1. Crop diversification: mandatory rotation between two and three crops depending on the size of the farm holding;
2. Permanent grassland: maintenance of permanent grassland based on national/regional ratios;
3. Ecological focus areas: maintenance of ecological focus areas of at least 5% of the arable land of the holding.

Once sustainable wheat is produced the proteins need to be extracted thereof. A huge advantage of the physicochemical behavior of wheat proteins is that upon hydration they agglomerate into a viscoelastic mass which can be extracted from the rest, with water as the only solvent. The wheat grain is separated into proteins, starch, and fiber-rich coproducts in a typical starch production plant. As such, the starch industry in Europe is evaluating its sustainability according to industry wide life cycle analysis (LCA). This LCA shows that the starch industry has:

1. A very wide application of combined heat and power generation (58% of generated electricity and heat);
2. A quite low impact on transport due to the close location of the production areas and the starch extraction plants;
3. Starch and protein extraction process is very resource efficient with less than 1% of processed crop not being sold as a product (Vercalsteren & Boonen, 2015).

4.2 PROTEINS FROM WHEAT

Wheat gluten is a natural protein derived from wheat or wheat flour. Once dried, it has a creamy color, neutral taste, and is free-flowing. Dried gluten is able to recover its unique viscoelastic structure when rehydrated. A typical composition for gluten is:

Protein	75–80%
Carbohydrates	15–17%
Fat	5–8%
Ash	0.6–1.2%

Three categories of wheat protein products are defined (CODEX Standard 163-1987):[13]

1. Vital wheat gluten—characterized by high viscoelasticity when hydrated, a protein content above 80% (N × 6.25), and declared as "vital wheat gluten" or "wheat gluten";
2. Devitalized wheat gluten—characterized by reduced property of viscoelasticity as hydrated due to denaturation, a protein content above 80% (N × 6.25), and declared as "devitalized wheat gluten" or "devital wheat gluten";
3. Solubilized wheat proteins—characterized by their reduced property of viscoelasticity as hydrated, due to partial hydrolysis of wheat gluten, a protein content above 60% (N × 6.25), and declared as "solubilized wheat protein" or "soluble wheat proteins."

Moisture content is determined by AOAC 925.09,[14] protein content by AOAC 979.09 for vital and devitalized wheat gluten,[15] and AOAC 920.87 for solubilized wheat protein.[16] In wheat, different types of proteins are found. They are differentiated by their structure as monomeric or polymeric and by their solubility or insolubility in water or alcohol. The monomeric proteins are albumins (soluble in water), globulins (soluble in salted solutions), and gliadins (soluble in alcohol). The polymeric proteins are mainly glutenins (insoluble). Gliadins and glutenins represent 75–80% of the proteins in wheat. When gluten is extracted from wheat flour albumins and globulins are mainly removed in

---

13. <http://www.fao.org/3/a-a1392e.pdf>.
14. <http://www.eoma.aoac.org/methods/info.asp?ID = 26685>.
15. <http://www.eoma.aoac.org/methods/info.asp?ID = 27450>.
16. <http://www.eoma.aoac.org/methods/info.asp?ID = 27076>.

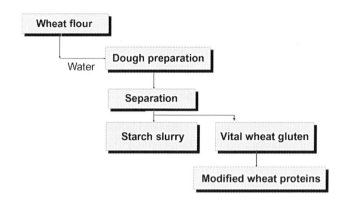

FIGURE 4.2 Production scheme for vital wheat gluten and modified wheat proteins. *From Tereos.*

the washing water (MacRitchie and Lafiandra, 1997). Glutenins are a combination of different chain length polymers. They vary largely by the proportion of different polymeric chain length and the internal and external disulfide bonds. The usual conversion factor from nitrogen percent to protein percent is 6.25 for vegetable proteins (average N content of proteins defined as 16%). However, for gluten the higher content of N in amino acids like glutamine leads to selecting a conversion factor of 5.7.[17] In terms of labeling, gluten and hydrolyzed wheat protein are considered as food ingredients.

4.2.1 Gluten Extraction From Wheat

Wheat grains are crushed and sieved in a dry mill. Bran and germs are removed from the flour. Flour is mixed with water and starch and gluten are separated. It is critical that the whole process does not to exceed a temperature of 70°C. Wheat proteins are extracted from wheat flour obtained by dry milling of wheat kernels. The unique agglomeration properties of gluten enable an efficient separation from the wheat starch. In starch production, wheat flour is blended with water and developed into a dough, enabling the gluten protein to form an elastic network. In this process, the starch is then washed out of the gluten network. Usually wheat gluten is dried and sold as vital wheat gluten or further transformed by hydrolyzing the gluten (Fig. 4.2).

Wheat gluten is composed of gliadin and glutenin proteins. An agglomeration process is utilized to obtain both high-quality gluten and high-quality starch in parallel. Intense mixing, high shear, good hydration, and operation at pH of isoelectric point are key parameters. Gluten differs widely in terms of properties due to the origin of the wheat, the extraction process, and drying conditions. Simple characterizations like water or protein content are not sufficient to predict the functionalities of the vital wheat gluten.

Soluble wheat protein isolates have superior properties in terms of foaming when compared to soy protein isolates or egg white, especially in ionic solutions. Water-holding capacity is also higher than sodium caseinates and egg white. Emulsification properties enable the use of soluble wheat protein in ice cream as a vegan-based alternative to caseinates (Ahmedna et al., 1999.

4.2.2 Protein Hydrolysis

As the insolubility of gluten in aqueous solutions is a major limitation for applications outside of bakery products, gluten can be hydrolyzed by enzymatic or acid means to increase solubility. Most of the commercially available solubilized wheat protein ingredients are made from enzymatic hydrolysis using one or several commercial proteases (Fig. 4.3).

The type of enzyme and the reaction conditions enable one to modulate the degree of hydrolysis and the molecular weight distribution. One of the most important properties is the increase in solubility as measured by the nitrogen solubility index (NSI) (Fig. 4.4).

The specific protein and polypeptide composition of the products can be determined by electrophoresis (SDS PAGE) and size exclusion chromatography (Kong et al., 2007).

---

17. <http://www.aaccnet.org/publications/cc/backissues/1969/documents/chem46_419.pdf>.

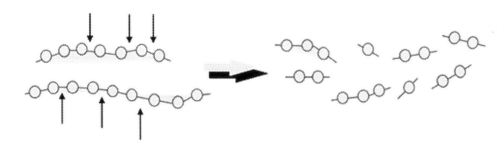

FIGURE 4.3 Hydrolysis of gluten. *From Tereos.*

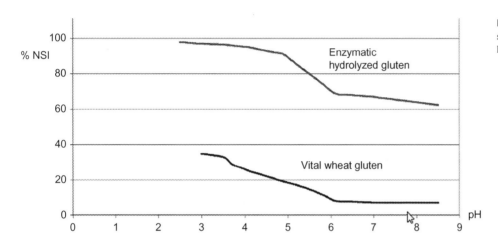

FIGURE 4.4 Change of nitrogen solubility index with pH for enzymatic hydrolyzed gluten. *From Tereos.*

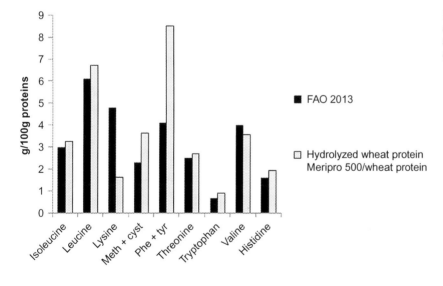

FIGURE 4.5 Composition of essential amino acids of hydrolyzed wheat proteins in comparison with reference protein for adults. *From FAO. (2013). Nutrition quality of proteins.*

4.3 NUTRITION AND DIGESTIBILITY, ALLERGEN, AND ANTINUTRITIVE ASPECTS

4.3.1 Amino Acid Composition

Similar to other cereals and most plant-based proteins, wheat lacks lysine but is rich in sulfur amino acids and contains enough branched-chain amino acids (BCAA) such as leucine, isoleucine, and valine in comparison to reference protein defined by FAO in 2013 (FAO, 2013; Fig. 4.5).

TABLE 4.1 Relative Percentage of Glutamine in Various Sources of Dietary Protein

Source of Protein	Glutamine Content (% of Protein)
Wheat gluten	36
Hydrolyzed wheat protein (Meripro 500)	36
Pea protein isolate	10–17
Soy protein	17–20
Whey protein	5–10
Casein	10–12

BCAAs represent around 35% of amino acids in muscle, therefore a proper BCAA intake is essential to reduce muscle damage after exercise and stimulate muscle protein synthesis (Negro, Giardina, Marzani, & Marzatico, 2008). Wheat proteins are also particularly rich in readily available glutamine in comparison to other dietary proteins (Table 4.1).

Glutamine acts on the structure and functioning of the small intestine and plays a role in the development of the intestinal mucosa. It constitutes the main energy substrate for enterocytes and plays a role in the development of intestinal mucosa (Ziegler, Evans, Fernandez-Estivariz, & Jones, 2003). Glutamine also acts on the immune system as it is an essential energy source for immunity cells like lymphocytes and macrophages that need to proliferate rapidly in order to induce an appropriate immune response (Ziegler et al., 2003).

L-Glutamine is also the most abundant amino acid in muscles and becomes an essential amino acid in the case of high-intensity training. Indeed, muscular levels of glutamine are sharply decreased after training and require adequate time to replenish. Dietary supplementation with glutamine is needed to accelerate the muscular repletion of this amino acid and support natural defenses that are impaired in the case of glutamine deficiency. Several studies have highlighted the potential benefits of glutamine-rich wheat protein fractions for sports nutrition. A study of half-marathon athletes has shown that hydrolyzed wheat proteins could help to reduce injury of active muscle fibers after exercise. One hour after completing the race, young athletes were randomly assigned to consume 0, 10, or 20 g of hydrolyzed wheat protein. It was shown that hydrolyzed wheat protein could dose-dependently reduce plasma activity of creatine kinase. The latter is an intramuscular protein and its circulation in the blood is a marker of muscle injury. The mechanism remains unknown but may be related to a unique combination of BCAA and glutamine concentration that is particularly high in hydrolyzed wheat protein (Koikawa et al., 2009; Sawaki, Takaoka, Sakuraba, & Suzuki, 2004). More recently, another study suggested that immediate consumption of 18 g of hydrolyzed wheat proteins suppresses delayed onset of muscle injury after soccer exercise (Aoki et al., 2012).

4.3.2 Digestibility Data and Mechanism

Wheat protein digestibility in humans is reported between 85% and 95% for true ileal digestibility (Bos et al., 2005; FAO, 2013; Juillet et al., 2008) and up to 99% for true fecal digestibility (Bodwell, Satterlee, & Hackler, 1980; Deglaire & Moughan, 2012). The difference observed in ileal digestibility may be explained by the study design and whether wheat proteins were tested as purified fractions alone or in complex food matrices (Smith et al., 2015). Gliadin fractions seem more readily digested than gluten proteins (Smith et al., 2015). Individual digestibility of essential amino acids from wheat gluten ranges from 86% for lysine to 99% for histidine (FAO, 2013). These values are consistent with those reported for plant proteins, excluding any antinutritional factors. Further studies also reported that biological utilization of wheat proteins is higher than expected from its composition in essential amino acids and more particularly its lack of lysine. Overall nutritional value is estimated around 90% of the nutritional value of milk proteins (Bos et al., 2005).

As mentioned above, food processing can significantly alter digestibility of proteins, including wheat proteins.[18] Studies are mostly available for applications where wheat is usually added, such as bakery products

---

18. <http://ir.canterbury.ac.nz/handle/10092/8403>.

and pasta. The baking process may reduce the digestibility of gluten proteins as demonstrated in vitro on purified protein fractions. However, in the real production of bread the presence of starch in the food may actually enhance digestibility because α-amylase will hydrolyze the gluten−starch complex formed during baking (Smith et al., 2015). Good overall digestibility of wheat proteins tested in biscotte (traditional French wheat toast) was confirmed in healthy adults (Bos et al., 2005). For pasta, it seems that high temperature (above 90−110°C) and low moisture content during drying can reduce digestibility of wheat proteins by around 10% due to the formation and presence of Maillard-type protein aggregates (De Zorzi, Curioni, Simonato, Giannattasio, & Pasini, 2007; Petitot et al., 2009). Therefore, the development of new food matrices incorporating wheat protein requires appropriate digestibility testing.

4.3.3 Allergenicity and Intolerance Mechanism

Three major forms of gluten adverse reactions are now defined: wheat allergy, celiac disease, and a newly introduced symptom of nonceliac gluten hypersensitivity (Sapone et al., 2012). Wheat allergy is defined as an adverse immunologic reaction to wheat proteins (Sapone et al., 2012). Wheat is one of the eight main food allergens listed in the United States (FDA, 2004) and one of the 14 listed in Europe (European Parliament, 2011). Allergenic proteins identified in wheat food allergy were found among different wheat protein fractions. However, based on an objectively verified food challenge the estimated prevalence of wheat allergy is around 0.1%, representing the lowest prevalence of common food allergies along with shellfish (Husby & Murray, 2015; Nwaru et al., 2014).

Food processing may have an impact on the allergenicity of wheat proteins. Similar to other food proteins (eg, milk), heating wheat proteins at high temperature in the presence of certain carbohydrates may induce the formation of protein aggregates with allergenic potential that are resistant to digestion. But other factors, like digestion of starch, enhance the extent of protein digestion and reduce the presence of allergenic structures (Smith et al., 2015; Verhoeckx et al., 2015). The type of hydrolysis of native gluten may also modify allergenicity. Acid hydrolysis may induce specific allergenicity in wheat-tolerant people, whereas enzymatic hydrolysis may reduce the allergenicity of wheat when specific proteolytic properties are present (Verhoeckx et al., 2015).

Gluten intolerance, also known as celiac disease, is an immune-mediated enteropathy triggered by consumption of gluten in genetically predisposed individuals carrying HLA-DQ2 or HLA-DQ8. The diagnosis of celiac disease is confirmed if at least four of the following criteria are fulfilled: (1) typical symptoms, (2) positivity of serum CD IgA class autoantibodies at high titer, (3) HLA-DQ2 and/or HLA-DQ8 genotypes, and (4) celiac enteropathy found on small bowel biopsy and response to a gluten-free diet (Sapone et al., 2012). Contrary to wheat allergy which induces an immediate reaction, the onset of symptoms in celiac disease is usually gradual (Sapone et al., 2012). The estimated prevalence of this disease is around 1% (Husby & Murray, 2015; Sapone et al., 2012).

The recent rise of gluten-free markets in the United States and Europe is sustained by individuals claiming "gluten sensitivity" and improvement of intestinal and extraintestinal symptoms on a gluten-free diet. However these symptoms are linked to neither allergic nor autoimmune responses characteristic of wheat allergy or celiac disease (Sapone et al., 2012). There is some evidence that nonceliac gluten sensitivity may exist but in a limited number of individuals (Biesiekierski & Iven, 2015; Husby & Murray, 2015). Further research is needed to improve the diagnosis and to identify the real cause of these symptoms. Whereas a gluten-free diet is also fashionable for sportsmen, a recent study showed no benefit on performance of gluten-free in nonceliac athletes (Lis, Stellingwerff, Kitic, Ahuja, & Fell, 2015).

4.3.4 Antinutritive Factors

Wheat and wheat proteins contain very limited amounts of antinutritional factors in comparison to other protein sources as suggested by its relatively high digestibility (Bos et al., 2005; Gilani, Xiao, & Cockell, 2012).

Phytic acid has been reported to interfere with the proteolytic action of pepsin in a number of proteins, possibly through the formation of phytate−protein interaction complexes at low pH (Gilani et al., 2012). Wheat gluten has a modest phytic acid content of 1.9 g/100 g, but has the lowest binding affinity when compared to soy and sunflower globulins. This might be explained by the lower number of cationic groups, especially in gliadin fractions (Hidvegi & Lasztity, 2002). D-amino acids but almost no lysinoalanine isomers (0.9% vs more than 4% in animal-origin proteins) due to its low content in lysine (Gilani et al., 2012), can be found in wheat.

4.4 PROTEIN FUNCTIONALITY

4.4.1 Solubility

Gluten is not soluble in water and therefore its major application will be found in flour-based products (bread, cereal-based products, extruded products for human or animal nutrition). However, proteins obtained by enzymatic modification have good solubility in water. This property enables their use in protein-enriched beverages and also for use in formulating high-protein products like biscuits with little to no impact on dough structure.

4.4.2 Foaming

Hydrolyzed wheat protein ingredients exhibit good foaming properties, especially when a mild degree of hydrolysis is applied (Drago et al., 2000). Improved foaming properties can be obtained when enzymatic hydrolysis is followed by a fractionation process of the obtained peptides (Linares, Larre, Meste, & Popineau, 2000).

4.4.3 Emulsification

Hydrolyzed wheat proteins exhibit good functionality in emulsification and are able to partially replace caseinates in numerous applications to achieve a more cost-efficient formulation. In a similar way to foam-forming properties the most efficient peptides are obtained after controlled hydrolysis followed by fractionation (Linares et al., 2000).

4.4.4 Satiety

Besides their functional properties, wheat proteins can also be used for protein-enriched foods, targeting a higher satiety effect than regular foods, especially in the context of calorie-reduced diets. Wheat proteins, tested as pure fractions alone (Bowen, Noakes, & Clifton, 2006) or included within a food matrix such as cereal-based bread enriched in protein (gluten and hydrolyzed wheat proteins) (Gonzalez-Anton et al., 2015), can significantly reduce satiety feeling in comparison to no- or less-protein intake in healthy lean adults. This confirms previous observations in rats which showed a higher potency of wheat proteins to reduce appetite compared to that of carbohydrate (Faipoux et al., 2006), and its effects were equivalent to those of milk proteins (Bensaïd et al., 2002; Faipoux et al., 2006).

4.5 APPLICATIONS IN FOOD AND FEED

About 80% of wheat gluten production is used in human nutrition, while the remaining 20% is used in animal nutrition.

4.5.1 Gluten in Bread Application

Bread is the primary food application that benefits from the unique viscoelastic property of gluten and its ability to absorb water. Gluten enables improved yields, softness, and shelf-life, and favorably impacts the volume and crumb regularity of bread. Vital wheat gluten is used in the milling and baking industries to standardize the level of protein in flours throughout the year due to variability in wheat supplies. This standardization is critical for bread dough machinability and processing. A trend in plant breeding, toward a reduction in protein content in wheat, also leads to a high demand for gluten in order to maintain required protein levels in flours and finished products.

Native or supplemented gluten provides the unique viscous and elastic properties specific to bread dough. The reason for these properties is the combined presence of gliadins and glutenins (high-molecular-weight polymeric proteins). The gliadins provide the viscosity to the dough whereas the glutenins provide the elasticity. Quality (such as size distribution and disulfide bonds) and quantity of glutenins determine the performance of gluten protein in bread making (Veraverbeke and Delcour 2002).

Gluten is able to form an extensible continuous network that is gas tight. It is the only protein with this viscoelastic film-forming property. The structure retains the gas formed during fermentation and baking of the bread and is the key parameter for the volume of bread and cell structure. A modification of the gluten type and quality might considerably affect the overall bread volume and the cell size and distribution. In addition to the use of gluten, supplementation of bread dough with hydrolyzed wheat proteins (0.5–1%) will increase the extensibility of the dough. Composition in gluten fraction has a significant impact on the optimal bread dough kneading time. Gliadin tends to reduce the optimal mixing time, whereas glutenin tends to increase the mixing time (MacRitchie, 1987).

Supplementation with vital wheat gluten is also typically used to provide high-protein flours to the bread industry. With the development of breads enriched in fibers, brans, whole grains and seeds, and cereals which cause a weakening of the native gluten structure, the need for a stronger and high-quality gluten network increases the levels of supplementation. Vital wheat gluten represents a good alternative to high-protein flours for cost-efficiency and availability.

4.5.2 Animal Nutrition

Gluten is used for nutritional protein content, improvement of digestibility, and as a functional binder in fish feed (Apper, Feneuil, Wagner, & Respondek, 2013). Gluten enables the improvement of cohesiveness and water stability of fish feed pellets. Hydrolyzed wheat proteins are used predominantly as an optimal choice for feeding piglets and calves (Ortigues-Marty et al., 2003). Gluten is also used in batters for its binding properties in crumbed meat and fish products.

4.5.3 Breakfast Cereals and Pasta

Wheat gluten provides the major source of protein and gluten and soluble hydrolyzed protein can be used to reinforce this contribution to early-morning intakes. Direct expanded breakfast cereals, as well as cereal flakes, can be formulated with up to 30% wheat proteins. In pasta application, gluten can reduce the stickiness of pasta.

4.5.4 Protein-Enriched Foods

Hydrolyzed wheat gluten is used for the formulation of protein-enriched foods in various flour-based products (breakfast cereals, biscuits, sweet breads, etc.), dairy products (yogurts, milks, ice cream, etc.), sports beverages (high-protein recovery drinks, etc.), soups, diet meals or meal alternatives, and many other foods. The hydrolyzed proteins lose their viscoelastic structure and become soluble in water, which enables easy incorporation (even at high incorporation levels) in high-moisture foods and in dough, without modification of the overall matrix. Limitations are mainly linked to the level of off-taste potentially present in the hydrolyzed proteins and to powder solubility. Combinations of wheat gluten and hydrolyzed wheat gluten can also be used in breakfast cereals, cereal bars, and snacks in order to reach high levels of protein. In addition, the foaming and emulsification properties enable hydrolyzed wheat proteins to be utilized as alternatives to caseinates in numerous food matrixes, ranging from nondairy creamers to chewy candies.

4.5.5 Uses in Vegetable-Based Meat Alternatives

In an attempt to consume vegetable proteins directly by humans, quite a large variety of meat alternatives have been developed. Besides soy, which is used for traditional products such as tofu and tempeh, wheat is used for a meat alternative called seitan. Seitan originated from China and is said to have been developed by monks in order to find an alternative to duck meat. Therefore, it is also called monk duck (duck made by monks) or mock duck (fake duck). Seitan consists of proteins that are extracted from wheat flour and then cooked in a vegetable soup or fried in oil. The main hurdle to broaden consumption of seitan is primarily related to its slightly soft and gummy texture. The production process for seitan allows the incorporation of spices and other taste-intense compounds into the product and cooking of the product in a vegetable soup which renders the product quite tasty.

Next to seitan, wheat proteins can also be texturized at a high temperature, high shear, and low moisture environment in an extruder. The structure formation of extrudate is believed to result from a complete restructuring of the polymeric material in an oriented pattern. The formation of the final molecular network involves the dissociation and unraveling of the macromolecules, which allows them to recombine and to crosslink through specific linkages in the high-temperature section of the extruder. Upon exiting the extruder die, the water evaporates and creates a layered and somewhat spongy structure (Areas, 1992). The main drawback of such technology is that the unraveling and recombining of the proteins happen within one processing step and therefore the control of structure and shape is very difficult, if not impossible. The shape is defined by the cross-section of the die and can only be decreased during further processing steps. No agglomeration of pieces is possible as the proteins are yet crosslinked. The obtained texturized wheat proteins are mostly used as meat extenders or in combination with other heat-gelling proteins, such as egg white or soy isolates.

One possibility to avoid a spongy structure of the texturized proteins is to increase moisture content during the extrusion step above 60% moisture and to cool down the protein melt below 100°C before exiting the die. This

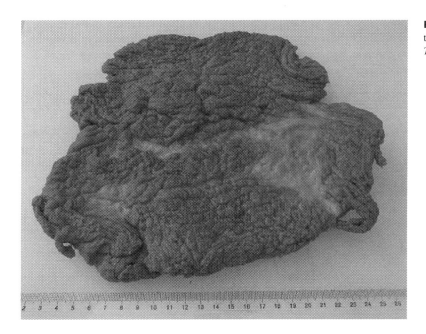

FIGURE 4.6 Vegetal meat pieces produce via low-temperature shear and static heating process. *From Tereos.*

so-called high-moisture extrusion process has been reviewed by Akdogan (1999). During the cooling of protein melt in the die a shear flow creates a fibrous or layered structure resulting in quite attractive meat analogs. The main difficulty of the process is to control the heat setting of the proteins and the flow pattern in the die.

Texturized wheat proteins are also produced by extrusion of wheat gluten (twin-screw extrusion process) and are typically used for crispy texture in cereal products, snacks, or fried food. These protein products absorb water for a meat-like texture, which is suitable for many food applications.

4.5.6 New Product and Technology for Wheat-Based Meat

A novel high-moisture shear process for soy protein in combination with wheat proteins has recently been developed by the research group of Atze Jan van de Goot (Grabowska, Tekidou, Boom, & van der Goot, 2014; Krintiras et al., 2016). In this process a mixture of protein isolate and gluten is subjected to shear in a couette cell during heating, which results in macroscopic orientation of protein fibrils that resemble meat fibers. Although the geometry of the pieces is larger than what can be obtained with an extrusion process, the size of the obtained pieces is determined by the shape of the shear cell and cannot be changed after.

Another recent process development aims to separate the unraveling of the native wheat protein and the formation of a protein network from the crosslinking step. The unraveling of the protein is done under shear conditions in low temperature, whereas the heat setting of the formed network is done without shear. In this way large meat-like pieces can also be formed (Fig. 4.6).

A precise control of shear parameters and heat-setting parameters enables control of the final texture without the difficulty of choosing between network creation and destruction as in a classical extrusion process.

4.6 CONCLUSION

Wheat is an important crop that can provide valuable protein and nutrition. From wheat, it is possible to produce different types of proteins with different functionalities, ranging from the unique viscoelastic behavior of gluten to the highly soluble hydrolyzed wheat proteins. They are used in numerous protein-enriched foods like cereal products but also as an alternative to dairy proteins in beverages and dairy products. The high content in glutamine is a key advantage for high-intensity training nutrition. Gluten and other wheat proteins are increasingly used in vegetal alternatives to meat, representing a sustainable and cost-effective option to fulfill the growing protein needs of the world populations.

REFERENCES

Ahmedna, M., Prinyawiwatkul, W., & Rao, R. M. (1999). Solubilized wheat protein isolate: functional properties and potential food applications. *Journal of Agricultural and Food Chemistry, 47*(4), 1340–1345.

Akdogan, H. (1999). High moisture food extrusion. *International Journal of Food Science and Technology, 34*, 195–207.

Aoki, K., Kohmura, Y., Suzuki, Y., Koikawa, N., Yoshimura, M., Aoba, Y., ... Sawaki, K. (2012). Post-training consumption of wheat gluten hydrolysate suppresses the delayed onset of muscle injury in soccer players. *Experimental and Therapeutic Medicine, 3*, 969–972.

Apper, E., Feneuil, A., Wagner, A., & Respondek, F. (2013). Use of vital wheat gluten in aquaculture feeds. *Aquatic Biosystems, 9*, 21.

Areas, J. A. G. (1992). Extrusion of food proteins. *Critical Reviews in Food Science and Nutrition, 32*(4), 365–392.

Bensaïd, A., Tomé, D., Gietzen, D., Even, P., Morens, C., Gausseres, N., & Fromentin, G. (2002). Protein is more potent than carbohydrate for reducing appetite in rats. *Physiology & Behavior, 75*(4), 577–582.

Biesiekierski, J. R., & Iven, J. (2015). Non-coeliac gluten sensitivity: Piecing the puzzle together. *United European Gastroenerololgy Journal, 3*(2), 160–165.

Bodwell, C. E., Satterlee, L. D., & Hackler, L. R. (1980). Protein digestibility of the same protein preparations by human and rat assays and by in vitro enzymic digestion methods. *American Journal of Clinical Nutrition, 33*(3), 677–686.

Bos, C., Juillet, B., Fouillet, H., Turlan, L., Dare, S., Luengo, C., ... Gaudichon, C. (2005). Postprandial metabolic utilization of wheat protein in humans. *American Journal of Clinical Nutrition, 81*(1), 87–94.

Bowen, J., Noakes, M., & Clifton, P. M. (2006). Appetite regulatory hormone responses to various dietary proteins differ by body mass index status despite similar reductions in ad libitum energy intake. *Journal of Clinical Endocrinology Metabolism, 91*(8), 2913–2919.

De Zorzi, M., Curioni, A., Simonato, B., Giannattasio, M., & Pasini, G. (2007). Effect of pasta drying temperature on gastrointestinal digestibility and allergenicity of durum wheat proteins. *Food Chemistry, 104*(1), 353–363.

Deglaire, A., & Moughan, P. J. (2012). Animal models for determining amino acid digestibility in humans – A review. *British Journal of Nutrition, 108*, 273–281.

Drago, S. R., & González, R. J. (2000). Foaming properties of enzymatically hydrolysed wheat gluten. *Innovative Food Science & Emerging Technologies, 1*(4), 269–273 , December

European Parliament. (2011). *Regulation (EU) No 1169/2011 of the European Parliament and of the Council of 25 October 2011 on the provision of food information to consumers.*

Faipoux, R., Tome, D., Bensaid, A., Morens, C., Oriol, E., Bonnano, L. M., & Fromentin, G. (2006). Yeast proteins enhance satiety in rats. *The Journal of Nutrition, 136*, 2350–2356.

FAO. (2013). *Nutrition quality of proteins.*

FDA. (2004). *Food Allergen Labeling and Consumer Protection Act of 2004.* 21 USC 301 note.

Gilani, G. S., Xiao, C. W., & Cockell, K. A. (2012). Impact of antinutritional factors in food proteins on the digestibility of protein and the bioavailability of amino acids and on protein quality. *British Journal of Nutrition, 108*, 315–332.

Gonzalez-Anton, C., Lopez-Millan, B., Rico, M. C., Sanchez-Rodriguez, E., Ruiz-Lopez, M. D., Gil, A., & Mesa, M. D. (2015). An enriched, cereal-based bread affects appetite ratings and glycemic, insulinemic, and gastrointestinal hormone responses in healthy adults in a randomized, controlled trial. *Journal of Nutrition, 145*(2), 231–238.

Grabowska, K. J., Tekidou, S., Boom, R. M., & van der Goot, A. J. (2014). Shear structuring as a new method to make anisotropic structures from soy–gluten blends. *Food Research International, 64*, 743–751.

Hidvegi, M., & Lasztity, R. (2002). Phytic acid content of cereals and legumes and interaction with proteins. *Periodica Polytechnica Ser. Chemical Engineering, 46*, 59–64.

Husby, S., & Murray, J. (2015). Non-celiac gluten hypersensitivity: What is all the fuss about? *F1000 Prime REPORTS, 7*, 54.

Juillet, B., Fouillet, H., Bos, C., Mariotti, F., Gausseres, N., Benamouzig, R., ... Gaudichon, C. (2008). Increasing habitual protein intake results in reduced postprandial efficiency of peripheral, anabolic wheat protein nitrogen use in humans. *American Journal of Clinical Nutrition, 87*(3), 666–678.

Koikawa, N., Nakamura, A., Ngaoka, I., Aoki, K., Sawaki, K., & Suzuki, Y. (2009). Delayed-onset muscle injury and its modification by wheat gluten hydrolysate. *Nutrition, 25*(5), 493–498.

Kong, X. Z., Zhou, H. M., & Qian, H. F. (2007). Enzymatic hydrolysis of wheat gluten by proteases and properties of the resulting hydrolysates. *Food Chemistry, 102*(3), 759–763.

Krintiras, G. A., Javier Gadea Diaz, J. G., van der Goot, A. J., Andrzej, I., Stankiewicz, A. J., & Stefanidis, G. D. (2016). On the use of the Couette Cell technology for large scale production of textured soy-based meat replacers. *Journal of Food Engineering, 169*, 205–213.

Linares, E., Larre, C. L. E., Meste, M., & Popineau, Y. (2000). Emulsifying and foaming properties of gluten hydrolysates with an increasing degree of hydrolysis: Role of soluble and insoluble fractions. *Cereal Chemistry*, 414–420.

Lis, D., Stellingwerff, T., Kitic, C. M., Ahuja, K. D., & Fell, J. (2015). No effects of a short-term gluten-free diet on performance in nonceliac athletes. *Medicine Science and Sports Exercise, 47*(12), 2563–2570.

MacRitchie, F. (1987). Evaluation of contributions from wheat-protein fractions to dough mixing and breadmaking. *Journal of Cereal Science, 6*(3), 259–268.

MacRitchie, F., & Lafiandra, D. (1997). Structure-function relationships of wheat proteins. In S. Damodaran, & A. Paraf (Eds.), *Food proteins and their applications* (pp. 293–323). New York: Marcel Dekker Inc.

Negro, M., Giardina, S., Marzani, B., & Marzatico, F. (2008). Branched-chain amino acid supplementation does not enhance athletic performance but affects muscle recovery and the immune system. *Journal of Sport Medicine Physical Fitness, 48*(3), 347–351.

Nwaru, B. I., Hickstein, L., Panesar, S. S., Roberts, G., Muraro, A., & Sheikh, A. (2014). Prevalence of common food allergies in Europe: A systematic review and meta-analysis. *Allergy, 69*(8), 992–1007.

Ortigues-Marty, I., Hocquette, J. F., Bertrand, G., Martineau, C., Vermorel, M., & Toullec, R. (2003). The incorporation of solubilized wheat proteins in milk replacers for veal calves: Effects on growth performance and muscle oxidative capacity. *Reproduction Nutrition Development, 43*, 57–76.

Petitot, M., Brossard, C., Barron, C., Larré, C., Morel, M. H., & Micard, V. (2009). Modification of pasta structure induced by high drying temperatures. Effects on the in vitro digestibility of protein and starch fractions and the potential allergenicity of protein hydrolysates. *Food Chemistry, 116*(2), 401–412.

Sapone, A., Bai, J. C., Ciacci, C., Dolinsek, J., Green, P. H. R., Hadjivassiliou, M., . . . Fasano, A. (2012). Spectrum of gluten-related disorders: Consensus on new nomenclature and classification. *BMC Medicine, 10*, 13.

Sawaki, K., Takaoka, I., Sakuraba, K., & Suzuki, Y. (2004). Effects of distance running and subsequent intake of glutamine rich peptide on biomedical parameters of male Japanese athletes. *Nutrition Research, 24*, 59–71.

Smith, F., Pan, X., Bellido, V., Toole, G. A., Gates, F. K., Wickham, M. S., . . . Mills, E. C. (2015). The digestibility of gluten proteins is reduced by baking and enhanced by starch digestion. *Molecular Nutrition and Food Research, 59*(10), 2034–2043.

Tilman, D., Kenneth, G., Cassman, K. G., Matson, P. A., Naylor, R., & Polasky, S. (2002). Agricultural sustainability and intensive production practices. *Nature, 418*, 671–677.

Veraverbeke, W. S., & Delcour, J. A. (2002). Wheat protein composition and properties of wheat glutenin in relation to breadmaking functionality. *Critical Reviews in Food Science and Nutrition, 42*(3), 179–208.

Verhoeckx, K. C., Vissers, Y. M., Baumert, J. L., Faludi, R., Feys, M., Flanagan, S., . . . Kimber, I. (2015). Food processing and allergenicity. *Food Chemistry and Toxicology, 80*, 223–240.

Vercalsteren, A., & Boonen, K. (2015). *Life Cycle Assessment study of starch products for the European starch industry association (Starch Europe): sector study* <http://www.starch.eu/wp-content/uploads/2015/05/LCA-study-summary-report-2015-update.pdf>.

Ziegler, T. R., Evans, M. E., Fernandez-Estivariz, C., & Jones, D. P. (2003). Trophic and cytoprotective nutrition for intestinal adaptation, mucosal repair and barrier function. *Annual Review of Nutrition, 23*, 229–261.

Chapter 5

Proteins From Sorghum and Millets

J.R.N. Taylor and J. Taylor
University of Pretoria, Hatfield, South Africa

5.1 INTRODUCTION

Sorghum (*Sorghum bicolor* (L.) Moench) and the millets are C4 (tropical) cereals (Fig. 5.1). Contrary to some literature, millet is not a single species but the collective name for several small-grain cereal species (Table 5.1). In descending order, quantitatively the most important millet species are pearl millet (*Pennisetum glaucum* (L.) R. Br.), foxtail millet (*Setaria italica* (L.) P. Beauv.), proso millet (*Panicum miliaceum* L.), and finger millet (*Eleusine coracana* (L.) Gaertn.). Teff (*Eragrostis tef* (Zuccagni) Trotter) and fonio (*Digitaria exilis* (Kippist) Stapf and *D. iburua* Stapf), which are also millets, are locally important staple food grains in Ethiopia and Eritrea, and the Sahel (Sahara desert margin) region of West Africa, respectively. Minor millets include little millet (*Panicum sumatrense* Roth), barnyard millet (*Echinochloa crus-galli* (L.) P. Beav.), and kodo millet (*Paspalum scrobiculatum* L.).

Sorghum and the millets are generally cultivated in the same geographical areas and have similar agronomic characteristics and hence they are often considered together. They are staple foods of smallholder farmer communities in Africa, India, and China and in some parts of central America. They are also widely cultivated in Africa for beverage production, for traditional beers and nonalcoholic fermented beverages, and today in the case of sorghum to produce commercial lager-type beers and nonalcoholic malt beverages. In China, sorghum is used to produce distilled spirit and vinegar. Sorghum is extensively cultivated as an animal feed grain in the US, Mexico, South America, and Australia. There is also considerable production of pearl millet and other millets as poultry, companion bird, and game bird feed grain in Brazil, the US, and elsewhere. Sorghum is used as a feedstock for grain bioethanol production in the US and production is commencing in other countries. An emerging use in Western countries for sorghum, proso millet and teff is for gluten-free baking flour and in the case of sorghum for gluten-free beer.

This chapter, which deals with sorghum and the major millet species in respect of their potential as sustainable protein sources, firstly considers sorghum and millet cultivation and their land, water, and energy use. It then examines their protein nutritive quality, the types, composition, and structure of their proteins, how they are isolated, and how protein products could be produced. Then, potential novel applications for the sorghum prolamin protein (kafirin) are examined. Following this, the effects of food and beverage-processing operations on their protein quality are considered. Lastly, current research into improving the nutritional quality of sorghum and millet proteins is explored. The concluding remarks identify challenges that need to be addressed to enable sorghum and millets to be major sustainable protein sources.

5.2 SORGHUM AND MILLET PRODUCTION: LAND, WATER, AND ENERGY USE

5.2.1 Production

Sorghum and the millets (collectively) are quantitatively the fifth and sixth most important cereal grains in terms of production after maize, wheat, rice, and barley (FAOSTAT3, 2013). They are generally cultivated in semiarid tropical and subtropical regions and are characterized by their water efficiency and tolerance to drought and poor soils. In several high-income and middle-income countries, sorghum and pearl millet are cultivated using mechanized, intensive agriculture where hybrid-type cultivars with high yield potential using inorganic fertilizer application are normally grown (ICRISAT/FAO, 1996). Traditional smallholder farming systems for sorghum and millets use open pollinated varieties (OPVs), which enable the farmer to keep the seed for replanting. However, even in traditional farming systems

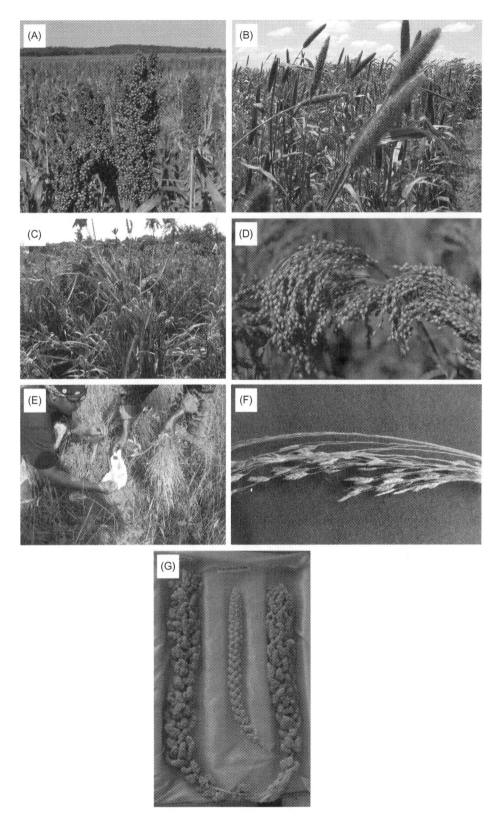

FIGURE 5.1 Sorghum and millet plants: (A) red (dark gray in print versions) sorghum in South Africa; (B) pearl millet in Kenya; (C) finger millet in Kenya; (D) proso millet; (E) white fonio in Nigeria; (F) teff—Ethiopia; (G) foxtail millet—China (center—traditional variety, right—hybrid). *For (D) Courtesy of Forestry Images—Dr. H.F. Schwartz, Colorado State University. (E) Courtesy of the late Dr. M.O. Edema, Federal University of Technology, Nigeria.*

TABLE 5.1 Sorghum and the Major Millet Species—Production, Grain Weight and Protein Content

Preferred English Name and Botanical Name[a]	Other English and Vernacular Names[a]	Major Producing Regions/Countries[b,c,d]	Approximate World Production (Million Tonnes)[b,c,e]	1000 Grain Weight (g)[f]	Protein Content (g/100 g db)[f]
Sorghum *Sorghum bicolor* (L.) Moench	Milo, jowar, durra, mabela, mtama	US, Northern Africa (Nigeria, Sudan, Ethiopia, Niger, Burkina Faso), Mexico, Argentina, China, Australia, Brazil	58	25–35	11.0 (7.3–15.6)
Pearl millet *Pennisetum glaucum* (L.) R. Br.	Bulrush millet, cattail millet, babala, bajra/bajira	West and Central Africa (Sahel regions of Niger, Mali, Burkina Faso, Nigeria), India, East and Southern Africa (Namibia, Botswana), US, Brazil	>24	8	14.5 (8.6–19.4)
Foxtail millet *Setaria italica* (L.) P. Beauv.	Italian millet, foxtail bristle grass, German millet, Hungarian millet	Eurasia, Southern Europe, tropical and subtropical Asia (China, India, Korea), US, Australia	10	5	11.7 (6.0–14.0)
Proso millet *Panicum miliaceum* L.	Common millet, broom millet, hog millet, panic millet	Eurasia (China, Kazakhstan, Afghanistan, India, Turkey, Romania), US, Australia	9	5	13.4 (6.4–15.9)
Finger millet *Eleusine coracana* (L.) Gaertn.	Ragi, wimbi	Eastern and Southern Africa (Uganda, Kenya, Zimbabwe) and Asia—Near East to Far East (India, Nepal, China)	7	2.5	8.0 (6.9–10.9)
Teff *Eragrostis tef* (Zuccagni) Trotter	Tef, teff grass, Abyssinian lovegrass	Ethiopia, Eritrea, South Africa, US, Australia	>4	0.3–0.4	10.9 (7.9–12.6)
White fonio *Digitaria exilis* (Kippist) Stapf	Fonio, acha, fonio millet, hungry rice	West Africa—mountainous regions (Guinea, Nigeria) (both fonio species)	0.1 (both species)	0.5 (both species)	8.7 (5.1–10.4) (both species)
Black fonio *Digitaria iburua* Stapf	Black acha, hungry rice				

[a]*Germplasm Resources Information Network (n.d.).*
[b]*FAOSTAT3 (2013).*
[c]*ICRISAT (n.d.).*
[d]*Obilana and Manyasa (2002).*
[e]*Demeke and Di Marcantonio (2013).*
[f]*Serna-Saldivar and Rooney (1995).*

improved varieties with better yield potential and disease resistance are rapidly replacing the local landraces. There are no genetically modified sorghum or millets under commercial cultivation.

Sorghum is cultivated worldwide (Table 5.1), generally in the same agro-ecological zones as maize. However, it requires less water and is more drought-tolerant. It can be grown with a seasonal rainfall as low as 400 mm and uses only 310 parts of water to produce 1 part compared to maize which uses 400 parts (Du Plessis, n.d.). Also, it can be cultivated in low-fertility shallow, heavy clay and alkaline soils (Du Plessis, n.d.; USDA, n.d.).

Pearl millet is cultivated for grain in hot, arid areas such as the Sahel region. It is very water-efficient and can be grown in areas with an annual rainfall as low as 250–400 mm (National Research Council, 1996; USDA, n.d.) or less.

although it cannot withstand drought as well as sorghum. It is mainly grown on well-drained sandy soil or light loam soils and can survive low pH and fertility (USDA, n.d.).

Foxtail millet is widely grown in marginal soil areas of temperate, subtropical, and tropical Asia and in southern Europe (ICRISAT, n.d.). It has only two-thirds the water requirement of maize and high tolerance to differing soil fertility. Proso millet is widely grown in Eastern Europe and Asia. It is a short season crop (60–90 days) and hence is grown further north than other millets and can be grown at higher altitudes (up to 3500 m in India) (ICRISAT, n.d.). It is heat- and drought-tolerant and has among the lowest water requirements of any cereal (ICRISAT, n.d.; USDA, n.d.).

Finger millet is primarily cultivated in India and East Africa. It requires slightly more water than other millets (annual rainfall 500–1000 mm) (Obilana & Manyasa, 2002) and can be grown at elevations up to 2000 m. Teff, which is closely related to finger millet, is cultivated primarily in Ethiopia, its center of origin (National Research Council, 1996). It is grown at high altitude (1700–2800 m), with widely varying rainfall (300–2500 mm) (Obilana & Manyasa, 2002). Fonio, of which there are two species (white and black) (Table 5.1), is cultivated almost exclusively in the highland regions of West Africa, primarily as a subsistence crop (Obilana & Manyasa, 2002). It is usually grown on poor sandy or ironstone soils, which are unsuitable for other cereals (National Research Council, 1996), under a very wide range of rainfall conditions (Obilana & Manyasa, 2002).

5.2.2 Land-Use Efficiency

With regard to land-use efficiency in terms of yield, maize yields are substantially higher than those for sorghum and the millets (Table 5.2). Concerning sorghum, yields for mechanized intensive agriculture, as practiced in, for example, Argentina, the US, and Australia, and for mainly nonmechanized intensive agriculture, as practiced in China, are substantially higher (>3 tonnes/ha) than in countries where agriculture is mainly nonmechanized and not as intensive such as India and in sub-Saharan African countries (≤2 tonnes/ha). However, with regard to millet yields (data primarily for pearl-, foxtail-, proso-, and finger millets), all with the exception of China are low (1–2 tonnes/ha) (FAOSTAT3, 2013). Fonio yields are very low, approximately 0.6 tonnes/ha. With teff, although yields in Ethiopia are still low (2011—1.26 tonnes/ha) they have increased dramatically, 33% in 6 years, driven by improved varieties in response to rapidly rising demand (Demeke & Di Marcantonio, 2013). An important factor which militates against dramatically increasing millet yields is the small size of the millet grains (Table 5.1 and Fig. 5.1). Hybrids and improved OPVs generally are of much larger grain size than traditional landraces, as is evident in the example of foxtail millet (Fig. 5.1(G)).

5.2.3 Water Efficiency

With regard to the effects of water availability on yield of sorghum and millets versus maize, in a semiarid tropical environment (Queensland, Australia) under fully irrigated high-fertility conditions using F1 hybrids, average yields for maize, sorghum, and pearl millet were 9.2, 5.6, and 2.9 tonnes/ha, respectively (Muchow, 1989a). However, under water-deficit conditions maize outyielded sorghum when the maize yield was ≥6 tonnes/ha, but sorghum yielded more than maize or pearl millet under water-deficit conditions that resulted in a maize yield of 1–2 tonnes/ha (Muchow, 1989b). Only when water deficit was so severe that maize did not produce a crop, did pearl millet yield the same as sorghum. However, importantly, although the pearl millet grain yield was low, it was stable under all water regimens. Unfortunately, such comparative data for other millet species are not available.

TABLE 5.2 Comparative Yields for Maize, Sorghum, Millet (Primarily Pearl-, Foxtail-, Proso-, and Finger Millets), and Fonio in Various Countries (Tonnes/ha)

Cereal	Country							
	Argentina	US	Australia	China	India	Ethiopia	Nigeria	Senegal
Maize	6.6	10.0	6.4	6.0	2.5	3.2	2.0	1.5
Sorghum	4.1	3.7	3.7	4.9	0.9	2.0	1.2	0.7
Millet	1.8	1.6	No data	2.4	1.2	1.9	1.3	0.8
Fonio	Not grown	Not grown	Not grown	Not grown	Not grown	Not grown	0.5	0.7

Source: Data from FAOSTAT3 (2013). Production, crops. Available at <http://faostat3.fao.org>. Accessed July 2015.

A more recent maize versus sorghum comparative yield study in a Mediterranean environment (north-eastern Spain), similarly revealed that although maize outyielded sorghum under well-irrigated conditions, sorghum outyielded maize under moderate and severe water deficit (Farré & Faci, 2006). The ability of sorghum to yield well under water-deficit conditions is attributed to its greater ability to extract water from deeper water layers due to its very extensive root system (National Research Council, 1996; USDA, n.d.) and better water use efficiency due to its leaf architecture (Blum, 2009).

5.2.4 Cultivation With Legumes

An important aspect of sustainable production of sorghum and millet is cultivation with legumes by rotation, green manuring, and intercropping. Data from ICRISAT (the International Crops Research Institute for the Semi-Arid Tropics), the international institute responsible for sorghum and pearl millet and peanut, chickpea, and pigeon pea agricultural research, shows that the residual effect of preceding grain legume (pulse) cultivation on sorghum yield is equivalent to some 68 kg N equiv./ha and for pearl millet 30–60 kg N equiv./ha (Wani, Rupela, & Lee, 1995). In an 8-year experiment in the semiarid tropics of Mali, crop rotation with cowpea increased sorghum and pearl millet yields (2 years sorghum followed by 6 years pearl millet) by 18% and 23% on loamy sand and loam soils, respectively, and green manuring with cowpea increased yields by 37% and 27% on these soils, respectively (Kouyaté, Franzluebbers, Jou, & Hossner, 2000).

With regard to sorghum intercropping with legumes, the effects on yield appear to be more complex. A two-season experiment in a semiarid region of Kenya evaluated several sorghum–cowpea intercropping parameters, but found no effect on harvest indices (Karanja, Kibe, Karogo, & Mwangi, 2014). Clearer results were obtained in a 3-year experiment in the Ethiopian highlands, which revealed that intercropping with the forage legume lablab yielded 27% more fodder compared to sole cereal cropping but slightly depressed grain yield (Mpairwe, Sabiiti, Ummuna, Tegegne, & Osuji, 2002). However, with manure fertilizer addition there was an average grain yield gain of 55.6% for sorghum intercropped with lablab compared to sorghum alone, and fodder yield was increased by 41.4%.

5.2.5 Sustainable Agriculture

Notwithstanding the differences in yield between mechanized intensive agriculture and more traditional agriculture, there is good on-farm evidence that sustainable-type agricultural systems for sorghum are more energy-efficient. Franzluebbers and Francis (1995) studied energy ouput:input ratios for a range of agricultural practices used in maize and sorghum cultivation in eastern Nebraska, US. They found that while full irrigation gave some 240% higher grain yield than dryland agriculture without herbicide and 190% higher for dryland agriculture with herbicide (not taking into account nitrogen (N) fertilizer use), the energy output:input ratio for dryland agriculture with broadcast herbicide use was 11.6:1, but only 4.1:1 for full irrigation with herbicide use. Furthermore, data from 45 studies across sub-Saharan Africa revealed that sustainable agriculture could increase sorghum/millet (presumably pearl millet and finger millet) yields by 30–100%, depending on rainfall and manure/fertilizer use (Pretty, 1995).

5.2.6 Cost of Grains

Regarding the relative cost of sorghum and millets, in international commodity trade and large-scale national trade the price of sorghum is always very similar to that of yellow maize, due to their similar feed value. A recent (2015) visit to Senegal revealed that the prices of maize, sorghum, and pearl millet in a street market were also very similar. Recent interactions through cereal projects in Ethiopia and Kenya, however, revealed that the prices of teff and finger millet were substantially higher than maize. This is due to the fact that they highly sought-after for making local staple food products, *injera* (flatbread) and *uji* (fermented gruel), respectively. Conversations with in-country experts and personal observations indicate that foxtail millet is priced as a commodity, whereas proso millet and fonio are higher-price speciality grains.

5.3 PROTEIN NUTRITIVE QUALITY

The protein content of sorghum and millet grains is typical of cereal grains in general, in the approximate range of 8–15% (dry basis) (Table 5.1). Pearl millet has among the highest protein contents of cereal grains, approximately 14.5%. This is because the pearl millet kernel has a proportionally very large protein-rich germ and consequently a relatively smaller endosperm (Serna-Saldivar & Rooney, 1995). Finger millet, in contrast, has a small germ, which is related to its relatively low-protein content (approximately 8.0%).

5.3.1 Protein Quality

With regard to protein quality, as with virtually all cereals, sorghum, and millets are all deficient in lysine when considered in terms of the indispensible (essential) amino acid requirements of growing children (Table 5.3). However, as a result of the revision of the amino acid requirements by the Joint WHO/FAO/UNU Expert Consultation (2007), it does not seem that they are deficient in other indispensible amino acids such as threonine and tryptophan. The great differences in reported values for the sulfur-containing amino acids (cystine and methionine) can be attributed to some laboratories not performing a performic acid oxidation step, without which there can be considerable destruction of these amino acids (Joint FAO/WHO Expert Consultation, 1991).

The lysine content of sorghum and millets varies considerably between the species, with finger millet, pearl millet, and teff protein having the highest protein lysine content (31–37 mg/kg), giving an amino acid score of 60–70% of the requirements of 1–2-year-olds (Table 5.3). Their high-protein lysine content is probably related to relatively higher proportions of the lysine-rich albumin and globulin or glutelin protein fractions in the grain (see Section 5.4). In contrast, the protein of sorghum, foxtail millet, and proso millet has the lowest lysine content (21–23 mg/kg protein), with an amino acid score of only approximately 40%. Their low protein lysine content is probably related to relatively higher levels of the lysine-poor prolamin protein fraction (Section 5.4.1). These lower lysine levels are similar to those in, for example, wheat (soft red winter) with a lysine content of approximately 23 mg/kg protein (USDA National Nutrient Database, 2014).

The protein of sorghum, pearl millet foxtail millet, proso millet, and finger millet is notably high in leucine (approximately 120–140 mg/kg protein) (Table 5.2). This compares to, for example, wheat (soft red winter) with 73 mg/kg protein (USDA National Nutrient Database, 2014). The high leucine content is due to its high content in their particular prolamin proteins, approximately 14.7 g/100 g in the case of the sorghum kafirins (Taylor & Schüssler, 1986). A possible concern with regard to the high level of leucine in cereals such as sorghum is that it may be involved in the etiology of pellagra through impairing the niacin-sparing effect of tryptophan (Klopfenstein & Hoseney, 1995). However, this is not proven.

5.3.2 Antinutrients

Some varieties of sorghum, properly referred to as tannin sorghums (GIPSA, 2013) (sometimes called brown, bitter, or bird-resistant types), and some varieties of finger millet (Siwela, Taylor, De Milliano, & Duodu, 2007) contain condensed tannins, proanthocyanidin or procyanidin oligomers, and polymers of flavonoid-type polyphenols. Tannin varieties of sorghum and finger millet are cultivated because the tannins protect the seeds from abiotic stresses (birds, insects, and mold) and hence reduce pre- and postharvest losses. It should be noted that in all probability there are no tannins in the other species of millet (Taylor & Duodu, 2015).

Many trials involving feeding tannin sorghum to chicks, rats, and various livestock animals have shown reduced digestibilities, growth rates, feed efficiencies, metabolizable energy, and amino acid bioavailability (Klopfenstein & Hoseney, 1995). For example, in two separate trials Cousins, Tanksley, Knabe, and Zebrowska (1981) fed noncannulated and cannulated pigs diets based on "low"-tannin (tannin-free) and high-tannin sorghums. With the noncannulated animals, dry matter, gross energy, and nitrogen digestibilities were significantly higher ($p < 0.01$) with the tannin-free sorghum diet. With the cannulated animals these parameters and the digestibility of all amino acids (with the exception of methionine) were significantly higher ($p < 0.01$) with the tannin-free sorghum diet. The major antinutritional effects of the tannins in tannin sorghum (and presumably in tannin finger millet) is through binding dietary proteins and hence reducing their digestibility (Bach Knudsen, Kirleis, Eggum, & Munck, 1988; Bach Knudsen, Munck, & Eggum, 1988) and probably also through their binding and inhibiting digestive enzymes such as the amylases (Daiber, 1975).

It is important not to overemphasize the antinutritional effects of tannins in sorghum and finger millet. Communities across sub-Saharan Africa have been consuming tannin sorghum and finger millet as staples for countless generations without any obvious adverse effects. It should also be noted that the great majority of varieties of sorghum and finger millet do not contain tannins and that in some major sorghum-growing countries, such as the US and Australia, tannin sorghums are not even cultivated. The presence of tannins in consignments of sorghum and finger millet can easily be detected by a simple bleach test which renders the tannin sorghum and finger millet kernels black in color (ICC, 2012).

TABLE 5.3 Indispensible Amino Acid Composition (mg/g Protein) of the Proteins of Sorghum and Millets Compared to the FAO/WHO/UNU Scoring Pattern for 1–2-year-Olds

Amino Acid	Sorghum[a]	Pearl Millet[b]	Foxtail Millet[b]	Proso Millet[b]	Finger Millet[b]	Teff[b]	Fonio[c]	FAO/WHO/UNU Pattern[d]
Histidine	24	22	23	22	26	26	22	18
Isoleucine	40	44	50	45	51	42	40	31
Leucine	140	122	133	129	135	79	99	63
Lysine	22 (42)[e]	33 (63)	21 (40)	22 (42)	37 (71)	31 (60)	24 (46)	52
	22[b]	30[f]	19[g]	17[g]	31[g]	37[h]	25[i]	
		58[f]	37[g]	33[g]	60	71[h]	48[i]	
Sulfur amino acids[j]	28	22	26	20	26	37	77	26
		37[c]		51[d]				
Aromatic amino acids[k]	82	52	53	52	62	51	50	46
Threonine	33	39	39	34	51	38	40	27
Tryptophan	11	16	15	9	13	14	35	7.4
Valine	53	57	52	51	57	54	58	42

[a]USDA National Nutrient Database (2014).
[b]Serna-Saldivar and Rooney (1995).
[c]Anuonye, Onuh, Egwim, and Adeyemo (2010).
[d]Joint WHO/FAO/UNU Expert Consultation (2007).
[e]Values in parentheses are the Amino Acid Score.
[f]Ejeta et al. (1987).
[g]Ravindran (1992).
[h]Lester and Bekele (1981).
[i]National Research Council (1996).
[j]Cystine + methionine.
[k]Phenylalanine + tyrosine.

The grains of sorghum (Kumari, Chandrashekar, & Shetty, 1992; Oukasha & El-latif, 2014) and millets (Chandrasekher, Raju, & Pattabiraman, 1982; Joshi, Sainani, Bastawade, Gupta, & Ranjekar, 1998; Ravindran, 1992) contain inhibitors of various protease enzymes. Some at least of these protease inhibitors are proteins (ie, true protease inhibitors) and seem to act as a defense against molds and insects. However, it appears doubtful whether they are major antinutrients as they are heat-labile and likely to be inactivated when the grains are thermally processed into foods.

5.3.3 Protein Toxicity

Sorghum and the millets are members of the Chloridoideae (finger millet and teff) and Panicoideae (sorghum and other millets) subfamilies of grasses and as such are only distantly related to wheat, barley, rye, and triticale, which are members of the Pooideae subfamily (Morrison & Wrigley, 2004). As a consequence, their prolamin storage proteins differ substantially from those of wheat and it relatives (Shewry, 2002; Shewry & Tatham, 1990). Hence, it has long been considered that sorghum and millets are safe foods for persons suffering from celiac disease and allergies to wheat-type proteins. With sorghum there is good evidence to support this. It has been shown that protein extracts from sorghum did not elicit any morphometric or immune-mediated changes of duodenal explants from celiac patients (Ciaccia et al., 2007). Furthermore, celiac patients did not experience any gastrointestinal or nongastrointestinal symptoms, nor was their level of antitransglutaminase antibodies affected when celiac patients were challenged with sorghum food products over 5 days. Similarly, Bergamo et al. (2011) found that alcohol-soluble protein fractions from teff and millet (species not stated) did not show any immune cross-reactivity with gliadin epitopes associated with triggering celiac disease, nor did they induce any early symptoms of celiac enteropathy in a mouse model.

There has been considerable interest in the use of kafirin and zein, the very similar prolamin protein of maize, as implantable biomaterials on account of their hydrophobicity, slow degradation, and the evidence of their nontoxicity when consumed by celiacs (Taylor, Anyango, & Taylor, 2013). However, recent work has indicated that when kafirin is implanted subcutaneously it can cause a chronic inflammatory response (Taylor et al., 2015).

5.3.4 Other Nutrients, Phytochemicals, and Nutritional Quality Issues

The protein nutritive quality of sorghum and the millets cannot be seen in isolation from the contribution that these grains can make to dietary requirements for other nutrients and health-promoting phytochemicals. The major nutrient in sorghum and millets, as with all other cereals, is starch, which is essentially only present in the kernel starchy endosperm. The starch content of sorghum and millets is typically in the range of 55–72% (dry basis) (Serna-Saldivar & Rooney, 1995). Importantly from the standpoint of providing sustainable energy and preventing hyperglycemia, it appears that the starch in wet-cooked sorghum foods is more slowly digested than in similar foods from other cereals (Taylor & Emmambux, 2010). This is believed to be on account of the endosperm protein matrix limiting starch granule expansion and availability to enzymic hydrolysis, and sorghum tannins (if present) inhibiting hydrolysis (see Section 5.3.2). There is also exciting recent evidence that traditional African foods prepared from sorghum and pearl millet show far slower gastric emptying than similar foods prepared from wheat, rice, and potatoes (Cisse, Erickson, Opekun, Nichols, & Hamaker, 2015).

The lipid content of sorghum and millets is typically in the range 1.5–5% (dry basis), with pearl millet probably having the highest lipid content and finger millet the lowest (Taylor & Kruger, 2016). The lipids are concentrated in the germ and are high in linoleic and oleic acids (Serna-Saldivar & Rooney, 1995). The germ oil is rich in tocopherols.

Whole-grain sorghum and millets are a good source of the B vitamins, thiamine, riboflavin, and niacin (National Research Council, 1996). These are concentrated in the aleurone layer and germ and in the case of niacin may be poorly available due to complexation with nonstarch polysaccharides (Serna-Saldivar & Rooney, 1995). The levels of provitamin A are very low in sorghum and millets, even in yellow endosperm types (Taylor, Belton, Beta, & Duodu, 2014). Vitamin C is absent from sorghum and millets.

With regard to essential minerals, these are also concentrated in the aleurone layer and germ of sorghum and millet grains and quantitatively may appear to be substantial. However, the iron and zinc contents in sorghum and millets are inadequate for people consuming an essentially plant-based diet (Taylor et al., 2014; Taylor & Kruger, 2016). This problem is exacerbated by the presence of antinutrients, in particular phytate (myoinositol hexaphosphate) which is present in these and all other grains. Phytate binds divalent minerals and greatly reduces their bioavailability. The level of calcium is also generally low in sorghum and millets. The exception is finger millet, which is much richer, at approximately 340 mg/100 g (Taylor & Kruger, 2016).

Sorghum and millet grains generally contain substantially higher levels of flavonoid-type polyphenols than other cereals and, as mentioned above, some sorghum and finger millet varieties contain substantial levels of condensed tannins. This is probably due to the fact that these grains have been less subject to intensive breeding to remove these strongly flavored and colored compounds. Much research, which has mainly been through in vitro and cell-line assay, has shown that the polyphenols from sorghum and millets have a wide range of important potentially health-promoting effects, which can be categorized into three broad areas: antidiabetic, antiinflammatory and cardiovascular disease prevention, and anticancer (Taylor et al., 2014; Taylor & Duodu, 2015). However, direct proof of these health-enhancing effects when these grains are actually consumed as foods and beverages is still lacking.

5.4 PROTEIN TYPES, COMPOSITION, AND STRUCTURE

A summary of what is known about the proteins of sorghum and millets and their properties is given in Table 5.4. The major storage proteins of these grains are the endosperm-specific prolamins, named kafirin in the case of sorghum and pennisetin in the case of pearl millet. The prolamins are rich in the proline and glutamine (hence their name) and the hydrophobic amino acids leucine, alanine, and cysteine. They are notably low in lysine, accounting for the low amino acid score of cereal proteins. The other protein fractions in sorghum and millets (and other cereal grains) are the albumins and globulins, which are concentrated in the germ, and the glutelins, of which the glutelin storage-type proteins are concentrated in endosperm. The former, in particular, are much richer in charged amino acids, such as glutamic acid and aspartic acid, and notably richer in lysine (Taylor & Schüssler, 1986).

5.4.1 Prolamin Proteins

Sorghum kafirin, which has been studied in much more detail than the millet prolamins, is composed of a number of subclasses, α-, β-,γ- (Shull, Watterson, & Kirleis, 1991) and δ- (Belton, Delgadillo, Halford, & Shewry, 2006). They are all small polypeptides (<28 kDa) that can polymerize through disulfide crosslinking, due to the high cysteine content of the β- and γ-subclasses. The kafirins are considered the most hydrophobic of the cereal prolamin proteins. However, they do have some hydrophilic characteristics (Belton et al., 2006). They are insoluble in water but soluble in aqueous ethanol. The exception is γ-kafirin, which is water-soluble in its monomeric form (Evans, Schüssler, & Taylor, 1987). γ-Kafirin is the only kafirin to contain a repeated amino acid sequence, a hexapeptide repeat of Pro-Pro-Pro-Val-His-Leu (Belton et al., 2006). The secondary structure of kafirin is predominately α-helical. There are no structural models for kafirin or any of its subclasses, but it is thought to be similar to those proposed for α-zein. The well-described "Argos" model for α-zein is based on a group of nine antiparallel α-helices arranged in a cylinder or hairpin shape (Argos, Pedersen, Marks, & Larkins, 1982). The polar amino acids are on the surface of the cylinder and are available to form intra- and intermolecular hydrogen bonds in the same plane, whereas the hydrophobic amino acids are hidden within the helices. The glutamine-rich turns at the ends of the cylinder of helices allow bonding between molecules in different planes. The Argos model was modified by Garratt, Oliva, Caracelli, Leite, and Arruda (1993) and extended to include all α-prolamins. A number of other models have since been proposed based on extended helical hairpin, rod, or ribbon-like structures, with clearly defined hydrophilic and hydrophobic domains (Bugs et al., 2004; Forato, Bicudo, & Colnago, 2003; Matsushima, Danno, Takezawa, & Izumi, 1997; Momany et al., 2006).

The proteins of the millet species have been studied far less than sorghum but it is evident that the major millet storage proteins are generally also prolamins (Shewry, 2002), and have similar amino acid compositions (Table 5.4). The exception is fonio, where the majority of the grain proteins appear to be glutelins (Carcea & Salvatorelli, 1999), which are richer in lysine. The millet prolamins have somewhat different solubility properties to kafirin, which is possibly a consequence of differences in polymerization or hydrophobicity. There is little information on the secondary structure of the millet prolamins, but they are considered to be similar to α-zein in structure (Bugs et al., 2004).

5.4.2 Protein Isolation and Functionality

The isolation of the various Osborne protein fractions from sorghum was investigated in detail by Taylor, Schüssler, and Van der Walt (1984) and has been extensively reviewed by Mesa-Stonestreet, Jhoe, Alavi, and Bean (2010), including the functions which the different reagents fulfill in the extraction processes. Since prolamins are the major protein group in sorghum and most millets and their relative hydrophobicity and crosslinking by disulfide bonding pose special challenges and also because extraction method affects the quality, type, and consequent functionality of the prolamins extracted (Schober, Bean, Tilley, Smith, & Ioerger, 2011), methods for prolamin extraction will be briefly reviewed.

TABLE 5.4 Composition and Structures of Sorghum and Millet Grain Proteins

Species	Osborne Protein Fraction	% of Total Protein	Polymerization	Subunit Molecular Weight (kDa)	Major Amino Acid Composition	Structural Model and Secondary Structure	Hydrophobicity	References
Sorghum	Albumins and globulins	18.3			Glutamine/glutamate, arginine, asparagine/aspartic acid, leucine, lysine			Taylor and Schüssler (1986)
	Prolamins (kafirin)	44.0			Glutamine/glutamate, leucine, alanine, proline			
	α-Kafirin (80% of total kafirin)		Polymerize through disulfide bonding with other β- and γ-kafirin	23–25	Glutamine/glutamate, leucine, alanine, proline, cysteine	Total kafirin (containing all prolamin subunits) similar secondary structure contents to α-zein, 40–60% α-helix (Belton et al., 2006)	More hydrophobic than gluten and zein, has some hydrophilic properties but is less hydrophilic than zein or gluten (Belton et al., 2006)	Belton et al. (2006), Shull et al. (1991), Watterson, Shull, and Kirleis (1993)
	β-Kafirin (7–8% of total kafirin)		Polymerize through disulfide bonding	16–20	Proline, glutamine/glutamate, alanine, leucine, methionine, cysteine	No structural models for kafirin or any of its subclasses but thought to be similar to zein		
	γ-Kafirin (9–12% of total kafirin)		Polymerize through disulfide bonding	28	Proline, glutamine/glutamate, histidine, cysteine	Only γ-kafirin contains repeated amino acid sequence, hexapeptide repeat of Pro-Pro-Pro-Val-His-Leu		
	δ-Kafirin				Methionine rich			
	Glutelins	33.3			Glutamine/glutamate, leucine, asparagine/aspartic acid, arginine, proline			Taylor and Schüssler (1986)

Pearl millet	Albumins and globulins	32		Glutamine/ glutamate, asparagine/aspartic acid, arginine, alanine	Ali, Tinay, Mohamed, and Babiker (2009), Okoh, Nwasike, and Ikediobi (1985)
	Prolamins (pennisetin)	43	22 and 20 and 10	Glutamine/ glutamate, leucine, alanine, phenylalanine, proline	72% α-helix, 15% β-turns and 9% β-sheet. Similar to α-zein, but slightly smaller, 14 nm ribbons of folded α-helical segments	Ali et al. (2009), Bugs et al. (2004), Okoh et al. (1985), Shewry (2002)
			Dimers 49–51			
	Glutelins	25		Glutamine/ glutamate, proline, leucine, tyrosine		Ali et al. (2009), Okoh et al. (1985)
Foxtail millet	Albumins and globulins	17.3[a]		Glutamine/ glutamate, asparagine/aspartic acid, arginine, leucine		Kumar and Parameswaran (1998), Monteiro, Virupaksha, and Rao (1982)
	Prolamins	76.3[a]	17–22 and 12	Glutamine/ glutamate, leucine, alanine, asparagine/ aspartic acid	Homologous to α-zein	Kohama et al. (1999), Kumar and Parameswaran (1998), Monteiro et al. (1982), Shewry (2002)
	Glutelins	22[a]	17–20	Glutamine/ glutamate, leucine, asparagine/aspartic acid, alanine	Homologous to γ-zein	Kohama et al. (1999), Kumar and Parameswaran (1998), Monteiro et al. (1982)

(Continued)

TABLE 5.4 (Continued)

Species	Osborne Protein Fraction	% of Total Protein	Polymerization	Subunit Molecular Weight (kDa)	Major Amino Acid Composition	Structural Model and Secondary Structure	Hydrophobicity	References
Proso millet	Albumins and globulins	20						Parameswaran and Sadasivam (1994)
	Prolamins	58		14–17 19–27	Glutamine/glutamate, alanine leucine, proline	Homologous to α-zein		Kohama et al. (1999), Shewry (2002), Parameswaran and Sadasivam (1994)
	Glutelins	12		17–20	Glutamine/glutamate, proline, alanine, methionine	Homologous to γ-zein		Kohama et al. (1999)
Finger millet	Albumins and globulins	11[b]			Glutamine/glutamate, arginine, asparagine/aspartic acid, alanine			Virupaksha, Ramachandra, and Nagaraju (1975)
	Prolamins	42[b]		21.9, 24.4, 25.7, 45.5, 60	Glutamine/glutamate, leucine proline, valine			Virupaksha et al. (1975)
	Glutelins	23[b]			Glutamine/glutamate, arginine, leucine, asparagine/aspartic acid			Virupaksha et al. (1975)
Teff	Albumins and globulins	11.2			Glutamine, asparagine/aspartic acid, arginine, glycine, leucine			Adebowale, Emmambux, Beukes, and Taylor (2011)
	Prolamins	40.7		22 and 25	Glutamine, proline, valine, leucine, alanine, isoleucine, phenylalanine	Single dominant sequence, high degree of homology with α-prolamins of maize and sorghum		Tatham et al. (1996)

	Glutelins	22.2		Adebowale et al. (2011)
Fonio	Albumins and globulins	5	Glutamic acid/glutamine, asparagine/aspartic acid, arginine, phenylalanine	Carcea and Salvatorelli (1999), Shewry (2002)
	Prolamins	35	19 and 17.5	Methionine, cysteine	
	Glutelins	60		Lysine	

[a]Mean value from three varieties.
[b]Mean value from two varieties.

Early work on kafirin extraction described one of the most efficient solvents as 60% aqueous tert-butanol with a reducing agent, either 0.6% 2-mercaptoethanol or 0.05% dithiothreitol (Taylor et al., 1984). A reducing agent is needed to break disulfide bonds present within and between the protein molecules, thus increasing the solubility of the protein and the amount of protein extractable (Wall & Paulis, 1978). An apparently more efficient extraction method using an alkaline buffer containing the anionic detergent sodium dodecyl sulfate and 2-mercaptoethanol, with the subsequent precipitation of nonprolamin proteins by addition of ethanol or 60% tert-butanol has been developed (Hamaker, Mohamed, Habben, Huang, & Larkins, 1995; Wallace, Lopes, Paiva, & Larkins, 1990). Using this method, 90–95% of the total grain protein was extracted, which comprised 77–82% kafirin when sorghum endosperm was used as the starting material (Hamaker et al., 1995).

However, these solvent systems are not food-compatible. A simple, food-compatible, one-stage extraction procedure based on a modified Carter and Reck (1970) patent has been widely used as a laboratory method for extraction of all the kafirin subclasses (Emmambux & Taylor, 2003; Wang, Tilley, Bean, Sun, & Wang, 2009). This method uses a 1-hour extraction at elevated temperature (70°C) with 70% aqueous ethanol containing 0.35% sodium hydroxide and 0.5% sodium metabisulfite. Another simple, food-compatible extraction procedure for kafirin involves the use of glacial acetic acid after a sodium metabisulfite soak (Taylor, Taylor, Dutton, & De Kock, 2005). The advantage of this method is that it can be carried out at ambient temperature.

Extraction methodology for millet prolamins has been limited to variations on the classical extraction procedure of Landry and Moureaux (1970), which employs an aqueous alcohol (usually 60–70% aqueous isopropanol) with a reducing agent (0.6–1.0% 2-mercaptoethanol) (Kohama, Nagasawa, & Nishizawa, 1999; Monteriro et al., 1982; Parameswaran & Thayumanavan, 1995). The optimization of millet prolamin extraction has been little investigated. Parameswaran and Thayumanavan (1995) found that 60% isopropanol plus 1% 2-mercaptoethanol extracted the most prolamin proteins from kodo millet.

The prolamin proteins of sorghum and millets are not produced commercially. There are several reasons for this. With the exception of sorghum, these grains are produced in relatively small quantities and generally consumed in the form of staple foods in many of the poorest areas of the world. Nutritionally and functionally there is no benefit in isolating these proteins. As described, the prolamins are very low in the indispensible amino acid lysine and have limited food functionally without modification (Mesa-Stonestreet et al., 2010). Consequently, it seems that they would provide little benefit as a nutritional food ingredient.

5.4.3 Potential Applications for Kafirin

Notwithstanding its poor nutritional quality, sorghum kafirin has some attributes that give it commercial potential. Industrial byproducts of the milling, brewing, and bioethanol industry could be used as high-protein feedstocks for kafirin extraction, improving the economics of the process and sparing grain for human consumption. Potential kafirin applications are as a functional protein in gluten-free products, since kafirin has been shown to be safe for celiac patients (Ciaccia et al., 2007). However, a major drawback is that kafirin does not form a viscoelastic wheat gluten-like dough when mixed with water (Schober et al., 2011), unlike the very similar maize zein (α-zein) (Lawton, 1992).

The inertness of kafirin in aqueous environments could, however, be advantageous in other applications, in particular as a high-value biodegradable bioplastic material because of its relative hydrophobicity. It could, for example, be used as an encapsulating agent for micronutrients and nutraceuticals. Recently, we demonstrated that microparticles comprising sorghum condensed tannins encapsulated in kafirin have potential as nutraceutical to inhibit digestive amylases and thereby attenuate postprandial hyperglycemia associated with the metabolic syndrome and type 2 diabetes (Links, Taylor, Kruger, & Taylor, 2015).

5.5 SORGHUM AND MILLET PROCESSING

Here the major technologies used to process sorghum and millet grains into foods (cooking, milling, malting, lactic acid fermentation, brewing, and bioethanol production) are considered in respect of their influence on protein composition and nutritional quality. Additionally, the effect of compositing (blending) legumes with sorghum and millets on protein quality is examined.

5.5.1 Effects of Cooking on the Proteins

A common feature of essentially all cereal food and beverage processing is that there is a cooking step, which serves to gelatinize the starch, giving the product a palatable texture and making it readily available for hydrolysis by amylases.

However, in the case of sorghum, wet cooking, as is used, for example, in porridge making and brewing, reduces the digestibility (susceptibility to hydrolysis by proteases) of the protein (Duodu, Taylor, Belton, & Hamaker, 2003). The average reduction in in vitro protein digestibility over a number of studies is some 33%. The phenomenon seems to be unique to sorghum as the reduction in protein digestibility caused by cooking is minimal in the major cereals, maize, rice, and wheat (Henley, Taylor, & Obukosia, 2010). This also seems to be the case with millets. For example, a reduction of only 4% was found with pearl millet (Ejeta, Hassen, & Mertz, 1987) and substantial increases were found with foxtail, proso, and finger millet (Ravindran, 1992). However, they have not been studied in any detail.

The reduction in protein digestibility in sorghum caused by wet cooking compounds the poor protein quality of sorghum foods, resulting from its low-lysine content. This results in wet-cooked sorghum having a calculated protein digestibility corrected amino acid score (PDCAAS) (protein digestibility × amino acid score) of only approximately 0.22, compared to wheat 0.44 and rice 0.60 (Henley et al., 2010). The poor protein quality of sorghum foods resulting from the combination of low-lysine and low-protein digestibility has been shown to impact negatively on its nutritional quality. MacLean, López de Romaña, Placko, and Graham (1981) in a study involving infants recovering from protein-energy malnutrition found that they showed poor weight gain (or even weight loss) and inadequate protein retention when receiving a sorghum-based diet. Nitrogen absorption and retention values were only 46% and 14% of intake, compared with 81% and 49%, respectively, with a preceding casein-based diet.

Regarding the cause of the reduction in sorghum protein digestibility, there is good evidence that it is primarily a result of disulfide bonded crosslinking of the kafirin and other proteins involving the cysteine-rich β- and γ-kafirin subclasses (Ezeogu, Duodu, & Taylor, 2005; Hamaker, Kirleis, Butler, Axtell, & Mertz, 1987; Rom, Shull, Chandrashekar, & Kirleis, 1992). The crosslinked proteins themselves are presumed to be resistant to digestion. It has also been proposed that they limit access of proteases to other more digestible proteins, in particular α-kafirin, the major kafirin subclass which is centrally located in the protein bodies (Oria, Hamaker, Axtell, & Huang, 2000), the organelles of kafirin storage in the grain endosperm.

Interestingly, "dry" cooking processes such as extrusion cooking (Hamaker, Mertz, & Axtell, 1994) and popping (Parker, Grant, Rigby, Belton, & Taylor, 1999) do not significantly reduce sorghum protein digestibility, presumably because there is insufficient moisture for extensive disulfide crosslinking.

5.5.2 Milling

Generally, milling cereal grains to produce flour does not simply involve reducing the kernel into a flour; it also involves removal of all or part of the outer "bran" layers of the kernel to obtain relative pure starchy endosperm. The outer components of the kernel comprise the pericarp, which is rich in insoluble dietary fiber, and the germ, which is oil-rich. Bran removal is done to improve palatability and shelf-life but it has a dramatic effect on the nutritional quality and protein composition. Sorghum and millet milling is generally done in two stages. The first involves mechanical dry abrasion using a dehuller, which progressively rubs off the outer layers. The second simply comprises reduction of the endosperm into a meal or flour. Alternatively, both steps can be achieved simultaneously using a break-type roller mill.

Table 5.5 shows the protein composition of the morphological components of sorghum grain. The general composition is similar with the millets. The vast majority of the protein in the kernel is in the endosperm (approximately 80%), but the concentration of protein in the endosperm is low (approximately 9%), similar to that in the whole kernel. Also, the lysine content of the protein in the endosperm (<2%) is very low due to the fact that the kafirin prolamin proteins are the major protein fraction in the endosperm. In fact, the prolamins are endosperm-specific proteins.

In contrast, the protein content of the germ (approximately 18%) is twice that of the endosperm. Further, the lysine content of the protein in the germ (approximately 6.7%) is similar to that in legume protein such as soy protein (USDA National Nutrient Database, 2014). This is due to the high proportion of low-molecular-weight nitrogen, and albumin and globulin proteins in the germ, some 77%. The pericarp is very low in protein, only approximately 5%. However, its lysine content is much higher than that of the endosperm. Thus, it can be seen that removal of the germ and pericarp to produce starchy endosperm flour is very detrimental to protein nutritional quality. Importantly, the bran components are also rich in dietary fiber, essential lipids, B vitamins, minerals, and phytochemicals (Stevenson, Phillips, O'sullivan, & Walton, 2012).

5.5.3 Malting

Malting is the limited controlled germination of grains in moist air, which results in the mobilization of amylases, proteases, and other enzymes which hydrolyze and modify the grain components and its structure. Across sub-Saharan

TABLE 5.5 Protein Composition of Sorghum Grain and Its Components

	Whole Kernel	Endosperm	Germ	Pericarp
Percent of kernel weight	100	86.1	8.4	5.6
Percent of protein in kernel	100	80.5	16.4	3.1
Protein content (g/100 g)	10.1	8.7	17.8	5.2
Lysine content (g/100 g protein)	2.6	1.7	6.7	5.0
Osborne-Type Protein Fraction Composition (Relative %)				
Low-molecular-weight nitrogen	3.4	1.8	44.2	13.7
Albumins + globulins	18.3	5.8	33.3	10.4
Prolamins	44.0	68.3	8.7	11.7
Glutelins	33.3	24.1	13.9	64.4

Average of Data from Red and White Non-Tannin Cultivars.
Source: Data from Taylor, J. R. N., & Schüssler L. (1986). The protein compositions of the different anatomical parts of sorghum grain. *Journal of Cereal Science, 4*, 361–369.

Africa and in India, sorghum and millets are malted for the production of traditional beers, nonalcoholic beverages, and gruels (Taylor & Dewar, 2000). In the 1980s there was considerable research into malting as a "simple" technology to improve the protein quality and availability of other nutrients in cereals (see Chavan & Kadam, 1989). Malted cereals were also promoted as a source of amylase to thin infant porridges through partial starch hydrolysis, so-called "Power Flour," which enables a porridge of high nutrient density to be produced (Mosha & Svanberg, 1990).

Regarding the effects of malting on sorghum and millet proteins, the malt has slightly increased protein content (Table 5.6) as a result of respiration of carbohydrate. However, if the protein-rich roots and shoots are removed from the malt there is a decrease in protein content. The lysine content of the protein is increased substantially, the extent also being affected by root and shoot removal. Similarly, the digestibility of the proteins is also substantially increased. In both cases, this is as a result of hydrolysis of the lysine-poor, insoluble prolamin storage proteins and their synthesis into new proteins. This is shown in Table 5.6 where over a 7-day malting period the proportion of sorghum kafirin prolamin proteins decreased from approximately 46% to 15%, while the proportion of albumin and globulin proteins, plus products of protein hydrolysis (low-molecular-weight nitrogen) increased from some 16–28% to 44–55%.

There are, however, significant drawbacks regarding malting as a technology to improve sorghum and millet nutritional quality. These have to be weighed against the benefits. The malting process takes up 1 week with hot air malt drying, and considerably longer with solar drying. There is a loss in dry matter of approximately 10% through grain respiration and substantially higher if the malt roots and shoots removed. Sorghum malting leads to the production of hydrogen cyanide in the malt, which can be at dangerous levels if the malt is not fully dried at 30°C or higher to drive off the cyanide gas (Aniche, 1990). Most importantly, if malting is not carried out properly there is great fungal growth on the malt and mycotoxins can be produced (Nkwe, Taylor, & Siame, 2005).

5.5.4 Lactic Acid Fermentation

Lactic acid bacteria (sourdough type) fermentation is also a traditional technology used for processing sorghum and millets across sub-Saharan Africa (Taylor & Dewar, 2000). Lactic acid fermentation is used in the production of traditional beers, nonalcoholic beverages, gruels, porridges, and flatbreads. Unlike malting, lactic fermentation is an invariably safe, fairly rapid (1–2 day), and simple process. The key to traditional lactic fermentation is the technique of "back-slopping" whereby a small portion of a previous successful fermentation, rich in active bacteria, is used to inoculate a new fermentation. Traditional lactic acid fermentation is so widely used because people like the sharp, sour taste imparted by the lactic acid and other fermentation products. Also, importantly, it renders the food safe from pathogenic bacteria and slows down the rate of microbial spoilage due to the low pH ($\leq$pH 4) and possible production of antimicrobial bacteriocins (Taylor & Duodu, 2015).

Additionally, as a result of the action of enzymes produced by the bacteria and present in the cereal flour, the cereal proteins and other components of the grain are modified, improving the product's nutritional quality

TABLE 5.6 Effects of Malting on Sorghum and Millet Protein Quality and Composition

	Sorghum		Pearl millet		Foxtail millet		Finger millet	
	Grain	Malt	Grain	Malt	Grain	Malt	Grain	Malt
Protein (g/100 g db)	8.9[a]	9.4[a] (7 days)	12.6[b]	12.6[b] (2 days)	11.4[b]	10.7[b] (2 days)	6.1[c]	7.9[c] (4 days)
							8.2[b]	7.5[b] (2 days)
								6.8[b] (4 days)
Lysine (g/100 g protein)	2.2[a]	2.8[a] (7 days)	3.7[b]	4.3[b] (2 days)	3.0[b]	3.3[b] (2 days)	3.5[b] (2 days)	4.0[b] (2 days)
	1.4[d]	4.5[d] (4 days)						5.3[b] (4 days)
	2.2[e]	3.1[e] (7 days)						
In vitro protein digestibility (%)	33.5[a]	57.7[a] (7 days)					33.9[c]	55.4[c] (4 days)
Osborne-Type Protein Fraction Composition (Relative %)								
Low-molecular-weight nitrogen	9.4[f]	36.6[f] (7 days)						
Albumin + globulins	17.4[f]	18.3[f] (7 days)						
	16[e]	44[e] (7 days)						
Prolamins	44.2[f]	14.1[f] (7 days)						
	48[e]	16[e] (7 days)						
Glutelins	28.7[f]	31.0[f] (7 days)						
	35[e]	35[e] (7 days)						

[a]Values with external roots and shoots, average of two cultivars (Dewar, 2003).
[b]Values after removal of external roots and shoots (Malleshi & Desikachar, 1986).
[c]Values with external roots and shoots, average of two cultivars (Mbithi-Mwikya, Van Camp, Yiro, & Huygebaert, 2000).
[d]Wang and Fields (1978).
[e]Wu and Wall (1980).
[f]Values after removal of external roots and shoots (Taylor, 1983).

(Taylor & Dewar, 2000). As with malting, lactic acid fermentation increases protein content as a result of respiration of carbohydrates and it also increases lysine and protein digestibility (Table 5.7) due to hydrolysis of storage proteins and synthesis of new proteins. However, the effects on the composition of the grain protein are much less than with malting. Data from sorghum and foxtail millet show that there were barely any changes in the relative proportions of albumins plus globulins, prolamins, and glutelins. This indicates that there is general protein hydrolysis of the grain proteins, and not just specific hydrolysis of the prolamins.

Importantly, the adverse effect of wet cooking on sorghum protein digestibility can be partially alleviated if the sorghum is subjected to a lactic acid fermentation before cooking as would take place in the production of a traditional fermented porridge (Table 5.7) (Taylor & Taylor, 2002). It is suggested that this is due to the fermentation causing structural changes in the kafirin and glutelin proteins, making them more susceptible to enzymic hydrolysis.

5.5.5 Brewing and Bioethanol Production

Commercial brewing of traditional opaque beer is a major industry in southern Africa (Daiber & Taylor, 1995). Over the past 30 years, lager-type beer brewing using sorghum has also developed across sub-Saharan Africa, and gluten-free lager-type beer brewing using sorghum is expanding worldwide (Taylor, Dlamini, & Kruger, 2013). Also, in the US, bioethanol production from sorghum grain is now a major industry (Stroade & Boland, 2013), and is also commencing in other countries. The brewing and bioethanol industries produce huge quantities of cereal coproduct called brewers' spent grain and distillers' dried grain, respectively. These coproducts are similar in that the concentration of protein has been increased several-fold compared to the grain, to some 21% and 33% (dry basis), respectively (Table 5.8). This increase is due primarily to the hydrolysis of the starch into fermentable sugars. The lysine content of the protein may

TABLE 5.7 Effects of Lactic Acid Fermentation on Sorghum and Millet Protein Quality and Composition

	Sorghum		Pearl millet		Foxtail millet		Finger millet	
	Grain	Fermented Product	Grain	Fermented Product	Grain	Fermented Product	Grain	Fermented Product
Protein (g/100 g db)	10.9[a]	11.8[a] (28 h)			10.2[b]	10.5[b] (48 h)	8.1[c]	8.3[c] (48 h)
Available lysine (g/100 g protein)	2.3[d]	4.0[d] (5 days)						
In vitro protein digestibility (%)	51.8[a] 27.7[f] 3.4[f] (5 days) 1.4[d] (5 days)	75.6[a] (28 h) 43.0[f] 22.0[f] (5 days) 8.3[d] (5 days)	61.2[e]	81.0[e] (36 h)	68.5[b] (protein extractability)	76.9[b] (48 h) (protein extractability)	59.9[c] (protein extractability)	76.2[c] (48 h) (protein extractability)
Osborne-Type Protein Fraction Composition (Relative %)								
Albumin + Globulins	14.8[a]	12.1[a] (28 h)			13.1[b]	17.0[b] (48 h)		
Prolamins	60.3[a]	66.9[a] (28 h)			61.1[b]	58.2[b] (48 h)		
Glutelins	26.0[b]	20.6[a] (28 h)			26.0[b]	24.8[b] (48 h)		

[a]Yousif and El Tinay (2001).
[b]Antony et al. (1996a).
[c]Antony et al. (1996b).
[d]Kazanas and Fields (1981).
[e]Average of two cultivars (Elyas, El Tinay, Yousif, & Elsheikh, 2002).
[f]Average of five cultivars, value in Italics are protein digestibilities after cooking (Taylor & Taylor, 2002).

TABLE 5.8 Protein Composition and Quality of Sorghum Brewers' Spent Grain and Distillers' Dried Grains and Solubles

	Brewers' Spent Grain	Distillers' Dried Grains and Solubles
Protein (g/100 g dry basis)	21.4[a]	32.7[b]
Lysine (g/100 g protein)	3.4[a]	2.1[b]
Kafirin (g/100 g protein)		≥40[c]

[a]Spent grains from 77% sorghum malt:23% maize grits brew, average of two sorghum cultivars (Adewusi & Ilori, 1994).
[b]Includes spent yeast (Urriola, Hoehler, Pedersen, Stein, & Shurson, 2009).
[c]Own data unpublished.

also be increased as a result of inclusion of spent yeast, and the product from the bioethanol industry is referred to as distillers' dried grains and solubles (DDGS). Currently, sorghum brewers' spent grain and DDGS are used solely as animal feed. However, as they are so protein-rich, they clearly have potential as a significant source of protein for human food.

5.5.6 Compositing With Legumes

As described in Section 5.2.4, the productivity of sorghum and millets can be considerably improved in a sustainable manner by cultivation with legumes. Legumes are consumed together with cereals worldwide. Such meals are referred to as composites, with the indispensible amino acid composition of the legume and cereal components complementing each other. The legume component provides the lysine, which is invariably the limiting indispensible amino acid in cereals, and the cereal component can enhance the level of the sulfur-containing amino acids cysteine and methionine if these are limiting in the particular legume (United Nations University, 1979).

The legume and cereal may also be composited together in a single food product, normally at a ratio of approximately 70:30 cereal:legume (FAO, 1995). Such products are also referred to as blends. The most widely produced example is the feeding intervention program food product known as corn soy blend (USAID, n.d.). Table 5.9 shows that composite foods of sorghum or millets plus legumes have almost twice the lysine content of the foods made from sorghum or millets alone. In fact in the case of the sorghum, pearl millet, and proso millet flatbreads, their protein lysine content of >50 mg/kg meets the scoring pattern for children of 1–2 years (WHO/FAO/UNU Expert Consultation, 2007). Also, the digestibility of the protein in the composite products is somewhat higher. Importantly, several different measures of protein quality, protein PDCAAS, protein efficiency ratio, and net protein utilization, are all substantially increased in the composite foods.

There can, however, be a drawback of inclusion of legumes into some foods, particularly those which are moist, such as porridges and flatbreads (Anyango et al., 2011a). The legume invariably introduces beany flavors, which are not normally associated with cereal foods. This does not seem to be so much of a problem with baked, dry foods such as biscuits (cookies). Young school-age children found sorghum−soy composite biscuits equally sensorially acceptable as inexpensive wheat biscuits (Serrem, De Kock, & Taylor, 2011).

5.6 DEVELOPMENTS IN IMPROVING SORGHUM AND MILLET PROTEIN QUALITY

5.6.1 Sorghum

There has been considerable research to improve sorghum protein quality over the past five decades. Several different approaches have been taken and protein lysine content and protein digestibility have been substantially improved. The agronomic and processing quality of the resulting lines has, however, been an on-going problem and up until now (2015) there are still no improved protein quality sorghum varieties under commercial cultivation.

Naturally high-lysine sorghum lines have been identified in Ethiopia, which are consumed as snacks (Singh & Axtell, 1973). However, the grains are shrunken and hence these lines have poor yield and processing quality. Chemical mutagenesis has been used to develop a high-lysine sorghum mutant called P721-*opaque* (Guiragossian et al., 1978). The grains have up to 60% higher lysine as result of reduced synthesis of kafirins. However, in the investigation referred to in Section 5.5.1, where infants recovering from protein-energy malnutrition received sorghum-based diets, it was found that there were no differences in parameters of protein digestibility between either of these types of high-lysine sorghums and normal sorghums (MacLean et al., 1981).

This research focused attention on the issue of the poor digestibility of sorghum protein when wet cooked during food processing. By crossing the P721-*opaque* sorghum with normal sorghums, lines were obtained that had some 25% higher cooked flour protein digestibility and somewhat higher than normal lysine content (Weaver, Hamaker, & Axtell, 1998). The improved protein digestibility appears to be due to a change in the shape of the kafirin protein bodies from spherical to folded (invaginated) (Oria et al., 2000). This results in the cysteine-rich γ-kafirin subclass involved in disulfide bonding being concentrated at the bottom of the folds. Hence, the crosslinked protein would not inhibit access of proteases to the digestible major α-kafirin subclass.

However, the grains of these high-digestibility lines are soft (Tesso et al., 2006), rendering them susceptible to mold and insect attack during cultivation and they have poor milling quality. Furthermore, feeding trials with pigs and broiler chickens did not show any improvement in important digestibility parameters compared to maize or normal sorghum (Nyannor, Adedokun, Hamaker, Ejeta, & Adeola, 2007). Notwithstanding these drawbacks, it has been found that these high-digestibility sorghum types could have application as gluten-free flour as they have improved dough and breadmaking quality compared to normal sorghums (Goodall, Campanella, Ejeta, & Hamaker, 2012). This is apparently because the kafirin protein is less entrapped in the protein bodies.

Improvement in sorghum protein quality using recombinant DNA genetically modified (GM) technology has also been investigated, notably through the Africa Biofortified Sorghum project (Africa Harvest Biotechnology Foundation International, 2010). Both sorghum protein lysine content and wet-cooked digestibility were improved using RNAi (RNA interference) technology to suppress the synthesis of specific combinations of kafirin subclasses and the catabolism of lysine by the enzyme lysine ketoreductase (Grootboom, 2010). Additionally, transgenes for lysine-rich proteins, such as an analog of barley hordothionin (Zhao et al., 2003), were expressed in some lines.

TABLE 5.9 Effects of Compositing Sorghum and Millets With Legumes on the Protein Quality of Food Products

	Sorghum		Pearl Millet		Proso Millet		Finger Millet	
	Alone	Legume Composite	Alone	Legume Composite	Alone	Legume Composite	Alone	Legume Composite
Lysine (g/kg protein) Unless stated otherwise	21[a] Unfermented porridge 16[a] Fermented porridge 23[a] Fermented flatbread 21[b] Unfermented flatbread 14[d] Biscuits	34[a] Unfermented porridge 30[a] Fermented porridge 39[a] Fermented flatbread 55[b] Unfermented flatbread 39[d] Biscuits	26[b] Unfermented flatbread	55[b] Unfermented flatbread	12[b] Unfermented flatbread	55[b] Unfermented flatbread	AAS 0.47[c] Malted, cooked, and fermented complementary food	AAS 0.84[c] Malted, cooked, and fermented complementary food
In vitro protein digestibility (%)	64.6[a] Unfermented porridge 68.3[a] Fermented porridge 76.4[a] Fermented flatbread 73.8[b] Unfermented flatbread 30.0[d] Biscuits	72.2[a] Unfermented porridge 77.0[a] Fermented porridge 79.8[a] Fermented flatbread 76.6[b] Unfermented flatbread 74.3[d] Biscuits	75.1[b] Unfermented flatbread	77.5[b] Unfermented flatbread	78.1[b] Unfermented flatbread	80.9[b] Unfermented flatbread		90.2[c] Malted, cooked, and fermented complementary food
Protein quality	PDCAAS 0.26[a] Unfermented porridge 0.21[a] Fermented porridge 0.34[a] Fermented flatbread PER 0.54[b] Unfermented flatbread PDCAAS 0.09[d] Biscuits	PDCAAS 0.48[a] Unfermented porridge 0.44[a] Fermented porridge 0.60[a] Fermented flatbread PER 1.75[b] Unfermented flatbread PDCAAS 0.61[d] Biscuits	PER 073[b] Unfermented flatbread	PER 1.94[b] Unfermented flatbread	PER 049[b] Unfermented flatbread	PER 1.93[b] Unfermented flatbread		NPU 74.0[c] Malted, cooked, and fermented complementary food

[a] 70:30 sorghum:cowpea composites (Anyango et al., 2011b).
[b] Approximately 70:30 cereal:soy composites (Lindell & Walker, 1984).
[c] Approximately 65:19:8:8 finger millet:kidney bean:peanut:mango composite (Mbithi-Mwikya et al., 2002).
[d] Approximately 71:29 sorghum:soy composite (Serrem et al., 2011).
AAS, amino acid score; PDCAAS, protein digestibility corrected amino acid score; PER, protein efficiency ratio.

The protein bodies of these GM sorghum lines were invaginated (Da Silva et al., 2011; Grootboom et al., 2014), like those of the high-protein digestibility mutant (Oria et al., 2000), and they were less densely packed in the endosperm than in normal sorghum. A significant problem was that the grains of the GM lines were soft and efforts to improve grain hardness by more limited suppression of kafirin synthesis resulted in lower improvement in protein digestibility (Da Silva et al., 2011). Nevertheless, with regard to protein quality, lines with cosuppression of several kafirin subclasses had double the lysine content (37–41 mg/kg protein) compared to their parent lines and the wet-cooked in vitro protein digestibility was some 81%, as compared to their controls (approximately 58%). Furthermore, when these sorghums were made into a range of traditional-type food products (couscous, nonfermented, fermented, and alkali cooked porridges, and nonfermented and fermented flatbreads) and also into biscuits, these products had almost double the PDCAAS as the same products made from their null control lines (Taylor & Taylor, 2011).

A recent non-GM approach has been to develop sorghum lines that have both high protein digestibility and waxy (high amylopectin) traits (Elhassan, Emmambux, Hays, Peterson, & Taylor, 2015; Jampala, Rooney, Peterson, Bean, & Hays, 2012). These sorghum lines have somewhat increased protein and starch digestibility compared to normal sorghum but their food/feed value is still to be determined. Notwithstanding this, like the high-protein digestibility only sorghum types (Goodall et al., 2012), these lines with the combined high-protein digestibility and waxy traits have better flour functional properties than normal sorghums (Elhassan et al., 2015).

5.6.2 Millets

There has been very little research into improving the protein quality of millets. With pearl millet, it has been found that among a hybrid population yield, lysine and tryptophan content are negatively correlated with protein content, offering the possibility of increasing both yield and protein quality (Mathur & Muthur, 1986). Furthermore, it was found that in pearl millet high-protein inbred lines there was a reduction in albumin proteins and an increase in prolamin proteins compared to normal protein lines, leading to a reduction in lysine protein content (Singh, Singh, Eggum, Kumar, & Andrews, 1987). Much more recently, quantitative trait loci (QTL) for the *Opaque2* trait modifier (*Opm*) and QTL of the related trait of tryptophan content have been identified in finger millet (Babu, Agrawal, Pandey, & Kumar, 2014). The *Opm* is responsible for restoring the hard endosperm phenotype in high-lysine maize and is expressed in quality protein maize (QPM).

5.7 CONCLUSION

In terms of sustainable cultivation in response to increasing pressures on land and water resources and climate change, sorghum and millets are advantageous on account of their capacity to produce a crop in harsh environments, and especially under drought conditions. However, their low yield relative to maize where sufficient water is available is a major drawback and needs to be addressed through intensified breeding. The cultivation of sorghum and millets together with legumes for nitrogen fertilization is an important technology for their sustainable production. Also, it will help meet the need for high-quality protein foods containing adequate levels of indispensible amino acids, especially lysine, through compositing sorghum and millets together with legumes.

The prolamin storage proteins of sorghum and millets differ substantially from those of wheat and its relatives and thus are suitable for celiacs and the grains can be categorized as being gluten-free. With regard to protein content and quality, pearl millet is probably the best, although its yield is generally lower than sorghum. Research has demonstrated that the protein quality of sorghum in terms of both lysine content and digestibility can be improved through conventional breeding and genetic engineering. However, problems remain with regard to grain softness, which need to be addressed before these lines can be commercialized.

Concerning processing, traditional sourdough-type lactic acid fermentation is a particularly useful technology as it improves sorghum and millet protein quality and is a simple and safe process. The availability of increasing quantities of protein-rich sorghum spent grain from expanding brewing and bioethanol production is a significant potential source of protein for human consumption and also for the isolation of kafirin protein for high-value applications.

REFERENCES

Adebowale, A.-R., Emmambux, N. M., Beukes, M., & Taylor, J. R. N. (2011). Fractionation and characterization of teff proteins. *Journal of Cereal Science*, 54, 380–386.

Adewusi, S. R., & Ilori, M. O. (1994). Nutritional evaluation of spent grains from sorghum malts and maize grit. *Plant Foods for Human Nutrition*, *46*, 41−51.

Africa Harvest Biotechnology Foundation International. (2010). *Africa biofortified sorghum project: 5 year progress report, 2010*. Available at <http://issuu.com/africaharvest> Accessed July 2015.

Ali, M. A., Tinay, A. H. E., Mohamed, I. A., & Babiker, E. E. (2009). Supplementation and cooking of pearl millet: Changes in protein fractions and sensory quality. *World Journal of Dairy and Food Sciences*, *4*, 41−45.

Aniche, G. N. (1990). Studies on the effect of germination and drying conditions on the cyanide content of sorghum sprouts. *Journal of Food Science and Technology*, *27*, 202−204.

Antony, U., Sripriya, G., & Chandra, T. S. (1996a). The effect of fermentation on the primary nutrients in foxtail millet (*Setaria italica*). *Food Chemistry*, *56*, 381−384.

Antony, U., Sripriya, G., & Chandra, T. S. (1996b). Effect of fermentation on the primary nutrients in finger millet (*Eleusine coracana*). *Journal of Agricultural and Food Chemistry*, *44*, 2616−2618.

Anuonye, J. C., Onuh, J. O., Egwim, E., & Adeyemo, S. O. (2010). Nutrient and antinutrient composition of extruded acha/soybean blends. *Journal of Food Processing and Preservation*, *34*, 680−691.

Anyango, J. O., De Kock, H. L., & Taylor, J. R. N. (2011a). Evaluation of the functional quality of cowpea-fortified traditional African sorghum foods using instrumental and descriptive sensory analysis. *LWT-Food Science and Technology*, *44*, 2126−2133.

Anyango, J. O., De Kock, H. L., & Taylor, J. R. N. (2011b). Impact of cowpea addition on the protein digestibility corrected amino score and other protein quality parameters of traditional African foods made from sorghum. *Food Chemistry*, *124*, 775−780.

Argos, P., Pedersen, K., Marks, D., & Larkins, B. A. (1982). A structural model for maize zein proteins. *The Journal of Biological Chemistry*, *257*, 9984−9990.

Babu, B. K., Agrawal, P. K., Pandey, D., & Kumar, A. (2014). Comparative genomics and association mapping approaches for opaque2 modifier genes in finger millet accessions using genic, genomic and candidate gene-based simple sequence repeat markers. *Molecular Breeding*, *34*, 1261−1279.

Bach Knudsen, K. E., Kirleis, A. W., Eggum, B. O., & Munck, L. (1988). Carbohydrate composition and nutritional quality for rats of sorghum tô prepared from decorticated white and whole grain red flour. *Journal of Nutrition*, *118*, 588−597.

Bach Knudsen, K. E., Munck, L., & Eggum, B. O. (1988). Effect of cooking, pH and polyphenol level on carbohydrate composition and nutritional quality of a sorghum (*Sorghum bicolor* (L.) Moench) food, ugali. *British Journal of Nutrition*, *59*, 31−47.

Belton, P. S., Delgadillo, I., Halford, N. G., & Shewry, P. R. (2006). Kafirin structure and functionality. *Journal of Cereal Science*, *44*, 272−286.

Bergamo, P., Maurano, F., Mazzarella, G., Iaquinto, G., Vocca, I., Rivelli, A. R., ... Rossi, M. (2011). Immunological evaluation of the alcohol-soluble protein fraction from gluten-free grains in relation to celiac disease. *Molecular Nutrition & Food Research*, *55*, 1266−1270.

Blum, A. (2009). Effective use of water (EUW) and not water-use efficiency (WUE) is the target of crop yield improvement under drought stress. *Field Crops Research*, *112*, 119−123.

Bugs, M. R., Forato, L. A., Bortoleto-Bugs, R. K., Fischer, H., Mascarenhas, Y. P., Ward, R. J., & Colnago, L. A. (2004). Spectroscopic characterisation and structural modeling of prolamin from maize and pearl millet. *European Biophysics Journal*, *33*, 335−343.

Carcea, M., & Salvatorelli, S. (1999). Extraction and characterisation of fonio (*Digitaria exilis* Stapf) proteins. *Les Colloques de l'INRA No. 91*, 51−58.

Carter, R., & Reck, D. R. (1970). Low temperature solvent extraction process for producing high purity zein. United States Patent and Trademark Office 3535305.

Chandrasekher, G., Raju, D. S., & Pattabiraman, T. N. (1982). Natural plant enzyme inhibitors: Protease inhibitors in millets. *Journal of the Science of Food and Agriculture*, *33*, 447−450.

Chavan, J. K., & Kadam, S. S. (1989). Nutritional improvement of cereals by sprouting. *Critical Reviews in Food Science and Nutrition*, *28*, 401−437.

Ciaccia, C., Maiuri, L., Caporaso, N., Bucci, C., Del Giudice, L., Massardo, D. R., ... Londei, M. (2007). Celiac disease: In vitro and in vivo safety and palatability of wheat-free sorghum food products. *Clinical Nutrition*, *26*, 799−805.

Cisse, F., Erickson, D., Opekun, A., Nichols, B., & Hamaker, B. (2015). Traditional foods made from sorghum and millet in Mali have slower gastric emptying than pasta, potatoes, and rice. *The FASEB Journal*, *29*(1 Suppl.), 898.37

Cousins, B. W., Tanksley, T. D., Knabe, D. A., & Zebrowska, T. (1981). Nutrient digestibility and performance of pigs fed sorghums varying in tannin concentration. *Journal of Animal Science*, *53*, 1524−1537.

Daiber, K. H. (1975). Enzyme inhibition by polyphenols of sorghum grain and malt. *Journal of the Science of Food and Agriculture*, *26*, 1399−1411.

Daiber, K. H., & Taylor, J. R. N. (1995). Opque beers. In D. A. V. Dendy (Ed.), *Sorghum and millets: Chemistry and technology* (pp. 299−323). St. Paul, MN: American Association of Cereal Chemists.

Da Silva, L. S., Jung, R., Zhao, Z., Glassman, K., Grootboom, A. W., Mehlo, L., ... Taylor, J. R. N. (2011). Effect of suppressing the synthesis of different kafirin sub-classes on grain endosperm texture, protein body structure and protein nutritional quality in improved sorghum lines. *Journal of Cereal Science*, *54*, 160−167.

Demeke, M., & Di Marcantonio, F. (2013). *Analysis of incentives and disincentives for teff in Ethiopia. Technical notes series*. Rome: MAFAP, FAO.

Dewar, J. (2003). Influence of malting on sorghum malting quality. In P. S. Belton, J. R. N. Taylor (Eds.), Afripro: Workshop on the proteins of sorghum and millets. Available at <www.afripro.org.uk> Accessed July 2015.

Duodu, K. G., Taylor, J. R. N., Belton, P. S., & Hamaker, B. R. (2003). Mini review: Factors affecting sorghum protein digestibility. *Journal of Cereal Science, 38,* 117–131.

Du Plessis, J. (n.d.). Sorghum production. South African National Department of Agriculture. Available at <www.nda.agric.za/docs/Infopaks/FieldCrops_Sorghum.pdf> Accessed July 2015.

Ejeta, G., Hassen, M. M., & Mertz, E. T. (1987). In vitro digestibility and amino acid composition of pearl millet (*Pennisetum typhoides*) and other cereals. *Proceedings of the National Academy of Sciences of the United States of America, 84,* 6016–6019.

Elhassan, M. S. M., Emmambux, M. N., Hays, D. B., Peterson, G. C., & Taylor, J. R. N. (2015). Novel biofortified sorghum lines with combined waxy (high amylopectin) starch and high protein digestibility traits: Effects on endosperm and flour properties. *Journal of Cereal Science, 62,* 132–139.

Elyas, S. H. A., El Tinay, A. H., Yousif, N. E., & Elsheikh, E. A. E. (2002). Effect of natural fermentation on nutritive value and in vitro protein digestibility of pearl millet. *Food Chemistry, 78,* 75–79.

Emmambux, N. M., & Taylor, J. R. N. (2003). Sorghum kafirin interaction with various phenolic compounds. *Journal of the Science of Food and Agriculture, 83,* 402–407.

Evans, D. J., Schüssler, L., & Taylor, J. R. N. (1987). Isolation of reduced-soluble protein from sorghum starchy endosperm. *Journal of Cereal Science, 5,* 61–65.

Ezeogu, L. I., Duodu, K. G., & Taylor, J. R. N. (2005). Effects of endosperm texture and cooking conditions on the in vitro starch digestibility of sorghum and maize flours. *Journal of Cereal Science, 42,* 33–44.

FAO. (1995). Sorghum and millets in human nutrition, FAO Food and Nutrition Series, No. 27. Available at <www.fao.org> Accessed July 2015.

FAOSTAT3. (2013). *Production, crops.* Available at <http://faostat3.fao.org>. Accessed July 2015.

Farré, I., & Faci, J. M. (2006). Comparative response of maize (*Zea mays* L.) and sorghum (*Sorghum bicolor* L. Moench) to deficit irrigation in a Mediterranean environment. *Agriculture Water Management, 83,* 135–143.

Forato, L. A., Bicudo, T. C., & Colnago, L. A. (2003). Conformation of α-zeins in solid state by Fourier transform IR. *Biopolymers, 6,* 421–426.

Franzluebbers, A. J., & Francis, C. A. (1995). Energy output:input ratio of maize and sorghum managements systems in eastern Nebraska. *Agriculture, Ecosystems and Environment, 53,* 271–278.

Garratt, R., Oliva, G., Caracelli, I., Leite, A., & Arruda, P. (1993). Studies of the zein-like α-prolamins based on an analysis of amino acid sequences: Implications for their evolution and three-dimensional structure. *Proteins: Structure, Function and Genetics, 15,* 88–99.

Germplasm Resources Information Network. (n.d.). *GRIN Taxonomy for Plants.* Available at <www.ars-grin.gov> Accessed July 2015.

GIPSA. (2013). *Grain inspection handbook II grain grading procedures.* Chapter 9 Sorghum. Available at: <www.gipsa.usda.gov> Accessed February 2015.

Goodall, M. A., Campanella, O. H., Ejeta, G., & Hamaker, B. R. (2012). Grain of high digestible, high lysine (HDHL) sorghum contains kafirins which enhance the protein network of composite dough and bread. *Journal of Cereal Science, 56,* 352–357.

Grootboom, A. W. (2010). *Effect of RNAi down-regulation of three lysine deficient kafirins on the seed lysine content of sorghum* [Sorghum bicolor *(L.) Moench*]. PhD thesis. South Africa: University of Pretoria.

Grootboom, A. W., Mkhonza, N. L., Mbambo, Z., O'Kennedy, M. M., Da Silva, L. S., Taylor, J., ... Mehlo, L. (2014). Co-suppression of synthesis of major α-kafirin sub-class together with γ-kafirin-1 and γ-kafirin-2 required for substantially improved protein digestibility in transgenic sorghum. *Plant Cell Reports, 33,* 521–537.

Guiragossian, V., Chibber, B. A. K., Van Scoyoc, S., Jambunathan, R., Mertz, E. T., & Axtell, J. D. (1978). Characteristics of proteins from normal, high lysine, and high tannin sorghums. *Journal of Agricultural and Food Chemistry, 26,* 219–223.

Hamaker, B. R., Kirleis, A. W., Butler, L. G., Axtell, J. D., & Mertz, E. T. (1987). Improving the in vitro protein digestibility of sorghum with reducing agents. *Proceedings of the National Academy of Sciences of the United States of America, 84,* 626–628.

Hamaker, B. R., Mertz, E. T., & Axtell, J. D. (1994). Effect of extrusion on sorghum kafirin solubility. *Cereal Chemistry, 71,* 515–517.

Hamaker, B. R., Mohamed, A. A., Habben, J. E., Huang, C. P., & Larkins, B. A. (1995). Efficient procedure for extracting maize and sorghum kernel proteins reveals higher prolamin contents than the conventional method. *Cereal Chemistry, 72,* 583–588.

Henley, E. C., Taylor, J. R. N., & Obukosia, S. D. (2010). The importance of dietary protein in human health: Combating protein deficiency in sub-Saharan Africa through transgenic biofortified sorghum. *Advances in Food and Nutrition Research, 60,* 21–52.

ICC. (2012). Standard no. 176. Estimation of sorghum grain endosperm texture, standard no. 177. Detection of tannin sorghum grain by the bleach test. ICC, Vienna.

ICRISAT. (n.d.). *ICRISAT mandate crops.* Available at <www.icrisat.org> Accessed July 2015.

ICRISAT/FAO. (1996). *The world sorghum and millet economies: Facts, trends and outlook.* Patancheru, India/Rome: ICRISAT, FAO.

Jampala, B., Rooney, W. L., Peterson, G. C., Bean, S., & Hays, D. B. (2012). Estimating the relative effects of the endosperm traits of waxy and high protein digestibility on yield in grain sorghum. *Field Crops Research, 139,* 57–62.

Joint FAO/WHO Expert Consultation. (1991). *Protein quality evaluation.* Rome: FAO.

Joint WHO/FAO/UNU Expert Consultation. (2007). *Protein and amino acid requirements in human nutrition.* Geneva: World Health Organization.

Joshi, B. N., Sainani, M. N., Bastawade, K. B., Gupta, V. S., & Ranjekar, P. K. (1998). Cysteine protease inhibitor from pearl millet: A new class of antifungal protein. *Biochemical and Biophysical Research Communications, 246,* 382–387.

Karanja, S. M., Kibe, A. M., Karogo, P. N., & Mwangi, M. (2014). Effects of intercrop population density and row orientation on growth and yields of sorghum – cowpea cropping systems in semi-arid Rongai, Kenya. *Journal of Agricultural Sciences, 6.* Available from http://dx.doi.org/10.5539/jas.v6n5p34.

Kazanas, N., & Fields, M. L. (1981). Nutritional improvement of sorghum by fermentation. *Journal of Food Science, 46*, 819–821.

Klopfenstein, C. F., & Hoseney, R. C. (1995). Nutritional properties of sorghum and the millets. In D. A. V. Dendy (Ed.), *Sorghum and millets: Chemistry and technology* (pp. 125–168). St. Paul, MN: American Association of Cereal Chemists.

Kohama, K., Nagasawa, T., & Nishizawa, N. (1999). Polypeptide composition and NH_2-terminal amino acid sequences of proteins in foxtail and proso millets. *Biosciences, Biotechnology and Biochemistry, 63*, 1921–1926.

Kouyaté, Z., Franzluebbers, K., Jou, A. S. R., & Hossner, L. R. (2000). Tillage, crop residue, legume rotation, and green manure effects on sorghum and millet yields in the semiarid tropics of Mali. *Plant and Soil, 225*, 141–151.

Kumar, K. K., & Parameswaran, K. P. (1998). Characterisation of storage protein from selected varieties of foxtail millet (*Setaria italica* (L.) Beauv. *Journal of the Science of Food and Agriculture, 77*, 535–542.

Kumari, S. R., Chandrashekar, A., & Shetty, H. S. (1992). Proteins in developing sorghum endosperm that may be involved in resistance to grain moulds. *Journal of the Science of Food and Agriculture, 60*, 275–282.

Landry, J., & Moureaux, T. (1970). Hétérogénéité des glutélines du grain de mais: Extraction selective et composition en acides aminés des trios fractions isolées. *Bulletin de la Société de Chimie Biologique, 52*, 1021–1037.

Lawton, J. W. (1992). Viscoelasticity of zein-starch doughs. *Cereal Chemistry, 69*, 351–355.

Lester, R. N., & Bekele, E. (1981). Amino acid composition of the cereal tef and related species of Eragrostis (Gramineae). *Cereal Chemistry, 58*, 113–115.

Lindell, M. J., & Walker, C. E. (1984). Soy enrichment of chapaties made from wheat and non-wheat flours. *Cereal Chemistry, 61*, 435–438.

Links, M. R., Taylor, J., Kruger, M. C., & Taylor, J. R. N. (2015). Sorghum condensed tannins encapsulated in kafirin microparticles as a nutraceutical for inhibition of amylases during digestion to attenuate hyperglycaemia. *Journal of Functional Foods, 12*, 55–63.

MacLean, W. C., Jr., López de Romaňa, G., Placko, R. P., & Graham, G. C. (1981). Protein quality and digestibility of sorghum in preschool children: Balance studies and plasma free amino acids. *Journal of Nutrition, 111*, 128–136.

Malleshi, N. G., & Desikachar, H. S. R. (1986). Nutritive value of malted pearl millet flours. *Plant Foods for Human Nutrition, 36*, 191–196.

Mathur, P. N., & Muthur, J. R. (1986). Combining ability for yield, protein, lysine and tryptophan in pearl millet (*Pennisetum americanum* L.). *Field Crops Research, 15*, 181–189.

Matsushima, N., Danno, G., Takezawa, H., & Izumi, Y. (1997). Three-dimensional structure of maize α-zein proteins studied by small-angle X-ray scattering. *Biochimica et Biopysica Acta, 1339*, 14–22.

Mbithi-Mwikya, S., Van Camp, J., Mamiro, P. R., Ooghe, W., Kolsteren, P., & Huyghebaert, A. (2002). Evaluation of the nutritional characteristics of a finger millet based complementary food. *Journal of Agricultural and Food Chemistry, 50*, 3030–3036.

Mbithi-Mwikya, S., Van Camp, J., Yiro, Y., & Huygebaert, A. (2000). Nutrient and antinutrient change in finger millet (Eleucine coracan) during sprouting. *LWT-Food Science and Technology, 33*, 9–14.

Mesa-Stonestreet, D., Jhoe, N., Alavi, S., & Bean, S. R. (2010). Sorghum proteins: The concentration, isolation, modification, and food applications of kafirins. *Journal of Food Science, 75*, R90–R104.

Momany, F. A., Sessa, D. J., Lawton, J. W., Selling, G. W., Hamaker, S. A. H., & Willett, J. L. (2006). Structural characterization of α-zein. *Journal of Agricultural and Food Chemistry, 54*, 543–547.

Monteiro, P. V., Virupaksha, T. K., & Rao, D. R. (1982). Proteins of Italian millet: Amino acid composition, solubility fractionation and electrophoresis of protein fractions. *Journal of the Science of Food and Agriculture, 33*, 1072–1079.

Morrison, L. A., & Wrigley, D. W. (2004). Taxonomic classification of grain species. In C. Wrigley, H. Corke, & C. E. Walker (Eds.), *Encyclopedia of grain science* (Vol. 3, pp. 271–280). Oxford: Elsevier.

Mosha, A. C., & Svanberg, U. (1990). The acceptance and intake of bulk-reduced weaning foods: The Luganga village study. *Food and Nutrition Bulletin, 12*, 69–74.

Mpairwe, D. R., Sabiiti, E. N., Ummuna, N. N., Tegegne, A., & Osuji, P. (2002). Effect of intercropping cereal crops with forage legumes and source of nutrients on cereal grain yield and fodder dry matter yields. *African Crop Science Journal, 10*, 81–97.

Muchow, R. C. (1989a). Comparative productivity of maize, sorghum and pearl millet in a semi-arid tropical environment I. Yield potential. *Field Crops Research, 20*, 191–205.

Muchow, R. C. (1989b). Comparative productivity of maize, sorghum and pearl millet in a semi-arid tropical environment II. Effect of water deficits. *Field Crops Research, 20*, 207–219.

National Research Council. (1996). *Lost crops of Africa, vol. 1: Grains*. Washington, DC: National Academy Press.

Nkwe, D. O., Taylor, J. E., & Siame, B. A. (2005). Fungi, aflatoxins, fumonisin B1 and zearalenone contaminating sorghum-based traditional malt, wort and beer in Botswana. *Mycopathologia, 160*, 177–186.

Nyannor, E. K. D., Adedokun, S. A., Hamaker, B. R., Ejeta, G., & Adeola, O. (2007). Nutritional evaluation of high-digestible sorghum for pigs and broiler chicks. *Journal of Animal Science, 85*, 196–203.

Obilana, A. B., & Manyasa, E. (2002). Millets. In P. S. Belton, & J. R. N. Taylor (Eds.), *Pseudocereals and less common cereals* (pp. 177–217). Berlin: Springer.

Okoh, P. N., Nwasike, C. C., & Ikediobi, C. O. (1985). Studies on seed proteins of pearl millets. 1. Amino acid composition of protein fractions of early and late maturing varieties. *Journal of Agricultural and Food Chemistry, 33*, 55–57.

Oria, M. P., Hamaker, B. R., Axtell, J. D., & Huang, C.-P. (2000). A highly digestible sorghum mutant cultivar exhibits a unique folded structure of endosperm protein bodies. *Proceedings of the National Academy of Sciences of the United States of America, 97*, 5065–5070.

Oukasha, A., & El-latif, A. (2014). In vivo and vitro inhibition of Spodoptera littoralis gut-serine protease by protease inhibitors isolated from maize and sorghum seeds. *Pesticide Biochemistry and Physiology, 116,* 40–48.

Parameswaran, K. P., & Sadasivam, S. (1994). Changes in carbohydrates and nitrogenous components during germination of proso millet, *Panicum miliaceum. Plant Foods for Human Nutrition, 45,* 97–102.

Parameswaran, K. P., & Thayumanavan, B. (1995). Homologies between prolamins of different minor millets. *Plant Foods for Human Nutrition, 48,* 119–126.

Parker, M. L., Grant, A., Rigby, N. M., Belton, P. S., & Taylor, J. R. N. (1999). Effects of popping on the endosperm cell walls of sorghum and maize. *Journal of Cereal Science, 30,* 209–216.

Pretty, J. (1995). Can sustainable agriculture feed Africa? New evidence on progress, processes and impacts. *Environment, Development and Sustainability, 1,* 253–274.

Ravindran, G. (1992). Seed protein of millets: Amino acid composition, proteinase inhibitors and in-vitro protein digestibility. *Food Chemistry, 44,* 13–17.

Rom, D. L., Shull, J. M., Chandrashekar, A., & Kirleis, A. W. (1992). Effects of cooking and treatment with sodium bisulfite on in vitro digestibility and microstructure of sorghum flour. *Cereal Chemistry, 69,* 178–181.

Schober, T. J., Bean, S. R., Tilley, M., Smith, B. M., & Ioerger, B. P. (2011). Impact of different isolation procedures on the functionality of zein and kafirin. *Journal of Cereal Science, 54,* 241–249.

Serna-Saldivar, S., & Rooney, L. W. (1995). Structure and chemistry of sorghum and millets. In D. A. V. Dendy (Ed.), *Sorghum and millets: Chemistry and technology* (pp. 69–124). St. Paul, MN: American Association of Cereal Chemists.

Serrem, C. A., De Kock, H. L., & Taylor, J. R. N. (2011). Nutritional quality, sensory quality and consumer acceptability of sorghum and bread wheat biscuits fortified with defatted soy flour. *International Journal of Food Science and Technology, 124,* 74–83.

Shewry, P. R. (2002). The major seed storage proteins of spelt wheat, sorghum, millets and pseudocereals. In P. S. Belton, & J. R. N. Taylor (Eds.), *Pseudocereals and less common cereals* (pp. 1–24). Berlin: Springer.

Shewry, P. R., & Tatham, A. S. (1990). The prolamin proteins of cereal seeds: Structure and evolution. *Biochemical Journal, 267,* 1–12.

Shull, J. M., Watterson, J. J., & Kirleis, A. W. (1991). Proposed nomenclature for the alcohol-soluble proteins (kafirins) of *Sorghum bicolor* (L. Moench) based on molecular weight, solubility and structure. *Journal of Agricultural and Food Chemistry, 39,* 83–87.

Singh, P., Singh, U., Eggum, B. O., Kumar, K. A., & Andrews, D. J. (1987). Nutritional evaluation of high protein genotypes of pearl millet (*Pennisetum americanum* (L.) Leeke). *Journal of the Science of Food and Agriculture, 38,* 41–48.

Singh, R., & Axtell, J. D. (1973). High lysine mutant gene (hl) that improves the quality and nutritional value of grain sorghum. *Crop Science, 13,* 535–539.

Siwela, M., Taylor, J. R. N., De Milliano, W. A. J., & Duodu, K. G. (2007). Occurrence and location of tannins in finger millet grain and antioxidant activity of different grain types. *Cereal Chemistry, 84,* 169–174.

Stevenson, L., Phillips, F., O'sullivan, K., & Walton, J. (2012). Wheat bran: Its composition and benefits to health, a European perspective. *International Journal of Food Sciences and Nutrition, 63,* 1001–1013.

Stroade, J., Boland, M. (2013). *Sorghum profile.* Available at <http://www.agmrc.org> Accessed July 2015.

Tatham, A. S., Fido, R. J., Moore, C. M., Kasarda, D. D., Kuzmicky, D. D., Keen, J. N., & Shewry, P. R. (1996). Characterisation of the major prolamins of tef (*Eragrostis tef*) and finger millet (*Eleusine coracana*). *Journal of Cereal Science, 24,* 65–71.

Taylor, J., Anyango, A. O., & Taylor, J. R. N. (2013). Developments in the science of zein, kafirin and gluten protein bio-plastic materials. *Cereal Chemistry, 90,* 344–357.

Taylor, J., Anyango, J. O., Potgieter, M., Kallmeyer, K., Naidoo, V., Pepper, M. S., & Taylor, J. R. N. (2015). Biocompatibility and biodegradation of protein microparticle and film scaffolds made from kafirin (sorghum prolamin protein) subcutaneously implanted in rodent models. *Journal of Biomedical Materials Research Part A, 103,* 2582–2590.

Taylor, J., & Taylor, J. R. N. (2002). Alleviation of the adverse effects of cooking on protein digestibility in sorghum through fermentation in traditional African porridges. *International Journal of Food Science and Technology, 37,* 129–138.

Taylor, J., & Taylor, J. R. N. (2011). Protein biofortified sorghum: Effect of processing into traditional African foods on their protein quality. *Journal of Agricultural and Food Chemistry, 59,* 2386–2392.

Taylor, J., Taylor, J. R. N., Dutton, M. F., & De Kock, S. (2005). Glacial acetic acid – a novel food-compatible solvent for kafirin. *Cereal Chemistry, 82,* 485–487.

Taylor, J. R. N. (1983). Effect of malting on the protein and free amino nitrogen composition of sorghum. *Journal of the Science of Food and Agriculture, 34,* 885–892.

Taylor, J. R. N., Belton, P. S., Beta, T., & Duodu, K. G. (2014). Review: Increasing the utilisation of sorghum, millets and pseudocereals: Developments in the science of their phenolic phytochemicals, biofortification and protein functionality. *Journal of Cereal Science, 59,* 257–275.

Taylor, J. R. N., & Dewar, J. (2000). Fermented products: Beverages and porridges. In C. Wayne Smith, & R. A. Frederiksen (Eds.), *Sorghum: Origin, history, technology, and production* (pp. 751–795). New York, NY: John Wiley & Sons.

Taylor, J. R. N., Dlamini, B. C., & Kruger, J. (2013). 125th anniversary review: The science of the tropical cereals sorghum, maize and rice in relation to lager beer brewing. *Journal of the Institute of Brewing, 119,* 1–14.

Taylor, J. R. N., & Duodu, K. G. (2015). Effects of processing sorghum and millets on their phenolic phytochemicals and the implications of this to the health-enhancing properties of sorghum and millet food and beverage products. *Journal of the Science of Food and Agriculture, 95,* 225–237.

Taylor, J. R. N., & Emmambux, M. N. (2010). Developments in our understanding of sorghum polysaccharides and their health benefits. *Cereal Chemistry, 87*, 263–271.

Taylor, J. R. N., & Kruger, J. (2016). Millets. In B. Cabellero, P. Finglas, & F. Toldrá (Eds.), *The encylopedia of food and health* (Vol. 3, pp. 748–757). Oxford: Academic Press.

Taylor, J. R. N., & Schüssler, L. (1986). The protein compositions of the different anatomical parts of sorghum grain. *Journal of Cereal Science, 4*, 361–369.

Taylor, J. R. N., Schüssler, L., & Van der Walt, W. H. (1984). Fractionation of proteins from low-tannin sorghum grain. *Journal of Agricultural and Food Chemistry, 32*, 149–154.

Tesso, T., Ejeta, G., Chandrashekar, A., Huang, C.-P., Tandjung, A., Lewamy, M., ... Hamaker, B. R. (2006). A novel modified endosperm texture in a mutant high-protein digestibility/high-lysine sorghum (*Sorghum bicolor* (L.) Moench). *Cereal Chemistry, 83*, 194–201.

United Nations University. (1979). Supplementary effect of beans for cereal grains and starchy foods, Vol. 1, No. 4. Available at <http://archive.unu.edu> Accessed July 2015.

Urriola, P. E., Hoehler, D., Pedersen, C., Stein, H. H., & Shurson, G. C. (2009). Amino acid digestibility of distillers dried grains with solubles, produced from sorghum, a sorghum-corn blend, and corn fed to growing pigs. *Journal of Animal Science, 87*, 2574–2580.

USAID. (n.d.). *Corn soy blend/plus commodity fact sheet*. Available at <www.usaid.gov> Accessed July 2015.

USDA National Nutrient Database. (2014). *National nutrient database for standard reference release 27*. Available at <http://ndb.nal.usda.gov> Accessed July 2015.

USDA. (n.d.). *Plants database*. Available at <http://plants.usda.gov> Accessed July 2015.

Virupaksha, T. K., Ramachandra, G., & Nagaraju, D. (1975). Seed proteins of finger millet and their amino acid composition. *Journal of the Science of Food and Agriculture, 26*, 1237–1246.

Wall, J. S., & Paulis, J. W. (1978). Corn and sorghum grain proteins. In Y. Pomeranz (Ed.), *Advances in cereal science and technology* (Vol. II, pp. 135–219). St Paul, MN: American Association of Cereal Chemists.

Wallace, J. C., Lopes, M. A., Paiva, E., & Larkins, B. A. (1990). New methods for extraction and quantitation of zeins reveal a high content of γ-zein in modified opaque-2 maize. *Plant Physiology, 92*, 191–196.

Wang, Y., Tilley, M., Bean, S., Sun, X. S., & Wang, D. (2009). Comparison of methods for extracting kafirin proteins from sorghum distillers dried grains with solubles. *Journal of Agricultural and Food Chemistry, 57*, 8366–8372.

Wang, Y.-Y. D., & Fields, M. L. (1978). Germination of corn and sorghum in the home to improve nutritive value. *Journal of Food Science, 43*, 1113–1115.

Wani, S. P., Rupela, O. P., & Lee, K. K. (1995). Sustainable agriculture in the semi-arid tropics though biological nitrogen fixation of grain legumes. *Plant and Soil, 174*, 29–49.

Watterson, J. J., Shull, J. M., & Kirleis, A. W. (1993). Quantitation of α-, β- and γ-kafirins in vitreous and opaque endosperm of *Sorghum bicolor*. *Cereal Chemistry, 70*, 452–457.

Weaver, C. A., Hamaker, B. R., & Axtell, J. D. (1998). Discovery of grain sorghum germ plasm with high uncooked and cooked in vitro protein digestibility. *Cereal Chemistry, 75*, 665–670.

Wu, Y. V., & Wall, J. S. (1980). Lysine content of protein increased by germination of normal and high-lysine sorghums. *Journal of Agricultural and Food Chemistry, 28*, 455–458.

Yousif, N. E., & El Tinay, A. H. (2001). Effect of fermentation on sorghum protein fractions and in vitro protein digestibility. *Plant Foods for Human Nutrition, 56*, 175–182.

Zhao, Z., Glassman, K., Sewalt, V., Wang, N., Miller, M., Chang, S., ... Jung, R. (2003). Nutritionally improved transgenic sorghum. In I. K. Vasil (Ed.), *Plant technology 2002 and beyond* (pp. 413–416). Dordrecht: Kluwer.

Chapter 6

Protein From Oat: Structure, Processes, Functionality, and Nutrition

O.E. Mäkinen, N. Sozer, D. Ercili-Cura and K. Poutanen
VTT Technical Research Centre of Finland, Espoo, Finland

6.1 INTRODUCTION

In today's food market, consumers demand high-protein or protein-enriched foods. Due to our constantly increasing understanding about the sustainability issues related to animal proteins, the demand for plants as protein sources is increasing. For example, according to a 2014 report, halving the consumption of meat and dairy in the European Union (EU) would decrease the nitrogen emissions by 40% and greenhouse gas emissions by 25−40% (Westhoek et al., 2014). Allergenicity and genetic modification (GMO) issues related to soybean, one of the most important plant-based protein sources, urge manufacturers to look for alternative proteins that have a high technological and nutritional quality.

Cereals are an important dietary protein source globally (Grigg, 1995). Oat (*Avena sativa*) belongs to the grass family *Gramineae* but not the *Triticeae* tribe like wheat, barley, and rye. The two main species for food are the common, covered white oat (*Avena sativa* L.) and a naked variety with loosely attached hulls (*Avena sativa* var. *nuda*) (Stewart & McDougall, 2014). Oat is a distinct cereal among others owing to its higher content of protein (15−20%), unsaturated fatty acids, soluble fiber (β-glucan), and antioxidants, as compared to the *Triticeae* cereals (Lásztity, 1998). The unique protein composition of oats which lacks gluten makes it a safe food ingredient for most individuals with celiac disease (Janatuinen et al., 1995; Størsrud et al., 2003). Moreover, oat proteins are mainly comprised of globulins that have a more balanced amino acid profile than other cereals. Despite the low significance of oat in human nutrition in the past, oat proteins have been well-studied because of their relevance in animal nutrition, particularly for horses (Shewry, 1999; Shotwell, 1999).

Oats are classically used as oat flour or flakes. Oat protein ingredients have only recently been developed to industrial-scale production. Today, technologies developed for fractionation of β-glucan (valuable due to its proven cholesterol-lowering effects) from oat grains provide concentrated protein fractions as a side stream, which can offer the food industry a new good-quality protein source. The climate and land-use impacts of oat protein evaluated as unprocessed grains are inarguably lower than those of animal-derived proteins, but subsequent processing into products is decisive in terms of the total farm-to-fork impact (González, Frostell, & Carlsson-Kanyama, 2011). Because of a potentially high-energy input, the production chain of a plant-based meat substitute product can be nearly as energy-consuming as that of an efficient pork chain (Apaiah, Linnemann, & van der Kooi, 2006). As large dilution and subsequent water removal constitute the main energy sink, it is evident that more energy-efficient dry fractionation processes are the future (Apaiah et al., 2006; Schutyser & van der Goot, 2011; Sibakov et al., 2011).

In this chapter, the present knowledge on the structure and nutritional properties, as well as the functional properties and processes for the enrichment of oat proteins are summarized.

6.2 OAT AS A PROTEIN CROP

6.2.1 Land Use

Oat is the seventh most abundant cereal produced in the world. It is nevertheless considered a minor cereal grain, as it falls far behind the production volumes of maize, rice, and wheat and accounts for less than 1% of cereal production (Faostat, 2014). Oat production started declining in the second half of the 20th century as farms mechanized and horse feed demand dropped, and when soy replaced oat as the primary protein feed for livestock (Strychar, Webster, & Wood, 2011). The worldwide production (22,965,903 tonnes in 2014) has remained fairly stable for the past 10 years (Faostat, 2014). The majority of oat (75%) is still used as animal feed, but food use has increased with the increased understanding of the benefits to human health (Stewart & McDougall, 2014).

Oat is a crop of northern regions—it grows optimally at moderate temperature and long day length (Stewart & McDougall, 2014). The biggest producers are Russia, Canada, Poland, and the Nordic countries (Faostat, 2014). Oat is robust and can tolerate wet weather and acidic soils relatively well. It is more resistant to plant diseases than other cereals, and can outgrow most weeds. Hence, oat requires lower agro-chemical and fertilizer inputs. This results in lower production costs and environmental burden. Oat also fits well in organic farming systems (Givens, Davies, & Laverick, 2004; Krimpen, van Bikker, Meer, van der Peet-Schwering, & van der Vereijken, 2013). The yield per hectare is 3–5 tonnes under European conditions. With 12–15% protein in the whole oat grain with hulls, this translates to a protein yield of 0.4–0.75 t/ha. Rapeseed and sunflower have similar yields, but legumes can produce up to 1.2 t/ha. Breeding for high yield, as has been done for wheat, could greatly increase the yield of oat (Krimpen et al., 2013). Oat prices in the biggest producer countries range from 162 to 166 USD/ton in Poland, Finland, and Canada, while Russian oat costs 132 USD/ton (Faostat, 2014).

6.2.2 Water Use

With 70% of the drinkable water on earth being used for agriculture, water will be an ever-increasing issue in food production (IWMI, 2007). The impact of water consumption during whole life cycles in food production, including water pollution, is critical for water conservation. The total water usage consists of green water, the natural water from precipitation and evapotranspiration, blue water, the fresh surface or ground water used for irrigation and processing, and gray water, the polluted water (Lindhol, 2012). According to an estimate, the global average green water footprint is 1479 m^3/ton for oat, and 1277 m^3/ton for wheat. When looking at the total water footprint, wheat has a slightly higher value with 1827 m^3/ton, when compared to oat with 1788 m^3/ton. Subsequent processing naturally influences the outcome: oat groats and flakes have a higher water footprint than wheat flour, bread, or pasta (Mekonnen & Hoekstra, 2011).

6.2.3 Energy Use

The composition of cereals can vary considerably between cultivars and due to different environmental factors. Protein is the most variable macronutrient, and can range from 11% to 24.5% in oat groats (Lásztity, 1998; Welch, 2011). Protein content is about equally influenced by environment and genotype (Doehlert, McMullen, & Hammond, 2001). Increased nitrogen supply as fertilizer increases the protein content and yield of oat, but otherwise higher protein content is related to lower yield (Doehlert, 2008; Redaelli et al., 2015; Welch, 2011). Environmental factors that influence yield also affect the protein content, for example, good water availability gives high yield but the grains have lower protein content (Welch, 2011).

Amino acid composition may vary with protein concentration, as higher protein content is generally linked to a relative increase of a certain protein fraction. In *Triticeae* cereals, the content of the prolamin fraction tends to increase when total protein content increases, which results in a poorer amino acid composition and nutritional quality. In oat on the other hand, mainly the globulin fraction increases with the total protein (Welch, 2011). Unlike in most cereals, the amino acid composition is not extensively altered by increased protein content, but slight decreases have been found in lysine, glycine, and alanine (Eppendorfer, 1977; Lásztity, 1998). Small differences in amino acid profiles do not greatly influence the nutritional value of oat proteins (Hischke, Potter, & Graham, 1968).

On a mass basis, the production of plant foods emits less greenhouse gases (GHG), and requires less land than animal-derived foods, but the varying nutritional profiles of foods complicate the comparison. González et al. (2011) related the amount of protein to the energy used in production and transport as well as related GHG emission. Per kg of carbon dioxide equivalent (CO_2-eq), 359 g domestic oat could be produced and transported. For comparison, the corresponding figures were 505 g for soybean and 31 g for milk protein.

6.2.4 Health Aspects of Oats

Oat is a nutritious grain, and besides protein, its soluble dietary fiber (β-glucan), lipids, vitamins, and antioxidants, as well as certain phytochemicals like avenanthramides, have been subject to many studies in relation to their potential health effects, as reviewed by Clemens and van Klinken (2014) and Sadiq Butt et al. (2008). Oat grain is also special in its suitability in the gluten-free diet of most celiac patients. Oat offers a nutritious source of plant protein, in addition to dietary fiber and associated phytochemicals which are often lacking in a gluten-free diet, and diversifies the range of cereal products in the diet (Pawlowska et al., 2013; Lee et al., 2009). The cholesterol-lowering effects of oat β-glucan have gained a great deal of interest and an array of human studies, leading to accepted health claims both in the US and in Europe. β-Glucans of oats can also be linked to health claims about glycemic control. Consumption of whole-grain cereals, such as whole-grain oat and flakes, has been shown in epidemiological studies to be associated with decreased risk of chronic diseases, such as type 2 diabetes and cardiovascular diseases, and also total mortality (Wu et al., 2015).

6.3 LOCALIZATION AND STRUCTURE OF OAT PROTEINS

6.3.1 Protein in the Oat Grain

Oat groat, the kernel after hull removal, contains 15–20% protein. Its content increases from the interior of the grain to the periphery: the starchy endosperm contains approximately 12% protein, while the bran (pericarp, testa, nucellus, aleurone, and some subaleurone) contains 18–26%, and the germ as much as 29–38% (Lásztity, 1998; Miller & Fulcher, 2011; Youngs, 1972). The distribution can be seen in Fig. 6.1, where protein is stained brownish red (gray in print versions).

The protein is deposited in protein bodies that range from 0.3 to 5 μm in diameter, the larger being more abundant in the subaleurone (Bechtel & Pomeranz, 1981; Miller & Fulcher, 2011). Unlike the *Triticeae* cereals (barley, rye, wheat) that mainly contain alcohol-soluble prolamins, the major oat storage proteins (70–80%) are salt-soluble globulins (Lásztity, 1998). The prolamin fraction present in oat, avenins, comprises merely 4–15% of the total protein. The 7S globulins are mainly located in the embryo, while 12S globulins and avenins are found in the endosperm (Burgess & Miflin, 1985; Draper, 1973). The globulin-to-avenin ratio is 26:1 on a mass basis (Boyer, Shotwell, & Larkins, 1992). Oat protein fractions and some of their properties are listed in Table 6.1.

6.3.2 Oat Protein Fractions

6.3.2.1 Oat Globulins

The major storage proteins in oat are salt-soluble globulins. From the total globulins, three fractions with sedimentation coefficients of 3S, 7S, and 12S have been identified (Shotwell, 1999). The 12S globulin is structurally similar to 11S globulins found in many dicotyledonous seeds—it is a 320-kDa hexamer that consists of subunits of 54 kDa held together by noncovalent interactions (Burgess, Shewry, Matlashewski, Aaltosaar, & Miflin, 1983; Casey, 1999; Shotwell, Afonso, Davies, Chesnut, & Larkins, 1988). These subunits consist of acidic (32 kDa) and basic (22 kDa) chains that are disulfide-bound (Burgess et al., 1983). The crystalline structure of 12S globulins has not been reported, but the organization of the subunits in the hexamer is presumed to be similar to relatively well-characterized soy

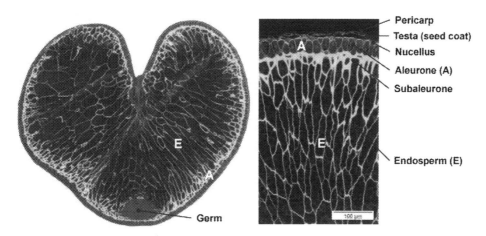

FIGURE 6.1 Cross-section of the oat grain. *Image courtesy of Dr. Ulla Holopainen-Mantila, VTT.*

TABLE 6.1 Oat Protein Fractions According to Osborne Protein Solubility (Klose & Arendt, 2012; Lásztity, 1998; Ma & Harwalkar, 1984; Peterson, 2011)

Osborne Class[a]	Protein (Function)	MW (kDa)	% of Protein[b]	pI
Globulins	12S (storage)	53–58	70–80	ca. 5.0
	α-Polypeptide	32–37	–	5.5
	β-Polypeptide	22–24	–	8.0–10.0
	7S (storage)	50–70	–	–
	3S (storage)	48–52	–	–
Prolamins	Avenins	17–34	4–14	5.0–9.0
Albumins	Various (metabolic)	14–17, 20–27, 36–47	1–12	4.0–7.5
Glutelins	Unextracted globulins and prolamins, minor polypetides	–	<10	–

[a]Albumins—water; globulins—salt; prolamins—aqueous ethanol; glutelins—dilute acid or alkali.
[b]Shows wide differences depending on the cultivar, growth conditions, and extraction method.

glycinins and other 11S globulins. The reported crystalline structure of soy glycinin is face-to-face stacking of two trigonal trimers forming the homohexamer (Adachi et al., 2003). The shape of the 12S oat globulin was predicted to be an oblate cylinder with a height of 8.5 nm using quasielastic light scattering. The cylinder is formed from two annular trimeric ring with diameters of 11.8 nm stacked on top of each other (Zhao, Mine, & Ma, 2004). A similar size was also obtained by atomic force microscopy; the particle size of dissolved oat protein isolate (OPI) that mainly consists of the 12S globulin ranges from 12 to 15 nm, depending on the concentration (Liu et al., 2009).

The tertiary structure of globulin is sensitive to alterations in pH and ionic strength that alter the association/dissociation behavior of the subunits (Marcone, 1999). Native 11S globulins are conformationally most stable at pH 6–9, where they exist as hexamers (Marcone, 1999; Molina, Petruccelli, & Añón, 2004). At acidic pH, they can lose their tertiary structure (Marcone, Yada, & Kakuda, 1997). Globulins from dicotyledonous plants undergo subunit dissociation at alkaline pH due to electrostatic repulsion between subunits, while oat and other monocotyledonous globulins do not show this behavior. Monocotyledonous globulins may have stronger forces holding the subunits together, or possess less acidic amino acid residues, aspartic (Asp) or glutamic acid (Glu) between the subunits, that would ionize at alkaline pH (Marcone, Kakuda, & Yada, 1998). In fact, heliathinin, the 11S globulin from sunflower seed (*Helianthus annuus*) that has a lower content of Asp and Glu, dissociates only partially into trimers at alkaline pH (Molina et al., 2004). Oat globulin contains even less Asp and Glu, which may explain its structural stability at high pH.

Oat globulin has a thermal denaturation temperature of 110°C, that is clearly higher than, for example, those of soy glycinin (91.5°C) and helianthinin (99.7°C) (Harwalkar & Ma, 1987; Molina et al., 2004). Compared to other proteins, globulins generally exhibit high denaturation temperatures. This may be caused by strong hydrophobic interactions between subunits that strengthen at higher temperatures (Gorinstein et al., 1996). For example, the difference between oat globulin and soy glycinin may be caused by differences in secondary and tertiary structures, charge, and surface hydrophobicity (Marcone, 1999). As a result of heating of oat globulins, partial denaturation, dissociation into subunits, formation of soluble aggregates followed by formation of large insoluble aggregates occur, depending on the extent of thermal treatment (Zhao et al., 2004).

The secondary structure of the 12S globulin has been reported to consist mainly of β-sheets (74%), followed by α-helices (19%) and β-turns (7%), as determined using FT-IR (Liu et al., 2009). A circular dichroism spectroscopy study also showed β-sheet as the dominant secondary structure with low α-helix content for oat globulin and another 21 seed globulin samples from similar plants (Marcone et al., 1997, 1998). Marcone (1999) has observed pH-induced changes in the secondary structure. Specifically, a transition from β-sheet structure at neutral pH to a random coil structure at acidic (pH 3) and alkaline (9–11) pH has been observed.

6.3.2.2 Oat Prolamins

Oat prolamins (avenins) belong to the sulfur-rich prolamins and contain high amounts of glutamic acid and glutamine, are low in proline compared to the prolamins of *Triticeae*, and are absent of tryptophan (Klose & Arendt, 2012; Shewry, 1999). Avenins can be extracted with 70% (v/v) ethanol without the reduction of disulfide bonds (Lásztity, 1998). In the oat grain, prolamin inclusions are present within a globulin matrix in the endosperm but not in the aleurone layer (Klose & Arendt, 2012; Lending, Chesnut, Shaw, & Larkins, 1989; Shewry, Napier, & Tatham, 1995). Avenins are polymorphic and consist of proteins with molecular weight between 20 and 30 kDa (group 2) and between 30 and 40 kDa (group 1). Also, a minor amount of lower-molecular-weight proteins may be present, but these differ from typical prolamins in terms of amino acid composition, and may in fact be enzyme inhibitors (Shewry, 1999).

Avenins contain four cysteine residues that form four intrachain disulfide bonds. Avenins are expected to have a conformation similar to the *Triticeae* prolamins: the nonrepetitive sequences are α-helix-rich globular structures, and proline-rich repeats found as two separate blocks, form β-reverse turns. Typically, prolamins contain low amounts of charged amino acid residues, resulting in a protein with a low net charge at any pH (Shewry, Tatham, & Halford, 1999).

6.3.2.3 Minor Protein Fractions

Proteins found in the oat grain in minor amounts include metabolically active proteins, mainly enzymes, proteinase inhibitors, and some structural proteins. Among the enzymes, the presence of proteases, maltase, α-amylase, lichenase, phenoxyacetic acid hydroxylase, phosphatase, tyrosinase, and lipases has been detected (Klose & Arendt, 2012; Lásztity, 1998). Proteinase inhibitors that are considered to be antinutrients are found in many oats, although at lower levels than many other seeds (Klose & Arendt, 2012). Albumins contain high levels of lysine, and the lowest levels of glutamine-glutamic acid among the other oat protein fractions.

Some proteins that are found in very small quantities, but have interesting roles, include oleosins and tryptophanins. Oleosins are 16-kDa proteins found on the surface of oil bodies that prevent the oil bodies from coalescing. Oleosin content in the oat endosperm is much lower than in the embryo, which leads to merging of lipid bodies, and formation of a fatty matrix around the protein bodies and starch granules (Heneen et al., 2008; Sibakov, 2014). Tryptophanins are similar to puroindolines, the grain softness proteins of wheat. They are basic, cysteine-rich proteins with a molecular weight of 14–16 kDa that also have a tryptophan-rich domain. The function of these proteins is unclear, but they have been suggested to be a part of the plant defense mechanism as a membrane-active toxin (Heneen et al., 2008; Tanchak, Schernthaner, Giband, & Altosaar, 1998). Tryptophanins appear to be highly concentrated in oat foams, and can be considered as an important surface-active component in oat (Kaukonen et al., 2011).

6.3.3 Nutritional Properties and Suitability for Celiac Patients

The most abundant amino acid in oat protein is glutamine-glutamic acid, that comprises nearly 25% of the total amino acid residues, followed by aspartic acid and leucine with 8.9% and 7.4%, respectively (Peterson, 2011). The different composition of oat protein compared to the *Triticeae* cereals is reflected as a proline content of 4.7%, less than half of that of wheat, barley, and rye. Oat contains more lysine, the first limiting amino acid in cereals other than the *Triticeae* (McKevith, 2004). Lysine is most abundant in the water-soluble albumin fraction. The lysine content is still lower than the FAO amino acid scoring pattern requirements for infants (Pedó, Sgarbieri, & Gutkoski, 1999; Peterson, 2011) (Table 6.2). Sulfur-containing amino acid and tryptophan contents are above the FAO pattern, making oat a good complementary protein source to legumes that are limiting in methionine. The storage globulins in many seeds are allergenic, but the only reported allergen in oat is avenin (Sathe, Kshirsagar, & Roux, 2005). Oat allergy is rare and limited to infancy (Gilissen, van der Meer, & Smulders, 2014; Sicherer & Sampson, 2010). Sensitization to oat proteins in topical creams can occur in young children with atopic dermatitis (Boussault et al., 2007).

The nutritional quality of proteins depends on their digestibility and amino acid profile. Several methods exist for the evaluation of the quality, including the in vivo method, protein efficiency ratio (PER), and amino acid chemical score based on comparison to a reference protein (Friedman, 1996). The method currently preferred by WHO/FAO is the protein digestibility-corrected amino acid score (PDCAAS), which compares the concentration of the first limiting amino acid to a reference pattern that is corrected for the digestibility (Schaafsma, 2000). The nutritional quality of plant proteins is generally lower than that of animal foods, but it also varies greatly within different plant foods. Oat PER values based on the weight gain of an experimental animal have been comparable to those of soy protein. Oat protein also has a high digestibility (Hischke et al., 1968; Stewart, Hensley, & Peters, 1943). Nevertheless, the reported PDCAAS values have been very low (45–51), while soy has values close to animal proteins (Table 6.2).

TABLE 6.2 Essential Amino Acids in Oat, Soy, and Casein Compared to the FAO Amino Acid Scoring Pattern Requirements (g/100 g), and Digestibility-Corrected Amino Acid Score (PCDAAS; Nontruncated Values), Digestibility, and Protein Efficiency Ratio (PER)

	Oat[a]	Wheat[b]	Soy[c]	Milk Protein[d]	FAO, Infant
Histidine	2.1–2.9	2.4	2.6	3.2	2.0
Isoleucine	3.8–4.1	2.7	4.9	5.0	3.2
Leucine	7.4–7.7	6.9	8.2	9.4	6.6
Lysine	4.1–4.5	2.4	6.3	7.6	5.7
Threonine	3.3–3.7	3.0	3.7	4.0	3.1
Tryptophan	0.8–0.9	1.4	1.3	n.r.	0.85
Valine	5.2–5.7	3.9	5.1	6.2	4.3
SAA	4.1[e]	3.5	2.6	3.5	2.7
AAA	8.4[e]	7.4	9.1	10.2	5.2
PDCAAS (%)	45–51[e]; 60[f]	42[e]; 37[f]	91–93[f,g]	112–120[f,g]	–
PER	2.3[h]	1.5[g]	0.46; 2.28[g]	3.1[g]	–
Digestibility (%)	>90[i]; 85[e]	77, 91[g]	95[g]	95[g]	–

[a]Pettersson et al. (1996).
[b]Abdel-Aal and Hucl (2002).
[c]Hughes et al. (2011).
[d]Rutherfurd and Moughan (1998).
[e]Pedó et al. (1999).
[f]Michaelsen et al. (2009).
[g]Schaafsma (2000).
[h]Hischke et al. (1968).
[i]Eggum and Gullord (1983).
Values in italics indicate heat-treated protein

It has been suggested that the PDCAAS method overestimates the nutritive value of casein in milk (Pedó et al., 1999). The bioavailability of threonine from oat is poor compared to other amino acids (Tang, Laudick, & Benton, 1958). Supplementation of the diet with lysine, methionine, and threonine is needed to obtain a growth rate equal to casein.

Celiac disease is an autoimmune condition with a worldwide prevalence of 1%. The condition is triggered in genetically susceptible individuals by the ingestion of cereal prolamins, and leads to mucosal inflammation in the small intestine, crypt hyperplasia, villous atrophy, and other symptoms. The immunotoxicity is suggested to originate from proline- and glutamine-rich peptide segments in partially digested prolamins, but other harmful sequences may exists (Catassi & Fasano, 2008; Qiao et al., 2004; Shan et al., 2002). The prevalence of the condition has increased in the past decade (Ludvigsson et al., 2013). Also, the gluten-free diet, the only treatment for celiac disease, has also become popular for nonceliac individuals. This trend has led to a massive and still ongoing growth of the market for gluten-free products.[1]

Oat is not only low in prolamins, but avenins contain less proline and glutamine than wheat, rye, and barley (Comino et al., 2011). In the past 20 years, a growing body of evidence has shown that oat can be tolerated by the majority of people with celiac disease at least in limited quantities (Hoffenberg et al., 2000; Janatuinen et al., 1995; Lundin, 2003; Rashid et al., 2007; Størsrud et al., 2003). The inclusion of oat products in the diet is recommended by many national celiac associations to bring variety and nutrition to gluten-free diets (Koerner et al., 2011; Peräaho et al., 2004). Regular oat is however nearly always contaminated with other cereals originating from other cereals in the fields, or from processing and storage facilities (Koerner et al., 2011). Oat from a gluten-free supply chain is marketed as "pure oats" in several countries. It has been suggested that varieties may vary in their toxicity for some celiac individuals unable to tolerate oat, and immunological screening of varieties could be utilized to find even safer oats (Comino et al., 2011).

---

1. http://www.foodnavigator-usa.com/Markets/Sales-of-gluten-free-products-will-continue-to-grow-double-digits/.

6.4 MANUFACTURE OF OAT PROTEIN ISOLATES AND CONCENTRATES

Protein-rich ingredients can be produced by enriching or isolating protein from the raw material. An established method for producing plant protein isolates is water or alkali extraction, followed by isoelectric precipitation or membrane filtration and drying (Mondor et al., 2009; Schutyser & van der Goot, 2011). The resulting isolate is high in protein (>80%), but the process requires a lot of water and energy, especially for the mixing and drying steps. Dry fractionation by milling and air classification produces concentrates with 30–60% protein, but the energy requirements are a lot lower. For example, the dry fractionation of wheat gluten-enriched flours requires 2 MJ/kg protein, while only the drying process of the wet process requires 14 MJ/kg protein (Schutyser & van der Goot, 2011).

In addition to laboratory-scale processes, oat protein production has been developed to an industrial scale in Finland (Kaukovirta-Norja, Myllymäki, Aro, Hietaniemi, & Pihlava, 2008) and Sweden. The process first commercialized by Biovelop in Sweden to produce an oat concentrate is now operated by Tate & Lyle (London, UK). In 2015, Fazer Group (Lahti, Finland) launched a series of oat ingredients, including a low-fat protein concentrate.[2] Low-fat content improves the shelf-life of oat protein products, as the presence of oat lipids can cause rancidity challenges.

6.4.1 Wet Methods

In wet methods the protein is extracted in liquid, separated by isoelectric precipitation or membrane filtration, and dried. Most of the scientific literature on this process is on laboratory-scale protein isolation (Guan, Yao, Chen, Shan, & Zhang, 2007; Ma & Harwalkar, 1984; Ma, Harwalkar, & Paquet, 1990; Wu, Sexson, Cluskey, & Inglett, 1977). The extraction liquid can be water, alkaline, or saline. Although salt extraction is a milder procedure compared to alkaline extraction, alkaline extraction (pH >9.5) gives the best yield. Moreover, alkaline-extracted OPIs showed better amino acid profile and comparable or even better functionality compared to salt extracts (Ma, 1983). A (near) complete extraction of the protein can only be accomplished using alkaline buffers containing detergents and reducing agents (Shotwell, 1999). The ratio of different proteins is influenced by the extraction method and medium. The content of globulins can be improved by increasing the ionic strength of the solvent: the highest amount of globulins can be extracted in 1 M NaCl at pH 8.5 (Lásztity, 1998). Alkaline treatments may alter the functional and nutritional properties of proteins (eg, as a result of amino acid racemization, peptide chain fragmentation, thiol oxidation, and β-elimination reaction) (Whitaker, Feeney, & Sternberg, 2009). Ma et al. (1990) tested the influence of alkaline treatment at a moderate temperature (pH 9.7, up to 96 h at 50°C) on the racemization of amino acid, but found no significant racemization of any amino acids (Ma et al., 1990). Also, the drying step can denature and aggregate proteins, leading to losses in solubility.

In the 1970s, industrial-scale wet milling processes were developed for the production of oat protein concentrates (OPCs), based on alkaline extraction of the defatted ground oat groats (Bell, Boocock, & Oughton, 1978; Cluskey, Wu, Wall, & Inglett, 1973; Hohner & Hyldon, 1975). After extraction at pH 9–11, the alkaline solutions were acidified and the protein concentrate recovered. More recently, Liu (2014) developed a process where β-glucan was first extracted from defatted oats with water, and protein, starch, and residual fiber were then fractionated using alkaline extraction. Protein contents of over 90% were obtained in this fractionation scheme.

The wet extraction yield can be improved by enzyme processing. Enzymatic pretreatment has been shown to be useful in the extraction of protein from oat bran (Guan et al., 2007; Liu, Guan, Zhu, & Sun, 2008). Defatted oat bran was hydrolyzed using a commercial enzyme mixture (Viscozyme L, containing β-glucanase activity) prior to extraction with 2 M NaOH at pH 9.5. The treatment increased protein extraction yield to 56.2% of the total protein as compared to the alkaline method without enzyme (14.8%) (Liu et al., 2009).

6.4.2 Dry Methods

In addition to conventional wet fractionation methods, dry fractionation has been applied for production of OPCs. Dry fractionation is typically based on milling fractionation. Development of milling technologies and use of air classification, where separation of different fractions is based on differences in density of particles, has led to better separation efficiency as reviewed recently for production of legume protein concentrates by Schutyser and van der Goot (2011). Another dry fractionation platform, based on milling and electrostatic separation, was reviewed by Barakat, Jérôme, & Rouau (2015). Here separation is based on charging by tribo-electricity and further by passing through high-voltage

---

2. http://www.bakervandsnacks.com/Ingredients/Fazer-secures-oat-extraction-license-from-VTT/.

electrodes (10,000 V), where the positively charged particles are separated from the negatively charged particles. Dry fractionation methods are usually economically more feasible than wet methods, as they avoid the need for energy-intensive drying steps. Dry fractionation also often results in better yields but only partial purification or enrichment, which often may be sufficient for food applications.

In the early work by Wu, Sexson, Cavins, and Inglett (1972), oats were dry-milled to conventional grain fractions, where the shorts and bran fractions had about double the protein content of whole oats. Protein and starch in oats are linked to lipids, which have been shown to be concentrated in subaleurone and endosperm in the vicinity of scutellum and embryo (Heneen et al., 2009). Removal of lipids can thus enable more efficient separation of the major oat components in dry fractionation (Knuckles, Chiu, & Betschart, 1992; Wu & Doehlert, 2002; Wu & Stringfellow, 1995) as compared to methods without lipid removal (Lehtomäki & Myllymäki, 2010; Mälkki, Myllymäki, Teinilä, & Koponen, 2001). Already in 1995 it was pointed out that air classification of defatted ground oats may have commercial potential for producing protein concentrate and enriched β-glucan fraction in a single process (Wu & Stringfellow, 1995). Hexane was used for lipid removal, and the combined fine fractions obtained contained about 30% protein, accounting for about 30% of the protein in the starting material.

In later work, removal of lipids from nonheat-treated oats by supercritical carbon dioxide (SC-CO_2) facilitated milling and air classification of oat to fractions enriched with starch, protein, and β-glucan (Kaukovirta-Norja et al., 2008; Sibakov et al., 2011). The protein content in the fine fraction after the third air classification step was 73% with a mass yield of 5%. When the mass yield was increased to 14.4%, the protein content of the corresponding fraction was 49.3% (Sibakov et al., 2011). The major nonprotein material in the fractions was starch.

6.5 FUNCTIONALITY AND POTENTIAL USES

6.5.1 Functional Characteristics of Oat Protein

The solubility dependence of oat protein is similar to other plant globulins, but oat protein generally has a lower solubility. It is especially limited around neutral or slightly acidic pH, which is the typical pH range for most food products. Solubility is critical for use of protein in food applications, as soluble proteins provide homogeneous dispersability in colloidal systems and enhance the interfacial properties. In accordance with solubility, foaming and emulsifying properties of OPIs were generally found to be low, at the pH range 4–7 (Ma, 1984). This restricts the use of plant proteins in food applications (Day, 2013).

The functional properties of proteins are based on their molecular size, structure (primary amino acid sequences, secondary and tertiary conformations), and the charge distribution, as well as the way in which proteins interact with carbohydrates, lipids and proteins, and small food components. Important functional properties of protein in foods include solubility, water- and fat-binding capacities, gel forming and rheological behaviors, emulsifying and foaming properties. As pointed out by Day (2013), apart from the dough properties of gluten, the physical and functional properties of plant proteins have not been studied as extensively as those from animal origin. It was suggested that one reason might lie in their presence as mixtures, and purified protein fractions have rarely been available for studies of functionality.

When exploring the literature on plant protein functionality, it should be kept in mind that the comparison of properties has its challenges, as the protein preparations differ in concentration, the presence of other compounds, and their processing history. OPI extracted from hexane-defatted oat flour has similar emulsifying capacity to that of soy protein isolate, but weaker emulsion stability (Wu et al., 1977). Mohamed, Biresaw, Xu, Hojilla-Evangelista, and Rayas-Duarte (2009) reported that protein in defatted oat flour produced very stable emulsions, and according to Heywood, Myers, Bailey, and Johnson (2002) attained nearly twice the emulsion activity index (EAI) of low-fat soy flour samples. Alkali-extracted OPI dispersed at pH 7 showed similar foaming capacity but twice higher foam stability compared to lupin protein isolate, whereas when compared with soy protein isolate it produced 30% less foam volume and significantly decreased foam stability (Mohamed et al., 2009). Alkali-extracted OPI dispersed at pH 7 showed 30% higher EAI value than acid-precipitated lupin protein, indicating superior emulsifying capacity. Firm gels can be formed at alkaline pH (pH 10) and high-temperature treatments around 90–100°C due to partial denaturation and proteolysis under alkaline pH (Ma et al., 1990; Ma, Rout, & Phillips, 2003; Mohamed et al., 2004).

The solubility difference between oat globulins and soy glycinins has been attributed partly to surface properties. Differently from all other seed-storage globulins and rice protein, oat globulin contains glutamine-rich repeats of eight amino acids near the C-terminus of the acidic polypeptide (in soy glycinin this region consists of acidic residues with different lengths). This region is located at the surface of the globulin, exposed to solvent, and renders oat globulins less hydrophilic compared to other globulins and partly explains the higher salt concentrations needed for oat globulin solubility (Shotwell et al., 1988).

The solubility and functional properties of proteins can be altered by hydrolysis and modification of amino acid residues. Amino acid modifications change the net charge and hydrophilicity of the protein, leading to changes in solubility, viscosity, and surface properties. Some of these modifications can be done enzymatically but acylation, an efficient way of altering the isoelectric point (pI) and functionality profiles, can only be carried out chemically. Acylation with acetic and succinic anhydride has been studied in a variety of food proteins, including oat. The reagents can react with all nucleophilic groups, but the ε-amino group of lysine is most readily acylated (Schwenke, 1997). Acetylation renders basic groups into neutral ones, but succinylation changes the positive charge to a negative charge. Both modifications render the net charge toward negative, leading to conformational changes and in the case of oligomeric plant proteins, subunit dissociation (Ma, 1984; Schwenke, 1997). The solubility, emulsifying properties, and fat-binding capacity of OPIs have been shown to improve by acylation (Ma, 1984). The effects are more pronounced with succinylation than acetylation (Ma, 1984; Schwenke, 1997). The introduction of more negatively charged groups results in increased electrostatic repulsion that efficiently prevents protein—protein interactions that lead to the loss of solubility and emulsion coalescence (Mirmoghtadaie, Kadivar, & Shahedi, 2009). Although the benefits of acylation are clear in terms of functionality, it has been shown to decrease the bioavailability of lysine in mice (Friedman & Gumbmann, 1981).

The conversion of amide groups of glutamine and asparagine residues into carboxyl groups by deamidation can greatly improve the functional properties of proteins, even at a low level of modification. This modification increases the negative charge of the protein, and leads to changes in conformation changes including the exposure of hydrophobic residues and increased disordered structures (Wong, Choi, Phillips, & Ma, 2009). Deamidated oat proteins show higher solubility, emulsifying activity, and emulsion stability, and altered structure-forming behavior (Jiang et al., 2015; Ma & Khanzada, 1987; Mirmoghtadaie et al., 2009). Deamidation can be done chemically by mild acid or alkaline treatments, physically with dry heat or enzymatically (Mirmoghtadaie et al., 2009; Wong et al., 2009; Yamaguchi & Yokoe, 2000). Protein deamidases have been found in germinating seeds and some microorganisms (Vaintraub, Kotova, & Shaha, 1992; Yamaguchi & Yokoe, 2000). Currently, the only deamidase that is produced industrially for food use is purified from *Chryseobacterium proteolyticum* (Jiang et al., 2015; Yamaguchi & Yokoe, 2000). Transglutaminase and some proteases can partially deamidate proteins under certain conditions: papain, chymotrypsin, and pronase (a commercial mixture from *Streptomyces griseus*) have been shown to deamidate a range of food proteins at alkaline pH and low temperature, where very limited proteolysis occurs (Kato, Tanaka, Matsudomi, & Kobayashi, 1987). Also transglutaminase, a protein crosslinking enzyme, can function as a deamidating enzyme at high enzyme-to-substrate ratios. Transglutaminase catalyzes the formation of an isopeptide linkage between a glutamine and the amino group of protein-bound lysine. In the absence of a lysine residue, water can serve as an acyl acceptor, leading to deamidation of the glutamine residue (Ercili-Cura et al., 2015; Griffin, Casadio, & Bergamini, 2002). In the case of transglutaminase-treated oat and faba protein isolates, the net charge increased as a function of transglutaminase dosage (Ercili-Cura et al., 2015; Nivala et al., 2016).

Limited hydrolysis can improve the solubility and especially the foaming activity of proteins (Guan et al., 2007; Ma & Khanzada, 1987). This, however, decreases the foam stability. When oat flour was hydrolyzed with commercial enzymes, Alcalase and Neutrase, proteolysis was shown to decrease the emulsion stability and fat-binding capacity, but the water hydration capacity increases with increasing degree of hydrolysis (Ponnampalam, Goulet, Amiot, & Brisson, 1987). Hydrolysis of oat bran protein concentrate with trypsin increased the solubility, water-holding capacities emulsifying activity, and foaming ability (Guan et al., 2007). Hydrolysis can also influence the structure-forming properties of proteins. Nieto-Nieto, Wang, Ozimek, and Chen (2014) hydrolyzed OPI using trypsin or Flavourzyme (a peptidase mixture from *Aspergillus oryzae*) (Merz et al., 2015), and prepared heat-set gels with the treated protein. The resulting gels were mechanically comparable or stronger than egg white gels when prepared at pH 5–7.

Lipids found in oat flour or OPIs or concentrates affect their foaming properties greatly. Kaukonen et al. (2011) showed that water extracts from supercritical CO_2 defatted oat flour contained only polar lipids and free fatty acids (FFA). Those extracts provided good foaming properties but addition of nonpolar lipids to the extract had a detrimental effect. Thus, foaming capacity is strongly affected by lipid composition of the oat flour used (Kaukonen et al., 2011). Such impurities in OPCs or isolates and various different extraction, preparation conditions, or environmental conditions (pH, ionic strength, etc.) used in published studies make it extremely challenging to make conclusive judgments and comparisons regarding the functional properties of oat proteins. However, according to the above-mentioned studies on functional properties of oat proteins, it is evident that the main limiting factor for their use in food systems is their low solubility at low and neutral pH. Modifications, especially enzymatic ones, can however improve the functionality and widen the applicability of oat proteins.

6.5.2 Applications of Oat Protein

The challenge in using oat and other plant protein ingredients for the manufacture of protein-rich foods is to accomplish the desired technical, sensory, and nutritional quality. Cereal and dairy foods are an important target for plant protein enrichment. Bread, pasta, or yogurt contain only 5–13% protein. In order to have a "source of protein" or "high-protein" claims in the EU, food products must have 12% or 20% of the energy content from proteins, respectively (EU Commission, 2006).

6.5.2.1 Baked Products

Baked products are an obvious application for oat and oat protein. The extraction method of oat proteins can influence baking properties due to protein denaturation occurring as a result of intensive heat treatment. Baking with 100% oat is challenging due to high β-glucan content and lack of viscoelastic properties of gluten. There are only a few reports on the physical and sensory properties of gluten-free oat breads (Flander, Holopainen, Kruus, & Buchert, 2011; Hager, Bosmans, & Delcour, 2014; Hüttner et al., 2011; Kim & Yokoyama, 2011). These breads were mainly starch-based and had quite low protein content. While improving the nutritional value and amino acid balance, protein incorporation in bread might alter the quality of crumb structure (Houben, Höchstötter, & Becker, 2012). OPC or isolate has been used as a part of a wheat-based formulation in some studies (D'Appolonia & Youngs, 1978; Lapveteläinen, 1994; Ma, 1983; Pastuszka et al., 2012). Addition of high-protein oat flour (51.6% protein, 28.0% fat) at levels of 3% and 6% of total flour weight (12% protein) increased the loaf volume of wheat bread (Lapveteläinen, 1994). More than 5% addition of OPI to wheat flour significantly lowered the volume and increased hardness and chewiness (Pastuszka et al., 2012). A recent study focused on gluten-free high-protein oat bread, which contained as high as 35% OPC of flour weight (Rekola, 2015). Increasing the amount of OPC from 15% to 35% decreased the hardness and chewiness of bread crumb and slowed down the rate of starch retrogradation. However, OPC did not have an effect on the specific loaf volume. Enzymes can be used to improve the baking quality of oat. Crosslinking the protein with laccase in oat flour (9.4% protein content) before baking led to increased loaf volume, decreased crumb hardness and chewiness (Renzetti, Courtin, Delcour, & Arendt, 2010). In contrast, Flander et al. (2011) reported an increase in crumb hardness as a result of laccase treatment due to the formation of phenoxy radicals that formed disulfide bonds between the proteins. Glucose oxidase treatment of oat flour promoted the formation of large protein aggregates due to formation of excessive protein polymerization, which further increased the crumb hardness (Renzetti et al., 2010). Beyond the optimal pH, disproportionate repulsive forces led to fewer protein interactions. Partial hydrolysis of OPI resulted in similar mechanical properties and water-holding capacity to that of egg white (Nieto-Nieto et al., 2014). This could enable the use of OPI as a texturizing and structure-forming ingredient to replace animal proteins.

6.5.2.2 Extruded Products

Extrusion is used to produce snacks and breakfast cereals. Sibakov (2014) utilized various oat bran fractions in extrudates made with defatted oats, mainly in an attempt to increase dietary fiber content. Addition of 10% water-insoluble oat bran concentrate (WIS-OBC) gave 17% protein in the final extrudate, whereas the addition of water-soluble oat bran concentrate (WS-OBC) at the same level gave only 14% protein. However, WIS-OBC had significantly decreased the expansion and increased hardness compared to WS-OBC, which was attributed to the high-protein content and high levels of insoluble dietary fiber.

6.5.2.3 Vegan Products

Plant-based dairy-style products have increased in popularity in the recent years. These include plant "milks," fermented yogurt-type products, thicker cream-like preparations for cooking, and frozen desserts. The protein content of commercial plant milks is significantly lower than of cow's milk (Mäkinen, Wanhalinna, Zannini, & Arendt, 2015). Increasing the solubility of oat protein could enable an increase in the protein content of such products. Oat proteins can heat gel at high concentrations, but they do not form structures upon acidification (Mäkinen, Uniacke-Lowe, O'Mahony, & Arendt, 2015; Mårtensson, Öste, & Holst, 2000; Nieto-Nieto et al., 2014). Loponen, Laine, Sontag-Strohm, and Salovaara (2007) studied the fermentation-induced changes in oat globulins in a lactic acid-fermented oat bran-based yogurt-type product. When fermented, the lowering pH of the yogurt decreases the solubility of oat globulins, which leads to aggregation and loss of solubility. A Finnish start-up has recently launched an oat-based meat analog, "pulled oats." The product consists of oat, faba bean, and pea proteins, and is produced using hydrothermal processing to yield a fibrous texture (Yle, 2016).

It is evident that significant improvements of functional properties, such as solubility, emulsifying, and foaming ability can be achieved by modification of oat proteins. However, systematic studies are lacking regarding the method of modification, resulting changes in structure, and functionality. Moreover, most of the studies have worked with oat flour or isolates, and gained different results due to the varying extraction methods and protein concentrations. The food ingredient market is lacking multifunctional, minimal processed, low-cost plant-based ingredients, where OPCs with tailored functionalities can find applications in the future.

6.6 FUTURE OUTLOOK

Oat protein properties are distinct, and unique among cereal proteins in their suitability for gluten-free products. Like with other plant proteins, food applications are limited by low solubility at neutral and acidic conditions. However, solubility increase by enzymatic proteolysis has been demonstrated, and improvement of functionality has also been achieved with other modifications. Oat protein has nutritionally good amino acid composition. It has also been shown to ameliorate exercise-induced fatigue in mice (Xu et al., 2013), suggesting its use to improve physiological condition.

OPCs have only recently become commercially available, and their properties, especially functionality and stability, are also dependent on the presence of other oat components, particularly lipids. Thus, the future applications of oat protein depend on the availability and type of oat protein-rich ingredients. The content of oat protein in oat brans high in oat β-glucan may range from 17% to 26%, which actually is at the same level or more than their β-glucan content (Sibakov, 2014). This means enrichment with oat protein, in addition to oat dietary fiber, in many oat-bran-enriched foods. Dry fractionation is a sustainable way of producing multifunctional plant protein ingredients, as reviewed by Schutyser et al. (2015), and defatting prior to dry fractionation facilitates separation and leads to more enriched ingredients (Sibakov et al., 2011). Systematic research to elucidate the parameters and to improve functionality of OPCs for new applications is underway. Oat is one of the new plant protein sources to pay attention to with respect to new applications in the coming years.

REFERENCES

Abdel-Aal, E.-S. M., & Hucl, P. (2002). Amino acid composition and in vitro protein digestibility of selected ancient wheats and their end products. *Journal of Food Composition and Analysis, 15*, 737–747.

Adachi, M., Kanamori, J., Masuda, T., Yagasaki, K., Kitamura, K., Mikami, B., & Utsumi, S. (2003). Crystal structure of soybean 11S globulin: Glycinin A3B4 homohexamer. *Proceedings of the National Academy of Sciences, 100*, 7395–7400.

Apaiah, R. K., Linnemann, A. R., & van der Kooi, H. J. (2006). Exergy analysis: A tool to study the sustainability of food supply chains. *Food Research International, 39*, 1–11.

Barakat, A., Jérôme, F., & Rouau, X. (2015). A dry platform for separation of proteins from biomass-containing polysaccharides, lignin, and polyphenols. *ChemSusChem, 8*, 1161–1166.

Bechtel, D. B., & Pomeranz, Y. (1981). Ultrastructural and cytochemistry of mature oat (*Avena sativa* L.) endosperm. The aleurone layer and starchy endosperm. *Cereal Chemistry, 58*, 61–69.

Bell, A., Boocock, J. R. B., & Oughton, R. W. (1978). *Extraction of protein food values from oats*. U.S. Patent 4,089,848.

Boussault, P., Léauté-Labrèze, C., Saubusse, E., Maurice-Tison, S., Perromat, M., Roul, S., ... Boralevi, F. (2007). Oat sensitization in children with atopic dermatitis: Prevalence, risks and associated factors. *Allergy, 62*(11), 1251–1256.

Boyer, S. K., Shotwell, M. A., & Larkins, B. A. (1992). Evidence for the translational control of storage protein gene expression in oat seeds. *The Journal of Biological Chemistry, 267*, 17449–17457.

Burgess, S. R., & Miflin, B. J. (1985). The localization of oat (*Avena sativa* L.) seed globulins in protein bodies. *Journal of Experimental Botany, 36*, 945–954.

Burgess, S. R., Shewry, P. R., Matlashewski, G. J., Aaltosaar, I., & Miflin, B. J. (1983). Characteristics of oat (*Avena sativa* L.) seed globulins. *Journal of Experimental Botany, 34*, 1320–1332.

Casey, R. (1999). Distribution and some properties of seed globulins. In P. R. Shewry, & R. Casey (Eds.), *Seed proteins* (pp. 159–169). Netherlands, Dordrecht: Springer.

Catassi, C., & Fasano, A. (2008). Celiac disease. *Current Opinion in Gastroenterology, 24*, 687.

Clemens, R., & van Klinken, J.-W. (2014). Oats, more than just a whole grain: an introduction. *British Journal of Nutrition, 112*(no. S2), S1–S3.

Cluskey, J. E., Wu, Y. V., Wall, J. S., & Inglett, G. E. (1973). Oat protein concentrates from a wet-milling process: Preparation. *Cereal Chemistry, 50*, 475–481.

Comino, I., Real, A., de Lorenzo, L., Cornell, H., López-Casado, M. Á., Barro, F., ... Sousa, C. (2011). Diversity in oat potential immunogenicity: Basis for the selection of oat varieties with no toxicity in coeliac disease. *Gut, 60*, 915–922.

D'Appolonia, B. L., & Youngs, V.-L. (1978). Effect of bran and high-protein concentrate from oats on dough properties and bread quality. *Cereal Chemistry*, *55*, 736−743.

Day, L. (2013). Proteins from land plants−potential resources for human nutrition and food security. *Trends in Food Science & Technology*, *32*, 25−42.

Doehlert, D. C. (2008). Quality improvement in oat. *Journal of Crop Production*, *5*, 165−189.

Doehlert, D. C., McMullen, M. S., & Hammond, J. J. (2001). Genotypic and environmental effects on grain yield and quality of oat grown in North Dakota. *Crop Science*, *41*, 1066.

Draper, S. R. (1973). Amino acid profiles of chemical and anatomical fractions of oat grains. *Journal of the Science of Food and Agriculture*, *24*, 1241−1250.

Eggum, B. O., & Gullord, M. (1983). The nutritional quality of some oat varieties cultivated in Norway. *Qualitas Plantarum*, *32*, 67−73.

Eppendorfer, W. H. (1977). Nutritive value of oat and rye grain protein as influenced by nitrogen and amino acid composition. *Journal of the Science of Food and Agriculture*, *28*, 152−156.

Ercili-Cura, D., Miyamoto, A., Paananen, A., Yoshii, H., Poutanen, K., & Partanen, R. (2015). Adsorption of oat proteins to air−water interface in relation to their colloidal state. *Food Hydrocolloids*, *44*, 183−190.

EU Commission. (2006). Regulation (EC) No 1924/2006 of the European Parliament and of the Council of 20 December 2006 on nutrition and health claims made on foods. *Official Journal of the European Union* L 404/9 49.

Faostat, F. (2014). *Food and Agricultural Organization of the United Nations*, Rome, Italy.

Flander, L., Holopainen, U., Kruus, K., & Buchert, J. (2011). Effects of tyrosinase and laccase on oat proteins and quality parameters of gluten-free oat breads. *Journal of Agricultural and Food Chemistry*, *59*, 8385−8390.

Friedman, M. (1996). Nutritional value of proteins from different food sources. A review. *Journal of Agricultural and Food Chemistry*, *44*, 6−29.

Friedman, M., & Gumbmann, M. R. (1981). Bioavailability of some lysine derivatives in mice. *The Journal of Nutrition*, *111*(8), 1362−1369.

Gilissen, L. J., van der Meer, I. M., & Smulders, M. J. (2014). Reducing the incidence of allergy and intolerance to cereals. *Journal of Cereal Science*, *59*(3), 337−353.

Givens, D., Davies, T., & Laverick, R. (2004). Effect of variety, nitrogen fertiliser and various agronomic factors on the nutritive value of husked and naked oats grain. *Animal Feed Science and Technology*, *113*(1), 169−181.

González, A. D., Frostell, B., & Carlsson-Kanyama, A. (2011). Protein efficiency per unit energy and per unit greenhouse gas emissions: Potential contribution of diet choices to climate change mitigation. *Food Policy*, *36*, 562−570.

Gorinstein, S., Zemser, M., Friedman, M., Rodrigues, W. A., Martins, P. S., Vello, N. A., ... Paredes-López, O. (1996). Physicochemical characterization of the structural stability of some plant globulins. *Food Chemistry*, *56*, 131−138.

Griffin, M., Casadio, R., & Bergamini, C. (2002). Transglutaminases: Nature's biological glues. *Biochemical Journal*, *368*, 377−396.

Grigg, D. (1995). The pattern of world protein consumption. *Geoforum*, *26*, 1−17.

Guan, X., Yao, H., Chen, Z., Shan, L., & Zhang, M. (2007). Some functional properties of oat bran protein concentrate modified by trypsin. *Food Chemistry*, *101*, 163−170.

Hager, A.-S., Bosmans, G. M., & Delcour, J. A. (2014). Physical and molecular changes during the storage of gluten-free rice and oat bread. *Journal of Agricultural and Food Chemistry*, *62*, 5682−5689.

Harwalkar, V. R., & Ma, C.-Y. (1987). Study of thermal properties of oat globulin by differential scanning calorimetry. *Journal of Food Science*, *52*, 394−398.

Heneen, W. K., Banaś, A., Leonova, S., Carlsson, A. S., Marttila, S., Debski, H., & Stymne, S. (2009). The distribution of oil in the oat grain. *Plant Signaling & Behavior*, *4*, 55−56.

Heneen, W. K., Karlsson, G., Brismar, K., Gummeson, P.-O., Marttila, S., Leonova, S., ... Stymne, S. (2008). Fusion of oil bodies in endosperm of oat grains. *Planta*, *228*, 589−599.

Heywood, A. A., Myers, D. J., Bailey, T. B., & Johnson, L. A. (2002). Functional properties of low-fat soy flour produced by an extrusion-expelling system. *Journal of the American Oil Chemists' Society*, *79*, 1249−1253.

Hischke, H. H., Potter, G. C., & Graham, W. R. (1968). Nutritive value of oat proteins. I. Varietal differences as measured by amino acid analysis and rat growth responses. *Cereal Chemistry*, *45*, 374−378.

Hoffenberg, E. J., Haas, J., Drescher, A., Barnhurst, R., Osberg, I., Bao, F., & Eisenbarth, G. (2000). A trial of oats in children with newly diagnosed celiac disease. *Journal of Pediatrics*, *137*, 361−366.

Hohner, G. A., & Hyldon, R. G. (1975). *Oat groat fractionation process*. Patent US 4028468A.

Houben, A., Höchstötter, A., & Becker, T. (2012). Possibilities to increase the quality in gluten-free bread production: An overview. *European Food Research and Technology*, *235*, 195−208.

Hughes, G. J., Ryan, D. J., Mukherjea, R., & Schasteen, C. S. (2011). Protein digestibility-corrected amino acid scores (PDCAAS) for soy protein isolates and concentrate: Criteria for evaluation. *Journal of Agricultural and Food Chemistry*, *59*, 12707−12712.

Hüttner, E. K., Bello, F. D., Zannini, E., Titze, J., Beuch, S., & Arendt, E. K. (2011). Physicochemical properties of oat varieties and their potential for breadmaking. *Cereal Chemistry*, *88*, 602−608.

IWMI (2007). *Water for food, water for life: A comprehensive assessment of water management in agriculture. IWMI standalone summary*. UK: Earthscan.

Janatuinen, E. K., Pikkarainen, P. H., Kemppainen, T. A., Kosma, V. M., Järvinen, R. M., Uusitupa, M. I., & Julkunen, R. J. (1995). A comparison of diets with and without oats in adults with celiac disease. *The New England Journal of Medicine*, *333*, 1033−1037.

Jiang, Z., Sontag-Strohm, T., Salovaara, H., Sibakov, J., Kanerva, P., & Loponen, J. (2015). Oat protein solubility and emulsion properties improved by enzymatic deamidation. *Journal of Cereal Science, 64*, 126–132.

Kato, A., Tanaka, A., Matsudomi, N., & Kobayashi, K. (1987). Deamidation of food proteins by protease in alkaline pH. *Journal of Agricultural and Food Chemistry, 35*, 224–227.

Kaukonen, O., Sontag-Strohm, T., Salovaara, H., Lampi, A.-M., Sibakov, J., & Loponen, J. (2011). Foaming of differently processed oats: Role of nonpolar lipids and tryptophanin proteins. *Cereal Chemistry, 88*, 239–244.

Kaukovirta-Norja, A., Myllymäki, O., Aro, H., Hietaniemi, V., & Pihlava, J.-M. (2008). *Method for fractionating oat, products thus obtained, and use thereof.* WO Pat. 2008/08096044 A1.

Kim, Y., & Yokoyama, W. H. (2011). Physical and sensory properties of all-barley and all-oat breads with additional hydroxypropyl methylcellulose (HPMC) β-glucan. *Journal of Agricultural and Food Chemistry, 59*, 741–746.

Klose, C., & Arendt, E. K. (2012). Proteins in oats; their synthesis and changes during germination: A review. *Critical Reviews in Food Science and Nutrition, 52*, 629–639.

Knuckles, B. E., Chiu, M. M., & Betschart, A. A. (1992). β-glucan-enriched fractions from laboratory-scale dry milling and sieving of barley and oats. *Cereal Chemistry, 69*, 198–202.

Koerner, T. B., Cléroux, C., Poirier, C., Cantin, I., Alimkulov, A., & Elamparo, H. (2011). Gluten contamination in the Canadian commercial oat supply. *Food Additives & Contaminants, 28*, 705–710.

Krimpen, M. M., van Bikker, P., Meer, I. M., van der Peet-Schwering, C. M. C., & van der Vereijken, J. M. (2013). In U. R. Wageningen (Ed.), *Cultivation, processing and nutritional aspects for pigs and poultry of European protein sources as alternatives for imported soybean products.* Lelystad, The Netherlands: Livestock Research Report 662.

Lapveteläinen, A. (1994). *Barley and oat protein products from wet processes: Food use potential. PhD thesis.* Finland: University of Turku.

Lásztity, R. (1998). Oat grain—A wonderful reservoir of natural nutrients and biologically active substances. *Food Reviews International, 14*, 99–119.

Lee, A. R., Ng, D. L., Dave, E., Ciaccio, E. J., & Green, P. H. R. (2009). The effect of substituting alternative grains in the diet on the nutritional profile of the gluten-free diet. *Journal of Human Nutrition and Dietetics, 22*(4), 359–363.

Lehtomäki, I., & Myllymäki, O. (2010). *New dry-milling method for preparing bran.* WO Pat. 2010/000935.

Lending, C. R., Chesnut, R. S., Shaw, K. L., & Larkins, B. A. (1989). Immunolocalization of avenin and globulin storage proteins in developing endosperm of *Avena sativa* L. *Planta, 178*, 315–324.

Lindhol, T. (2012). *Water footprint assessment for water stewardship in the agri-food sector. MSc thesis.* Sweden: Lund University.

Liu, G., Li, J., Shi, K., Wang, S., Chen, J., Liu, Y., & Huang, Q. (2009). Composition, secondary structure, and self-assembly of oat protein isolate. *Journal of Agricultural and Food Chemistry, 57*, 4552–4558.

Liu, J., Guan, X., Zhu, D., & Sun, J. (2008). Optimization of the enzymatic pretreatment in oat bran protein extraction by particle swarm optimization algorithms for response surface modeling. *LWT - Food Science and Technology, 41*, 1913–1918.

Liu, K. (2014). Fractionation of oats into products enriched with protein, beta-glucan, starch, or other carbohydrates. *Journal of Cereal Science, 60*, 317–322.

Loponen, J., Laine, P., Sontag-Strohm, T., & Salovaara, H. (2007). Behaviour of oat globulins in lactic acid fermentation of oat bran. *European Food Research and Technology, 225*, 105–110.

Ludvigsson, J. F., Rubio-Tapia, A., van Dyke, C. T., Melton, L. J., Zinsmeister, A. R., Lahr, B. D., & Murray, J. A. (2013). Increasing incidence of celiac disease in a North American population. *The American Journal of Gastroenterology, 108*, 818–824.

Lundin, K. E. A. (2003). Oats induced villous atrophy in coeliac disease. *Gut, 52*, 1649–1652.

Ma, C. Y. (1984). Functional properties of acylated oat protein. *Journal of Food Science, 49*, 1128–1131.

Ma, C. Y. (1983). Chemical characterization and functionality assessment of protein concentrates from oats. *Cereal Chemistry, 60*, 36–42.

Ma, C. Y., & Harwalkar, V. R. (1984). Chemical characterization and functionality assessment of oat protein fractions. *Journal of Agricultural and Food Chemistry, 32*, 144–149.

Ma, C. Y., Harwalkar, V. R., & Paquet, A. (1990). Physicochemical properties of alkali-treated oat globulin. *Journal of Agricultural and Food Chemistry, 38*, 1707–1711.

Ma, C.-Y., & Khanzada, G. (1987). Functional properties of deamidated oat protein isolates. *Journal of Food Science, 52*, 1583–1587.

Ma, C.-Y., Rout, M. K., & Phillips, D. L. (2003). Study of thermal aggregation and gelation of oat globulin by Raman spectroscopy. *Journal of Spectroscopy, 17*, 417–428.

Mäkinen, O. E., Uniacke-Lowe, T., O'Mahony, J. A., & Arendt, E. (2015). Physicochemical and acid gelation properties of commercial UHT-treated plant-based milk substitutes and lactose free bovine milk. *Food Chemistry, 168*, 630–638.

Mäkinen, O. E., Wanhalinna, V., Zannini, E., & Arendt, E. K. (2015). Foods for special dietary needs: Non-dairy plant based milk substitutes and fermented dairy type products. *Critical Reviews in Food Science and Nutrition.* In press. <http://dx.doi.org/10.1080/10408398.2012.761950>

Mälkki, Y., Myllymäki, O., Teinilä, K., & Koponen, S. (2001). *A method for preparing an oat product and a foodstuff enriched in the content of beta-glucan.* Patent WO 01/26479 A1.

Marcone, M. F. (1999). Biochemical and biophysical properties of plant storage proteins. *Food Research International, 32*, 79–92.

Marcone, M. F., Kakuda, Y., & Yada, R. Y. (1998). Salt-soluble seed globulins of various dicotyledonous and monocotyledonous plants—I. Isolation/purification and characterization. *Food Chemistry, 62*, 27–47.

Marcone, M. F., Yada, R. Y., & Kakuda, Y. (1997). Evidence for a molten globule state in an oligomeric plant protein. *Food Chemistry, 60*, 623–631.

Mårtensson, O., Öste, R., & Holst, O. (2000). Lactic acid bacteria in an oat-based non-dairy milk substitute: Fermentation characteristics and exopolysaccharide formation. *LWT - Food Science and Technology, 33,* 525–530.

McKevith, B. (2004). Nutritional aspects of cereals. *Nutrition Bulletin, 29,* 111–142.

Mekonnen, M. M., & Hoekstra, A. Y. (2011). The green, blue and grey water footprint of crops and derived crop products. *Hydrology and Earth System Sciences, 15,* 1577–1600.

Merz, M., Eisele, T., Berends, P., Appel, D., Rabe, S., Blank, I., ... Fischer, L. (2015). Flavourzyme, an enzyme preparation with industrial relevance: Automated nine-step purification and partial characterization of eight enzymes. *Journal of Agricultural and Food Chemistry, 63,* 5682–5693.

Michaelsen, K. F., Hoppe, C., Roos, N., Kaestel, P., Stougaard, M., Lauritzen, L., ... Prinzo, Z. W. (2009). *Choice of foods and ingredients for moderately malnourished children 6 months to 5 years of age. WHO/UNICEF/WFP/UNHCR consultation on the management of moderate malnutrition in children under 5 years of age* (pp. S343–S404). Geneva, Switzerland: United Nations University Press, 30 September–3 October, 2008.

Miller, S. S., & Fulcher, R. G. (2011). Microstructure and chemistry of the oat kernel. In F. H. Webster, & P. J. Wood (Eds.), *Oats: Chemistry and technology* (pp. 77–94). St. Paul, MN: American Association of Cereal Chemists, Inc (AACC).

Mirmoghtadaie, L., Kadivar, M., & Shahedi, M. (2009). Effects of succinylation and deamidation on functional properties of oat protein isolate. *Food Chemistry, 114,* 127–131.

Mohamed, A., Biresaw, G., Xu, J., Hojilla-Evangelista, M. P., & Rayas-Duarte, P. (2009). Oats protein isolate: Thermal, rheological, surface and functional properties. *Food Research International, 42,* 107–114.

Mohamed, A., Peterson, S. C., Hojilla-Evangelista, M. P., Sessa, D. J., Rayas-Duarte, P., & Biresaw, G. (2004). Effect of heat treatment and pH on the physicochemical properties of lupin protein. *Journal of the American Oil Chemists' Society, 81,* 1153–1157.

Molina, M. I., Petruccelli, S., & Añón, M. C. (2004). Effect of pH and ionic strength modifications on thermal denaturation of the 11S globulin of sunflower (*Helianthus annuus*). *Journal of Agricultural and Food Chemistry, 52,* 6023–6029.

Mondor, M., Aksay, S., Drolet, H., Roufik, S., Farnworth, E., & Boye, J. I. (2009). Influence of processing on composition and antinutritional factors of chickpea protein concentrates produced by isoelectric precipitation and ultrafiltration. *Innovative Food Science and Emerging Technologies, 10,* 342–347.

Nieto-Nieto, T. V., Wang, Y. X., Ozimek, L., & Chen, L. (2014). Effects of partial hydrolysis on structure and gelling properties of oat globular proteins. *Food Research International, 55,* 418–425.

Nivala, O., Mäkinen, O. E., Nordlund, E., Kruus, K., & Ercili-Cura, D. (2016). Structuring colloidal oat and faba bean protein particles via enzymatic modification. *Manuscript in preparation*.

Pastuszka, D., Gambuś, H., Ziobro, R., Mickowska, B., Buksa, K., & Sabat, R. (2012). Quality and nutritional value of wheat bread with a preparation of oat proteins. In: *Biotechnology and quality of raw materials and foodstuffs. 7th international scientific conference, manor house Mojmírovce, Slovakia, 1–2 February 2012.* (pp. 980–987). Faculty of biotechnology and food sciences, Slovak University of Agriculture.

Pawlowska, P., Diowksz, A., & Kordialik-Bogacka, E. (2013). Gluten-free oat malt as brewing raw material. *Zywnosc: Nauka, Technologia, Jakosc, 20,* 181–190.

Pedó, I., Sgarbieri, V. C., & Gutkoski, L. C. (1999). Protein evaluation of four oat (*Avena sativa* L.) cultivars adapted for cultivation in the south of Brazil. *Plant Foods for Human Nutrition, 53,* 297–304.

Peräaho, M., Collin, P., Kaukinen, K., Kekkonen, L., Miettinen, S., & Mäki, M. (2004). Oats can diversify a gluten-free diet in celiac disease and dermatitis herpetiformis. *Journal of the American Dietetic Association, 104,* 1148–1150.

Peterson, D. M. (2011). Storage proteins. In F. H. Webster, P. J. Wood (Eds.), *Oats: Chemistry and technology*, (123–142). St. Paul, MN: American Association of Cereal Chemists.

Pettersson, Å., Lindberg, J. E., Thomke, S., & Eggum, B. O. (1996). Nutrient digestibility and protein quality of oats differing in chemical composition evaluated in rats and by an in vitro technique. *Animal Feed Science and Technology, 62,* 203–213.

Ponnampalam, R., Goulet, G., Amiot, J., & Brisson, G. J. (1987). Some functional and nutritional properties of oat flours as affected by proteolysis. *Journal of Agricultural and Food Chemistry, 35,* 279–285.

Qiao, S.-W., Bergseng, E., Molberg, O., Xia, J., Fleckenstein, B., Khosla, C., & Sollid, L. M. (2004). Antigen presentation to celiac lesion-derived T cells of a 33-mer gliadin peptide naturally formed by gastrointestinal digestion. *The Journal of Immunology, 173,* 1757–1762.

Rashid, M., Butzner, D., Burrows, V., Zarkadas, M., Case, S., Molloy, M., ... Switzer, C. (2007). Consumption of pure oats by individuals with celiac disease: A position statement by the Canadian Celiac Association. *The Canadian Journal of Gastroenterology, 21,* 649–651.

Redaelli, R., Scalfati, G., Ciccoritti, R., Cacciatori, P., De Stefanis, E., & Sgrulletta, D. (2015). Effects of genetic and agronomic factors on grain composition in oats. *Cereal Research Communications, 43,* 144–154.

Rekola, K. (2015). *Development of high protein gluten-free oat bread. MSc thesis*. Finland: University of Helsinki.

Renzetti, S., Courtin, C. M., Delcour, J. A., & Arendt, E. K. (2010). Oxidative and proteolytic enzyme preparations as promising improvers for oat bread formulations: Rheological, biochemical and microstructural background. *Food Chemistry, 119,* 1465–1473.

Rutherfurd, S. M., & Moughan, P. J. (1998). The digestible amino acid composition of several milk proteins: Application of a new bioassay. *Journal of Dairy Science, 81,* 909–917.

Sadiq Butt, M., Tahir-Nadeem, M., Khan, M. K. I., Shabir, R., & Butt, M. S. (2008). Oat: unique among the cereals. *European journal of nutrition, 47*(2), 68–79.

Sathe, S. K., Kshirsagar, H. H., & Roux, K. H. (2005). Advances in seed protein research: A perspective on seed allergens. *Journal of Food Science, 70*(6), r93–r120.

Schaafsma, G. (2000). The protein digestibility-corrected amino acid score. *Journal of Nutrition, 130,* 1865S–1867S.

Schutyser, M. A. I., & van der Goot, A. J. (2011). The potential of dry fractionation processes for sustainable plant protein production. *Trends in Food Science & Technology, 22*, 154–164.

Schutyser, M. A. I., Pelgrom, P. J. M., van der Goot, A. J., & Boom, R. M. (2015). Dry fractionation for sustainable production of functional legume protein concentrates. *Trends in Food Science & Technology, 45*(2), 327–335.

Schwenke, K. D. (1997). Enzyme and chemical modification of proteins. In S. Damodaran, & A. Paraf (Eds.), *Food proteins and their applications* (pp. 393–423). New York, NY: Marcel Dekker.

Shan, L., Molberg, Ø., Parrot, I., Hausch, F., Filiz, F., Gray, G. M., ... Khosla, C. (2002). Structural basis for gluten intolerance in celiac sprue. *Science, 297*, 2275–2279.

Shewry, P. R. (1999). Avenins: The prolamins of oats. In P. R. Shewry, & R. Casey (Eds.), *Seed proteins* (pp. 79–92). Netherlands, Dordrecht: Springer.

Shewry, P. R., Napier, J. A., & Tatham, A. S. (1995). Seed storage proteins: Structures and biosynthesis. *Plant Cell, 7*, 945–956.

Shewry, P. R., Tatham, A. S., & Halford, N. G. (1999). The prolamins of the triticeae. In P. R. Shewry, & R. Casey (Eds.), *Seed proteins* (pp. 35–78). Netherlands, Dordrecht: Springer.

Shotwell, M. A. (1999). Oat globulins. In P. Shewry, & R. Casey (Eds.), *Seed proteins* (pp. 389–400). Dordrecth: Kluwer Academic Publishers.

Shotwell, M. A., Afonso, C., Davies, E., Chesnut, R. S., & Larkins, B. A. (1988). Molecular characterization of oat seed globulins. *Plant Physiology, 87*, 698–704.

Sibakov, J. (2014). *Processing of oat dietary fibre for improved functionality as a food ingredient*. PhD thesis. Espoo, Finland: Aalto University.

Sibakov, J., Myllymäki, O., Holopainen, U., Kaukovirta-Norja, A., Hietaniemi, V., Pihlava, J. M., ... Lehtinen, P. (2011). Lipid removal enhances separation of oat grain cell wall material from starch and protein. *Journal of Cereal Science, 54*, 104–109.

Sicherer, S. H., & Sampson, H. A. (2010). Food allergy. *Journal of Allergy and Clinical Immunology, 125*(2), S116–S125.

Stewart, D., & McDougall, G. (2014). Oat agriculture, cultivation and breeding targets: Implications for human nutrition and health. *British Journal of Nutrition, 112*(Suppl. 2), S50–S57.

Stewart, R. A., Hensley, G. W., & Peters, F. N. (1943). The nutritive value of protein I. The effect of processing on oat protein. *Journal of Nutrition, 26*, 519–526.

Størsrud, S., Olsson, M., Arvidsson Lenner, R., Nilsson, L. A., Nilsson, O., & Kilander, A. (2003). Adult coeliac patients do tolerate large amounts of oats. *European Journal of Clinical Nutrition, 57*, 163–169.

Strychar, R., Webster, F. H., & Wood, P. J. (2011). World oat production, trade, and usage. In F. H. Webster, P. J. Wood (Eds.), *Oats: Chemistry and technology* (pp. 1–10). St. Paul, MN: American Association of Cereal Chemists.

Tanchak, M. A., Schernthaner, J. P., Giband, M., & Altosaar, I. (1998). Tryptophanins: Isolation and molecular characterization of oat cDNA clones encoding proteins structurally related to puroindoline and wheat grain softness proteins. *Plant Science, 137*, 173–184.

Tang, J. J., Laudick, L. L., & Benton, D. A. (1958). Studies of amino acid supplementation and amino acid availability with oats. *Journal of Nutrition, 66*, 533–543.

Vaintraub, I. A., Kotova, L. V., & Shaha, R. (1992). Protein deamidase from germinating wheat grains. *FEBS Letters, 302*, 169–171.

Welch, R. W. (2011). Nutrient composition and nutritional quality of oats and comparisons with other cereals. In F. H. Webster, & P. J. Wood (Eds.), *Oats: Chemistry and technology* (pp. 95–107). St. Paul, MN: American Association of Cereal Chemists, Inc (AACC).

Westhoek, H., Lesschen, J. P., Rood, T., Wagner, S., De Marco, A., Murphy-Bokern, D., ... Oenema, O. (2014). Food choices, health and environment: Effects of cutting Europe's meat and dairy intake. *Global Environmental Change, 26*, 196–205.

Whitaker, J. R., Feeney, R. E., & Sternberg, M. M. (2009). Chemical and physical modification of proteins by the hydroxideion. *Critical Reviews in Food Science and Nutrition, 19*, 173–212.

Wong, H.-W., Choi, S.-M., Phillips, D. L., & Ma, C.-Y. (2009). Raman spectroscopic study of deamidated food proteins. *Food Chemistry, 113*, 363–370.

Wu, Y., & Doehlert, D. (2002). Enrichment of β-glucan in oat bran by fine grinding and air classification. *LWT - Food Science and Technology, 35*, 30–33.

Wu, Y. V., Sexson, K. R., Cavins, J. F., & Inglett, G. E. (1972). Oats and their dry-milled fractions: Protein isolation and properties of four varieties. *Journal of Agricultural and Food Chemistry, 20*, 757–761.

Wu, Y. V., Sexson, K. R., Cluskey, J. E., & Inglett, G. E. (1977). Protein isolate from high protein oats: Preparation, composition and properties. *Journal of Food Science, 42*, 1383–1386.

Wu, Y. V., & Stringfellow, A. C. (1995). Enriched protein- and beta-glucan fractions from high-protein oats by air classification. *Cereal Chemistry, 72*, 132–134.

Wu, Y., Qian, Y., Pan, Y., Li, P., Yang, J., Ye, X., & Xu, G. (2015). Association between dietary fiber intake and risk of coronary heart disease: A meta-analysis. *Clinical Nutrition, 34*, 603–611.

Xu, C., Lv, J., You, S., Zhao, Q., Chen, X., & Hu, X. (2013). Supplementation with oat protein ameliorates exercise-induced fatigue in mice. *Food & Function, 4*, 303–309.

Yamaguchi, S., & Yokoe, M. (2000). A novel protein-deamidating enzyme from *Chryseobacterium proteolyticum* sp. nov., a newly isolated bacterium from soil. *Applied and Environmental Microbiology, 66*, 3337–3343.

Yle- Finnish Broadcasting Company. (2016). Forget pulled pork, Helsinki firm looks to export 'pulled oats'. <http://yle.fi/uutiset/forget_pulled_pork_helsinki_firm_looks_to_export_pulled_oats/8579348> January 21, 2016.

Youngs, V. L. (1972). Protein distribution in the oat kernel. *Cereal Chemistry, 49*, 407–411.

Zhao, Y., Mine, Y., & Ma, C.-Y. (2004). Study of thermal aggregation of oat globulin by laser light scattering. *Journal of Agricultural and Food Chemistry, 52*, 3089–3096.

Chapter 7

Hemp Seed (*Cannabis sativa* L.) Proteins: Composition, Structure, Enzymatic Modification, and Functional or Bioactive Properties

R.E. Aluko

University of Manitoba, Winnipeg, MB, Canada

7.1 GENERAL OVERVIEW

Hemp (*Cannabis sativa* L.) is an annual herbaceous plant that belongs to the Cannabinaceae family and has traditionally been grown for the bast fiber (also called phloem fiber) in its stalk (Turner, El Sohly, & Boeren, 1980). The seed is economically important as an edible oil source and has long been used as foodstuff in the Old World and especially in Asian countries (Callaway, 2004; Odani & Odani, 1998; Xiaozhai & Clarke, 1995; Zias et al., 1993). The hemp fiber is a very valuable raw material for the manufacture of durable fabrics and specialty papers. However, the high level of THC (tetrahydrocannabinol) has long hindered widespread use of hemp seed as food in other parts of the world. About two decades ago, industrial hemp with low-THC levels (<0.3%) became available in several countries, especially China and Canada, which has led to increased commercialization of foods formulated with hemp seeds. Postharvest hemp seed processing involves drying to reduce moisture content to ≤10%, which helps to prevent sprouting during storage. The dried seeds are extracted for edible oil by feeding them into a hydraulic screw press at a pressure of ∼500 bars to limit excessive temperature increases (Deferne & Pate, 1996). The first pass through the mechanical press leaves a crushed residue with high oil levels (up to 30%). Therefore, the crushed residue is sometimes passed through the mechanical press again to squeeze out more oil but the extraction yield is still less than that of techniques where solvents or high temperatures are used. However, the low temperature employed during the mechanical press has the advantage of minimizing oil degradative changes. Oil bottling occurs quickly, usually under nitrogen into opaque bottles, which is then followed by refrigeration to protect against light and oxidation-induced oil degradation. In some cases antioxidants may be added to extend shelf-life, especially if the product is to be stored at room temperature. The crushed residue contains the valuable proteins and is then ground, sieved, and sold for human and animal food uses.

7.1.1 Growing Regions and Yield

Hemp grows well in a variety of climates and soil types with a superior ability to grow without fungicides, herbicides, and pesticides (MAFRD, 2015c). The hemp plant absorbs carbon dioxide up to five times more efficiently (reduces global warming) than the same acreage of forest trees and has a very short maturity period of 3–4 months. Hemp fiber processing also reduces environmental toxin load because the plant has a low lignin content, which can be converted into pulp using less chemicals than regular wood. Hemp fiber is also naturally brighter than regular wood and can be bleached with hydrogen peroxide instead of chlorine dioxide, which reduces the amount of extremely toxic dioxin that ends up in streams. For experienced growers, it has been estimated that an average of 800 kg of seed (250–2200 kg range) can be obtained from one hectare of hemp; this seed yield translates into an average of ∼200 L of oil and 600 kg of protein-rich (up to 35%) meal. However, for new growers the seed yield may be lower at 449–561 kg/ha (MAFRD, 2015c). Hemp is naturally pest-resistant, and requires little or no pesticide use, making hemp an exceptionally environmentally friendly crop. Similarly, hemp cultivation requires minimal herbicide use because of the rapid growth and high plant density, which basically leads to weed smothering. However, because hemp plant density is lower when grown for seed production, some minimal use of herbicide may be required, unlike fiber hemp cultivation. Hemp can return up to 60–70% of the nutrients taken from the soil when dried and allowed to be composted in the field for the next cropping season (MAFRD, 2015c). This is because approximately 42% of hemp plant biomass is returned to the soil in the form of leaves, roots, and tops, which represents over half of the nutrients applied to the crop. Many of these nutrients will be available to help feed the following year's crop. Its deep root system is also very beneficial as it is effective in preventing erosion, cleaning the ground, providing a disease break, and helping the soil structure by aerating the soil for future crops, when it is grown in rotation with other crops.

7.1.2 Land Use

Due to the regulatory limitations placed on hemp cultivation, information on land use is very scarce. However, it was estimated that approximately 66,000 acres of land were cultivated in Canada in 2013, specifically for hemp seed production (MAFRD, 2015a). Hemp plant grows well on loosely packed soils and will establish tap roots that are 15–30 cm long. In compacted or poorly drained soils, the plant fibrous roots grow in a more lateral but shallow direction. In contrast, hemp grows well in a well-drained, loam soil with reduced acidity (pH > 6.0), preferably neutral to slightly alkaline (pH 7.0–7.5). Establishment of this deep root system is beneficial to the environment because it prevents erosion, cleans the ground, and helps create a properly aerated soil structure, which is beneficial for future crops when hemp is grown in rotation with other crops. The higher the clay content of the soil, the lower the yield of fiber or grain produced. Clay soils are easily compacted and hemp is very sensitive to soil compaction. Similarly, optimal growth of the hemp plant cannot be achieved in poorly structured, drought-prone sandy soils because of the very low amount of natural fertility or nutrient support for the plant. In such poor soils, extra nutrients and water (irrigation) are required to achieve maximum yields.

7.1.3 Water Use

Hemp thrives best in areas with moderate rainfall (30–40 cm) and good soil fertility; 80–120 days to maturity is common but depends on variety and seeding date. In particular, high soil moisture content is needed during the first 6 weeks, during germination and until the plant has become well-rooted and established. For maximum grain yields, approximately half of the hemp plant's moisture requirement is during flowering and seed set. Drought during this stage reduces seed set and produces poorly developed grain heads. But it should be noted that hemp will not grow well under persistently water-logged conditions and may actually turn yellow, cease to grow, and eventually die.

7.1.4 Energy Use and Cost

It has been estimated that hemp may require total nutrient levels (field plus fertilizer nutrients) of 89–135 kg nitrogen/ha, 45 kg phosphorus/ha, 67 kg potassium/ha, and 17 kg sulfur/ha (MAFRD, 2015c). Soil testing to determine soil nutrient levels is recommended prior to fertilizer application. Previous works have shown increases in seed yield, biomass, plant height, and protein content can be achieved when the nitrogen fertilizer application dosage was increased up to 120 kg/ha. Estimated seed and treatment cost is ~US$32/acre, while fertilizer costs ~US$42/acre and chemical use costs ~US$28/acre according to recent estimates (MAFRD, 2015b). Based on these productions costs, estimated contract price ranges from US$0.75 to US$0.84 per pound for clean high-quality commercial grain. For organic hemp seed, the price is generally 30–40% higher depending on the contractor.

7.1.5 Plant and Seed

Most *Cannabis* plant varieties are adapted to grow at temperate or equatorial climates; however, the short daylight limits flowering time, which in turn reduces seed production. In contrast, early blooming varieties grown at high latitudes can take advantage of the long summer days in Jun. and Jul. to produce abundant amounts of seed (Callaway, 2002). In addition, cropping at high latitudes enhances production of seeds that have higher profiles of essential unsaturated fatty acids, especially γ-linolenic acid and stearidonic acid. One such early blooming variety is Finola, a short-stature plant (<2m when cultivated at latitude 62°N), which was developed in Finland specifically as a low-THC seed for food use. Finola has been commercialized in Europe and Canada with seed yields reported in the 1700−2000 kg/ha range (Callaway, 2002). Finola matures in less than 115 days, has been reported to be frost-tolerant at all growth stages, and can grow without herbicides or pesticides at high altitudes. Finola produces flowers with 0.04−0.16% THC, which is less than the 0.3% cut-off level established by Canadian and EU regulatory authorities. The cannabinoid/THC ratio of Finola is >10:1, which is higher than the 2:1 EU requirement, which ensures that this hemp variety is useful only for food and cannot be used as a recreational drug. As a plant, hemp is an open pollinated crop that requires no insects during seed production. However, Finola is known to produce large amounts of pollen that could assist apiarists in raising bees because the copious availability of pollen enables increased honey yields. Generally, highly branched varieties are usually preferred and male plants are sometimes removed after pollination has occurred, in order to leave more space for female plants during seed production (Deferne & Pate, 1996). Unlike fiber hemp, maximum seed yield requires that hemp be sown at a much lower density, though excessive weed growth can occur if planting density is too sparse (Reichert, 1994).

Hemp seeds are actually achene fruits that consist of a single seed within a hard shell (Clarke, 2007). The seeds are 2.5−3.5 mm in length and have a brown color with darker brown stripes that are usually rubbed off during threshing such that the cleaned seeds have a light brownish-gray color. The seeds are consumed raw, cooked, or roasted while the oil has also been used as medicine. In some countries the roasted seeds are ground into flour and added to cooked dishes to provide a distinct flavor. For example, in Nepal and some parts of India, the condiment called *bhang chortney* (chutney) is made fresh daily and consumed along with beans and rice (dhal bhat). To prepare *bhang chortney* the dried hemp seeds are first crushed with a pestle on a stone slate slab and then other ingredients such as onion, garlic, ginger, spices, and chillies are added followed by mashing into a smooth paste (Clarke, 2007). The dried seeds can also be mixed with popped amaranth grains and honey added to make them stick together to be consumed as a snack. In Eastern European countries, a butter substitute is produced using hemp seed oil and consumed by the poor who cannot afford dairy products. In Canada, commercial hemp seed products include oil, dehulled hemp seeds or nut, milk, flour, toasted hemp seed, coffee, butter, and protein powder. Hemp seed is also used to make nonfood products such as shampoo, conditioner, hand lotion, and lip balm. A recent estimation suggests that the North America hemp seed industry is now worth ∼US$35 million.

7.1.6 Seed Composition and Protein Quality

Hemp seeds contain ∼30% oil and ∼25% protein, both of high nutritional quality, in addition to 10−15% insoluble fiber (Deferne & Pate, 1996). The oil is especially rich in polyunsaturated fatty acids, especially the omega-3 and omega-6 types that constitute ∼80% of the fatty acids, while the protein has high levels of essential amino acids and arginine (Malomo, He, & Aluko, 2015; Tang, Wang, & Yang, 2009). Specifically, the oil is rich in oleic acid, linoleic acid, α-linolenic acid, γ-linolenic acid, and stearidonic acid, with only about 10% of saturated fatty acids. Fresh hemp seed oil is green in color because of the chlorophyll present in the mature seed. Hemp seed contains mainly storage proteins, which consist of albumin (25−37%) and the legumin called edestin (67−75%), and no protease inhibitors. The absence of protease inhibitors is believed to contribute to enhanced protein digestibility properties. The essential amino acid content of hemp seed proteins is superior to that of soybean and is sufficient for humans who are 10 years of age or older. House, Neufeld, and Leson (2010) reported in vitro protein digestibility and protein digestibility-corrected amino acid score (PDCAAS) values of up to 92% and 66%, respectively, for dehulled hemp seed. Lysine and tryptophan are the main limiting amino acids in the hemp seed, which probably contributed to the low PDCAAS value when compared to the 92% reported for soybean protein isolate (House et al., 2010). High arginine content makes hemp seed protein especially valuable as a nutritional ingredient to formulate foods that enhance cardiovascular health. This is because arginine is a precursor of nitric oxide, the vasodilating agent that enhances blood flow and contributes to maintenance of normal blood pressure (Wu & Meininger, 2002).

7.2 MAJOR SEED PROTEINS

7.2.1 Globulin

Also called edestin, the legumin (globulin) protein fraction is the main (∼75%) storage protein of hemp seed. Hemp seed legumin consists of mainly the 11S and 7S protein types, which can be separated using pH shifts as described by Wang, Tang, Yang, and Gao (2008). The defatted flour was extracted for 1 h at room temperature with alkaline water at pH 10 followed by centrifugation to isolate the solubilized proteins in the supernatant. Approximately 0.98 g/L of sodium bisulfite was added to the supernatant and adjusted to pH 6.4 with 1 M HCl; the slurry was kept at 4°C overnight to facilitate 11S precipitation. After centrifugation, the 11S precipitate was mixed with water, adjusted to pH 7.0, dialyzed, and then freeze-dried. The supernatant obtained after 11S precipitation was adjusted to pH 4.6, which precipitated the 7S protein. The 7S precipitate was mixed with water, adjusted to pH 7.0, dialyzed, and freeze-dried. Gel electrophoresis suggested a 300-kDa molecular mass for the hexameric hemp seed edestin (globulin). The high level of aggregation between the polypeptide chains was reflected as the insoluble high-intensity bands that did not enter the gel under nonreducing conditions. Wang et al. (2008) also showed that the 7S protein had no thermal transition, while the 11S protein had 91.9°C denaturation temperature, which was similar to the 92.0°C obtained for the hemp seed protein isolate (HPI). Therefore, the HPI thermal property was due mainly to the 11S component. However, the enthalpy change for 11S protein was significantly less than that of the HPI, which suggests some protein denaturation occurred during the 11S isolation protocol in comparison to the highly ordered native protein structure. The absence of thermal transition signals suggests that the isolated 7S protein was already denatured and lacked an ordered structure. The 11S protein also had superior nutritional value as shown by the higher levels of sulfur-containing amino acids, arginine, and essential amino acids. Protein digestibility of the hemp seed protein products was similar after a 4-h digestion but the high nutritional value of the hemp seed protein products was also evident in superior protein digestibility values that were up to 20% higher than those of soybean proteins.

A globulin isolate was produced through salt extraction of hemp seed meal followed by dialysis against water; the precipitate was collected and freeze-dried (Malomo & Aluko, 2015a). Amino acid composition analysis indicated an arginine/lysine ratio of 4.37, which is significantly higher than the 1.74 for albumin. The high arginine/lysine ratio indicates strong potential for the globulin to be used in the formulation of cardiovascular health-promoting food products. Fluorescence intensity (FI) data showed almost no structural conformation at pH 5.0, which is consistent with an aggregated or amorphous protein structure at the isoelectric point environment. However, FI increased above and below pH 5.0 as the globulin formed more compact conformations. Consistent with the FI results, circular dichroism showed higher levels of secondary and tertiary structure conformations at pH 7.0 and 9.0, when compared to the acidic pH values. The globulin was least soluble in the acidic pH range with values <20% but increased up to ~50% at pH 8.0 and 9.0. Foaming capacity of the globulin was very poor and inferior to that of the albumin; however, the emulsion-forming ability was similar with oil droplet sizes <0.8 μm and similar to those of milk emulsions. The strong emulsifying ability (small oil droplet sizes) suggests a hydrophobic character that makes the globulin interact well with the oil phase and indicates a potential ingredient to formulate various high-quality oil-in-water food emulsions.

7.2.2 Albumin

Dialysis of a salt extract of hemp seed meal led to precipitation of the water-insoluble globulin while the albumin remained in solution (Malomo & Aluko, 2015a). The albumin constitutes ~25% of hemp seed storage proteins and has very little compact structure as evident in the low FI values at different pH. This is consistent with a flexible hydrophilic structure that prevents extensive protein folding and hence most of the residues are in contact with the environment. Therefore, the albumin has greater flexibility and less compact structure than the globulin. However, the secondary structure of albumin showed a more ordered polypeptide arrangement than that of the globulin. The albumin had very little tertiary conformation at pH 3.0 but increased at pH 7.0 and 9.0. Protein solubility of the albumin ranged from ~57% at pH 3.0 to ~84% at pH 8.0, which is significantly superior to those of the globulin. Foaming capacity reflected the high albumin solubility with ~90% increase in volume at pH 3.0, 5.0, 7.0, and 9.0 in comparison to <40% for globulin. The high degree of flexibility and ordered secondary structure are probably structural factors that contribute to the high solubility and foaming capacity of albumin in comparison to the more compact or aggregated globulin. The albumin also produced high-quality emulsions (small oil droplet sizes) with oil droplet sizes of <0.8 μm just like those of globulin emulsions. The results indicate strong emulsifying properties for the albumin and globulin fractions, which may be used to fabricate high-quality emulsified foods.

7.2.3 Sulfur-Rich Proteins

Using several purification protocols, a 10-kDa protein (2S albumin) was isolated from hemp seeds and shown to consist of two polypeptide chains (small and large) with 27 and 61 amino acid residues, respectively (Odani & Odani, 1998). The two polypeptide chains contain 18% by weight of sulfur-containing amino acids (cysteine and methionine) and are held together by two disulfide bonds. As shown in Fig. 7.1, the small subunit contains five sulfur-containing amino acids (residues 7, 17, 19, 21, and 25) while the larger subunit contains 11 (residues 8, 9, 19, 21, 26, 39, 40, 49, 50, 52, and 57).

```
                              1      7        17 19  21    25 27
         Small subunit       SGSEQECRRQRQDNLHCRMYMREKMHG


                              1         8 9            19 21      26
         Large subunit       YSQHLDQCCSQLRNVNERCRCPALEMEIQK
                             31         39 40          49 50 52       57      61
                             EQGQDKQRMMESARNIPSMCGMQPRTCQFHS
```

FIGURE 7.1 Amino acid sequence of the small and large subunits of the hemp seed 10-kDa 2S albumin. Sulfur-containing amino acid residues are shown in bold font. *Reproduced with permission from Odani, S., & Odani, S. (1998). Isolation and primary structure of a methionine- and cysteine-rich seed protein of* Cannabis sativa. *Bioscience, Biotechnology and Biochemistry, 62, 650–654. Copyright © Japan Society for Bioscience and Agrochemistry, reprinted by permission of Taylor & Francis Ltd, www.tandfonline.com on behalf of the Japan Society for Bioscience and Agrochemistry.*

This sulfur-rich protein had no inhibitory activity against trypsin and could serve as a rich thiol source to formulate highly nutritious foods. This is important since several plant food proteins, especially leguminous crops such as soybean, peas, and beans, are deficient in sulfur. Therefore, the hemp seed 10-kDa protein could be extracted and used to fortify foods formulated with legumes, especially as a nutritional tool to boost the antioxidant capacity of the human body. This is because cysteine is a critical component of reduced glutathione, the powerful cellular antioxidant. The high sulfur content could also enhance liver-detoxifying capacity since enzyme-catalyzed sulfurylation of toxins confers hydrophilic properties and improves their elimination through the urine. In addition to the high sulfur content, the lack of trypsin inhibitory activity makes the protein desirable in food formulations since extensive heat processing will not be required to make the protein digestible.

7.2.4 Allergenicity

Proteins that belong to the 2S albumin family are known to elicit allergenic reactions upon consumption. Therefore, information on the allergenic properties of 2S albumin isolated from hemp seed is required before food use can be recommended. However, currently there is no information on ability of hemp seed 2S albumin to induce allergic reactions. In fact, one of the advertising points of hemp seed product manufacturers is the claim that the protein is nonallergenic.

7.3 FUNCTIONAL PROPERTIES OF HEMP SEED PROTEIN PRODUCTS

7.3.1 Defatted Flour

A hemp seed defatted meal that contained ~44% protein content was recently evaluated for structural and functional properties in comparison to a purer protein isolate obtained through isoelectric pH precipitation (Malomo, He et al., 2015). Gel electrophoresis under reducing conditions confirmed the presence of typical hemp seed polypeptides such as the 47, 33, 20, and 10 kDa. The 33, which is the acidic subunit (AS), and 20 kDa, the basic subunit (BS), were the most abundant polypeptides. FI spectra showed increased intensity of the tryptophan peak as the environment changed from pH 3.0 to 9.0. These changes in FI reflect a protein structural rearrangement that moved the tryptophan residues into the hydrophobic core and away from the hydrophilic environment. However, the presence of nonprotein materials could have influenced the observed spectra, especially if these materials become very hydrophilic at pH >5.0. The meal proteins showed more compact structural conformation at pH 5.0–9.0 as reflected in the bigger tryptophan peak. The results indicate the presence of denatured protein molecules in the isolate, probably due to the strong effect of pH shifts used during preparation. The FI results were confirmed by circular dichroism data, which showed very little secondary structure conformation for the meal at pH 3.0 but increased gradually as pH was increased to 7.0 and then 9.0. In contrast, the protein isolate had compact secondary structure at pH 3.0 but was significantly reduced and less than that of the meal proteins at pH 7.0 and 9.0. The hemp seed meal had a low (3.35) arginine/lysine ratio, which is superior to the 2.65 for whole seeds (House et al., 2010) but inferior to the 5.52 obtained for a protein isolate (Malomo, He et al., 2015). Therefore, the potential cardiovascular-protective value (arginine/lysine ratio) of the hemp seed proteins seems to be higher when protein purity increases. In terms of functionality, the hemp seed meal had similar water-holding capacity (WHC), but oil-holding capacity (OHC) was inferior when compared to the protein isolate. The least gelation concentration (LGC) of the meal (12%) was significantly lower (better gel-forming ability) than the

22% for the purer protein isolate. Contributions from nonprotein materials, especially sugars and polysaccharides, may have contributed to the superior LGC of the hemp seed meal. Foaming capacity of the meal improved as the environment changed from pH 3.0 to 9.0, which suggests increased interaction with water and protein unfolding at neutral and alkaline pH values. The foaming capacity and stability of the meal was inferior when compared to the purer HPI. Interference from nonprotein materials may have reduced the ability of meal proteins to form and stabilize foams. However, the hemp seed meal formed higher-quality emulsions (smaller oil droplet sizes) than the purer protein isolate. It is possible that nonprotein components enhanced the emulsion-forming ability of the meal in addition to the less-denatured state as revealed by FI data.

7.3.2 Protein Concentrates

Additional processing steps are usually applied to hemp seed meals for removal of nonprotein materials to produce protein concentrates with protein contents that range from 50% to 75% on a wet weight basis. The higher protein content makes the concentrates attractive for food formulations, especially where protein functionality determines food product properties and consumer acceptability. In a recent work, the functional properties of commercial and laboratory-processed hemp seed protein concentrates were compared (Malomo & Aluko, 2015b). The lab protein concentrate was produced by digestion of the polysaccharides with cellulase followed by removal of the digested fragments through membrane ultrafiltration. This digestion coupled with ultrafiltration enabled protein isolation in its native form without the adverse effects of pH-shift treatment. Gel electrophoresis showed that the membrane process enabled better recovery of the <14-kDa proteins, which may not have been susceptible to precipitation during the normal pH-shift protocol. However, overall, the gel electrophoresis patterns of the commercial protein concentrate (cHPC) were similar to those of membrane concentrate (mHPC) and the original seed meal. Protein solubility of the protein concentrates was significantly higher than that of the meal and protein isolate (produced by pH-shift protocols) at pH 3.0–9.0. A remarkable difference is the high solubility (>60%) in the pH 3–6 range for the protein concentrates when compared to <20% for the meal and protein isolate (Fig. 7.2). The mHPC had superior protein solubility with minimum 74% at pH 4.0–5.0 when compared to the 60% for cHPC. The mHPC also had significantly higher foaming capacity, WHC, OHC, and protein digestibility when compared to the cHPC. However, at most pHs and concentrations studied, the cHPC formed better emulsions (smaller oil droplet sizes) than the mHPC. Overall, the results suggest that the membrane process used to produce mHPC led to isolation of proteins with least denaturation when compared to the cHPC and protein isolate. In particular, the high acid solubility of the mHPC is novel and could permit formulation of free-flowing beverages fortified with hemp seed proteins for improved nutritional value. The commercial product (cHPC) was produced using a proprietary method and hence it is difficult to compare processing effects.

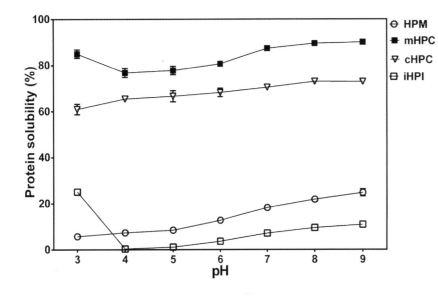

FIGURE 7.2 Protein solubility profile of hemp seed protein products at different pH values: cHPC, commercial hemp seed protein concentrate; iHPI, isoelectric pH-precipitated protein isolate; mHPC, membrane ultrafiltration protein concentrate; HPM, hemp seed protein meal. *Reproduced with permission from Malomo, S.A., & Aluko, R.E. (2015b) Conversion of a low protein hemp seed meal into a functional protein concentrate through enzymatic digestion of fiber coupled with membrane ultrafiltration. Innovative Food Science and Emerging Technologies, 31, 151–159. copyright with permission from Elsevier.*

7.3.3 Protein Isolates

In general, protein isolates have >85% protein content on a wet basis and are, therefore, purer forms of protein than the concentrates. HPI (80% edestin and 20% albumin) is traditionally produced by the pH-shift method, which first involves alkaline extraction of defatted flour followed by recovery of the solubilized proteins in the supernatant after centrifugation (Tang, Ten, Wang, & Yang, 2006; Yin et al., 2008). However, acid solubilization at pH 2.0 followed by centrifugation has also been used for hemp seed protein extraction, though yield and dark color (but not functionality) of the HPI were reported to be lower than the alkaline solubilization method (Teh, Bekhit, Carne, & Birch, 2014). Overall, the amino acid composition (especially arginine and branched-chain) of the alkaline-extract HPI was reported to be superior to that of acid-extracted HPI (Teh et al., 2014). Second, adjustment of the alkali- or acid-extracted supernatant to pH 5.0 with HCl will precipitate most of the storage proteins, which are then recovered as a precipitate after centrifugation. The acidic pH adjustment produces intense protein–protein interactions during precipitation; therefore, the precipitate is normally dispersed in water and adjusted to pH 7.0 prior to freeze-drying in order to improve HPI solubility. Even with the pH 7.0 adjustment, the HPI still has poor solubility and functional properties. On a wet basis, Yin et al. (2008) determined HPI protein content to be 91.2%, while Tang et al. (2006) reported an 86.9% value both using the Kjeldahl method ($N \times 6.25$). Hemp seed protein is composed of three main polypeptide chains, a 48-kDa β-chain (similar to soybean β-subunit of β-conglycinin), a 33-kDa AS, and a 20-kDa BS as shown in Fig. 7.3. Hemp seed proteins do not contain β-conglycinin α and α'-subunits like soybean. Other minor polypeptides such as those in the 10–18-kDa (albumins) and 20–33-kDa ranges are also present in the seed (Tang et al., 2006).

In an attempt to improve protein functionality, HPI was heat-pretreated (75°C, 80°C, and 90°C) and then subjected to limited (10 min) trypsin hydrolysis in comparison with a nonpretreated sample. Heat pretreatment at 75°C and 80°C led to improved proteolysis at various points, while 90°C pretreatment actually caused decreased proteolysis (Yin et al., 2008). These effects are believed to be due to protein unfolding at 75°C and 80°C, which led to increased exposure of susceptible peptide bonds. In contrast, the results suggest protein aggregation occurred at 90°C, which produced a compact structure with reduced exposure of peptide bonds and hence less proteolysis when compared to the 75°C and 80°C pretreated HPI. During trypsin hydrolysis, the edestin BS was less susceptible than the AS. The differences in digestibility may be because the BS is usually located within the interior of the edestin quaternary structure and hence less accessible to proteases, while AS is located on the outside with better accessibility. Size exclusion chromatography (SEC) showed the presence of two main protein peaks within the HPI in addition to a high-molecular-weight aggregate peak that eluted with the void volume. Heat treatment led to reductions in both the first protein and protein aggregate peaks, which confirms heat-induced formation of insoluble proteins that did not enter the gel. Trypsin hydrolysis and production of soluble peptides were reflected as increased size of the second protein peak, which is a confirmation of size reduction during proteolysis.

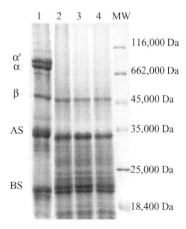

FIGURE 7.3. SDS-PAGE profiles of hemp and soy proteins: lane 1, soy protein isolate; lane 2, defatted hemp seed meal; lane 3, whole hemp seed protein isolate (HPI); lane 4, precipitate of HPI at pH 7.0; AS, acidic subunit; BS, basic subunit. *Reprinted with permission from Tang, C.-H., Ten, Z., Wang, X.-S., Yang, X.-Q. (2006). Physicochemical and functional properties of hemp* (Cannabis sativa L.) *protein isolate. Journal of Agricultural and Food Chemistry, 54, 8945–8950. Copyright (2006) American Chemical Society.*

As expected, the HPI was least soluble (<5%) at pH 5.0–6.0 while solubility increased at pH <5.0 and >6.0 (Yin et al., 2008). Heat treatment worsened HPI solubility when compared to the raw HPI at all the pH values, which confirms heat-induced formation of insoluble aggregates as indicated by the SEC data. Trypsin proteolysis led to improved HPI solubility at all the pH values with up to 85% value at pH 7.0 and above. Protein solubility at pH <6.0 was positively related to degree of hydrolysis (DH), which is consistent with greater release of soluble peptides from the increased digestion of insoluble protein aggregates. Thermal analysis revealed significant differences between the HPI samples in terms of denaturation temperature (T_d) and enthalpy change (ΔH). For example, the heat-treated HPI showed no thermal transition, which is consistent with a totally denatured protein. In contrast, the raw HPI had a T_d of 95.1°C (edestin) with 11.9 J/g ΔH (Yin et al., 2008), which reflects a highly ordered protein structure. However, trypsin digestion produced protein hydrolysates with higher T_d and less ΔH values, which reflects hydrophobic interactions between the digested peptides and less ordered structure, respectively. WHC, and FAC (fat absorption capacity) were significantly reduced by trypsin hydrolysis of HPI; with the exception of FAC at 6.7% DH, which was similar to that of the raw sample and higher than the heat-treated sample. The decreased WHC and FAC values after protein hydrolysis were attributed to protein interactions, which may have reduced exposure of hydrophilic and hydrophobic groups. However, at 6.7% DH, the results suggest formation of protein aggregates with hydrophobic core that can properly entrap oil molecules.

Emulsion-forming ability of HPI, determined as emulsification activity index (EAI), was significantly improved by heat treatment when compared to the raw or trypsin-digested samples (Yin et al., 2008). The improved EAI may be due to increased exposure of hydrophobic groups in the heat-treated HPI, which enhances protein interactions with oil droplets. In contrast, the protein hydrolysates contained protein aggregates that enhanced formation of large-size, coalescence-prone emulsified oil droplets due to limited interfacial activity in terms of formation of a viscoelastic membrane. Moreover, EAI values were higher at pH 7.0 and 9.0 when compared to pH 3.0 and 5.0. Foaming capacity was also reduced by trypsin hydrolysis but not by heat treatment. The decreased chain length after hydrolysis may have limited the interfacial membrane strength and hence led to production of poor foams.

The poor functionality of native HPI has also been improved using acylation methods such as succinylation and acetylation. These HPI modifications shifted minimum protein solubility from pH 5.0–6.0 for the native protein to pH 4.0–5.0 for the acylated protein (Yin, Tang, Wen, & Yang, 2009). At pH 6.0 and above, succinylation or acetylation led to significantly improved protein solubility when compared to the native HPI. However, at pH 2.0 and 3.0, only succinylation improved protein solubility, which decreased for acetylated HPI in comparison to the native protein. Improved protein solubility for the succinylated HPI was attributed to the enhanced electrostatic repulsions that arise from introduction of negatively charged succinate groups. Similarly, at low degrees of acetylation, introduction of electrostatic charges contributed to improved protein solubility. However, at higher acetylation degrees, there is increased hydrophobic character because of the acyl group, which reduces protein–water interactions and hence lower protein solubility. EAI was significantly improved by acylation and was positively related to the degree of succinylation or acetylation, although the former was more effective. The improved EAI of the acylated samples is believed to be due to increased protein unfolding from the greater number of electrostatic charges. The unfolded proteins then have more exposed hydrophobic groups that can interact more efficiently with oil droplets when compared to the more compact native HPI proteins. FI measurement showed both acylation methods had substantial effects in structurally modifying the HPI, especially by promoting protein unfolding. Interestingly, only succinylation led to an improved in vitro protein digestibility, while acetylation had no measurable effect.

7.4 BIOACTIVE PROPERTIES OF HEMP SEED PROTEINS AND PEPTIDES

7.4.1 Renal Disease Modulation

Using an animal model of human polycystic kidney disease, a HPI has been reported to ameliorate some of the disease-associated pathological symptoms (Aukema et al., 2011). The work involved feeding Han:SPRD-cy rats (polycystic kidney disease model) with diets that contained 17% protein from soybean, yellow field pea, hemp seed, or casein. The authors reported that kidneys from diseased rats fed soybean or hemp seed protein-containing diets were less enlarged, had lower fluid content, smaller cyst volumes, less fibrosis, lower chemokine receptor 2 levels, and normalized serum creatinine levels in comparison to rats that consumed casein-based diet. The ability of hemp seed proteins to attenuate disease symptom progression suggests a role for the prevention and treatment of human chronic kidney disease (CKD). Heart size, which was enlarged in diseased rats, was normalized by soybean and hemp protein diets when compared with rats that consumed the casein diet. The cardiovascular-protective effects of hemp seed proteins are highly significant since the majority of CKD patients die from cardiovascular complications. Therefore, hemp seed proteins could be an important therapeutic ingredient to formulate nutritionally effective diets that limit the pathological intensity of CKD.

7.4.2 Antioxidant

In one of the earlier works to examine the antioxidant properties of hemp seed peptides, six protein hydrolysates were produced through enzymatic hydrolysis of the protein with alcalase, flavourzyme, pepsin, neutrase, protamex, or trypsin (Tang et al., 2009). Protein hydrolysis was conducted separately for 2 and 4 h, followed by testing for antioxidant activities such as 2,2-diphenyl-1-picrylhydrazyl (DPPH) radical scavenging, iron (III) reduction, and iron chelation. Pepsin was the most active in digesting the hemp seed proteins, which was attributed to protein subunit dissociation at the acidic pH of digestion. The dissociated proteins then become more susceptible to proteolysis than the native aggregated form. Overall, gel electrophoresis showed that most of the edestin molecules were completely digested into low-molecular-weight peptides. The hydrolysates exhibited varying degrees of antioxidant activities but the protamex hydrolysate showed an overall stronger effect. Peptide yield and surface hydrophobicity (H_o) of the protein hydrolysates were positively related to DPPH radical scavenging and iron-chelating abilities. Finally, the effect of peptide is obvious since more peptides means increased availability of scavenging and chelating groups, while H_o contributes to better interactions with the lipophilic DPPH radical.

Digestion of hemp seed proteins with a combination of pepsin and pancreatin produced a hydrolysate that showed antioxidant properties during in vitro and in vivo tests. The in vitro tests also involved a comparison of the antioxidant properties of the protein hydrolysate with those of membrane-fractionated peptides. Using a sequential method that involved permeate collection and ultrafiltration of the retentate with a higher-molecular-weight membrane, the hemp seed protein hydrolysate (HPH) was separated into peptides with <1, 1−3, 3−5, and 5−10 kDa sizes (Girgih, Udenigwe, & Aluko, 2011). Amino acid composition analysis showed that the <1 kDa contained significantly higher hydrophobic and aromatic amino acid levels. In contrast, the level of negatively charged amino acids was low in the <1-kDa peptide fraction but increased significantly in the 3−5-kDa and 5−10-kDa fractions. The membrane fractions significantly enhanced DPPH radical scavenging activity (DRSA) of the peptides with <5% for the protein hydrolysate compared to 18−24% for the peptide fractions. Among the peptide fractions, DRSA was highest for <1 kDa and decreased as peptide size increased to 5−10 kDa. The high DRSA for the <1-kDa fraction was attributed to the significantly higher level of hydrophobic and aromatic amino acids, which enhanced interactions with the hydrophobic DPPH radical (Girgih, Udenigwe, & Aluko, 2011). Moreover, aromatic amino acids are efficient electron or hydrogen atom donors due to the ability to assume a stable postdonation resonance structure. Membrane fractionation also significantly enhanced hydroxyl radical scavenging ability of the peptides as is evident in the zero value of the hydrolysate while fractions had 16−24%. However, there was no significant difference in the hydroxyl radical scavenging ability of the peptide fractions, which indicates lack of amino acid composition effect. In contrast to the DRSA, metal chelation and ferric iron reduction were positively related to peptide size, which suggests an additive effect of amino acids; hence longer chains had better properties. Similarly, the ability to inhibit lipid peroxidation was dependent on peptide chain length and reflects additive contributions of the amino acids. The HPH was then tested for ability to attenuate oxidative stress development in spontaneously hypertensive rats (SHR). Girgih et al. (2014) showed that supplementation of young growing SHR diet or adult rat diet with HPH led to significantly improved plasma superoxide dismutase (SOD) and catalase activities (CAT). As part of the efficient plasma antioxidant enzymes, SOD is a superoxide radical detoxifying factor, while CAT neutralizes hydrogen peroxide. Both enzymes constitute important physiological molecules for oxidative stress prevention or elimination, which limits oxidative damage to critical cellular biopolymers such as enzymes and DNA. The findings are consonant with the observed SOD and CAT upregulation by HPH, where plasma total peroxide level was lower in the treated SHR when compared to the control rats. Interestingly, SHR feeding with unhydrolyzed hemp seed protein also provided similar but weaker effects as the HPH, which confirms that bioactive peptides could be liberated in vivo during protein digestion. However, the longer digestion and absorption times required for the unhydrolyzed hemp seed protein within the gut may be responsible for the weaker in vivo antioxidant effects when compared to the predigested HPH. Thus, the HPH could serve as a more efficient nutritional aide than the whole protein for oxidative stress reduction in mammalian systems.

7.4.3 Antihypertensive

The HPH and peptide fractions were also tested for in vitro and in vivo antihypertensive effects in order to determine potential use as a bioactive agent. In vitro tests were performed by determining the ability of the peptide samples to inhibit renin and angiotensin-converting enzyme (ACE) activities, the two enzymes implicated in human hypertension pathogenesis (Aluko, 2015). Excessive activities of the two enzymes lead to high plasma levels of angiotensin II (product of ACE action), which cause excessive blood vessel contractions without adequate relaxation and contribute to the development of hypertension. Results showed that the HPH had stronger ACE and renin-inhibitory activities when compared to the peptide fractions (Girgih, Udenigwe, Li, Adebiyi, & Aluko, 2011). For example, HPH had 0.67 and 0.81 mg/mL inhibitory concentration that reduced 50% activity (IC_{50}) of ACE and renin, respectively. In contrast, the IC_{50} values for <1-kDa peptide fraction were 1.05 and 2.52 mg/mL, while the 1–3-kDa peptide fraction had 1.17 and 1.89 mg/mL, respectively, against ACE and renin. Kinetic analysis indicated a mixed-type pattern of inhibition for HPH and peptide fractions against both ACE and renin. Therefore, the results suggest that the hemp seed peptides bind to both the active and nonactive sites to reduce renin and ACE enzymatic catalysis. During a 24-h test period, the HPH and peptide fractions were orally administered to SHR and blood pressure measured periodically. The results indicated membrane fractionation led to reduced efficiency of the hydrolysate as an antihypertensive agent (Fig. 7.4). This is because the HPH had significantly stronger systolic blood pressure (SBP)-reducing effects at 2 h (−20 mmHg), 4 h (−20 mmHg), 6 h (−23 mmHg), 8 h (−30 mmHg), and 24 h (−17 mmHg) after oral administration when compared to the peptide fractions. In contrast, the <1 and 1−3 kDa had SBP-reducing effects, respectively, at 2 h (−2 and −8 mmHg), 4 h (−7 and −10 mmHg), 6 h (−13 and −15 mmHg), 8 h (−12 and −10 mmHg), and 24 h (+10 and −1 mmHg). The unhydrolyzed protein was also administered but had no measurable antihypertensive effect during the 24-h period. Therefore, the results suggest that protein digestion into bioactive peptides facilitated the antihypertensive effects observed for HPH and peptide fractions. The weaker antihypertensive effects of the <1-kDa and 1–3-kDa peptide fractions suggest strong synergistic activities between peptides of different sizes in the HPH. Separation into defined peptide units reduced these synergistic activities and led to weakening of the antihypertensive effects of <1-kDa and 1−3-kDa peptide fractions. A short-term feeding experiment was also used to evaluate the SBP-lowering effects of HPHs that were hydrolyzed with different enzymes and to varying degrees of hydrolysis. In vitro assay showed that the protein hydrolysates produced with 2% papain or 2% alcalase were the most active against ACE and renin with IC_{50} values <1.0 mg/mL (Malomo, Girgih, Onuh, & Aluko, 2015). However, during in vivo tests in SHR, the strongest SBP-reducing effect was by 1% alcalase (−33 mmHg) followed by the 2% papain (−31 mmHg) and then the 2% pepsin + pancreatin (−28 mmHg) hydrolysates. But the 2% pepsin and 4% pepsin caused the most persistent effects, with up to −22 mmHg 24 h after oral administration when compared to only −15 mmHg or less for the

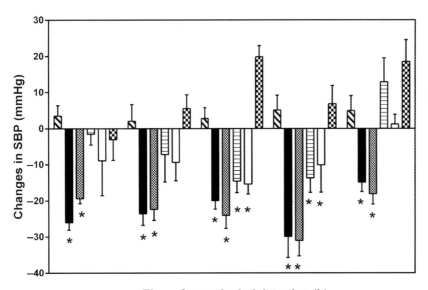

FIGURE 7.4 Time-dependent changes in systolic blood pressure (SBP) of spontaneously hypertensive rats after oral administration of 200 mg/kg body weight each of hemp seed protein isolate (HPI), unfractionated protein hydrolysate (HPH) from pepsin-pancreatin digestion of HPI and membrane ultrafiltration fractions of HPH (<1 and 1–3 kDa) in comparison to 3 mg/kg body weight of captopril. Bars with asterisks (*) have mean values that are significantly lower ($p < 0.05$) than the mean values for saline and HPI bars. *With kind permission from Springer Science + Business Media: Girgih, A.T., Udenigwe, C.C., Li, H., Adebiyi, A.P., & Aluko, R.E. (2011) Kinetics of enzyme inhibition and antihypertensive effects of hemp seed* (Cannabis sativa L.) *protein hydrolysates. Journal of the American Oil Chemists Society, 88,1767–1774, Fig. 4.*

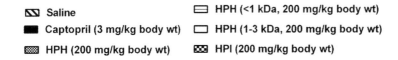

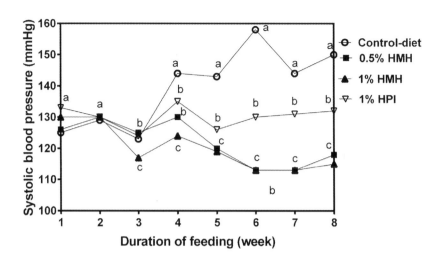

FIGURE 7.5 Effects of casein-only diet or casein diet that contained hempseed products on the systolic blood pressure of young growing spontaneously hypertensive rats. *With kind permission from Springer Science + Business Media: Girgih, A.T., Alashi, A.M., He, R., Malomo, S.A., Aluko, R.E. (2014). Preventive and treatment effects of hemp seed (Cannabis sativa L.) meal protein hydrolysate against blood pressure in spontaneously hypertensive rats. European Journal of Nutrition, 53, 1237–1246, Fig. 2A.*

other hydrolysates. Similar to the results reported by Girgih, Udenigwe, Li et al. (2011), oral administration of the unhydrolyzed hemp seed protein did not produce significant antihypertensive effects. This was probably due to insufficient digestion time within the 24-h experimental period to ensure release of an adequate level of antihypertensive peptides from the hemp seed proteins during passage through the SHR gut.

The long-term preventive or treatment effect of the HPH was also determined by feeding young growing or adult SHR for 8 or 4 weeks, respectively. In the young rats, inclusion of 0.5% or 1.0% (w/w) of HPH in the diet led to complete prevention of hypertension development (Girgih, Alashi, He, Malomo, & Aluko, 2014). After 8 weeks, rats on the control diet had 148 mmHg SBP compared to ~118 mmHg for HPH-fed rats (Fig. 7.5). The unhydrolyzed hemp seed protein was also effective but produced a weaker −130 mmHg SBP after 8 weeks. Therefore, unlike the short-term experiments, the 8 weeks provided adequate time for digestion of hemp seed proteins and absorption of the antihypertensive peptides within the rat gut. However, weaker antihypertensive effect of the unhydrolyzed protein reflects the superior absorption properties of predigested peptides. The results indicate that consumption of these hemp seed products, especially the HPH early in life, could be used as a preventive tool against hypertension development. The HPH also had similar SBP-reducing effects when administered in the diet of adult rats that have already developed hypertension, which is an indication of treatment potential for this product. The mechanism of action of the hemp seed products was confirmed through measurement of plasma ACE and renin activities. Results showed significant reductions in plasma ACE activity with 0.047 and 0.059 U/mL for 0.5% and 1% HPH diets, respectively, after the 8-week feeding trial when compared to the unhydrolyzed protein (0.072 U/mL) and control (0.123 U/mL) diets (Girgih, Alashi, He, Malomo, & Aluko, 2014). Similarly, there were significant reductions in plasma renin activities with 0.040 and 0.054 μg/mL for 1% and 0.5% diets, respectively, when compared to the significantly higher levels obtained for rats that consumed the unhydrolyzed protein (0.095 μg/mL) or control (0.151 μg/mL) diets. The results suggest that hemp seed peptides were absorbed from the SHR gastrointestinal tract and transported through the blood circulatory system where they interacted with ACE and renin to cause negative modulation of catalytic activities. Reduced renin and ACE activities would have led to less production of angiotensin II (the vasopressive compound), which resulted in less contractile action of the blood vessels as reflected in the lower SBP values observed in SHR fed hemp seed protein or protein hydrolysate.

7.5 CONCLUDING REMARKS

Hemp seed is becoming an emerging food crop and a critical contribution to the global economy is expected to increase in the next decade. The attraction to hemp seed has manifold factors. First, because it is mainly an organic crop and hence is compatible with the dietary choices of people who prefer pesticide-free food materials. Second is the high nutritional value of the seed, especially the oil that is rich in omega-3 fatty acids while the proteins have high digestibility. The high arginine level is particularly desirable to health-conscious people who can use the hemp seed protein as a dietary tool to maintain cardiovascular health. Third, many of the hemp seed products contain high levels of dietary fiber and polyphenolic compounds. The fiber content is compatible with maintenance of a healthy colon where it serves as a prebiotic to promote probiotic growth. As antioxidants, the hemp seed polyphenols provide nutritional sources of compounds that can reduce oxidative stress, which reduces the risk of chronic diseases such as cancer, hypertension, renal impairment, and neurodegenerative disorders. However, additional research is required to fully determine the potential food uses and health benefits of individual protein fractions such as the 11S and 7S. While preliminary works have established antihypertensive properties of various HPHs, human intervention trials are required to confirm health benefits and obtain specific health claims that would allow commercialization of these products as functional foods and nutraceuticals.

REFERENCES

Aluko, R. E. (2015). Antihypertensive peptides from food proteins. *Annual Reviews in Food Science and Technology*, 6, 235–262.

Aukema, H. M., Gauthier, J., Roy, M., Jia, Y., Li, H., & Aluko, R. E. (2011). Distinctive effects of plant protein sources on renal disease progression and associated cardiac hypertrophy in experimental kidney disease. *Molecular Nutrition and Food Research*, 55, 1044–1051.

Callaway, J. C. (2002). Hemp as food at high latitudes. *Journal of Industrial Hemp*, 7, 105–117.

Callaway, J. C. (2004). Hempseed as a nutritional resource: An overview. *Euphytica*, 140, 65–72.

Clarke, R. C. (2007). Traditional *Cannabis* cultivation in Darchula district, Nepal—seed, resin and textiles. *Journal of Industrial Hemp*, 12, 19–42.

Deferne, J.-L., & Pate, D. W. (1996). Hemp seed oil: A source of valuable fatty acids. *Journal of the International Hemp Association*, 3, 1–7.

Girgih, A. T., Alashi, A. M., He, R., Malomo, S. A., & Aluko, R. E. (2014). Preventive and treatment effects of hemp seed (*Cannabis sativa* L.) meal protein hydrolysate against high blood pressure in spontaneously hypertensive rats. *European Journal of Nutrition*, 53, 1237–1246.

Girgih, A. T., Alashi, A. M., He, R., Malomo, S. A., Raj, P., Netticadan, T., & Aluko, R. E. (2014). A novel hemp seed meal protein hydrolysate reduces oxidative stress factors in spontaneously hypertensive rats. *Nutrients*, 6, 5652–5666.

Girgih, A. T., Udenigwe, C. C., & Aluko, R. E. (2011). In vitro antioxidant properties of hempseed (*Cannabis sativa* L.) protein hydrolysate fractions. *Journal of the American Oil Chemists Society*, 88, 381–389.

Girgih, A. T., Udenigwe, C. C., Li, H., Adebiyi, A. P., & Aluko, R. E. (2011). Kinetics of enzyme inhibition and antihypertensive effects of hemp seed (*Cannabis sativa* L.) protein hydrolysates. *Journal of the American Oil Chemists Society*, 88, 1767–1774.

House, J. D., Neufeld, J., & Leson, G. (2010). Evaluating the quality of protein from hemp seed (*Cannabis sativa* L.) products through the use of the protein digestibility-corrected amino acid score method. *Journal of Agricultural and Food Chemistry*, 58, 11801–11807.

MAFRD. (2015a). *Industrial hemp production*. <http://www.gov.mb.ca/agriculture/crops/production/hemp.html> Accessed December 8, 2015.

MAFRD. (2015b). *Guidelines for estimating crop production costs 2016*. Manitoba: Manitoba Agriculture, Food and Rural Development.

MAFRD. (2015c). Industrial hemp production and management. <http://www.gov.mb.ca/agriculture/crops/production/hemp-production.html> Accessed December 8, 2015.

Malomo, S. A., & Aluko, R. E. (2015a). A comparative study of the structural and functional properties of isolated hemp seed (*Cannabis sativa* L.) albumin and globulin fractions. *Food Hydrocolloids*, 43, 743–752.

Malomo, S. A., & Aluko, R. E. (2015b). Conversion of a low protein hemp seed meal into a functional protein concentrate through enzymatic digestion of fibre coupled with membrane ultrafiltration. *Innovative Food Science and Emerging Technologies*, 31, 151–159.

Malomo, S. A., Girgih, A. T., Onuh, J. O., & Aluko, R. E. (2015). Structural and antihypertensive properties of enzymatic hemp seed protein hydrolysates. *Nutrients*, 7, 7616–7632.

Malomo, S. A., He, R., & Aluko, R. E. (2015). Structural and functional properties of hemp seed protein products. *Journal of Food Science*, 79, C1512–C1521.

Odani, S., & Odani, S. (1998). Isolation and primary structure of a methionine- and cysteine-rich seed protein of *Cannabis sativa*. *Bioscience, Biotechnology and Biochemistry*, 62, 650–654.

Reichert, G. (1994). Government of Canada report on hemp. *Bi-weekly Bulletin*, 7(23), 1–8.

Tang, C.-H., Ten, Z., Wang, X.-S., & Yang, X.-Q. (2006). Physicochemical and functional properties of hemp (*Cannabis sativa* L.) protein isolate. *Journal of Agricultural and Food Chemistry*, 54, 8945–8950.

Tang, C.-H., Wang, X.-S., & Yang, X.-Q. (2009). Enzymatic hydrolysis of hemp (*Cannabis sativa* L.) protein isolate by various proteases and antioxidant properties of the resulting hydrolysates. *Food Chemistry*, 114, 1484–1490.

Teh, S.-S., Bekhit, A. E.-D., Carne, A., & Birch, J. (2014). Effect of the defatting process, acid and alkali extraction on the physicochemical and functional properties of hemp, flax and canola seed cake protein isolates. *Food Measure*, 8, 92–104.

Turner, C. E., El Sohly, M. A., & Boeren, E. G. (1980). Constituents of *Cannabis sativa* L. XVII. A review of natural constituents. *Journal of Natural Products*, 43, 169–234.

Wang, X.-S., Tang, C.-H., Yang, X.-Q., & Gao, W.-R. (2008). Characterization, amino acid composition and in vitro digestibility of hemp (*Cannabis sativa* L.) proteins. *Food Chemistry*, 107, 11–18.

Wu, G., & Meininger, C. J. (2002). Regulation of nitric oxide synthesis by dietary factors. *Annual Reviews of Nutrition*, 22, 61–86.

Xiaozhai, L., & Clarke, R. C. (1995). The cultivation and use of hemp (*Cannabis sativa* L.) in ancient China. *Journal of International Hemp Association*, 2, 26–33.

Yin, S.-W., Tang, C.-H., Cao, J.-S., Hu, E.-K., Wen, Q.-B., & Yang, X.-Q. (2008). Effects of limited enzymatic hydrolysis with trypsin on the functional properties of hemp (*Cannabis sativa* L.) protein isolate. *Food Chemistry*, 106, 1004–1013.

Yin, S.-W., Tang, C.-H., Wen, Q.-B., & Yang, X.-Q. (2009). Functional and structural properties and in vitro digestibility of acylated hemp (*Cannabis sativa* L.) protein isolates. *International Journal of Food Science and Technology*, 44, 2653–2661.

Zias, J., Stark, H., Sellgman, J., Levy, R., Werker, E., Breuer, A., & Mechoulam, R. (1993). Early medicinal use of cannabis. *Nature*, 363, 215.

Chapter 8

Protein From Flaxseed (*Linum usitatissimum* L.)

H.K. Marambe[1] and J.P.D. Wanasundara[2]

[1]*Agriculture Research Branch, Saskatchewan Ministry of Agriculture, Regina, SK, Canada,* [2]*Agriculture and Agri-Food Canada, Saskatoon, SK, Canada*

8.1 INTRODUCTION

Flax (*Linum usitatissimum* L.) is an annual crop belonging to family Linnaceae and is one of the oldest arable crops with the origin going back to the high Asia or Caucasus region, later spreading to China and India. Archeological evidence supports that the flax cultivation in ancient civilizations was to obtain fiber (Van Sumere, 1992). With the adoption of cotton as a fiber crop for cloth preparation, fiber flax production declined and the major use of flax was switched from stem fiber to seed oil. Traditionally, the flax (or linseed) oil was used in the manufacture of paints, varnishes, and linoleum mainly because of the drying and hardening properties upon exposure to air and sunlight owing to the abundance of polyunsaturated fatty acids (PUFA) (Coskuner & Karababa, 2007). As indicated by the Latin name *usitatissimum*, which means "most useful," different parts of flax plant, the stem and seeds are utilized for various purposes. Use of flax seeds in various forms as a food ingredient, medicinal purposes, and a source of oil dates back to 5000 BC (Amin & Thakur, 2014; Oomah & Mazza, 1998a).

8.1.1 Plant and Seeds

Domesticated *Linum* species plant, *L. usitatissimum* L. throughout cultivation has evolved into two ecotypes. The type that grows for seed oil extraction has a fairly short plant with many secondary branches compared to the type that is grown for the stem fiber (Gill, 1987). Today, the term flaxseed is used to describe the seeds of flax when consumed by humans, while linseed is used to describe the seed of flax when it is used for industrial and feed purposes (Morris, 2007). Flax plant grows to 12–36″ in height and has a typical life cycle of 45–60 days of vegetative period, followed by 15–25 days of flowering period, and 30–40 days of maturation period. The plant produces flowers of blue, white, pink, or violet depending on the variety. The mature fruit of the flax plant is a dry boll or capsule with five segments. Each segment of the boll contains two seeds, therefore a capsule carries up to 10 (average of 6–8) flaxseeds (Saskatchewan Flax Development Commission; Oplinger, Oeleke, Doll, Bundy, & Schuler, 1989).

Seeds of oil flax varieties are larger in size than fiber flax (Green & Marshall, 1981). The physical components of flaxseed include seed coat (testa, true hull, or spermoderm), embryo or the germ, thin endosperm, and two large, flattened cotyledons. The cotyledons form the bulk of the seed weight (57%) followed by the seed coat (38%) and the endosperm (5%) (Wanasundara & Shahidi, 1998). The seed coat has five distinct layers. The epidermal layer or the mucilage layer and the testa, consisting of pigmented cells responsible for the color of flaxseed, are the two important layers of the seed coat. The seeds are reddish to deep brown or smoky yellow in color (Saskatchewan Flax Development Commission, http://www.saskflax.com/ Accessed June 2015; Oplinger et al., 1989). The seed of flax is small, flat, oval-shaped, and pointed at one end with a smooth glossy surface. The seed color ranges from medium, reddish brown to a light yellow (Freeman, 1995). Of these, brown flaxseed is the most common. The seed color is determined by the amount of tannin pigments in the pigment cells of seed coat and brown flaxseeds contain more pigments compared to yellow seeds. In yellow-seeded flax, these pigment cells are often absent or may be present without any pigments (Diederichsen & Richards, 2003). Solin (Linola) is a yellow-seeded commercial flaxseed variety released and marketed in Canada (Muir & Westcott, 2003).

8.1.2 Chemical Composition

Flaxseeds are rich in oil (42–46% by seed weight) with a healthy fatty acid profile. This oil consists of ~73% PUFA, ~9% saturated fatty acids, 52–57% (mean value for Canadian varieties during 2004–13. http://www.grainscanada.gc.ca/flax-lin/harvest-recolte/2014/hqf14-qrl14-en.pdf/ Accessed November 3, 2015.) α-linolenic acid (ALA) and an ω-3/ω-6 ratio of 1:0.3 (Madhusudhan, 2009). Linola is low in ALA (5% or less) compared to brown flaxseed. Thus, the oil of Linola seeds are more stable for oxidation compared to that of brown flaxseed and is suitable for many culinary uses such as for cooking, salads, margarines, and shortenings (Muir & Westcott, 2003).

Most importantly, flaxseed is rich in proteins; 22.4% N-based protein in whole dry seed (mean value for Canadian varieties during 2004–2013, http://www.grainscanada.gc.ca/flax-lin/harvest-recolte/2014/hqf14-qrl14-en.pdf/ Accessed November 3, 2015.) with a range of 10.5–31.0% (Oomah & Mazza, 1993). According to Sammour (1999), the protein level of defatted flaxseed meal (DFM) may range from 35% to 40%. Seed protein level may be influenced by genetic and environmental factors. Flaxseed proteins are mainly located in the cotyledons (Wanasundara & Shahidi, 1998) and the majority is composed of two major protein fractions; a predominantly salt-soluble fraction with high molecular weight (11–12S globulin, 18.6% nitrogen) and a water-soluble basic component with low molecular weight (1.6–2S albumin, 17.7% nitrogen) (Dev, Sienkiewicz, Quensel, & Hansen, 1986; Madhusudhan & Singh, 1983; Sammour, 1999; Vassel & Nesbit, 1945). According to Madhusudhan and Singh (1983) globulins comprise 70–85% of flaxseed proteins. Oomah and Mazza (1993) and Chung Lei and Li-Chan (2005) identified major storage proteins of flaxseed as linin (11–12S) and conlinin (2S) with molecular masses of 252–298 kDa and 16–17 kDa, respectively. Total dietary fiber level of flaxseed is about 400 g/kg which is rich in pentosans. The hull or seed coat contains 2–7% mucilage that is composed of soluble polysaccharides (Venglat et al., 2011).

Among the minor compounds in flaxseed, cyanogenic glycosides (CG), phytates, lignans, and antipyridoxin factors are reported. Flaxseed contains the lignan secoisolariciresinol diglucoside, at levels 75–800 times greater than any other crops or vegetables currently known (Madhusudhan, 2009). The lignan level of flaxseed varies from 0.9% to 3% (Muir & Westcott, 2003) and flaxseed is the richest source of this mammalian lignan precursor. Flax lignan exhibits weak estrogenic and antiestrogenic activity and may prevent estrogen-dependent cancer growth. Hypercholestrolemic, antiartherosclerotic, antidiabetic, and antioxidative properties of flaxseed lignans have been reported (Muir & Westcott, 2003).

Currently, several flaxseed-derived products are commercially available and marketed for their functional food and nutraceutical properties. They include whole seeds, ground or milled flaxseed (flour), oil extracted (by pressing; cold-pressed or not) flax meal, seed coat, partially removed seed, flaxseed hull, cyclic peptides (orbitides) from flaxseed oil, and lignan extracts from flaxseed hull (Shim, Gui, Wang, & Reaney, 2015).

8.2 SUSTAINABILITY OF FLAX: LAND, WATER, AND ENERGY USE

The current trend in crop production is to utilize more environmentally friendly and ecologically sound practices that reduce carbon emission and pollution, enhance energy and resource use efficiency, and to minimize loss of biodiversity and ecosystem. Flax fits well with this trend toward using environmentally and ecologically sound practices meeting the demand for sustainability while reducing production losses.

8.2.1 Land Use

To date, flax is cultivated as a commercial or subsistence crop in more than 30 countries around the world and genetically modified flax is not an available option for the producers. Flax thrives in fertile, fine-textured soil with high water-holding capacity, such as alluvial and loam, but not in coarse-textured sandy soils (Chen, Liu, & Bharat, 2010; Oplinger et al., 1989). Poorly drained land or land subjected to excessive drought or erosion are not suitable for flax cultivation. In 2013, flax cultivation covered 2.3 million ha around the world, producing 2.2 million tons seed, in which Canada contributed 0.7 million tons. Currently, the major flaxseed producers in the world are Canada, China, Russia, Kazakhstan, India, and the United States, contributing more than 70% of world flaxseed production (FAO, http://faostat.fao.org. Accessed May 2015). As the world leading flaxseed producer, Canada contributes ~40% to global flaxseed production (Saskatchewan Flax Development Commission, http://www.saskflax.com/ Accessed June 2015).

8.2.2 Water Use

On average, a flax plant requires 200–215 g of water for every 0.5 kg of dry matter accumulated (Chen et al., 2010). The critical water requirement period for flax is from flowering to just prior to seed ripening. Therefore, to maximize yield and oil content, adequate soil moisture must be maintained during that period (Flax Council of Canada, http://flaxcouncil.ca/ Accessed May 2015). However, according to Canadian Grain Commission reports, cool and wet growing conditions produce flaxseed with higher oil content but lower protein content (Canadian Grain Commission, http://www.canadagrainscouncil.ca/ Accessed May 2015). Flax is considered as an excellent crop for irrigated crop rotation with cereals, corn, sugarcane, and legumes less prone to *Sclerotinia* stem rot that affects canola, sunflower, peas, and beans (Flax Council Canada, http://flaxcouncil.ca/ Accessed May 2015). Energy usage data related to flaxseed production are not available.

8.2.3 Energy Use

Most of the data available on flaxseed cultivation are related to the production in Canadian prairies (provinces of Saskatchewan and Manitoba) and the state of North Dakota of the United States. In crop rotations, flax yields are higher when cultivated after wheat than canola. Flax plant responds to nitrogen (N) when the soil N level is low. Excessive N fertilizer input than the recommended rates (45–110 kg/ha depending on the situation) has no positive influence on increasing seed yield (http://www.agannex.com/field-crops/flax-production-revisited; http://flaxcouncil.ca/growing-flax/introduction). The flax plant is less responsive to phosphorous (P) fertilizer and prefers to have soil residual P coming from the previous crop. When no P fertilizer is added, the flax plant can still maintain high seed yield while showing a high infection rate of arbuscular mycorrhizal fungi (these fungi help to mobilize soil P and transfer to host plant) (http://flaxcouncil.ca/growing-flax/introduction; Franzen, 2004). No direct P fertilization is recommended for flax due to inadequate yield increase with P fertilizer application, however, depending on soil P and potassium (K) levels, adequate amounts should be supplemented from appropriate sources. Equal or better yields can be obtained from flax under reduced tillage (minimum or zero till) than a conventional tillage system. Minimum and zero tillage also help in reducing early weed emergence, improved soil organic matter, increased soil moisture availability and improved mucorrhiza colonization of flax cultivation (http://flaxcouncil.ca/growing-flax/introduction).

8.3 PROCESSING OF PROTEINS AND TYPES OF PRODUCTS FROM FLAXSEED

Flaxseed use in food products escalated with the accumulating scientific evidence on the health benefits of its components, mainly ALA, soluble dietary fiber, and lignan. As the global protein market was valued at US $24.5 billion in 2015, and global plant protein use is expected to reach 2.3 million tons by 2018, as an emerging plant protein, flaxseed has a special place owing to its current acceptability in the health food sector. Currently, there are few companies manufacturing flaxseed protein concentrate and other flaxseed products for food uses, but their product lines do not include isolated flaxseed protein (Table 8.1).

The DFM is the coproduct of flaxseed oil extraction and has protein content ranging from 35% to 40%, soluble and insoluble dietary fiber (20:80–40:60), and lignans (Rabetafika, Van Remoortel, Danthine, Paquot, & Blecker, 2011; Singh, Mridula, Rehal, & Barnwal, 2011) and is considered as an ideal source for recovering protein. Several studies have been conducted on extraction processes for flaxseed protein, however the isolated form of flaxseed protein is not still available on a commercial scale. A major impediment in obtaining protein from DFM using aqueous processes is the mucilage that remains intact with the seed coat as part of the seed meal. Water-soluble mucilage makes highly viscous aqueous extracts and reduces protein extraction efficiency. Due to the viscous nature of protein extract and possible interaction between solubilized protein and polysaccharides, recovery of protein in high purity is difficult. According to Oomah, Mazza, and Cui (1994), extensive process steps are required to remove or reduce mucilage from the extracts or final products, therefore obtaining protein products containing a high level of protein (>75% protein) does not seem viable on a commercial scale. However, several studies at a laboratory scale have shown improved flaxseed protein extraction processes that can bring highly protein-enriched products.

The very first scientific reporting on isolation of flaxseed protein was by Osborne in 1892. Similar to many other seed meals, the solubility of protein in seeds after defatting (DFM) is dependent on pH, solvent-to-meal ratio, solvent composition, salt concentration, and heat treatment employed (Madhusudhan & Singh, 1983). The presence of seed coat polysaccharides (mucilage) increases viscosity of protein extraction medium and affects protein extractability. Moreover protein–polysaccharide interactions cause settling down of proteins during isolation, yielding products with

TABLE 8.1 Commercially Available Flaxseed Products and Flaxseed Protein Products

Commercial Entity	Product Name	Product Type, Description	Special Features	Applications
Glanbia Nutritionals (http://www.glanbianutritionals.com)	Bargain700EF	Blend of pea, chia, and flaxseed protein	80% protein, vegan, non-GMO, gluten-free, enhanced texture, flavor, and shelf-life	Extruded and baked bars, clusters
	Bargain701EF	Blend of soy and flaxseed proteins		
	Harvestpro Flaxprotein 35 flax protein concentrate	Heat-treated natural flax protein concentrate	35% protein, non-GMO, hormone-free, allergen-free, gluten-free	Beverages, foods
	LinPro 140	Flax protein powder	Allergen-free	Protein fortification, bars, clusters, cereals, beverages
Shape Foods Inc. (http://www.shapefoods.com/ Accessed June 2015)	Flax meal	Flax powder	Rich in ω-3 fatty acids, lignin, protein, and fiber, gluten-free	Flax bread, muffins
Natunola Health Inc. (http://www.natunola.com)	Natunola ω-3 flax meal	Large-particle flax powder	20% protein, kosher-certified, non-GMO, gluten-free	Bread, muffin, cookies, cereals, snack foods, bars
	Natunola ω-3 milled flax	Medium-particle flax powder	18% protein, kosher-certified, non-GMO, gluten-free	Crackers, bread, cake, cereal, cookies, snack foods, bars
	Natunola ω-3 flax flour	Fine flax powder	20% protein, non-GMO, gluten-free	Bread, muffin, cookies, cereal, snacks, pasta
Bobs Red Mill (https://www.bobsredmill.com/ Accessed June 2015)	Whole-ground golden flaxseed meal	Milled flaxseed	Freshly milled flaxseed	Bread, pancakes, muffin, bars, cookies

low protein content through aqueous extraction processes. Therefore, several procedures including physical, chemical, or enzymatic methods have been described in the literature to reduce seed mucilage as a step prior to protein extraction (Wanasundara & Shahidi, 1997). The easiest physical way is to remove seed coat as a front-end processing step of oil extraction process. Canada-based ingredient company Natunola (http://www.natunola.com/ Accessed June 2015) produces partially dehulled flaxseed and seed coat and the products are available for food product application. Another way of obtaining mucilage-free seed meal is by treating the whole seed to reduce mucilage in the outermost mucilage-laden seed coat epidermis cells.

Wanasundara and Shahidi (1997) reported that soaking of flaxseed in water or $NaHCO_3$ solutions (or treatment with commercially available carbohydrases; Celluclast 1.5L, Pectinex Ultra SP, and Viscozyme L) reduced the amount of mucilage remaining in the seeds. Low-mucilage-containing seeds prepared via $NaHCO_3$ soaking (0.10 M, 12 h) and treatment with Viscozyme L (22.5 mg enzyme protein per 100 g, 3 h) showed a remarkable improvement in protein extractability of flaxseed seeds. Use of polysaccharide-degrading enzymes, alone or in combination, can also reduce seed coat polysaccharides. According to Wanasundara and Shahidi (1997) protein recovery of 70% can be obtained when Viscozyme (Novozyme, 100 Fungal β glucanase/g) was used in the soaking solution (0.2 g/mL in 0.01 M acetate buffer, seed:solvent 1:10) that is maintained at pH 4.0 and 40°C. This pretreatment for 3 h resulted in the same protein extraction levels as the seed pretreatment of 0.10 M $NaHCO_3$ for 12 h at 30°C. Slominski, Meng, Campbell, Guenter, and Jones (2006) also showed that treatment of DFM with a mixture of cellulase, mannase, and pectinase can reduce mucilage content by 34.7%.

Different extraction methods have been employed for isolation of proteins from flaxseed. These include alkali solubilization followed by acid precipitation, buffered salt (NaCl) extraction, polyphosphate extraction, and micellization. Of these, alkali extraction is popular, as the majority of the proteins go into solution at alkaline pH, so high recovery of protein from meal is reported. According to the literature, flaxseed protein has been extracted from defatted meal under alkaline pH values ranging from 8.5 to 11.0 or in the presence of Na salts (Table 8.2). Similar to many other seed proteins, use of strong alkaline conditions causes undesirable protein modifications such as protein denaturation, chemical changes in amino acids, protein–carbohydrate interactions (Maillard reaction) resulting in formation of dark pigments, and loss of nutritive value. Among the amino acids that modify during strong alkaline conditions are destruction of cysteine and formation of dehydroalanine, which reacts with the epsilon amino group of lysine to produce lysinoalanine. Although the toxicity of lysinoalanine in humans is not reported, this compound has caused the formation of kidney lesions in rats (Masters & Friedman, 1980). Therefore, solubilization of seed proteins in the alkaline pH range (7.5–9.0) is preferred (Berk, 1992). In order to recover protein from alkali extracts of flaxseed meal, several authors have used lowering of pH of the extracts down to the values between 3.5 and 4.4 (Table 8.2). For oil-free flaxseed meal, the minimum N solubility is reported between pH 3.5 and 4.0 (Madhusudhan & Singh, 1983), whereas for demucilaged, defatted, and dehulled flaxseed it occurs at a broad range of pH (3.0–6.0). Membrane filtration followed by diluting the extract with water to form protein micelles is another way to recover

TABLE 8.2 Processes Described for Flaxseed Protein Extraction

Pretreatment of Seed	Protein Obtaining Conditions		Product Protein Content	References
	Extraction	Recovery		
No mucilage removal	pH 6.8, with 1.28 M NaCl (solvent:meal ratio of 16)	No precipitation	82%	Oomah et al. (1994)
No mucilage removal	With 0.15 M NaCl, 13°C	Ultrafiltration (30,000 Da MWCO) + dilution to form micelles	92% (wt)	Green et al. (2003)
No mucilage removal	pH 12	Precipitation at pH 4.4	0.782 albumin eq/g of isolate	Guttierez et al. (2010)
Wash seeds after incubation with 0.1 M NaHCO$_3$ for 12 h (1:8 w/v)	pH 4.98–10.02, with Na hexametaphosphate	Precipitation at pH 3.55	78.1%	Wanasundara and Shahidi (1996)
Wash seeds after incubation with 0.5 M NaHCO$_3$ for 1 h (1:8 w/v; 50°C)	pH 8.5, meal to solvent ratio of 1:10 w/v	Precipitation at pH 3.8	80.2%	Marambe et al. (2008)
Wash seeds after incubation with 0.5 M NaHCO$_3$ (1:8 w/w at 40°C for 1 h)	pH 8.5	Precipitation at pH 3.8	Not reported	Tehrani, Batal, Kamalinejad, and Mahbubi (2014)
Defatted meal slurry (pH 5.0, 37°C) treated with cellulase (1% w/w, 1.44 U/mg) for 4 h	pH 10	Precipitation at pH 4.2	78.9%	Udenigwe, Lu, Han, Hou, & Aluko (2009)
Defatted meal	pH 9, water to meal ratio of 210 mL/g at 160°C	No precipitation	67.9%	Ho et al. (2007)

protein from flaxseed extracts (Green, Martens, Tergesen, & Milanova, 2003). The final product obtained as either a curd/precipitate (acid precipitation) or micelles is dried to generate flaxseed protein isolate.

According to Oomah et al. (1994) under optimum conditions, (1.28 M NaCl, pH 6.8, meal-to-solvent ratio of 1:16 (w:v) at ambient temperature), up to 82% seed protein can be solubilized. Although the highest protein solubility was seen at a solvent-to-meal ratio of 1:10 (pH: 8.0, ionic strength: 0.8 M NaCl), protein extraction under these conditions cannot be considered practical due to the viscous nature of the resulting extract (Oomah et al., 1994). In general, protein-rich products obtained from flaxseed meal are lighter in color.

8.4 NUTRITIVE VALUE OF FLAXSEED PROTEINS

8.4.1 Amino Acids and Proteins

Flaxseed protein has an amino acid composition similar to soy (Madhusudhan, 2009; Thompson & Cunnane, 2003). Table 8.3 shows the amino acid composition of brown-seeded (var. CDC Valour, NorLin) and yellow-seeded (var. Foster, Omega) flaxseed proteins. Similar to other seed storage proteins (SSP), the major protein of flaxseed has high contents of Arg, Glu/Gln, and Asp/Asn (Marambe, Shand, & Wanasundara, 2011; Oomah, 2001; Oomah & Mazza, 2000). The amino acids Lys, Thr, and Tyr are the limiting amino acids of flax protein (Oomah & Mazza, 1995). The essential amino acid index of flaxseed meal is 69 compared to 79 and 75 that were reported for soybean and canola

TABLE 8.3 Amino Acid Composition of Flaxseed Protein From Four Different Canadian Cultivars

Amino Acid	g/100 g Protein				Amino Acid Requirement for Adults (mg/kg/day)
	CDC Valour[a]	NorLin[b]	Foster[b]	Omega[b]	
Essesntial					
His	1.6	2.2	2.1	2.3	8–10
Ile	3.4	4.0	4.1	4.0	12
Leu	4.7	5.8	6.0	5.9	14
Lys	2.1	4.0	4.0	3.9	12
Met + Cys	3.7	2.6	3.2	2.5	13
Phe + Tyr	6.0	6.9	7.2	7.0	14
Thr	2.8	3.6	3.8	3.7	7
Trp	1.1	NR	NR	NR	3.5
Val	3.8	4.6	5.1	4.7	10
Nonessential					
Ala	3.8	4.4	4.7	4.5	
Arg	9.7	9.2	10.0	9.4	
Asp	9.0	9.3	10.0	9.7	
Glu	19.8	19.6	20.0	19.7	
Gly	5.2	5.8	5.9	5.8	
Pro	2.5	3.5	3.8	3.5	
Ser	4.5	4.5	4.7	4.6	

[a]Marambe et al. (2011).
[b]Oomah and Mazza (1993).

meals, respectively (Oomah & Mazza, 2000). Similarly, the protein score based on the most limiting amino acid relative to the Food and Agriculture Organization (FAO) requirement is 82 for flaxseed meal and 67 for soybean meal (Sosulski & Sarwar, 1973). According to Marambe et al. (2011), the total content of essential amino acids in flaxseed protein is 34.3%. The Lys to Arg ratio that determines the cholesterolemic and atherogenic effects of a protein (Czarnecki & Kritchevsky, 1992) is 0.22–0.37 for flaxseed, suggesting that it is less lipidemic and atherogenic compared to soybean or canola proteins, which have Lys to Arg ratios of 0.88 and 0.7–0.9, respectively (Marambe et al., 2011; Oomah, 2001; Oomah & Mazza, 2000; Tan, Mailer, Blanchard, & Agboola, 2011).

Essential amino acid composition of egg protein is superior to flaxseed protein except for Trp content (Udenigwe & Aluko, 2011). Moreover, flaxseed protein satisfies the amino acid requirements of adults, but not for infants and older children due to the limited amounts of Leu and Lys (Udenigwe & Aluko, 2011).

Several studies have been conducted to determine the digestibility of flaxseed protein in vivo and in vitro. An apparent in vivo protein digestibility of 81.4–85.8% is reported when fish species were fed with a diet containing flaxseed meal as the source of protein (Hossain & Jauncy 1989; Hossain, Nahar, & Kamal, 1997; Hossain, Nahar, Kamal, & Islam, 1992), similar to soybean protein (84–85%) (Hossain et al., 1997) and biological value (BV) ranging from 66.4% (El-Kady, 2000) to 77.4% (Frank, 1987; Martinchik, Baturin, Zubtsov, & Molofeev, 2012). In comparison to soybean meal, flaxseed meal has a slightly lower net protein utilization and protein efficiency ratio but higher protein score (Oomah & Mazza, 1995). In vitro digestibility of flaxseed protein is affected by the matrix components, especially mucilage and oil, and the prior processing that seeds receive (Marambe, Shand, & Wanasundara, 2013). For example, the mucilage and lipids in flaxseed can enhance the viscosity of digestive media and decrease the accessibility of digestive enzymes to flaxseed protein, decreasing the protein digestibility, therefore removal of these components improves flaxseed protein digestibility. Removal of mucilage, and mucilage together with oil, has improved in vitro protein digestibility of flaxseed meal up to 51.0% and 66.8%, respectively, compared to 12.6% for full-fat and mucilage containing ground flaxseed (Marambe et al., 2013). Heat treatment that is similar to homestyle baking (31.8%) and boiling (28.0%) also improves in vitro protein digestibility of raw flaxseed (12.6%). The extrusion process increases the nutritional quality and digestibility of flaxseed protein (Giacomino et al., 2013; Wang et al., 2008), resulting in a BV of 80% and a true protein digestibility of 73%. According to Ahmad Khan, Booker, and Yu (2015), in ruminants, the moist heat treatment decreases soluble protein content of flaxseed from 56.5% to 25.9%, lowers the α-helix to β-sheet ratio of containing proteins, and increases the intestinal digestibility of protein, whereas dry heating and microwave irradiation showed no significant impact on the above parameters.

8.4.2 Allergenicity of Flaxseed Proteins

Allergy to flaxseed is rarely reported. In medical literature, the few reported cases are for uncommonly induced symptoms of food allergy in sensitized individuals. However, increased exposure to flaxseed can be a concern due to the escalating number and variety of foods containing flaxseed. Although potent allergens from flaxseed (linseed) are described, no characterized allergens are reported. In two cases of flaxseed allergy, five allergens with molecular weights of 38, 35, 30, 22, and 20 kDa have been detected by Alonso et al. (1996). Lezaun et al. (1998) reported intensive binding of IgE to disulfide bond intact polypeptides with molecular weight of 150–175 kDa. It was identified that a 56-kDa allergen, supposedly a dimer corresponding to a 28-kDa subunit could be allergenic. A malate dehydrogenase was proposed as a candidate molecule that corresponds to a 25-kDa protein (León, Rodriguez, & Cuevas, 2002). Investigation of 1317 patients (54% of them with food or respiratory allergy) using a positive prick test, Fremont et al. (2010) extrapolated that among the French population, flaxseed sensitization is in the range of 0.54–1.08%. Patient allergic to flaxseed showed a positive reaction to heated and extruded flaxseed, indicating the thermostable nature of the allergenic protein. Structural changes in the protein secondary components were also noted due to heat treatment. Flaxseed storage proteins may show cross-reactivity because of the shared homology with other SSP, such as from hemp, lupine, rape, soy, and wheat (Fremont et al., 2010).

8.5 USES AND FUNCTIONALITY OF FLAXSEED PROTEIN

Most of the flaxseed protein functionality evaluations are in model systems and in lab scale. Also, the functional properties vary with the method used for protein extraction. Flaxseed proteins have exhibited water absorption, oil absorption, emulsifying, and foaming properties comparable to those of other oilseed proteins. The presence of mucilage associated with flaxseed protein is reported to enhance the observed functionalities (Rebetafika et al., 2011). Solubility is the most important functional property of a protein as it determines several other functionalities. Flaxseed protein isolates prepared by alkali solubilization followed by acid precipitation have shown greater acid and alkali solubility compared to soy protein isolates and moderate to high solubility in low and high concentrations of NaCl. The presence of salts such as NaCl can shift the minimum solubility pH of flaxseed protein to much lower pH values (Oomah & Mazza, 1993; 1998b). The solubility of isoelectrically precipitated flaxseed protein is reported to be lower compared to that prepared by micellization (Krause, Schultz, & Dudek, 2002) that goes through extraction with salt.

Alkali-extracted and acid-precipitated flaxseed protein has demonstrated a high level of water (WAC) and oil absorption capacities (OAC), with four times more OAC compared to soy protein (Dev & Quensel, 1989). OAC is important for flavor retention and mouthfeel (Martinez-Flores et al., 2006). Due to such OAC values, incorporation of flaxseed protein in emulsion-type meat products is advantageous and reduces fat losses, that is, it reduces product weight loss during cooking. According to Martinez-Flores et al. (2006), flaxseed protein concentrate shows WAC similar to other oilseed protein concentrates and isolates such as that of sunflower seed, and higher than that of bean protein concentrate (Mizubuti, Júnior, de Oliveira Souza, & Ida, 2000) or oat protein concentrate (Ma, 1985). Flax protein concentrate has also exhibited OAC higher than that of amaranth protein concentrate (Martinez-Flores et al., 2006) but lower than bean protein concentrate (Mizubuti et al., 2000). According to Oomah and Mazza (1998b), flax protein concentrate with varying levels of mucilage (changed by removing mucilage at different levels) showed favorable WAC, OAC, emulsifying activity, and emulsion stability compared to soy protein. Using hexametaphosphate-assisted flaxseed protein extracts, Wanasundara and Shahidi (1997) reported the possibility of improving solubility and emulsifying properties by attaching acyl (acetyl or succinyl) groups. A low degree of acetylation improved the oil-binding capacity of flax protein isolates compared to the unmodified (Wanasundara & Shahidi, 1997). Similar to any other protein, flaxseed protein acts as a good emulsifier when the pH is away from isoelectric pH (Martinez-Flores et al., 2006). Several studies report high emulsifying capacity (EC) for alkali-solubilized flaxseed protein (Mueller, Eisner, & Kirchhoff, 2010; Yoshie-Stark et al., 2011). Mueller et al. (2010) also showed poor EC of acid-soluble flaxseed protein fractions in comparison to commercial soy protein isolate, whereas alkaline-soluble protein fraction showed an EC comparable to whole egg. According to the evaluation by Yoshie-Stark et al. (2011) alkaline-soluble flaxseed protein fractions have an EC (535 mL/g) greater than whole egg (495 mL/g) but lower than egg white (800 mL/g), whereas the acid-soluble fraction provided high viscosity of the medium. Flaxseed protein products have shown emulsion stability comparable to that of gelatin (Dev & Quensel, 1989). The studies of Wang, Li, Wang, and Özkan (2010) showed flaxseed protein concentrate generated stable emulsions against droplet aggregation and creaming but was less effective as an emulsifier compared to soy protein concentrate due to its low emulsion viscosity. Therefore, flaxseed protein concentrate is suggested to be more effective in fairly viscous emulsions (Wang et al., 2010).

Flaxseed protein is reported to generate foams when whipped, because they are surface-active. Martines-Flores et al. (2006) showed that at pH 6 flaxseed protein concentrate produced a highly stable foam but with low foam volume. The foam capacity was high at extreme pH conditions (pH 2 and 10) but the stability was poor. In contrast, Mueller et al. (2010) showed poor foaming capacity in acid-soluble flaxseed protein. The addition of flaxseed protein into icecream mixes can increase the product viscosity, specific gravity, and overrun, but decreases meltdown time when the level of addition is increased from 0.5% to 1%. The functionalities shown by flaxseed protein suggests that it is an ideal ingredient to be used in various food formulations including bakery products, salad dressings, mayonnaise, hamburgers, etc. Incorporation of flaxseed protein at 3% (w/w) level has generated a smooth, creamy fish sauce devoid of any undesirable flavors (Dev & Quensel, 1989).

8.6 APPLICATION AND CURRENT PRODUCTS

Currently, whole flaxseeds and milled flaxseed are available to the consumer in the health, functional food product category. These products are marketed as rich sources of ω-3 fatty acids, dietary fiber, and lignans. Whole flaxseeds are found in many regular food products such as muffins, bread, crackers, tortilla, cereals, and snack bars. Very few flaxseed products are commercially marketed as protein sources for food use. *Glanbia Nutritionals* (http://www.glanbianutritionals.com/ Accessed June 2015) is the major manufacturer of flaxseed protein products ranging from concentrates to protein blends. These products can be used as ingredients in baked goods, bars, beverages, cereals, etc. and are listed in Table 8.1. Off-flavor notes of flaxseed are mostly from the oxidized lipids when ground seed is not properly stored. High ALA content makes oil-containing disintegrated seeds highly prone to oxidation upon exposure to air and heat. Whole flaxseed is known to have a nutty, pleasant aroma and taste in baked products.

8.7 POTENTIAL NEW USES, ISSUES, AND CHALLENGES

Whole and milled flaxseed has "Generally Recognized as Safe" status (Flax Focus, 2009), therefore food manufacturers use these flax products in a variety of food formulations. Currently, whole and ground flaxseed are incorporated into cereal and bakery products to provide a pleasant nutty flavor and to increase the health benefits of the final product. Due to its gluten-free nature and promising functional properties, flaxseed products including ground seed, defatted meal, and protein products are tangible solutions for gluten-free ingredients in products for celiac patients. Several attempts have been made to fortify breads with flaxseed flour. For example, replacement of more than 15% wheat flour with flax flour resulted in poor texture, crumb color, graininess, volume, and crust color (Conforti & Davis, 2006). Use of bleaching agents to decolorize flax flour would avoid this limitation. Aider and Martel (2011) evaluated the ability of hydrogen peroxide to decolorize brown flaxseed meal. The product whiteness and yellowness were improved at pH 9 with 3% v/w hydrogen peroxide. The bleachability of flaxseed meal under these conditions was enhanced by increasing temperature but as meal content increased the effectiveness was reduced. Use of 30–50% ground flaxseed is reported to produce acceptable oatmeal cookies and banana nut muffins with only a slight difference in sensory attributes compared to those made with all-purpose flour (Alpers & Sawyer-Morse, 1996).

Flaxseed oil consists of PUFA. Due to the same reason, when using flaxseed products in bakery formulations, unsaturated fatty acid oxidation and compounds such as malonaldehyde (MDA) generation is highly possible. According to Cunnane et al. (1993) normal cooking temperature and time do not increase MDA to a notable level in flaxseed. A major challenge in using flaxseed products in food applications is the presence of antinutritional factors. CG found in flaxseed are linustatin, neolinustatin, and linamarin (Newkirk, 2015). When the cell structure is disrupted, these compounds are degraded by β-glucosidases releasing small amounts of hydrogen cyanide, which is a powerful respiratory inhibitor. Wanasundara, Amarowicz, Kara, and Shahidi (1993) showed that defatting ground flaxseed with methanol—ammonia—water (95:10:5 v:w:v)/hexane, extracted oil and reduces CG (most likey degraded). According to the authors, extraction of flaxseed meal 2–3 times with methanol—ammonia—water (95:10:5 v:w:v) and then with hexane was able to reduce CG by over 90%. Heat treatment is also considered as a suitable method to reduce CG in flaxseed (Madhusudhan & Singh, 1985). For example, heating flaxseeds at 177°C for 1 h resulted in an 80% reduction of CG level in seeds (Chadha, Lawrence, & Ratnayake, 1995). Boiling of flaxseed for 5 min in water, dry and wet autoclaving, and acid treatment followed by autoclaving are the other reported methods for reduction of CG levels in flaxseed (Madhusudhan & Singh, 1985). According to Imran, Anjum, Butt, Siddiq, and Sheikh (2013) a significant reduction of HCN levels in flaxseed is achieved by extrusion even without using a die.

Flaxseed also contains a vitamin B6 (pyridoxine) antagonist, linatine. The concentration of linatine typically ranges from 20 to 100 mg/kg. Heat processing may be necessary to remove these antinutritional factors before consumption (Newkirk, 2015).

Flaxseed proteins contain bioactive peptide sequences that can be liberated by controlled hydrolysis catalyzed by food-grade proteolytic enzymes or gastrointestinal (GI) digestive enzymes (Marambe et al., 2008, 2011). Flaxseed protein-derived bioactive peptides with in vitro antihypertensive, antidiabetic, and antioxidant activities have been reported previously (Doyen et al., 2014; Marambe et al., 2008; Udenigwe & Aluko, 2010; Udenigwe et al., 2009). The most studied bioactivity of flaxseed-derived peptides is the antihypertensive activity, which occurs due to angiotensin 1-converting enzyme inhibition (ACEI) or renin inhibition. The ability of flaxseed protein to release ACEI peptides during simulated GI digestion was reported by Marambe et al. (2011). Abundance of Arg in flaxseed protein is important for cardiovascular health. Arg is an NO precursor in the vascular endothelium. Thus, Arg-rich peptides generated from flaxseed protein can act as potential inhibitors of vasodilators and have hypertension-mitigating ability. Oral administration (200 mg/kg body weight) of flaxseed protein-derived cationic peptides generated by the hydrolytic action of trypsin and Pronase caused a rapid decrease in systolic blood pressure (SBP) in spontaneously hypertensive rats (SHR) compared to that of isolated flaxseed protein. Nwachukwu, Girgih, Malomo, Onuh, and Aluko (2014) also showed that oral administration of Thermoase-digested flaxseed protein to SHR led to lowering of SBP.

Flaxseed protein hydrolysates have also exhibited calmodulin (CaM)binding activity (Omoni & Aluko, 2006). The CaM-dependent neuronal nitric oxide synthase (nNOS) catalyzes production of NO, which in excessive amounts can lead to acute and chronic neurogenerative diseases, stroke, Alzheimer disease, Parkinson disease, headache, convulsion, and pain. Thus, CaM-binding activity of flaxseed protein hydrolysate can inhibit nNOS activity and can be used to prevent/treat pathological conditions caused by the action of nNOS. Recently, using chemical-induced colonic injury in a mouse model, Zarepoor et al. (2014) showed that flaxseed components without mucilage can pose an enhancing effect on colonic injury which warrants further investigation.

The in vivo efficacy of flaxseed protein-derived bioactive peptides enhances the value of flaxseed protein not only as a bulk protein source but also in functional food and nutraceutical applications. The flax protein hydrolysates are suggested as a good source of amino acids as well as bioactive peptide-rich ingredients that will provide physiological benefits when incorporated in to foods. Almost all the studies on bioactive peptide generation have been conducted using isolated protein from flaxseed. In a study on the effects of seed matrix components on flaxseed protein digestibility, Marambe et al. (2013) identified that flaxseed meal with no oil or mucilage and the protein isolated from flaxseed have similar digestibility values. Digestibility is a good indicator of the ability to release bioactive peptides. Thus, DFM upon mucilage removal will be an ideal protein source that can provide the health benefits from bioactive peptides.

8.8 CONCLUDING REMARKS

Flaxseed meal is a rich source of protein but its food uses are limited. Production of flaxseed protein isolate from the oil-extracted flax meal, which is a coproduct of oil extraction, opens more avenues for flaxseed protein incorporation into food. According to the literature, flax protein isolates may be used in protein fortification of processed foods covering a wide range of functions needed in food systems, such as oil emulsification, body formation in baked goods, and foam formation. In addition, the protein isolate may be formed into protein fibers, useful in meat analogs, may be used as an egg white substitute, or an extender in food products where egg white is used as a binder. The flax protein isolate can also be used as a nutritional supplement and the accumulating body of scientific evidence supports health benefits of flaxseed protein-derived peptides.

REFERENCES

Ahmad Khan, N., Booker, H., & Yu, P. (2015). Effect of heating method on alteration of protein molecular structure in flaxseed: Relationship with changes in protein subfraction profile and digestion in dairy cows. *Journal of Agricultural and Food Chemistry, 63*, 1057–1066.

Aider, M., & Martel, A. A. (2011). Bleaching of defatted flaxseed meal to improve its usage as ingredient in food applications. *International Journal of Food Science and Technology, 46*, 2297–2304.

Alonso, L., Marcos, M. L., Blanco, J. G., Navarro, J. A., Juste, S., del Mar Garces, M., ... Carretero, P. J. (1996). Anaphylaxis caused by linseed (flaxseed) intake. *Journal of Allergy & Clinical Immunology, 98*, 469–470.

Alpers, L., & Sawyer-Morse, M. K. (1996). Eating quality of banana nut muffins and oatmeal cookies made with ground flaxseed. *Journal of the American Dietetic Association, 96*, 794–796.

Amin, T., & Thakur, M. (2014). *Linum usitatissimum* L. (flaxseed) a multifarious functional food. *Online International Interdisciplinary Research, IV*, 220–238.

Berk, Z. (1992). Isolate soybean proteins. In Z. Berk (Ed.), *Technology of production of edible flours and protein products from soybeans* (pp. 82–95). Rome: FAO of the United Nations.

Chadha, R. K., Lawrence, J. F., & Ratnayake, W. M. N. (1995). Ion chromatographic determination of cyanide released from flaxseed under autohydrolysis conditions. *Food Additives and Contaminants, 12*, 527–533.

Chen, J. Y., Liu, F., & Bharat, P. S. (2010). Bast fibres: From plants to products. In B. P. Singh (Ed.), *Industrial crops and uses* (pp. 308–325). USA: CAB International.

Chung, M. W. Y., Lei, B., & Li-Chan, E. C. Y. (2005). Isolation and structural characterization of the major protein fraction from NorMan flaxseed (*Linum usitatissimum* L.). *Food Chemistry, 90*, 271–279.

Conforti, F. D., & Davis, S. F. (2006). The effect of soya flour and flaxseed as a partial replacement for bread flour in yeast bread. *International Journal of Food Science and Technology, 41*, 95–101.

Coşkuner, Y., & Karababa, E. (2007). Some physical properties of flaxseed (*Linum usitatissimum* L.). *Journal of Food Engineering, 78*, 1067–1073.

Cunnane, S. C., Ganguli, S., Menard, C., Liede, A. C., Hamadeh, M. J., Chen, Z. Y., & Jenkins, D. J. (1993). High α-linolenic acid flaxseed (*Linum usitatissimum*): Some nutritional properties in humans. *British Journal of Nutrition, 69*, 443–453.

Czarnecki, S. K., & Kritchevsky, D. (1992). Dietary protein and atherosclerosis. In G. U. Liepa, D. C. Bietz, A. C. Beynen, & M. A. Gorman (Eds.), *Dietary proteins: How they alleviate disease and promote better health* (pp. 42–56). American Oils Chemists Society Champaign Il.

Dev, D. K., & Quensel, L. (1989). Functional properties of linseed protein products containing different levels of mucilage in selected food systems. *Journal of Food Science, 54*, 183–186.

Dev, D. K., Sienkiewicz, T., Quensel, E., & Hansen, R. (1986). Isolation and partial characterization of flaxseed (*Linum usitatissimum* L.) proteins. *Food/Nahrung, 30*, 391–393.

Diederichsen, A., & Richards, K. (2003). Cultivated flax and the genus *Linum* L. In A. Muir, & N. Westcott (Eds.), *Flax: The genus Linum* (pp. 22–54). NW: CRC Press.

Doyen, A., Udenigwe, C. C., Mitchell, P. L., Marette, A., Aluko, R. E., & Bazinet, L. (2014). Anti-diabetic and antihypertensive activities of two flaxseed protein hydrolysate fractions revealed following their simultaneous separation by electrodialysis with ultrafiltration membranes. *Food Chemistry, 145*, 66–76.

El-Kady, E. A. (2000). *Chemical and technological studies on seed of some field crops of agriculture*. PhD thesis. Tanta University.

FAO, http://faostat.fao.org. Accessed May 2015.

Flax Focus. (2009). http://www.ameriflax.com/UserFiles/File/FF_Apr09_R2.pdf.

Frank, A. W. (1987). Food uses of cottonseed protein. In B. J. Hudson (Ed.), *Development in food proteins-5* (pp. 30−80). London: Elsevier Applied Science Publishers.

Franzen, D. (2004). *Fertilizing flax. NDSU Extension Service document SF-717*. https://www.ag.ndsu.edu/pubs/plantsci/soilfert/sf717.pdf.

Freeman, T. P. (1995). Structure of flaxseed. In L. C. Cunnane, & L. U. Thompson (Eds.), *Flaxseed in human nutrition* (pp. 11−21). Champaign Illinois: AOCS Press.

Fremont, S., Moneret-Vautrin, P., Morisset, Fm, Croizier, A., Codreanu, F., & Kanny, G. (2010). Prospective study of sensitization and food allergy to flaxseed in 1,317 subjects. *European Annals of Allergy and Clinical Immunology, 42*, 103−111.

Giacomino, S., Peñas, E., Ferreyra, V., Pellegrino, N., Fournier, M., Apro, N., & Frías, J. (2013). Extruded flaxseed meal enhances the nutritional quality of cereal-based products. *Plant Foods for Human Nutrition, 68*, 131−136.

Gill, K. S. (1987). *Linseed*. New Delhi, India: Indian Council of Agricultural Research.

Green, A. G., & Marshall, D. R. (1981). Variation for oil quantity and quality in linseed (*Linum usitatissimum*). *Crop and Pasture Science, 32*, 599−607.

Green, B. E., Martens, R. W., Tergesen, J. F., Milanova, R. (2003). U.S. Patent No. 20,030,109,679. Washington, DC: U.S. Patent and Trademark Office.

Gutiérrez, C., Rubilar, M., Jara, C., Verdugo, M., Sineiro, J., & Shene, C. (2010). Flaxseed and flaxseed cake as a source of compounds for food industry. *Journal of Soil Science and Plant Nutrition, 10*, 454−463.

Ho, C. H. L., Cacace, J., & Mazza, G. (2007). Extraction of lignans, proteins and carbohydrates from flaxseed meal with pressurized low polarity water. *LWT- Food Science & Technology, 40*, 1637−1647.

Hossain, M. A., & Jauncey, K. (1989). Studies on the protein, energy and amino acid digestibility of fish meal, mustard oilcake, linseed and sesame meal for common carp (*Cyprinus carpio* L.). *Aquaculture, 83*, 59−72.

Hossain, M. A., Nahar, N., & Kamal, M. (1997). Nutrient digestibility coefficients of some plant and animal proteins for rohu (*Labeo rohita*). *Aquaculture, 151*, 37−45.

Hossain, M. A., Nahar, N., Kamal, M., & Islam, M. N. (1992). Nutrient digestibility coefficients of some plant and animal proteins for tilapia (*Oreochromis mossambicus*). *Journal of Aquaculture in the Tropics, 7*, 257−266.

Imran, M., Anjum, F. M., Butt, M. S., Siddiq, M., & Sheikh, M. A. (2013). Reduction of cyanogenic compounds in flaxseed (*Linum usitatissimum* L.) meal using thermal treatment. *International Journal of Food Properties, 16*, 1809−1818.

Krause, J. P., Schultz, M., & Dudek, S. (2002). Effect of extraction conditions on composition, surface activity and rheological properties of protein isolates from flaxseed (*Linum usitativissimum* L). *Journal of the Science of Food and Agriculture, 82*, 970−976.

León, F., Rodriguez, M., & Cuevas, M. (2002). The major allergen of linseed. *Allergy, 57*, 968.

Lezaun, A., Fraj, J., Colas, C., Duce, F., Dominguez, M. A., Cuevas, M., & Eiras, P. (1998). Anaphylaxis from linseed. *Allergy, 53*, 105−106.

Ma, C. Y. (1985). Functional properties of oat concentrate treated with linoleate or trypsin. *Canadian Institute of Food Science and Technology Journal, 18*, 79−84.

Madhusudhan, B. (2009). Potential benefits of flaxseed in health and disease − A perspective. *Agriculturae Conspectus Scientificus (ACS), 74*, 67−72.

Madhusudhan, K. T., & Singh, N. (1983). Studies on linseed proteins. *Journal of Agricultural and Food Chemistry, 31*, 959−963.

Madhusudhan, K. T., & Singh, N. (1985). Effect of detoxification treatment on the physicochemical properties of linseed. *Journal of Agricultural and Food Chemistry, 33*, 1219−1222.

Marambe, P. W. M. L. H. K., Shand, P. J., & Wanasundara, J. P. D. (2008). An *in vitro* investigation of selected biological activities of hydrolyzed flaxseed (*Linum usitatissimum* L.) proteins. *Journal of American Oil Chemists' Society, 85*(12), 1155−1164.

Marambe, H. K., Shand, P. J., & Wanasundara, J. P. (2011). Release of angiotensin I-converting enzyme inhibitory peptides from flaxseed (*Linum usitatissimum* L.) protein under simulated gastrointestinal digestion. *Journal of Agricultural and Food Chemistry, 59*, 9596−9604.

Marambe, H. K., Shand, P. J., & Wanasundara, J. P. (2013). In vitro digestibility of flaxseed (*Linum usitatissimum* L.) protein: Effect of seed mucilage, oil and thermal processing. *International Journal of Food Science and Technology, 48*, 628−635.

Martinchik, A. N., Baturin, A. K., Zubtsov, V. V., & Molofeev, V. (2012). Nutritional value and functional properties of flaxseed. *Voprosy Pitaniia, 81*, 4−10.

Martínez-Flores, H. E., Barrera, E. S., Garnica-Romo, M. G., Penagos, C. J. C., Saavedra, J. P., & Macazaga-Alvarez, R. (2006). Functional characteristics of protein flaxseed concentrate obtained applying a response surface methodology. *Journal of Food Science, 71*, C495−C498.

Masters, P. M., & Friedman, M. (1980). Amino acid racemization in alkali treated food proteins-Chemistry, toxicology and nutritional consequences. In J. R. Whitaker, & M. Fujimaki (Eds.), *Chemical Deterioration of Proteins* (Volume 123, pp. 165−194). ACS Symposium Series.

Mizubuti, I. Y., Júnior, O. B., de Oliveira Souza, L. W., & Ida, E. I. (2000). Response surface methodology for extraction optimization of pigeon pea protein. *Food Chemistry, 70*, 259−265.

Morris, D. H. (2007). *Flax − A health and nutrition primer*. <http://www.flaxcouncil.ca> Accessed August 2015.

Mueller, K., Eisner, P., & Kirchhoff, E. (2010). Simplified fractionation process for linseed meal by alkaline extraction − Functional properties of protein and fibre fractions. *Journal of Food Engineering, 99*, 49−54.

Muir, A. D., & Westcott, N. D. (2003). Current regulatory status of flaxseed and commercial products. In A. Muir, & N. Westcott (Eds.), *Flax: The genus Linum* (pp. 292−298). NW: CRC Press.

Newkirk, R. (2015). *Flax feed industry guide*. Flax Canada 2015 Inc.

Nwachukwu, I. D., Girgih, A. T., Malomo, S. A., Onuh, J. O., & Aluko, R. E. (2014). Thermoase-derived flaxseed protein hydrolysates and membrane ultrafiltration peptide fractions have systolic blood pressure-lowering effects in spontaneously hypertensive rats. *International Journal of Molecular Sciences, 15*(10), 18131−18147.

Omoni, A. O., & Aluko, R. E. (2006). Mechanism of the inhibition of calmodulin-dependent neuronal nitric oxide synthase by flaxseed protein hydrolysates. *Journal of the American Oil Chemists' Society, 83*, 335—340.

Oomah, B. D. (2001). Flaxseed as a functional food source. *Journal of the Science of Food and Agriculture, 81*, 889—894.

Oomah, B. D., & Mazza, G. (1993). Flaxseed proteins—A review. *Food Chemistry, 48*, 109—114.

Oomah, B. D., & Mazza, G. (1995). Functional properties, uses of flaxseed protein. *Inform, 6*, 1246—1252.

Oomah, B. D., & Mazza, G. (1998a). Compositional changes during commercial processing of flaxseed. *Industrial Crops and Products, 9*, 29—37.

Oomah, B. D., & Mazza, G. (1998b). Flaxseed products for disease prevention. In G. Mazza (Ed.), *Functional foods: Biochemical and processing aspects (vol. 1)* (pp. 91—138). PA: CRC Press.

Oomah, B. D., & Mazza, G. (2000). Bioactive components of flaxseed: Occurrence. In F. Shahidi, & C. Ho (Eds.), *Phytochemicals and phytopharmaceuticals* (pp. 106—121). The American Oil Chemists Society.

Oomah, B. D., Mazza, G., & Cui, W. (1994). Optimization of protein extraction from flaxseed meal. *Food Research International, 27*, 355—361.

Oplinger, E., Oeleke, E., Doll, J., Bundy, L., & Schuler, R. (1989). *Alternative field crops manual: Flax. Online.* Purdue University Center for New Crops and Plants Products.

Osborne, T. B. (1892). Crystallised vegetable proteids. *American Chemistry Journal, 14*, 662—689.

Rabetafika, H. N., Van Remoortel, V., Danthine, S., Paquot, M., & Blecker, C. (2011). Flaxseed proteins: Food uses and health benefits. *International Journal of Food Science & Technology, 46*, 221—228.

Sammour, R. H. (1999). Proteins of linseed (*Linum usitatissimum* L.), extraction and characterization by electrophoresis. *Botanical Bulletin of Academia Sinica, 40*, 121—126.

Shim, Y. Y., Gui, B., Wang, Y., & Reaney, M. J. (2015). Flaxseed (*Linum usitatissimum* L.) oil processing and selected products. *Trends in Food Science & Technology, 43*, 162—177.

Singh, K. K., Mridula, D., Rehal, J., & Barnwal, P. (2011). Flaxseed: A potential source of food, feed and fibre. *Critical Reviews in Food Science and Nutrition, 5*, 210—222.

Slominski, B. A., Meng, X., Campbell, L. D., Guenter, W., & Jones, O. (2006). The use of enzyme technology for improved energy utilization from full-fat oilseeds. Part II: Flaxseed. *Poultry Science, 85*, 1031—1037.

Sosulski, F. W., & Sarwar, G. (1973). Amino acid composition of oilseed meals and protein isolates. *Canadian Institute of Food Science and Technology Journal, 6*, 1—5.

Tan, S. H., Mailer, R. J., Blanchard, C. L., & Agboola, S. O. (2011). Canola proteins for human consumption: Extraction, profile, and functional properties. *Journal of Food Science, 7*, R16—R28.

Tehrani, M. H. H., Batal, R., Kamalinejad, M., & Mahbubi, A. (2014). Extraction and purification of flaxseed proteins and studying their antibacterial activities. *Journal of Plant Sciences, 2*, 70—76.

Thompson, L. U., & Cunnane, S. C. (2003). *Flaxseed in human nutrition.* AOCS Press.

Udenigwe, C. C., & Aluko, R. E. (2010). Antioxidant and angiotensin converting enzyme-inhibitory properties of a flaxseed protein-derived high fischer ratio peptide mixture. *Journal of Agricultural and Food Chemistry, 58*, 4762—4768.

Udenigwe, C. C., & Aluko, R. E. (2011). Another side of flaxseed proteins and peptides. *Agro Food Industry Hi Tech, 22*, 50—53.

Udenigwe, C. C., Lu, Y. L., Han, C. H., Hou, W. C., & Aluko, R. E. (2009). Flaxseed protein-derived peptide fractions: Antioxidant properties and inhibition of lipopolysaccharide-induced nitric oxide production in murine macrophages. *Food Chemistry, 116*, 277—284.

Van Sumere, C. (1992). Retting of flax with special reference to enzyme-retting. In S. H. Shekher Sharms, & C. Van Sumere (Eds.), *The biology and processing of flax* (pp. 153—193). Ireland: M Publications.

Vassel, B., & Nesbitt, L. L. (1945). The nitrogenous constituents of flaxseed II. The isolation of a purified protein fraction. *Journal of Biological Chemistry, 159*, 571—584.

Venglat, P., Xiang, D., Qiu, S., Stone, S. L., Tibiche, C., Cram, D., ... Datla, R. (2011). Gene expression analysis of flax seed development. *BMC Plant Biology, 11*, 74—88.

Wanasundara, P. K. J. P. D., Amarowicz, R., Kara, M. T., & Shahidi, F. (1993). Removal of cyanogenic glycosides of flaxseed meal. *Food Chemistry, 48*, 263—266.

Wanasundara, P. K. J. P. D., & Shahidi, F. (1996). Optimization of hexametaphosphate-assisted extraction of flaxseed proteins using response surface methodology. *Journal of Food Science, 61*, 604—607.

Wanasundara, P. K. J. P. D., & Shahidi, F. (1997). Functional properties of acylated flax protein isolates. *Journal of Agricultural and Food Chemistry, 45*, 2431—2441.

Wanasundara, P. K. J. P. D., & Shahidi, F. (1998). Process-induced compositional changes of flaxseed. In F. Shahidi, & T. C. Ho (Eds.), *Process-induced chemical changes in food* (pp. 307—325). New York: Plenium Press.

Wang, Y., Li, D., Wang, L. J., Chiu, Y. L., Chen, X. D., Mao, Z. H., & Song, C. F. (2008). Optimization of extrusion of flaxseeds for in vitro protein digestibility analysis using response surface methodology. *Journal of Food Engineering, 85*, 59—64.

Wang, B., Li, D., Wang, L. J., & Özkan, N. (2010). Effect of concentrated flaxseed protein on the stability and rheological properties of soybean oil-in-water emulsions. *Journal of Food Engineering, 96*, 555—561.

Yoshie-Stark, Y., Mueller, K., Kawarada, H., Futagawa, K., Nakada, R., & Tashiro, Y. (2011). Functional properties of linseed meal fractions: Application as nutraceutical ingredient. *Food Science and Technology Research, 17*, 301—310.

Zarepoor, L., Lu, J. T., Zhang, C., Wu, W., Lepp, D., Robinson, L., ... Power, K. A. (2014). Dietary flaxseed intake exacerbates acute colonic mucosal injury and inflammation induced by dextran sodium sulfate. *American Journal of Physiology, Gastrointestinal and Liver Physiology, 306*, G1042—G1055.

Chapter 9

Pea: A Sustainable Vegetable Protein Crop

M.C. Tulbek, R.S.H. Lam, Y.(C.) Wang, P. Asavajaru and A. Lam
AGT Foods, Saskatoon, SK, Canada

9.1 INTRODUCTION

Pea (garden pea, field pea, spring pea, English pea, common pea, green pea (*Pisum sativum* L. ssp. *sativum*) and Austrian winter pea (*Pisum sativum* L. ssp. *sativum* var. *arvense*)) are cool-season pulse crops primarily grown for protein and feed purposes around the world (Pavek, 2012). Several types of pea genotypes are available and cultivated for select end-use markets. Snap pea and fresh garden pea are harvested fresh (72–80% moisture) for the canning and frozen food industries, whereas field pea and Austrian pea are harvested dry (10–15% moisture) for global feed (Elzebroek & Wind, 2008) and food industries. Peas are also a major raw material for the whole, split, and flour ingredient marketplace (Pavek, 2012).

Peas are cultivated primarily in Canada, Russia, the United States, France, and Australia within variable growing and soil zones (Table 9.1). Since the 1970s, major initiatives provided by Canadian government have increased dry pea production in western Canada, which consequently assisted producers with the improved cereal and oilseed yield benefits as part of a rotational crop. In addition, Canadian producers observed benefits such as increased land use, reduced summer fallow acreage, improved soil aggregation, and breaking the disease cycle by adding peas to their rotations (AGT Foods).

Similar growth patterns of pea cultivation and production have been observed in US agriculture since the 2000s. As peas were introduced to the US food aid programs, US growers increased dry pea production in western North Dakota and eastern Montana. Peas have been serving as a rotational crop with cereal and oilseed crops, assisting in disease management and increasing organic matter and fixing nitrogen in the soil, improving soil aggregation and conservation of water (Biederbeck, Zenter, & Campbell, 2005; Chen et al., 2006; Lupwayi, Rice, & Clayton, 1998). Overall, peas became a major sustainable crop for their nitrogen-fixation benefits and as a protein source for global protein supply for the last three decades in North America (Pavek, 2012).

Most of the North American dry pea production (estimated 70%) was destined for export, while a relatively small amount of dry pea is used for domestic consumption. India and China are the leading export markets for North American peas, primarily as a staple food and for milling purposes in India and as a vermicelli noodle in China.

9.1.1 Cultivation

Pea crop can grow within several climate and soil zones. However, pea plants grow best on fertile, light, well-drained, and humus-rich soils. Soil salinity and extreme acidity can be detrimental for pea production whereby the ideal soil pH for pea production is 6.5–7.0. Precipitation may significantly affect pea production where a range between 14 and 40 inches is desirable for cultivation. Unnecessary tillage in the spring may dry out soils and cause problems because peas require more moisture during germination than other crops such as cereals. In terms of temperature, pea plants can tolerate −25°F if covered with snow. However, newer cold-hardy varieties can tolerate even lower temperatures where further research is underway to expand the production region further north (Saskatchewan Pulse Growers, 2016).

Soil micronutrient levels ideally should be high in potassium, phosphorus, and manganese for optimal growth and nitrogen fixation. Producers are encouraged to inoculate the pea seed with an appropriate nitrogen-fixing bacterium

TABLE 9.1 Major Pea-Producing Countries of the World (FAO, 2015)

Country	5-Year Average (Metric Tons)	2014 (Metric Tons)
Canada	3,217,800	3,300,000
Russia	1,580,000	2,197,000
United States	578,000	729,000
France	686,600	575,000
Australia	356,000	334,000
World	10,268,000	11,164,000

called *Rhizobia*. *Rhizobia* application significantly increases yield and nitrogen fixation, which will increase the nitrogen content within the plant and in the soil. If inoculation is applied properly, nitrogen fixation will occur approximately 4 weeks after germination and continue through seeding (Saskatchewan Pulse Growers, 2016).

Factors such as growing region, climate, rainfall, growing season, disease pressures, and soil health dictate pea production management. Each region will have its unique production techniques and management tools. Depending on the cultivar, climate, and growing conditions there can be 850–3000 pea seeds/pound after harvest, which is influenced by the seed size and bulk density. The average yield of peas can be variable, between 15 and 70 bushels/acre. The ideal test weight for field peas is 60 lb./bushel. Peas should be harvested at physiological maturity, when most pods have changed from a green to yellow color. Harvesting might be difficult if the plants are not sufficiently dry, but seed damage is possible if growers delay harvest until peas are too dry and brittle (Pavek, 2012).

9.1.2 Cultivars

Several fresh, garden, and dry pea cultivars are globally available for pea cultivation. Agriculture and Agri-Food Canada (AAFC), the United States Department of Agriculture (USDA), Crop Development Centre in Saskatoon Saskatchewan; North Dakota State University in Fargo, ND; Montana State University in Bozeman, MT, Washington State University, International Center for Agricultural Research in the Dry Area (ICARDA), Consortium of International Agricultural Research Center (CGIAR) and several seed companies are the major research institutes that are actively working on global dry pea seed development and genomics. The breeders primarily select pea plants for height, vegetative growth form, season of maturity, disease resistance, pod shape and length, seed color, tenderness, sweetness, seed shape, number of seeds per pod, and pod production per node (Elzebroek & Wind, 2008; Hartmann, Kofranek, Rubatzky, & Flocker, 1988).

Canadian growers primarily grow CDC Golden and CDC Meadow yellow pea cultivars and as of 2015 these varieties represent 65% of the total yellow pea production. In terms of green pea production, producers primarily grow CDC Striker, CDC Patrick, CDC Sage, and CDC Cooper cultivars, which constitute 70% of production (AGT Foods). As new cultivars with enhanced traits are introduced to the market, older cultivars will lose their market share, which is a part of the life cycle of a cultivar. US producers primarily grow Ariel, Arcadia, Cruiser, Banner, Columbia, CDC Striker, and K-2 green pea cultivars and CDC Meadow, CDC Golden, DS Admiral, CDC Agassiz, Delta, and Bridger yellow pea cultivars. These varieties constitute about 65–70% of total pea production in the United States.

It is imperative to understand that crop yield, disease resistance, and other agronomic factors are the most influential attributes for the long life expectancy of cultivars. Protein content, cooking quality, color, and taste are considered as secondary attributes which affect the penetration of these varieties into the global marketplace.

9.2 SUSTAINABILITY, ENERGY, AND WATER USE

Since the 1990s, food companies have come to value the sustainable supply of food and ingredients, whereby their focus is on the energy and water usage required for production. As raw materials are analyzed for their total water and energy use per unit raw material, transportation energy use and greenhouse emission use; food companies have become increasingly interested in determining a product's footprint in detail so that they may have a positive impact on our global environment. Unilever (2002) reported that sustainable agriculture is productive, competitive, and efficient while at the same time protecting the natural environment and conditions of local communities. Primary principles of sustainable agriculture are based on (Unilever, 2002):

- Producing crops with high yield and nutritional quality to meet existing and future needs while keeping resource inputs as low as possible;
- Ensuring that any adverse effects on soil fertility, water, and air quality and biodiversity from agricultural activities are minimized and positive contribution will be made where possible;
- Optimizing the use of renewable resources while minimizing the use of nonrenewable resources;
- Sustainable agriculture should enable local communities to protect and improve their wellbeing and environments.

Pea plants have a symbiotic relationship with soil microorganisms such as *Rhizobia* which enable peas to fixate nitrogen from atmospheric nitrogen into soil, therefore reducing the need for energy-intensive synthetic nitrogen.

Zentner et al. (2004) reported that, based on 12 years of field data (1987–98), growing pea crops required half the energy input of spring wheat in western Canada. In terms of efficiency, peas produced almost twice the amount of grain per unit of energy input as spring wheat. Spring wheat grown after pea requires 8% less energy than spring wheat grown after a cereal (Zentner et al., 2004). When 1 year of pea was included in a 4-year crop rotation cycle, the total energy requirement of the entire system was reduced by 13% (http://www.pulsecanada.com/environment/sustainability/non-renewable-energy/whats-the-pulse-impact). A life cycle analysis conducted by the Saskatchewan Research Council (2011) demonstrated that replacing 1 year of spring wheat in a 4-year crop rotation (canola-spring wheat-spring wheat-spring wheat) with pea or lentil crop, reduced the nonrenewable energy use of the entire rotation by 24% and 22%, respectively. This was attributed to the lower energy requirement of the nitrogen-fixing pulses, and the reduced fertilizer requirement of the wheat grown after the pulse crop. The Sarecon Sustainability Report (2011) demonstrated a 20% improvement in the energy index for peas from 1981 to 2006 and a 33% improvement for lentils from 1986 to 2006 in western Canada.

In terms of water usage, Hoekstra (2015) reported that the water footprint per gram of protein for milk, eggs, and chicken meat is about 1.5 times larger than for pulses and in beef, the water footprint per gram of protein is six times larger than for pulses. When comparing vegetable versus animal protein sources, there is ample evidence that vegetable proteins utilize much less water during production and within the consumer supply chain.

9.3 PROCESSING OF PEAS

Pea crop (both green and yellow) have been traditionally processed based on cleaning and splitting mechanical steps. Cleaning is the first step in which impurities such as chaff, soil, dirt, and other seeds are removed from whole peas. Canola seed, wheat, mustard, wild oats, and barley seed should be cleaned from whole pea for purity compliance in addition to allergen control. Wheat, barley, and rye contain gluten, thus pea crops have to be cleaned in order to support gluten-free claims in food formulations. Equipment such as indent cleaners can be used in removing impurities (Fig. 9.1).

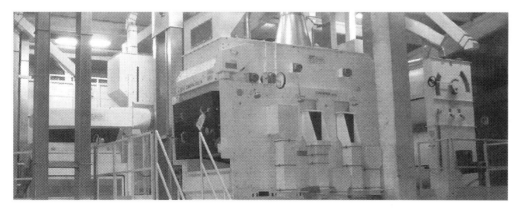

FIGURE 9.1 Indent cleaner. *Courtesy of Cimbria Corporation.*

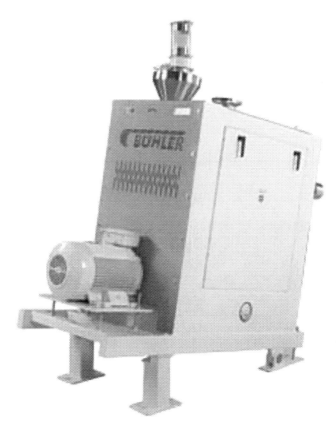

FIGURE 9.2 Dehuller. *Courtesy of Buhler AG.*

The cleaning process is followed by splitting and dehulling, which splits the pea seed and removes the hull portion of whole peas, respectively. These processes were designed primarily to reduce cooking time and prepare split peas for the traditional soup industry. Dehullers can be used to produce split peas and remove hulls (Fig. 9.2).

Split peas may be further processed into flour, protein, and starch fractions based on dry milling and air classification or wet milling technologies. These technologies will define the purity level of each ingredient in terms of protein and starch concentrations.

Dry milling technology is a traditional mechanical process used to reduce the particle size of split or whole peas into coarse or fine flours. The main goals of dry milling are to create appropriate particle sizes for end-product functionality and to create a free-flowing material. Desired particle size distribution and milling efficiency are important factors to consider in choosing milling technology, capacity, and process design. Roller mills combined with sifter technologies can be used in coarse pea meal production, whereas pin mills (Fig. 9.3) can be used to produce finely ground particles. Roasting and precooking technologies have been used to inactivate lipoxygenase and improve taste and flavor attributes (Tulbek, Simsek, & Hall, 2009).

Dry milling and air classification technology is a clean label milling and separation technology which can be used to produce fine flour, coarse flour, protein concentrate, and starch concentrate products. In this process, finely ground, pin-milled flour is air-classified with reverse-pressure air stream. Starch and protein fractions are removed based on particle size distribution, bulk density, size, shape, and powder characteristics. Protein fractions are separated as fine particles (2–25 μm) and starch fractions (25–70 μm) are collected as heavy particles. In its final form, protein fractions may be labeled as protein concentrates or air-classified pea protein (Fig. 9.4) while starch fractions may be labeled as a starch concentrate or an air-classified pea starch (Fig. 9.5). Proximate analyses of pea protein and pea starch concentrates are provided in Table 9.2.

Scanning electron micrograph (SEM) analyses clearly show the mechanical separation of protein and starch fractions by the dry milling and air classification processes. This technology can be used as a clean label and natural process by the industry. Tyler and Panchuk (1982), Han and Khan (1992a, 1992b), and Wu and Nichols (2005) reported the fundamentals of dry milling and air classification on the functional attributes of peas and edible beans. Pea protein concentrate produced in this process will be over 48%, which is twice the protein content in the seed.

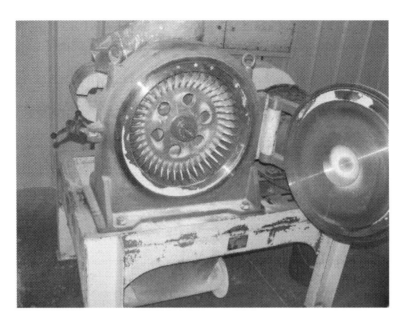

FIGURE 9.3 Pin mill. *Courtesy of Particle Control LLC.*

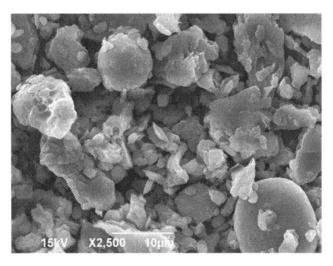

FIGURE 9.4 Scanning electron micrograph of air-classified pea protein ($\times 2500$).

Pea seeds can be processed into protein and starch isolates through wet fractionation/milling processes. Wet-milled pea proteins and starches can be processed according to the technologies listed below (Tulbek, 2014):

- Process based on traditional Chinese vermicelli noodle production
  - Pulse protein (over 72% protein)
  - Pulse starch (90–99% starch);
- Isoelectric precipitation and extraction
  - Pulse protein (over 77% protein)
  - Pulse starch (90–99% starch);
- Water/salt-based extraction
  - Pulse protein (over 75% protein)
  - Pulse starch (90–99% starch);
- Enzymatically assisted isoelectric precipitation and extraction
  - Pulse protein (over 85% protein)
  - Pulse starch (90–99% starch).

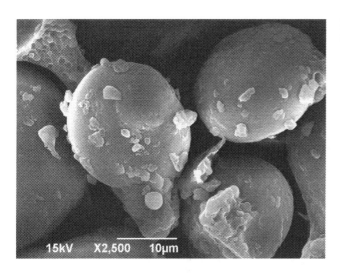

FIGURE 9.5 Scanning electron micrograph of air-classified pea starch ($\times 2500$).

TABLE 9.2 Proximate Analysis of Pea Protein and Pea Starch Concentrates

	Protein (% dm)	Starch (% dm)	Fat (% dm)	Ash (% dm)
Whole pea	21–24	42–46	1.5–2.0	1.9–2.2
Split pea	25–27	46–52	1.5–2.0	2.3–2.5
Pea protein concentrate	48–55	5–10	2.5–3.0	2.7–3.1
Pea starch concentrate	10–15	65–75	0.9–1.3	1.2–1.4

dm, dry matter.

Wet fractionation technology for peas was first developed by Chinese vermicelli noodle manufacturers in Qingdao, China, as a part of a traditional vermicelli noodle-manufacturing process. Whole peas are soaked and lactic acid bacterial fermentation is applied until a soaked pea slurry forms. Following a 96-h fermentation process starch is removed from fiber and protein fractions for vermicelli production. Protein and inner and outer fiber fractions are separated as coproducts (AGT Foods).

Schoch and Maywald (1968) published their pioneering work on the extraction of starch from split yellow peas and other pulse sources. This process involves the preparation of a slurry in alkaline solution followed by centrifugation and drying. Alkali neutralization and salt removal may also be required based on the process design and end-product specifications. Since the 1970s there have been well-established pea protein isolation processes established in the European Union and Canada. Protein isolates are produced according to the solubilization of proteins at alkaline pH 9.5–10.5 followed by isoelectric precipitation at pH 4.0–5.0, neutralization of the slurry at pH 7.0, and a drying process. SEM revealed the purity of the isolated pea starch granules by the absence of protein fragments on the surface of the starch granules (Fig. 9.6). Simsek, Tulbek, Yao, and Schatz (2009) reported the isolated pea starch morphologies and attributes. Most of the granules were oval, however round, spherical, elliptical, and irregularly shaped granules were also observed (Simsek et al., 2009). Based on SEM analysis, the surfaces of pea starch granules were observed to be smooth and displayed no fissures or compound granules. Proteins and starch fractions demonstrate variable functional properties based on extraction technology, chemicals used, retention time, separation process (ie, centrifugation, filtration) and drying technology (ie, spray-drying, flash-drying, drum-drying). These factors influence the ingredient attributes, such as water-binding capacity, oil-binding capacity, emulsification, foaming, whippability, gelling, solubility, and adhesion.

9.4 NUTRITIVE VALUE OF PEAS

9.4.1 Major Components

Peas are an excellent source of proteins, carbohydrates, dietary fiber, minerals, vitamins, and phytochemicals. Researchers have demonstrated that pea seeds have considerable genetic variability in their composition. Moreover,

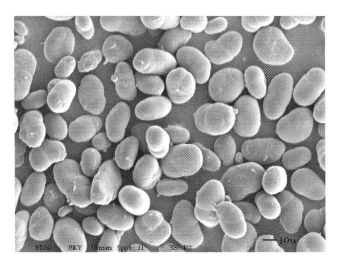

FIGURE 9.6 Scanning electron micrograph of wet fractionated pea starch of Cruiser cultivar ($\times 2500$).

TABLE 9.3 Proximate Composition Analysis of Peas Compared to Wheat (Tulbek, 2014)

Parameters (% as is)	Pea	Wheat
Protein	23.4	13.5
Fat	1.2	1.3
Carbohydrate	60.1	75.4
Total dietary fiber	21.2	11.7
Sugars	6.5	1.6
Starch	49.0	67.0

seed chemical composition is modified by environmental factors, genotype, and growing regions. Peas provide a unique supply of complementary protein to cereal proteins, and thus can be used to improve the overall nutritional status of food products. Table 9.3 illustrates the proximate composition of peas compared to wheat.

Pea seeds have higher protein, total dietary fiber, and total sugar content compared to whole wheat, while wheat and other cereals have higher starch content compared to peas. This natural phenomenon elevates the significance of peas as a protein and dietary fiber source for developing and underdeveloped countries. Pea seeds accumulate large amounts of protein during development and these protein bodies accumulate in the seed cotyledons. Protein content varies from 18% to 30% depending on environment factors and the cultivar. Unlike animal proteins, pea proteins contain essential amino acids in the essential proportions, whereby methionine is the limiting amino acid in peas. Pea proteins have five protein fractions which are albumins (water soluble), globulins (soluble in dilute salt solution), prolamins (soluble in 70% ethanol solution), glutelins (soluble in dilute alkaline solution), and residue protein (left over protein) based on the Osborne classification (Osborne, 1924). The most abundant class of proteins in peas is globulins, which consists of 7S (vicilin) and 11S (legumin) globulin proteins. In food applications, such as beverages, sauces, and custards, albumins and globulins are the main protein fractions attributing to the functionality of pea proteins.

Pea seeds contain 60—65% carbohydrates mainly composed of monosaccharides, disaccharides, oligosaccharides, and polysaccharides. The major carbohydrate fraction in peas is starch, which is the major storage carbohydrate in the cotyledons. Starch is composed of amylose (25—45%) and amylopectin (55—75%) (Hoover, Hughes, Chung, & Liu, 2010). Starch fractions in peas can be further classified according to slowly digestible, rapidly digestible and resistant starch (Zhang & Hamaker, 2009). Englyst et al. (1992) reported resistant starch as the indigestible fraction of starch in the gastrointestinal tract. Pea seeds contain 2—10% of resistant starch depending on processing, cultivar, and region (Dostalova, Horacek, Hasalova, & Trojan, 2009; Tulbek, Simsek, Yao, & Hall, 2008).

Pea seeds have higher total dietary fiber levels compared to wheat and other cereals. Dietary fiber has been defined by American Association of Cereal Chemists (AACC, 2001) as "the edible parts of plants or analogous carbohydrates that are resistant to digestion and absorption in the human small intestine with complete or partial fermentation in the large intestine (AACC, 2001)." Dietary fiber consists of hemicellulose, cellulose, pectin, gums, mucilage, resistant starches, and lignin. Dry pea has 17–27% dietary fiber depending on their cultivar, environment, and global growing region (Tulbek, 2014).

In terms of sugars, pea seeds contain 5–6% sucrose and raffinose. Sucrose ranges from 2.2% to 2.6%, whereas oligosaccharides, such as raffinose have a range of 0.2–1.0%, stachyose 1.3–3.2%, and verbascose 1.2–4.0% depending on cultivar and environment.

The fat content of pea seeds ranges from 1.2% to 1.8% depending on the cultivar and about 25% of fatty acids are composed of oleic acid (18:1) and 50% of linoleic acid (18:2), which is similar to other pulse crops. Due to the low levels of fat in peas, lipid oxidation and shelf-life issues are not observed in whole peas, split peas, and pea ingredients.

9.4.2 Minerals and Vitamins

Pea seeds are a rich source of minerals and vitamins. Compared to wheat and other cereals, peas contain higher levels of calcium, magnesium, phosphorus, iron, zinc, and copper (Table 9.4). In addition, peas are a rich source of folic acid, niacin, thiamine, riboflavin, pyridoxamine, pyridoxal, and pyridoxine. Peas may be used in combination with other cereals to provide a balanced mineral and vitamin composition which may improve the nutritional health in developing and underdeveloped nations.

9.4.3 Antinutritive Factors

Antinutritive factors in peas lower the nutritional value of foods by reducing their digestibility and bioavailability. This may reduce the health benefits of peas such as anticarcinogenicity, cardiovascular health diseases, and risk factors of menopause (Champ, 2002). The antinutritive factors of peas, pea ingredients, and soybeans are given in Table 9.5. Results indicated that pea seeds have lower phytic acid, trypsin inhibitor, saponins, total polyphenols, and stachyose levels compared to soybean, whereas phenolics (percentage of tannins acid), raffinose, and verbascose levels were observed to be higher than soybeans.

Phytic acid (myo-inositol hexakisphosphate or phytates) is a major phosphorus storage component in plant tissues. Phytates bind to minerals in the stomach, reducing protein digestibility and act as a metal-chelating antioxidant (Hall, 2008). Phytates are primarily found in protein bodies and the hull fraction of whole peas (Table 9.5). Soaking, fermentation, and germination may be used to reduce phytic acid levels in pea seeds.

Trypsin and chymotrypsin inhibitors are small protein bodies (MW 6–20 kDa) found in pea cotyledon and are responsible for reducing protein digestibility and bioavailability. Trypsin inhibitors are part of a plant's defense system (Hall, 2008). Thermal treatment and germination may be used to reduce trypsin and chymotrypsin inhibitors in peas.

Lectins (hemagglutinins) are small protein bodies (MW 10–120 kDa) of nonimmune origin that specifically interact with carbohydrates and sugar molecules without modifying them. Lectins are found in pea cotyledons and are associated with proteins (Table 9.5). Lectins are known to agglutinate red blood cells, disrupt brushborder enzymes, reduce

TABLE 9.4 Mineral Composition and Folic Acid Content of Pea Compared to Wheat (Tulbek, 2014)

Parameters	Pea	Wheat
Calcium (ppm)	850	340
Magnesium (ppm)	1450	1380
Phosphorus (ppm)	5500	3500
Iron (ppm)	60	38
Zinc (ppm)	43	29
Copper (ppm)	7	4
Folate (μg/100 g)	350	40

TABLE 9.5 Antinutritive Factors of Whole Pea, Pea Ingredients, and Soybeans (Tulbek, 2014)

	Whole Peas	Pea Starch Concentrate	Pea Protein Concentrate	Pea Fiber	Soybeans
Phytic acid (%)	0.54	0.42	1.60	2.80	1.32
Trypsin inhibitor (TIU/g)	2100	1300	2300	<1000	49,450
Lectin (g/kg)	5.77	5.98	23.2	3.78	5.88
Phenolics (as tannic acid % w/w)	1.12	0.47	1.79	2.97	0.46
Total saponins (mg/g)	0.0087	<0.05	0.28	<0.05	0.0714
Urease activity/pH rise (unit)	0.07	0.06	0.02	0.02	1.83
Free urea (g/kg)	<0.05	<0.05	<0.05	<0.05	<0.05
Total polyphenols (mg/kg)	1000	762	1440	3750	4800
Raffinose (%)	0.82	1.6	2.8	0.2	0.68
Stachyose (%)	1.62	0.4	0.9	N/D[a]	5.67
Verbascose (%)	3.72	3.4	7.0	0.1	0.52
Nitrogen digestibility (%)	74	92	93	N/A[a]	77

[a]N/D, not determined; N/A, not available.

viable epithelial cells, and provide insecticidal activity (Hall, 2008). Lectins can be inactivated with thermal treatment of peas.

Polyphenols and tannins are astringent and bitter-tasting plant compounds which bind to and precipitate proteins. Tannins originate from the "tanning" of animal hides into leather. This term is widely applied to any large polyphenolic compound containing sufficient hydroxyl and carboxyl moieties to form strong complexes with proteins and other macromolecules. Polyphenols and tannins are found in the seed coat and bind to protein and minerals, which reduces their bioavailability, inhibiting trypsin, alpha-amylase, and lipase enzymes (Hall, 2008). Polyphenols and tannins can be partially inactivated with soaking, dehulling, and thermal treatment.

Saponins are glycosides of steroids, steroid alkaloids and triterpenes which are found in plants, especially plant skins, where they form a waxy protective coating. The word saponin is derived from the word *sapon* meaning soap. Saponins may trigger the lysis of erythrocytes, which can deteriorate intestinal mucosal membranes, and bind to cholesterol and lipids. Due to its bitter taste it serves as an insecticide in peas (Hall, 2008). Saponins are primarily found in cotyledon and associated with protein bodies of legumes. The accumulation of saponins can be observed in pea protein concentrates produced by dry milling and air classification (Table 9.5). Thermal treatment and fermentation may be used in reducing saponin levels in peas.

Raffinose-type sugars (alpha-galactosides) are saccharide polymers containing a small number (3–10) of monosaccharides. Raffinose-type sugars can cause flatulence and diarrhea in humans, and reduce protein digestibility when they are fermented by microflora in the intestine. Germination, soaking, and fermentation processes can reduce the levels of raffinose-type sugars in peas.

9.4.4 Bioavailability

Bioavailability is the amount of a nutrient (ie, proteins, starches, and minerals) which is absorbed when consumed. Bioavailability accounts for the difference between exposure and dose. Bioavailability is determined by the amount of a substance that is absorbed by the intestinal tract. There are several factors affecting bioavailability (Hall, 2008):

- Type of nutrient and their associated levels of antinutrient components;
- Health of the consumer;
- Types of food consumed along with peas;
- Preparation of food product.

Habiba (2002) reported that both cooking time and the method of cooking (ie, boiling, autoclave, and microwave) influence the digestibility of a protein, whereby an increase in cooking time increases protein digestibility. Extrusion technology can increase protein digestibility from 74% to 78% (El-Hady & Habiba, 2003). Soaking did not significantly influence protein digestibility. In terms of mineral availability, Habiba (2002) did not observe any significant differences in boiling and autoclave processes depending on cooking time, whereas microwave slightly increased percentage of HCl extractable ash level. Alonso et al. (2001) investigated the effect of extrusion technology on the mineral availability in peas. Extrusion did not significantly affect mineral content (21 kg/h, 25% moisture, 150°C, and 100 rpm) but it did increase the absorption of iron, copper, and phosphorus. Periago, Englyst, and Hudson (1996) reported on the starch digestion in boiling and canning systems where starch digestion was observed to be higher in canned peas compared to boiled peas. Extrusion, germination, boiling, canning, and enzyme treatments significantly reduce trypsin inhibitor levels of peas, while improving the palatability and texture (Alonso, Orue, & Marzo, 1998; Habiba, 2002; Periago et al., 1996).

9.4.5 Allergenicity

Pea proteins have been widely consumed in the European Union and North America since the 1970s as an alternative vegetable protein because of their nutraceutical attributes. However, pea proteins may be a potential food allergen (Sanchez-Monge et al., 2004; Sathe, Kshirsagar, & Roux, 2005; Szymkiewicz, Jędrychowski, & Wagner, 2007). Green pea allergen was first determined by Malley, Baecher, Mackler, and Perlman (1975), and is attributed to the pea globulin fraction legumin and vicilin proteins (Szymkiewicz et al., 2007) and the proteins of albumin fraction (Croy, Hoque, Gatehouse, & Boulter, 1984; Sell, Steinhart, & Paschke, 2005; Vioque et al., 1998). Vioque et al. (1998) reported on cytosolic albumins which are stable during the germination process and caused allergic reactions in chickpea-sensitive individuals.

Sanchez-Monge et al. (2004) investigated the allergenicity of crude pea extracts and IgE immune-detection of extracts showed that convicilin and vicilin and one of its proteolytic fragments, reacted with more than 50% of the individuals in the panel ($n = 18$). Sell et al. (2005) reported on the impact of maturation of pea seeds with respect to allergenicity. They observed that as the seed maturity progressed, allergenic activity increased, which was primarily triggered by the albumins as opposed to the legumin and vicillin fractions (Sell et al., 2005). Troszynska, Szymkiewicz, and Wołejszo (2007) reported on the relationship between germination process (3 days at 20°C) and allergenic activity in peas and soybean seeds. Germination was found to reduce immunoreactivity and was suggested as a technology to produce products for people who suffer from food allergic disorders (Troszynska et al., 2007). Currently peas and pea proteins are not included in the "Big-8" in the Codex Alimentarius allergen labeling recommendations, however research projects are globally underway to understand the allergenic activities of food legumes and fractions derived from them.

9.4.6 Off-Tastes

Peas and pea ingredients have a unique taste and flavor profile due to the nature of their intrinsic compounds. Aroma and flavor compounds of peas and sensory attributes of peas have been extensively reported (Azarnia, Boye, Warkentin, & Malcolmson, 2011a, 2011b; Azarnia, Boye, Warkentin, Malcolmson, Sabik, et al., 2011; Heng et al., 2006; Malcolmson, Frohlich, Boux, Bellido, & Warkentin, 2014). Azarnia et al. (2011b) reported the volatile flavor profile of pea cultivars grown in Canada at variable storage conditions. At high-temperature storage conditions (22°C and 37°C) aldehydes were detected as primary components, whereas at low-temperature storage conditions (4°C) 1-hexanol, hexanal, and butanone were detected as major flavor compounds indicating the presence of alcohols, aldehydes, and ketones. Azarnia, Boye, Warkentin, Malcolmson, Sabik, et al. (2011) investigated the impact of crop year and processing of Canadian pea cultivars and observed that the aromatic volatile composition significantly varied within cultivars and growing conditions. Cooking significantly reduced the presence of aldehydes, alcohols, and ketones compared to milling and dehulling processes, indicating that thermal treatment influenced the aroma and flavor profile of peas. Taste and bitterness attributes of peas are related to inherent saponin content. A study on the effect of two saponins, saponin B and DDMP (2,3-dihydro-2,5-dihydroxy-6-methyl-4H-pyran-4-one) saponin, was investigated in 16 pea cultivars where DDMP saponin was found to be more bitter than saponin B (Heng et al., 2006). Malcolmson et al. (2014) conducted a sensory panel and investigated the aroma and flavor properties of cooked pea cultivars grown in Canada. Panelists observed the significant differences in sensory attributes among pea market classes and crop year (Malcolmson et al., 2014).

Pea ingredients can influence aroma, flavor, and overall acceptability of food products where the inclusion rate was found to be the main controlling factor. When peas and pea protein ingredients are used in pasta formulations over 5%, sensory panelists observed beany and earthy flavor notes in cooked pasta (Tulbek, 2011). Saponin content and volatiles are the major contributors in pasta sensory attributes. Therefore cooking, precooking, roasting, wet fractionation, and drying may be used as technologies to improve the acceptability of pea flours, pea proteins, and pea starches in food systems, so that inclusion rates may be increased. Precooking and roasting technologies may reduce aldehydes, ketones, and alcohol compounds, while increasing pyrazines which can contribute to roasted, toasted, and creamy notes in pea flour and ingredient aroma and flavor (Tulbek et al., 2009).

9.5 USES AND FUNCTIONALITY

Whole pea seeds, split peas, and pea ingredients are globally utilized in food, companion animal, and feed industries in several forms. Depending on value proposition and applied technologies they can exhibit variable functionalities.

9.5.1 Whole Peas

Whole peas are utilized in a broad range of applications and processed by cooking, canning, frying, or milling processes. Size, color, shape, uniformity, soaking quality, unsoaked seed percentage, and canning properties are key attributes for whole peas. Size, color, shape, and uniformity are desired quality factors for end-users, whereas color, soaking quality, and unsoaked seed percentage are required attributes for fried pea snack manufacturers (Fig. 9.7).

A high percentage of unsoaked seeds can influence the texture of roasted and fried snack products, which can be detrimental for end-users. In terms of canning quality color (greenness), soaking, unsoaked seed percentage, and texture are desired factors for canning quality. Although there have been different regulatory requirements for canned products of dry peas versus fresh peas, there is increasing interest in using dry green peas for canning due to seasonal and logistical challenges of fresh garden pea production (Fig. 9.8).

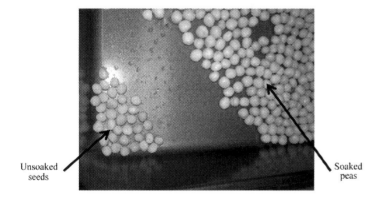

FIGURE 9.7 Soaking quality of yellow peas (breakdown of unsoaked peas vs soaked peas).

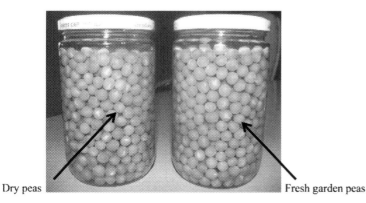

FIGURE 9.8 Canning quality of dry green peas versus fresh garden peas.

9.5.2 Split Peas

Split peas are produced by dehulling of whole pea seeds and primarily used in soup, canned soup, and global food aid supply. Size, color, shape, uniformity, soaking and cooking quality are important factors for split peas. Broken pieces, dust, off-colored seeds, adhering hull particles, and uniformity of cotyledons are additional quality attributes required for soup and the packing dry pea industry (Fig. 9.9).

9.5.3 Pea Flour

Pea flour is manufactured from whole or split peas into several different granulations based on end-product use, such as snacks, baked goods, savory, batters, breading, pasta, and extruded and canned pet food. Pea flour contains 22–28% protein, 40–53% starch, and 6–20% dietary fiber based on cultivar, processing technology, and particle size distribution. Pea flour is commonly used as a protein component in combination with cereal flour (Huisman & van der Poel, 1994). The major attributes of pea flour are water-binding, oil-binding, emulsification, gelation, and texturizing, which can be uniquely utilized in cereal, pulse, meat, and gluten-free formulations. A typical 15-min Rapid Visco Analyzer (RVA) profile of pea flour (milled through 100 mesh) is given in Fig. 9.10. Pea flour can withstand longer cooking times, shear, and thermal stability and does not show any breakdown during extensive cooking. Following starch retrogradation pea flour generates a firm gel due to its amylose content.

9.5.4 Pea Proteins

Pea proteins can be produced based on dry-milling and wet-milling technologies which will have protein content ranging from 48% to 90%. Nutritional benefits, water-binding capacity, oil-binding capacity, foam expansion, foam stability, whippability, gelation, emulsion stability and emulsion ability ratio are major functional properties of pea protein concentrates and isolates. Recent studies regarding pea protein functionalities have revealed unique properties compared to soybean protein isolates (Kaur, Sandhu, & Singh, 2006; O'Kane, Vereijken, Gruppen, & Van Boekel, 2005; Periago et al., 1998; Rangel, Domont, Pedrosa, & Ferreira, 2003; Shand, Ya, Pietrasik, & Wanasundara, 2007, 2008; Sun & Arntfield, 2011a, 2011b).

In terms of functionality, gels made from pea protein isolates are weaker than soybean protein isolates (Bildstein, Lohmann, Hennigs, Krause, & Hilz, 2008). Pea proteins are a better emulsifier and foaming agent at pH 7.0 compared to soy protein isolates (Bildstein et al., 2008). Recent studies have shown that the functional properties of pea proteins can be improved by applying enzymatic treatments (Shand et al., 2008; Sun & Arntfield, 2011a). Transglutaminase treatment improved the gel strength (Shand et al., 2008; Sun & Arntfield, 2011a), while acid proteases increased its emulsification capacity (Periago et al., 1998). These enzymatic treatments help transform pea protein isolates into functional proteins comparable to egg-white proteins and soy protein isolates. Typical 15 min RVA profiles of pea protein

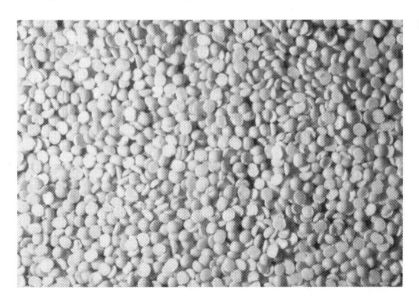

FIGURE 9.9 Split peas.

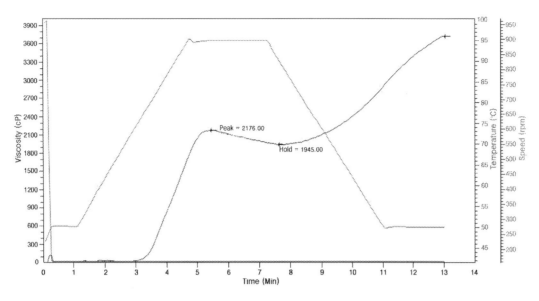

FIGURE 9.10 Typical Rapid Visco Analyzer profile of pea flour (100% milled through 100 mesh).

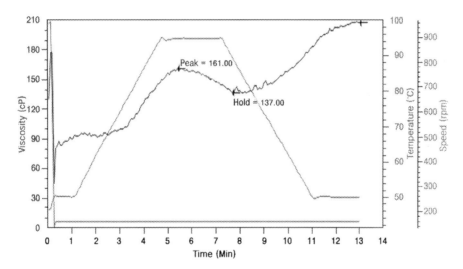

FIGURE 9.11 Typical Rapid Visco Analyzer profile of pea protein isolate (100% milled through 100 mesh).

isolate and pea protein concentrates are given Figs. 9.11 and 9.12, respectively. Since most of the carbohydrates are removed in manufacturing pea protein isolates, the RVA profile is much flatter compared to pea protein concentrates, even though both products have similar final viscosity values.

Current research indicates that pea protein products tend to exhibit weaker gel strength, viscosity, and texture compared to egg, soy, and meat proteins, however new extraction and drying technologies can improve the functional attributes of pea proteins.

9.5.5 Pea Starch

Pea starch produced by dry-milling and wet-milling technologies will have starch content ranging from 60% to 99%. Extensive studies have been conducted on the functionality of corn, wheat, potato, and rice starches due to their global availability; however, pea starches have only been studied since the 1960s for their functionalities, and their effects on different food systems (Chen, Liu, Chang, Cao, & Anderson, 2009; Ma, Chang, & Yu, 2008; Ratnayake, Hoover, & Warkentin, 2002; Ring, 1983; Simsek et al., 2009; Tan, Li, & Tan, 2009).

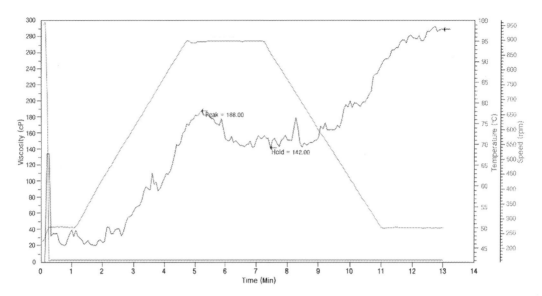

FIGURE 9.12 Typical Rapid Visco Analyzer profile of pea protein concentrate (100% milled through 100 mesh).

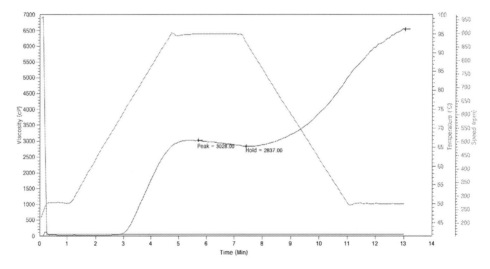

FIGURE 9.13 Typical Rapid Visco Analyzer profile of pea starch concentrate (100% milled through 100 mesh).

Pea starches are stable against thermal and mechanical shear, in addition, they provide a good source of resistant starch (4–20%) which makes them an appealing ingredient for the food industry. Pea starches have key functional attributes such as texturizing, gel formation, and pasting properties greatly desired by the food industry. Isolated pea starch may have slightly different properties compared to dry-fractionated pea starch products due to its wet chemical extraction and their extensive washing processes. However, both dry- and wet-fractionated starch products provide cooking stability and gel formation due to high amylose content and intrinsic properties. A typical 15 min RVA profile of pea starch concentrate (65% protein) is given in Fig. 9.13. Pea starch concentrate exhibits similar starch pasting and gel formation properties compared to rice, wheat, and corn flour, which may potentially be used as replacements for gluten-free and grain-free food and the pet food industry.

9.5.6 Pea Fiber

Pea fiber is produced using both dry- and wet-milling processing technologies and contains variable levels of total dietary fiber ranging from 50% to 90%. Water-binding capacity and total dietary fiber content are the key functional

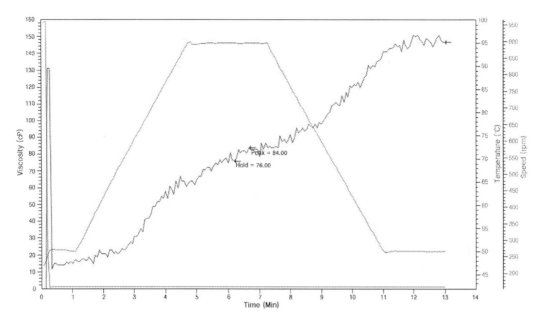

FIGURE 9.14 Typical Rapid Visco Analyzer profile of pea fiber with 80% dietary fiber (100% milled through 100 mesh).

attributes of pea fiber. Pea hull fiber products manufactured by milling pea hulls into fine powder contain over 90% insoluble and 10% soluble dietary fiber, whereas inner pea fiber products manufactured by wet fractionation have 50% soluble and 50% insoluble dietary fiber. Pea hull fibers bind approximately 3.5–4.0 g water per 1 g fiber, whereas inner pea fibers can bind up to 9.0 g water per 1 g fiber. Pea fibers help provide structure in food systems, primarily in baked good and extruded snacks, thus providing texturizing properties. A typical 15 min RVA profile of pea hull fiber is given in Fig. 9.14 indicating a low-viscosity development in cooking systems.

9.6 APPLICATIONS AND CURRENT PRODUCTS

9.6.1 Baked Goods

Pea ingredients can be used in baked goods as nutritional supplements, as bread improvers, and to replace allergens such as soy or egg. Pea flour and pea starch concentrates naturally have lipoxygenase enzymes which can be used in premixes as a soy flour replacement. Since lipoxygenase is required in these applications, the pea flour used should have a high protein dispersibility index (PDI) and not be exposed to any heat treatments. Due to the taste and flavor challenges of pea ingredients, precooked or deflavored pea flours are required for uses at higher inclusion rates, typically to increase protein content, for applications such as breads, donuts, cookies, muffins, tortillas, and cakes. Precooked pea flours may be used in bread formulations up to 30%; in tortillas, 20%; in hamburger buns, 30%; in whole wheat breads, 15%; and in donuts, 50%. Since pea flour and proteins are rich in lysine amino acid, wheat flour blended with precooked pea flour formulations may possibly be used as natural, complete protein baked goods into the food industry. In addition to pea flour and proteins, pea fiber ingredients can be utilized to increase water-binding in baked goods due to its water-binding capacity. Depending on bread type, formulation and baking technology pea fiber may be included at 1–2% for dough yield enhancement.

9.6.2 Pasta and Noodle

Pea ingredients can be used in pasta and noodle applications as base ingredients, such as pea flour and pea proteins in traditional-style durum wheat-based pasta and pea starch in Chinese vermicelli noodle. Pasta products are traditionally manufactured from durum wheat semolina, based on a low-temperature low-shear extrusion process followed by drying. Use of yellow and green pea flour (5–20%) in durum wheat pasta processing and texture has been investigated (Tulbek, 2007). Pea flour inclusion in durum wheat pasta did not change water addition rate in extrusion process (330–350 mL/min).

TABLE 9.6 Effects of Yellow Pea Flour on Spaghetti Quality (Tulbek, 2007)

Pasta Attributes	Control	5%	10%	15%	20%
Cooking Quality (al dente)					
Cooked weight (g)	75.8	75.3	77.7	77.2	76.3
Cooking loss (%)	5.9	5.6	5.9	6.1	6.3
Cooked firmness (g cm)	12.9	12.4	12.5	13.4	14.4
Cooking Quality (Overcook 6 min)					
Cooked weight (g)	87.4	86.7	87.9	88	88
Cooking loss (%)	7.2	6.6	7.3	7.2	7.3
Cooked firmness (g cm)	9.3	9	9.1	9.6	10.2

Extruder screw current and wet product output attributes were stable. Extruder die pressure increased from 650 to 794 psi when 20% pea flour was added in durum wheat pasta. Pasta quality attributes were variable, based on type and inclusion rate of the raw material. Green pea flour influenced pasta color and significantly reduced brightness and yellowness scores, whereas yellow pea flour did not change pasta color at a 10% inclusion rate. Pea flour inclusion improved cooked pasta texture and significantly increased pasta firmness, which can be attributed to higher protein content (Table 9.6). Similar trends in pasta were observed in the literature (Bahnassey & Khan, 1986; Zhao, Manthey, Chang, Hou, & Yuan, 2005), which showed increased pasta firmness with pea, lentil, chickpea, and edible bean flour fortification in spaghetti.

Pea starch is an ingredient which is widely used in vermicelli noodle manufacturing. Pea starch has become a major ingredient for Chinese noodle manufacturers due to the decline in mung bean production and reduced mung bean starch supply. High pea starch purity level (over 98% starch content) and unique starch pasting properties are required for vermicelli noodle quality which has to be further investigated.

Pea flour and proteins can be used as a nutritional additive in the production of specialty and functional spaghetti and pasta products made with durum wheat semolina. Deflavored or precooked flours and proteins can be added to improve sensory attributes of pasta and noodle products at higher ($>20\%$) ingredient inclusion rates.

9.6.3 Extruded Snacks

Pea ingredients can be used in expanded snacks and breakfast cereals. Extrusion cooking is a continuous process by which starchy and proteinaceous materials are plasticized and cooked by a combination of moisture, pressure, temperature, and mechanical shear. During extrusion cooking starch is gelatinized, protein is denatured, and more than 90% of the antinutritional components are inactivated. Corn, rice, and potato ingredients have been the major ingredients used in the snack and breakfast cereal industries which lack protein, dietary fiber, and micronutrients. Pea flour exhibits similar properties to corn or rice flour in the extrusion process with comparable expansion ratio and bulk density. Extrusion technology can influence final product quality based on raw material selection. Coarse pea flours can be used in both single- and twin-screw systems, whereas fine pea flour products will be more applicable for twin-screw extrusion process.

Several researchers reported the use of peas and other pulse ingredients in extruded snack applications (Hood-Niefer & Tyler, 2010; Simons et al., 2014; Simons, Hall, & Tulbek, 2012; Vadukapuram, Hall, Tulbek, & Niehaus, 2014). Hood-Niefer and Tyler (2010) investigated the protein and carbohydrate levels suitable for pea flour extrusion and low starch ingredients showed less expansion. Similar trends were observed by Vadukapuram et al. (2014). Combinations of bean flours were fortified with different levels (0–20%) of milled flaxseed and extruded in a twin-screw extruder. As the starch content decreased in formulations, the expansion ratio and sensory attributes decreased. Simons et al. (2012, 2014) observed lower glycemic index scores for the products obtained at low-speed extrusion conditions, which can be attributed to less shearing and depolymerization due to low extrusion conditions and specific mechanical energy. At higher speeds, extrudates reduced their capacity to expand and to hold structure firmly. In addition, this could be associated with a significant reduction in water activity and texture attributes.

During extrusion cooking, protein solubility increases while amino acid losses occur. Lysine, an amino acid sensitive to heat and mechanical shear is reduced depending on extrusion process conditions. Lysine loss in pea proteins was observed to be much lower than faba bean proteins in the extruded snacks and crisps (Tulbek, unpublished data). In addition, lysine losses may be attributed to their participation in Maillard reactions which occur due to the interactions of free amino acids and reducing sugars.

Pea flours and ingredients can be used as nutritious ingredients in extruded snacks and breakfast cereals as a major alternative for traditional ingredients to increase protein, micronutrient, and dietary fiber levels. There is limited information on the complete protein profile and blending potential of pulse ingredients with cereals which have to be studied further.

9.6.4 Meat and Meat Analogs

Peas and pea ingredients can be used in meat and meat analog applications in several forms based on formulation, technology, and regulatory compliance. Pea proteins and flours can bind water and fat and generate firm texture after thermal process due to amylose content, starch retrogradation, gel formation, and protein gelation properties. These attributes enable peas and pea ingredients as unique and effective ingredients as binders, fillers, and functional improvers. Several researchers have reported the use of pulse flours in meat applications (Dzudie, Scher, & Hardy, 2002; Modi, Mahendrakar, Narasimha Rao, & Sachindra, 2003; Serdaroglu, Yildiz-Turp, & Abrodimov, 2005). Common observations were related to the interaction of pulse flours with meat components, improved fat binding, reduced weight loss, and increased water retention in meat products. Major challenges in using pea proteins and pea flours in meat products are the taste and flavor which detrimentally influence processed meat sensory attributes. Thus, use of pea protein isolates, deflavored and thermally stabilized pulse ingredients can be suggested as alternative ingredients. Stabilized pea ingredients, such as deflavored flours and pea protein isolates, contain no lipoxgenase enzyme which can negatively affect processed meat quality. Der (2010) reported the use of micronized lentil flours in low-fat beefburgers and demonstrated the detrimental impact of lipoxygenase enzyme.

Peas and pea ingredients can also be used in veggie meat analogs such as pakoras, matzah balls, and falafel products. Pea flour and starch can be used as a base ingredient in these formulations, which are produced with forming and frying processes. In addition, pea ingredients can be used in extruded meat analogs and texturized proteins in developing countries.

9.7 HEALTH BENEFITS OF PEAS

Health benefits of peas have been reviewed and the levels of concentrations of protein, starch, fiber, vitamins, minerals, and phytochemical components have been suggested as major factors influencing health impact with regards to physiological attributes of each fraction (Dahl, Foster, & Tyler, 2012). Epidemiological, in vitro, and interventional studies demonstrated that peas and pea ingredients can influence glycemic response and insulin resistance, cardiovascular health, gastrointestinal health, and weight management. Based on the literature review, the impact of fiber and indigestible carbohydrates was observed with experimental and clinical trials (Dahl et al., 2012).

Marinangeli, Kassis, and Jones (2009) reported the impact of the blood glucose response curve in whole pea flour fortified banana bread, biscotti, and pasta products. They observed that the blood glucose response curve was reduced in banana bread and biscotti, however it was increased in pasta. Glycemic response and insulin resistance were also investigated in hypercholesterolemic overweight patients in a 56-day study. It was observed that whole pea flour reduced fasting insulin more than split pea flour which was related to the presence of the pea hull fiber (Marinangeli & Jones, 2011).

Recent studies published by the University of Toronto, Canada, state that pea protein reduced the blood glucose response curve more than the pea fiber fraction (Mollard, Luhovyy, Smith, & Anderson, 2014). Smith, Mollard, Luhovyy, and Anderson (2011) reported that pea protein isolate suppressed short-term energy intake and postprandial glycemia in young healthy males and reduced pre- and post-meal blood glucose.

The potential benefits of frequent consumption of peas may be attributed to their effects on satiety, food intake, and blood glucose (Dahl et al., 2012). The appetite-suppressing effects of peas may be related to high amounts of protein and dietary fiber, which may delay gastric emptying, attenuate glucose absorption and concentration and stimulate the release of appetite-regulating hormones.

9.8 CONCLUSION

In this chapter, production, cultivars, sustainability, energy use, processing, composition, nutrition, end-use attributes, and health benefits of peas and pea ingredients were reviewed. Peas are gluten-free and a conventionally bred crop which provides an abundant source of energy, proteins, carbohydrates, and micronutrients. Due to the growing (production) sustainability, low carbon footprint, non-GMO, allergen-free, clean label, and single-ingredient trends in the global marketplace, peas and pea ingredients are becoming major alternative ingredients, which present opportunities to add value for the food industry. Peas and pea ingredients can be successfully use in pasta, noodle, meat, bakery, extruded snack, breakfast cereal, and pet food ingredients for functional and nutritional value propositions. Taste, flavor, and overall sensory attributes are the leading challenges for restricting pea ingredient use in major food applications.

In order to overcome the challenges in utilizing pea ingredients, regulatory compliance with regards to nutritional claims, health claims, and labeling have to be addressed. Breeding research efforts for improved taste and flavor, enhanced protein content and quality, reduced energy use, increased yield attributes will be the targets for the future of peas. Research efforts focusing on fortification, minimal processing of pea ingredients with improved sensory profiles will address consumer interests with regards to convenience, health, and nutrition.

REFERENCES

AACC. (2001). *Web*: <http://www.aaccnet.org/initiatives/definitions/documents/dietaryfiber/dfdef.pdf>.
Alonso, R., Orue, E., & Marzo, F. (1998). Effects of extrusion and conventional processing methods on protein and antinutritional factor contents in pea seeds. *Food Chemistry, 63*, 505–512.
Alonso, R., Rubio, L. R., Muzquiz, M., & Marzo, F. (2001). The effect of extrusion cooking on mineral bioavailability in pea and kidney bean seed meals. *Animal Feed Science and Technology, 94*(1), 1–13.
Azarnia, S., Boye, J. I., Warkentin, T., & Malcolmson, L. (2011a). Market class, cultivar, location, and crop year effects on the volatile flavour composition of field pea cultivars. In A. M. Comstock, & B. E. Lothrop (Eds.), *Peas: Cultivation, varieties and nutritional uses* (pp. 49–82). Hauppauge, NY: Nova Science Publishers Inc.
Azarnia, S., Boye, J. I., Warkentin, T., & Malcolmson, L. (2011b). Changes in volatile flavour compounds in field pea cultivars as affected by storage conditions. *International Journal of Food Science and Technology, 46*, 2408–2419.
Azarnia, S., Boye, J. I., Warkentin, T., Malcolmson, L., Sabik, H., & Bellido, A. S. (2011). Volatile flavour profile changes in selected field pea cultivars as affected by crop year and processing. *Food Chemistry, 124*, 326–335.
Bahnassey, Y., & Khan, K. (1986). Fortification of spaghetti with edible legumes. II. Rheological, processing and quality evaluation studies. *Cereal Chemistry, 63*, 216–219.
Biederbeck, V. O., Zenter, R. P., & Campbell, C. A. (2005). Soil microbial populations and activities as influenced by legume green fallow in a semiarid climate. *Soil Biology and Biochemistry, 37*, 1775–1784.
Bildstein, M., Lohmann, M., Hennigs, C., Krause, A., & Hilz, H. (2008). An enzyme-based extraction process for the purification and enrichment of vegetable proteins to be applied in bakery products. *European Food Research and Technology, 228*, 177–186.
Champ, M. M. (2002). Non-nutrient bioactive substances of pulses. *British Journal of Nutrition, 88*, 307–319.
Chen, C., Miller, P., Muehlbauer, F., Neill, K., Wichman, D., & McPhee, K. (2006). Winter pea and lentil response to seeding date and micro and macro-environments. *Agronomy Journal, 98*, 1655–1663.
Chen, Y., Liu, C., Chang, P. R., Cao, X., & Anderson, D. P. (2009). Bionanocomposites based on pea starch and cellulose nanowhiskers hydrolyzed from pea hull fiber: Effect of hydrolysis time. *Carbohydrate Polymers, 76*, 607–615.
Croy, R. D., Hoque, M. S., Gatehouse, J. A., & Boulter, D. (1984). The major albumin proteins from pea (*Pisum sativum* L.). *Biochemistry Journal, 218*, 795–803.
Dahl, W. J., Foster, L. M., & Tyler, R. T. (2012). Review of the health benefits of peas (*Pisum sativum* L.). *British Journal of Nutrition, 108*, 3–10.
Der, T. (2010). *Evaluation of micronized lentil and its utilization in low-dat beef burgers*. Master thesis. Department of Food and Bioproduct Sciences, University of Saskatchewan.
Dostalova, R., Horacek, J., Hasalova, I., & Trojan, R. (2009). Study of resistant starch (RS) content in peas during maturation. *Czech Journal of Food Science, 27*, 120–124.
Dzudie, T., Scher, J., & Hardy, J. (2002). Common bean flour as an extender in beef sausages. *Journal of Food Processing, 52*, 143–147.
El-Hady, E. A. A., & Habiba, R. (2003). Effect of soaking and extrusion conditions on antinutrients and protein digestibility of legume seeds. *Lebensmittel Wissenschaft and Technology, 36*, 285–293.
Englyst, H. N., Kingman, S. N., & Cummings, J. H. (1992). Classification and measurement of nutritionally important starch fractions. *European Journal of Clinical Nutrition, 46*(Supplement 2), S33–S50.
Elzebroek, T., & Wind, K. (2008). *Guide to cultivated plants*. Oxfordshire, UK: CAB International.
FAO. (2015). *Food and agriculture organization statistics*.
Habiba, R. A. (2002). Changes in anti-nutrients, protein solubility, digestibility, and HCl extractability of ash and phosphorus in vegetable peas as affected by cooking methods. *Food Chemistry, 77*, 187–192.
Hall, C. (2008). Antinutrients, digestibility and antigenicity of pulses. In: *Pulse quality and utilization short course, October, 2008, Fargo, ND*.
Han, J. Y., & Khan, K. (1992a). Physicochemical studies of pin milled and air classified dry edible bean fractions. *Cereal Chemistry, 67*, 384–390.
Han, J. Y., & Khan, K. (1992b). Functional studies of pin milled and air classified dry edible bean fractions. *Cereal Chemistry, 67*, 390–394.

Hartmann, H. T., Kofranek, A. M., Rubatzky, V. E., & Flocker, W. J. (1988). *Plant science: Growth, development and utilization of cultivated plants* (2nd ed.). Englewood Cliffs, NJ: Prentice Hall Career and Technology.

Heng, L., Vincken, J. P., van Koningsveld, G., Legger, A., Gruppen, H., van Boekel, T., ... Voragen, F. (2006). Bitterness of saponins and their content in dry peas. *Journal of the Science of Food and Agriculture, 86*, 1225–1231.

Hoekstra, A. J. (2015). The water footprint: The relation between human consumption and water use. In M. Antonelli, & F. Greco (Eds.), *The water we eat*. Switzerland: Springer International Publishing. <http://waterfootprint.org/media/downloads/Hoekstra-2015_1.pdf>.

Hood-Niefer, S. D., & Tyler, R. T. (2010). Effect of protein, moisture content and barrel temperature on the physicochemical characteristics of pea flour extrudates. *Food Research International, 43*, 659–663.

Hoover, R., Hughes, T., Chung, H. J., & Liu, Q. (2010). Composition, molecular structure, properties, and modification of pulse starches: A review. *Food Research International, 43*, 399–413.

Huisman, J., & van der Poel, A. F. B. (1994). *Aspects of the nutritional quality and use of coolseason food legumes in animal feed. Expanding the production and use of cool season food legumes* (pp. 53–76). Dordrecht, The Netherlands: Kluwer Academic Publishers.

Kaur, M., Sandhu, K., & Singh, N. (2006). Comparative study of the functional, thermal, andpasting properties of flours from different field pea (*Pisum sativum* L.) and pigeon pea (*Cajanus cajan* L.). *Food Chemistry, 104*, 259–267.

Lupwayi, N. Z., Rice, W. A., & Clayton, G. W. (1998). Soil microbial diversity and community structure under wheat as influenced by tillage and crop rotation. *Soil Biology and Biochemistry, 30*, 1733–1741.

Ma, X., Chang, P. R., & Yu, J. (2008). Properties of biodegradable thermoplastic pea starch/carboxymethyl cellulose and pea starch/microcrystalline cellulose composites. *Carbohydrate Polymers, 72*, 369–375.

Malcolmson, L., Frohlich, P., Boux, G., Bellido, A. S., & Warkentin, T. D. (2014). Aroma and flavour properties of Saskatchewan grown field peas (*Pisum sativum* L.). *Canadian Journal of Food Science, 94*, 1419–1426.

Malley, A., Baecher, L., Mackler, B., & Perlman, E. (1975). The isolation of allergens from the green pea. *Journal of Allergy and Clinical Immunology, 56*, 282–290.

Marinangeli, C. P., & Jones, P. J. (2011). Whole and fractionated yellow pea flours reduce fasting insulin and insulin resistance in hypercholesterolaemic and overweight human subjects. *British Journal of Nutrition, 105*, 110–117.

Marinangeli, C. P., Kassis, A. N., & Jones, P. J. (2009). Glycemic responses and sensory characteristics of whole yellow pea flour added to novel functional foods. *Journal of Food Science, 74*, 385–389.

Modi, V. K., Mahendrakar, N. S., Narasimha Rao, D., & Sachindra, N. M. (2003). Quality of buffalo meat burger containing legume flours as binders. *Meat Science, 66*, 143–149.

Mollard, R. C., Luhovyy, B. L., Smith, C. E., & Anderson, G. H. (2014). Acute effects of pea protein and hull fibre alone and combined on blood glucose, appetite, and food intake in healthy young men – A randomized crossover trial. *Applied Physiology Nutrition and Metabolism, 12*, 1–6.

O'Kane, F. E., Vereijken, J. M., Gruppen, H., & Van Boekel, M. A. J. S. (2005). Gelation behavior of protein isolates extracted from 5 cultivars of *Pisum sativum* L. *Journal of Food Science, 70*, 132–137.

Osborne, T. B. (1924). *The vegetable proteins*. London: Longmans, Green and Co.

Pavek, P. L. S. (2012). *Plant guide for pea (*Pisum sativum* L.)*. Pullman, WA: USDA-Natural Resources Conservation Service.

Periago, M. J., Englyst, H. N., & Hudson, G. J. (1996). The influence of thermal processing on the non-starch polysaccharide (NSP) content and in vitro digestibility of starch in peas (*Pisum sativum* L.). *Lebensmittel Wissenschaft und Technologie, 29*, 33–40.

Periago, M. J., Vidal, M. L., Ros, G., Rincon, F., Martinez, C., Lopez, G., ... Martinez, I. (1998). Influence of enzymatic treatment on the nutritional and functional properties of pea flour. *Food Chemistry, 63*, 71–78.

Rangel, A., Domont, G. B., Pedrosa, C., & Ferreira, S. T. (2003). Functional properties of purified vicilins from cowpea (*Vigna unguiculata*) and pea (*Pisum sativum*) and cowpea protein isolate. *Journal of Agriculture and Food Chemistry, 51*, 5792–5797.

Ratnayake, W. S., Hoover, R., & Warkentin, T. (2002). Pea starch: Composition, structure and properties – A review. *Starch, 54*, 217–234.

Ring, S. G. (1983). *Pea starch gels*. University of Leeds.

Sanchez-Monge, R., Lopez-Torrejon, G., Pascual, C. Y., Varela, J., Martin-Esteban, M., & Salcedo, G. (2004). Vicilin and convicilin are potential major allergens from pea. *Clinical Experimental Allergy, 34*, 1747–1753.

Sarecon Management Consulting Report. (2011). *Application of sustainable agriculture metrics to selected Western Canadian field crops*.

Saskatchewan Pulse Growers. (2016). *Web*: <http://saskpulse.com/growing/peas/>.

Saskatchewan Research Council. (2011). *Life cycle and socio-economic analysis of pulse crop production and pulse grain use in Western Canada*. Saskatchewan Research Council Publication No. 12135-1E11, March 2011.

Sathe, S. K., Kshirsagar, H. H., & Roux, K. H. (2005). Advances in seed protein research: A perspective on seed allergens. *Journal of Food Science, 70*, 93–120.

Schoch, T. J., & Maywald, E. C. (1968). Preparation and properties of various legume starches. *Cereal Chemistry, 45*, 564–573.

Sell, M., Steinhart, H., & Paschke, A. (2005). Influence of maturation on the alteration of allergenicity of green pea (*Pisum sativum* L.). *Journal of Agriculture and Food Chemistry, 53*, 1717–1722.

Serdaroglu, M., Yildiz-Turp, G., & Abrodimov, K. (2005). Quality of low-fat meatballs containing legume flours as extenders. *Meat Science, 70*, 99–105.

Shand, P., Ya, H., Pietrasik, Z., & Wanasundara, P. K. J. P. D. (2007). Physicochemical and textural properties of heat–induced pea protein isolate gels. *Food Chemistry, 102*, 1119–1130.

Shand, P., Ya, H., Pietrasik, Z., & Wanasundara, P. K. J. P. D. (2008). Transglutaminase and treatment of pea proteins. Effect on physicochemical and rheological properties of heat induced protein gels. *Food Chemistry, 107*, 692–699.

Simons, C., Hall, C., & Tulbek, M. C. (2012). Effects of extruder screw speeds on physical properties and in vitro starch hydrolysis of pre-cooked pinto, navy, red and black bean extrudates. *Cereal Chemistry, 89*(3), 176–181.

Simons, C. W., Hall, C., III, Tulbek, M. C., Mendis, M., Ogunyemi, S., & Heck, T. (2014). Acceptability and characterization of extruded pinto, navy and black beans. *Journal of the Science of Food and Agriculture, 95*(11), 2287–2291.

Simsek, S., Tulbek, M., Yao, Y., & Schatz, B. (2009). Starch characteristics of peas (*Pisum sativum* L.) grown in the USA. *Food Chemistry, 115*, 832–838.

Smith, C. E., Mollard, R. C., Luhovyy, B. L., & Anderson, G. H. (2011). Isolated yellow pea protein, but not fiber, suppresses short-term energy intake and postprandial glycemia in young healthy males. *Canadian Journal of Plant Science, 91*, 377.

Sun, X. D., & Arntfield, S. D. (2011a). Gelation properties of salt−extracted pea protein isolate catalyzed by microbial transglutaminase cross−linking. *Food Hydrocolloids, 25*, 25–31.

Sun, X. D., & Arntfield, S. D. (2011b). Gelation properties of salt−extracted pea protein isolate induced by heat treatment: Effect of heating and cooling rate. *Food Chemistry, 124*, 1011–1016.

Szymkiewicz, A., Jędrychowski, L., & Wagner, A. (2007). Effect of thermal treatment and enzymic hydrolysis on allergenicity of pea proteins. *Zywnosc, 14*, 147–158.

Tan, H. Z., Li, Z. G., & Tan, B. (2009). Starch noodles: History, classification, materials, processing, structure, nutrition, quality evaluating and improving. *Food Research International, 42*, 551–576.

Troszynska, A., Szymkiewicz, A., & Wołejszo, A. (2007). The effects of germination on the sensory quality and immunoreactive properties of pea (*Pisum sativum* L.) and soybean (*Glycine max*). *Journal of Food Quality, 30*, 1083–1100.

Tulbek, M. C. (2007). Use of dry peas in pasta and noodle: Technology and quality issues. In: *Pea flour utilization in pasta and noodle making short course, May 21–25, 2007, Northern Crops Institute Fargo, ND*.

Tulbek, M. C. (2011). Beyond wheat – Review of pasta products made with multigrain, pulses, fibres, and other ingredients. In: *2011 AACC international annual meeting, Palm Springs, CA*.

Tulbek, M. C. (2014). Pulse flours as functional ingredients. In: *IUFOST annual conference, Montreal QC, Canada*.

Tulbek, M. C., Simsek, S., & Hall, C. (2009). Precooked pulse flour: Processing, quality and end product utilization. In: *Oral presentation at AACC international annual meeting, Baltimore, MD*.

Tulbek, M. C., Simsek, S., Yao, Y., & Hall, C. (2008). Characterization of pre-cooked split and whole dry edible pea flours. In: *AACC international annual meeting, Honolulu, HI*.

Tyler, R. T., & Panchuk, B. D. (1982). Effect of moisture content on the air classification of field peas and faba beans. *Cereal Chemistry, 53*, 928–936.

Unilever. (2002). *Web*: <https://www.unilever.com/Images/2002--in-pursuit-of-the-sustainable-pea_tcm244-409704_1_en.pdf>.

Vadukapuram, N., Hall, C., III, Tulbek, M. C., & Niehaus, M. (2014). Physicochemical properties of flaxseed fortified extruded bean snack. *International Journal of Food Science, 2014*. Hindawi Publishing Co. Article ID 478018 <http://www.hindawi.com/journals/ijfs/2014/478018/ref/>.

Vioque, J., Clemente, A., Sanchez-Vioque, R., Pedroche, J., Bautista, J., & Milan, F. (1998). Comparative study of chickpea and pea PA2 albumins. *Journal of Agriculture Food Chemistry, 46*, 3609–3613.

Wu, Y. V., & Nichols, N. N. (2005). Fine grinding and air classification of field peas. *Cereal Chemistry, 82*, 341–344.

Zentner, R. P., Lafond, G. P., Derksen, D. A., Nagy, C. N., Wall, D. D., & May, W. E. (2004). Effects of tillage method and crop rotation on non-renewable energy use efficiency for a thin Black Chernozem in the Canadian Prairies. *Soil & Tillage Research, 77*, 125–136.

Zhang, G., & Hamaker, B. R. (2009). Slowly digestible starch: Concept, mechanism, and proposed extended glycemic index. *Critical Reviews in Food Science and Nutrition, 49*, 852–867.

Zhao, Y., Manthey, F. A., Chang, S. K. C., Hou, H. J., & Yuan, S. H. (2005). Quality characteristics of spaghetti as affected by green and yellow pea, lentil, and chickpea flours. *Journal of Food Science, 70*, 371–376.

Chapter 10

Lupin: An Important Protein and Nutrient Source

M. van de Noort

MFH Pulses, Rotterdam, The Netherlands

10.1 INTRODUCTION

Plant-based foods can provide good nutrition for a healthy life. Our ancestors ate a primarily plant-based diet and many cultures around the globe still do. In recent times, meat and other animal-based foods have increased in importance in many countries. On a fundamental level, meat became a food of choice for a society that could afford to feed animals with plants (grains, pulses, and roots). Soon, meat was valued as a protein-rich food source and became entrenched in Western countries, while relegating grain, fruit, and vegetables to a minor role in daily food options. Vegetables and fruit became sources that required consumption to provide vitamins, minerals, and as a source of fiber. Today, we have gained a lot of insight into the role of plant-based foods in reducing the risk for chronic and systemic diseases by providing critical nutrients. Continuing research is uncovering new beneficial components leading to increased consumption of plant-based foods. In addition, trends are supporting this move toward plant-based diets as consumers are making choices to eat and live in a sustainable manner for the greater good of the planet.

Among grain legumes, lupin holds an important place. Lupin has a long history in agriculture that traces back more than 4000 years (Kurlovich, 2002). Domestication occurred first in the Mediterranean region, followed by cultivation in the American continent. However, the real breakthrough that made lupin a modern agricultural crop occurred in Europe and Australia. The history of lupin domestication is discussed in the following paragraph (Clements et al., 2005; Kurlovich, 2002).

Lupin (*Lupinus* spp.) was cultivated in ancient Greece and Egypt before 2000 BC, to produce grain for human and animal consumption, as well as for cosmetics and medicine. Around 1000–800 BC, *Lupinus albus* was utilized as green manure in ancient Rome and, subsequently, in other Mediterranean countries. Two centuries later (700–600 BC), Andean pearl lupine (*Lupinus mutabilis*) was domesticated on the American continent. In the 1860s, *Lupinus luteus* and *Lupinus angustifolius* were used for green manure production in Baltic countries and later in Germany. Methods for selecting low-alkaloid lupin mutants were developed in Germany in the late 1920s. Later, sweet lupin varieties were developed in the 1930s–70s, followed by permeable seeds from *L. luteus*, *L. albus*, *L. angustifolius*, and *L. mutabilis* in Germany, Sweden, and Russia. In the 1980s–90s, several lupin varieties including *Lupinus cosentinii* species (*Lupinus atlanticus*, *Lupinus pilosus*, and *Lupinus polyphyllus* Lindl.) were cultivated in Australia and Russia.

Older varieties of lupin tasted bitter due to the presence of alkaloids. This required soaking the beans in saltwater to remove the bitter alkaloid components, for a more consumable form. Classical breeding techniques have generated sweet lupin varieties with low alkaloid content without the need for soaking the beans. The high protein content of lupin (30–40%) along with its content of complex carbohydrates, without digestible starch, makes lupines unique among the pea, beans, and lentil.

10.1.1 Cultivation of *Lupinus* Species

Lupinus is a diverse genus in the legume family with both annual and perennial species. Lupin have a long history as ornamental plants in gardens and as an agricultural crop. Four lupin species have gained agricultural importance, *L. angustifolius*, *L. albus*, *L. luteus*, and *L. mutabilis*. The cultivated main species are blue narrow leaf lupin

(*L. angustifolius*), white broad leaf lupin (*L. albus*), and yellow lupin (*L. luteus*). These three listed species comprise sweet lupin and are annual crops. The tolerance for human and animal consumption for the alkaloids is 0.02% (Cowling, Buirchell, & Tapia, 1998) and these three varieties are typically within this alkaloid-level specification.

When choosing a landrace of lupin to grow, factors including the type of lupin (blue narrow leaf, white broad leaf lupin, or yellow lupin), the growing type (debranching or not), and the alkaloid number are the considerations. Seed supply is critical and, for Europe, the main addresses to buy lupin seed are Saatsucht Steinach (http://www.saatzucht-steinach.de/english/index.html) in Germany and SoyaUK (http://www.soya-uk.com/). In the optimization tests done at Louis Bolk Institute (the Netherlands) (http://www.louisbolk.org/), the following landraces were found suitable for cultivation in Europe: *L. angustifolius* (Iris, Primadonna, Regent, Boruta) and *L. albus* (Dieta and Boros).

For lupin cultivation, sowing starts by Mar. in the Netherlands, though early sowing may increase the risk of seed exposure to low temperatures. Blue lupin are more resistant to freezing ($-8°C$ to $-10°C$) in comparison with white lupin. The amount of seeds required per square meter is around 80–100. In the first stage, sprouts are visible in 1–3 weeks. From the day of sowing, seeds germinate within an average of 12 days. Flowering starts about 62 after sowing. Harvest for the blue lupin debranching (Race Iris) is around 165 days after sowing, while harvest for the white lupin debranching is around 190 days after the sowing (Azo, Lane, Davis, & Cannon, 2012).

Lupin can grow on poor soil and under extreme circumstances. However, the lupin crop is susceptible to mold at high moisture levels. The pH of the soil must be below 6.8 for cultivation of *L. angustifolius* and below pH 6 for *L. luteus*. Normally, lupin does not tolerate high calcium levels, though *L. albus* is most tolerant to higher pH (up to 7 or 8) and up to 10% calcium.

Pulses and lupin are not very sensitive for weeds compared to grains like wheat. In addition, chemical-based weed control is not allowed in Europe, thus requiring mechanical weed disposal. In Jun. and Jul., moisture availability is important for the lupin plant. With adequate moisture, each lupin plant can produce 4–5 pods. Lupin is sensitive for diseases during germination and the growth phase of the plant. Pathogenic mold in the soil can damage lupin plants, requiring the use of crop rotation and healthy seeds to provide a good start. Later, during the growth phase, diseases such as brown leaf spot caused by *Pleiochaeta setosa* and brown spot disease due to anthracnose can occur (Luckett, Cowley, Richards, & Roberts, 2008). Blue lupin is more resistant to anthracnose. Hares and roe deer like to eat lupin plants. Although partly eaten plants can still grow back, flowering and seed production will be delayed.

Harvest of branching blue lupin is between late Aug. and mid-Sep. and between early Sep. and mid-Oct. for branching white lupin. For winnowing lupin, a grain thresher can be used by adjusting the parameters of the sieves and straw cutter. Harvested lupin is sensitive for mold growth and they need immediate drying to a maximum of 14% moisture (http://www.pulseaus.com.au/storage/app/media/crops/2007_Lupins-SA-Vic.pdf). Air-drying in wooden boxes is an effective method.

10.2 SUSTAINABILITY

10.2.1 Land Use

Western Australia is the largest producer of lupin (90%) in the world with *L. angustifolius* being the dominant species. Annual production of lupin is over 2 million pounds. Besides Australia, other lupin-producing countries include Chile, Russia, Poland, Morocco, South Africa, and Spain (http://www.lupins.org/lupins/). Lupin is mainly used as animal feed, and to a lesser extent, for human consumption in some European and South American countries. An average 41% of the annual Australian lupin production was exported during the 5-year to 2005–2006. Over this period, exports averaged 430,000 tons, with an annual value of nearly $100 million (Lawrence, 2007). In 2007, the main destinations for Australia's lupin exports were South Korea, the European Union, Japan, and Chinese Taipei. A recent figure shows that South Korea, Japan, the Netherlands, Malaysia, and Germany were the top five western Australian lupin export markets in 2010–2011 (DAFWA, 2012; https://www.agric.wa.gov.au/crops/grains/lupins). Lupin seeds are currently receiving increasing international interest as an alternative source of human food ingredients due to their high-quality protein and dietary fiber (Figs. 10.1 and 10.2).

10.2.2 Water Use

Lupin is cultivated in areas receiving less than 500 mm annual rainfall in Australia (French & Buirchell, 2005). Sowing occurs between late Apr. and early Jun. and the optimal sowing times depend on rainfall zones and soil types. As a

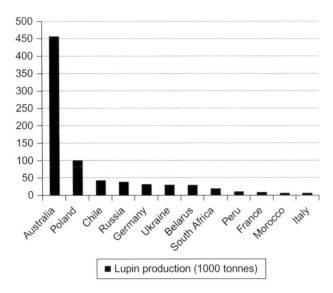

FIGURE 10.1 Annual production of lupin globally (1000 tonnes). *Adapted from http://www.factfish.com/statistic/lupins,%20production%20quantity/pie-chart.*

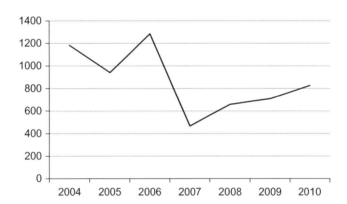

FIGURE 10.2 Production of lupins in Australia (1000 tonnes) (http://www.grdc.com.au/uploads/documents/GRDC_ImpAss_LupinBreeding.PDF). *Adapted from ABARES (2010).*

rule, the sowing times on sandy soils are mid-Apr. to early May, early to mid-May, and mid-May for zones with yearly rainfall below 350, 350−450, and above 450 mm, respectively. Cultivated lupins begin flowering from late Jul. to early Sep. with harvesting in Oct. or Nov. Like in Northern Europe, lupins grow well on well-drained soils, with reasonable depth and slightly acidic or neutral pH. Water stress during the growing season (too much or too little moisture) can raise the alkaloid level (Gershenzon, 1984).

10.2.3 Energy Use

Farmers can choose from a large variety of lupins to cultivate. In addition, the crops are able to fix nitrogen (150−200 kg N/ha) and mobilize soil-bound phosphate. Addition of nitrogenous fertilizers is not required, thus reducing the demand for fossil energy-dependent manufacture of nitrogenous fertilizers. Phosphate can be mobilized out of the soil by the plant and hence potassium is the only fertilizer required (Schulze, Temple, Temple, Beschow, & Vance, 2006). The addition of potassium sulfate was found to lower the alkaloid content in the beans, which is an added benefit (Prins and Nuijten: http://www.louisbolk.org/downloads/3043.pdf).

10.3 FOOD (PROTEIN) DEPENDENCE OF THE EU

There is an ongoing debate on the food sovereignty and food dependence of the European Union (EU) (Hospes, 2008). Changes in the geopolitical situation in the EU, such as the recent food boycott by Russia (2015: http://www.ibtimes.com/russia-food-crisis-russian-boycott-european-fruit-vegetable-imports-helps-turkey-1827946), highlight the importance of food security. Nevertheless, the EU is highly dependent on the import of protein crops. Soy protein in the form of soy cake (second) and as soybeans (fifth) is the most imported crop of the EU, while wheat is the primary import. Protein crops are mainly used for animal feed and, to a lesser degree, for human consumption in different products. An alternative use for soy in Europe is biodiesel production, using the oil from the bean instead of the protein (2011: http://gain.fas.usda.gov/Recent%20GAIN%20Publications/Biofuels%20Annual_The%20Hague_EU-27_6-22-2011.pdf). Without these imported soybeans, the EU would not be able to maintain its level of livestock production (http://www.gmo-compass.org/eng/grocery_shopping/crops/19.genetically_modified_soybean.html). Furthermore, the import of protein crops is projected to rise even further, which will only increase the food dependency of the EU (Ruitenberg, 2014).

To make the EU less dependent on food imports, several projects have been launched to stimulate the cultivation of more protein crops in the EU (Legato: http://www.legato-fp7.eu/; European Commission Research-Biosociety, 2007). However, the main problem for growing protein crops in the EU is that it is not yet financially attractive. There are various reasons behind the unprofitability of crops such as soy and lupines (AgManager, 2014: http://www.agmanager.info/marketing/outlook/newletters/All.asp). They can be listed as:

1. Competitive disadvantage to GM crops produced in the Americas;
2. Low world market prices;
3. Challenging climate conditions;
4. Expensive land and labor.

The following agricultural research and policy initiatives can aid farmers in improving their crop yields and make it financially viable:

1. Plant breeding practices to develop new varieties with higher yield, high protein content, and low alkaloid levels;
2. Cross-pollinating existing high-yielding cultivars of blue lupin;
3. Development of new safer alternatives to combat weeds and plant pests that affect lupin growth and yields;
4. Improve strategies to empower farming communities, such as cooperatives, contract farming, farmer-owned brand, price premiums;
5. Funding or subsidies from various countries and government involvement;
6. EU funding to offset losses due to crop failure;
7. Fair prices for food based on an alternate system.

10.4 PROCESSING OF LUPIN

10.4.1 Flour

The process to produce lupin flour starts in most cases with dry cleaning and dehulling (http://www.lupin.fr/en/production/), followed by sieving and sorting seeds by specific weight. Lupin's thick skin is removed by cutting the seed into two halves, followed by polishing. After that, the two lupin halves can be milled and/or fractionated. Milling the dehulled lupin gives native flour. This process is nonthermal and as such natural enzyme activity (lipoxygenase) will remain.

10.4.2 Concentrate

Milling lupin followed by fractionating produces a high-protein concentrate and high-carbohydrate portion. These are dry processes and typically done by pin milling, hammer milling, or jet milling and air classification. The product must be milled into very fine particles (100%; $<60\,\mu m$) to get the best results. Tyler and Panchuk (1982) comprehensively studied wheat processing in the 1980s, which aided in the production of protein concentrates by several means. Air classifying and protein-starch fractionation are similar in all pulses except for chickpea (Han & Khan, 1990) and lupin. Chickpea and lupin are exceptions due to their inherently high fat content (5–8% in chickpea and 7–10% in lupine). The fat portion ends up in the protein fraction. After milling, fractionating occurs based on particle size in a fluidized tower system with cyclones and sieves.

In a typical process, from 940 kg of pea, 84.6 kg pea hulls, 513.24 kg starch concentrate, and 342.16 kg protein concentrate (55–60% of protein) can be obtained (Tulbek, 2010). Similarly, a 1000-kg lupin batch provides 24 kg hulls, 150 kg protein concentrate, and 600 kg carbohydrate fraction (Blonk Milieu Advies, 2011: http://blonkconsultants.nl/upload/pdf/Bijlagendocument%20EDVV%20D5.0.pdf). An alternative process is milling, followed by sieving without any separation through cyclones. Lower yields are obtained for the protein concentrate with more of the carbohydrate fraction. This product can be used as normal lupin flour.

10.4.3 Isolates

A wet process involving alkali extraction produces isolates. Proteins, fats, and sugars are present in the alkali solutions of lupin. The extraction is followed by isoelectric precipitation of two classical storage globulins (conglutins α and β) and one albumin (conglutin δ). The supernatant contains conglutin γ, another main lupin protein. Further purification of conglutin γ can be by selective Zn^{2+} precipitation via resuspension of this isoelectric precipitate in saline water/ethanol solution to yield conglutin δ, a 2S sulfur-rich lupin protein (Duranti, Consonni, Magni, Sessa, & Scarafoni, 2008).

After the completely wet process, the protein fraction (and carbohydrate fraction) can be spray-dried. Fraunhofer (http://www.ivv.fraunhofer.de/en/geschaeftsfelder/funktionelle-zutaten/plantsprofood.html) developed a process optimization for the production of lupin protein isolates (LPIs) with improved water solubility while reducing thermal damage. Two types of protein products were obtained; LPI type E with better emulsifying capacity and LPI type F with an improved foam formation and stabilization.

Ultrafiltration followed by diafiltration can further separate lupin proteins to improve their functional properties (Hojilla-Evangelista, Sessa, & Mohamed, 2004). This process produces protein fractions with better surface hydrophobicity and emulsifying properties. In general, lupin proteins are soluble, have good emulsification, and moderate gelation properties in comparison to soy proteins.

The application of the lupin products in food is limited, largely due to a greeny and bean-like flavor (Bader, Czerny, Eisner, & Buettner, 2009). The Fraunhofer Institute tried to improve lupin products by dehulling followed by flacking the kernels. Lupin oil was removed by extraction with hydrocarbons of alcohols or supercritical carbon dioxide (https://www.fraunhofer.de/en/press/research-news/2014/september/fraunhofer-researchers-nominated-for-german-future-prize-2014-lupine-proteins.html). After aqueous extraction and isoelectric precipitation of the proteins, the yield, functionality, and sensory properties were studied. The conclusion was that extraction with supercritical carbon dioxide (at 285 bars) gave better yields and improved sensory properties. Protein solubility and emulsifying properties were unchanged.

10.5 NUTRITIVE VALUE

Among the pulses, pea, beans, and lentil, lupin has the highest amount of protein and dietary fiber (see Fig. 10.3).

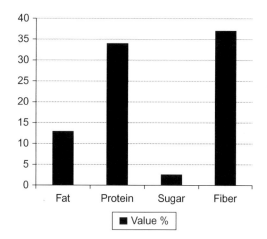

FIGURE 10.3 Nutritional value of white lupin (*Lupinus albus*) seeds (Martínez-Villaluenga, Frías, & Vidal-Valverde, 2006).

TABLE 10.1 Amino Acid Composition of Lupin Varieties

Amino Acid	L. albus g/16 g N	L. angustifolius g/16 g N	L. luteus g/16 g N
Histidine	3.30	3.10	2.70
Isoleucine	4.30	3.80	3.50
Leucine	7.80	6.60	6.80
Lysine	4.90	4.70	4.50
Threonine	3.50	3.10	2.90
Tryptophan	0.60	0.70	0.60
Valine	4.10	3.80	3.20
Meth. + cysteine	2.50	2.10	2.80
Phe + tyrosine	5.60	5.30	4.90

Source: Adapted from Sujak, A., Kotlarz, A., & Strobel, W. (2006). Compositional and nutritional evaluation of several lupin seeds. *Food Chemistry*, 98(4), 711–719 (Sujak, Kotlarz, & Strobel, 2006).

10.5.1 Protein

Protein delivers energy and is important for building and maintenance of the body functions. It is recommended that people obtain 10% of their daily energy from proteins. For vegetarians and vegans, the value increases by a further 20–30%. In addition, it is also important that people do not overconsume protein and limit their energy intake from proteins to 25% of daily caloric consumption. Higher protein intake is thought to increase stress on renal function (Martin, Armstrong, & Rodriguez, 2005) (Table 10.1).

Lupinus angustifolius contains about 34% protein. In all lupin species (and other legumes), the amino acids cysteine and methionine are limited. Ileal digestibility measures the actual break down of amino acids. When ileal digestibility of lupin protein is compared to milk, soy, pea, and wheat proteins, lupin may be considered a very beneficial plant protein (Tome, 2013).

10.5.2 Fats

Fats are a source of energy, vitamins A, D, and E, and essential fatty acids. For a healthy diet, fat should provide 20–35% of the daily energy needs (http://www.mayoclinic.org/healthy-lifestyle/nutrition-and-healthy-eating/in-depth/how-to-eat-healthy/art-20046590). Limiting consumption of saturated fats, and transfat is correlated with a reduction in risk for heart diseases. Lupin oil contains 75% of unsaturated fatty acids, while the linoleic:linolenic acid ratio in *L. angustifolius* is 6:1. In addition, the oil has high natural antioxidant capacity and is stable for 3 months. The omega-6 and omega-3 fatty acids content in lupin have similar health benefits as they have in soy oil (Fig. 10.4).

10.5.3 Carbohydrates

Dietary fibers are indigestible carbohydrates. Humans cannot digest dietary fibers in the small intestine, while in the colon, dietary fibers are important for normal functioning of the intestinal system. Food fiber is a group of substances like pectin, psyllium, inulin, cellulose, and resistant starch. Dietary fiber can be divided into soluble and insoluble based on the ability of microorganisms in the colon to ferment them. Lupin hulls consist of cellulose, hemicellulose, and pectin. In the cotyledons (inside the lupin) there is no starch but polysaccharides composed of galactose, arabinose, and uronic acid. These polysaccharides can bind large quantities of water. Cell walls are built up with pectin-like material, which can provide a hypocholesterolemic effect (Viveros, Centeno,

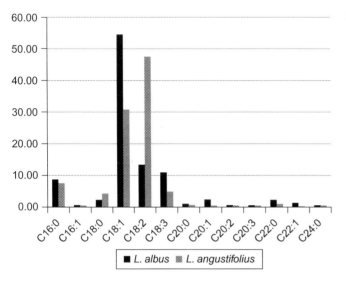

FIGURE 10.4 Fatty acid profiles of lupin oil (Hansen, 1976).

Arija, & Brenes, 2007). The oligosaccharides raffinose, stachyose, and verbascose, can cause flatulence, but also have a beneficial role in osmotic regulation of the gastrointestinal tract.

10.5.4 Minerals and Vitamins

10.5.4.1 Heavy Metals

Cadmium content in lupin was found to be below the proposed Codex Alimentarius limit of 0.1 mg/kg. The lead content should always be below the National Food Authority (Australia) limit of 2.0 mg/kg for legume foods. In *L. luteus*, accumulation of cadmium can occur because of the root architecture of this lupine variety. This does not happen in *L. angustifolius* (Brennan & Mann, 2005).

10.5.4.2 Minerals

Pulses contain mainly potassium and phosphorus. Typical calcium content in lupin is 1.5–2.2 g/kg, which is higher than in pea and lower in comparison with soya. The phosphorus content in lupin is 3.0–5.1 g/kg, which is equal with pea and lower than in soybean (Hung et al., 1988). Magnesium content (1.4–2.1 g/kg) is similar to pea and soybean and potassium (8.1–9.8 g/kg) is similar to peas but much lower than in soybean meal.

10.5.5 Evaluation of the Protein Quality and Digestibility of Lupin

A study by Monteiro et al. (2013) assessed protein quality and digestibility of *L. albus* and *L. angustifolius* in comparison with casein in a rat feeding study. The protein efficiency ratio (PER), net efficiency ratio and digestibility, average percentage of adequate casein, as measured by relative PER (R-PER), relative NPR (R-NPR), and relative digestibility (R-DV) were determined. Both lupin types had a high digestible protein, despite lower PER, NPR, and net protein utilization than for casein. There was no statistical difference between the two lupin species in relation to protein quality indexes evaluated in this research, although the amount of fiber in *L. angustifolius* was higher in comparison to that present in *L. albus* (Fig. 10.5).

Based on the above study, the authors concluded that lupin proteins were suitable for human consumption. An earlier study on rats also found that lupin proteins are potentially a useful protein source for humans. Though proteins from *L. mutabilis* had a lower PER, the addition of 0.2% methionine greatly improved the PER (Schoeneberger, Gross, Cremer, & Elmadfa, 1982) (Table 10.2).

Lupin is a good alternative source of protein, allowing the nutritional enrichment of foods and making them economically viable for underserved populations. Thus, there is a great potential for use of lupin by the food industry.

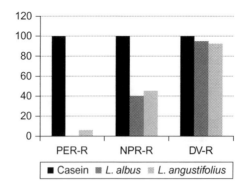

FIGURE 10.5 Comparison of protein qualities of lupin versus casein (Monteiro et al., 2013).

TABLE 10.2 Protein Efficiency Ratio of *L. mutabilis* Compared to Casein (Schoeneberger et al., 1982)

Protein Source	PER	Digestiblity (%)
L. mutabilis (raw)	1.34	80
L. mutabilis (debittered)	1.59	81
L. mutabilis + 0.2% DL methionine	3.05	85
Casein	3.09	87

10.6 ANTINUTRITIVE FACTORS AND ALLERGENICITY

10.6.1 Antinutritive Factors

Unlike other legumes, lupin does not need to be cooked before consumption because it is so low in antinutritional factors (especially the proteinaceous factors) in comparison with soybean and pea (Table 10.3).

10.6.1.1 Phytates and Lectins

Lupin is low in phytates, which can bind minerals such as calcium and zinc, leading to lower bioavailability (Mohamed & Rayas-Duarte, 1995). Trypsin inhibitors can reduce protein digestibility but are also low in lupin. In addition, lectins (gastric irritants that can cause agglutination of red blood cells) were not detected. Fermentation of lupin can further lower the phytate content and the concentration of oligosaccharides (De Silva, Trugo, da Costa Terzi, & Couri, 2005). Tannins are astringent and can precipitate proteins. A negligible amount of tannin was found in lupin. However, tannins can increase with added fertilizers (Lampert-Szczapa, Korczak, Nogala-Kalucka, & Zawirska-Wojtasiak, 2003).

10.6.1.2 Alkaloids

Alkaloid concentration in *L. angustifolius* is 200 mg/kg but these alkaloids have low toxicity. Germination can lower the alkaloid content by 80% and up to 85% by fermentation (de Cortes Sanchez et al., 2005). There are several alkaloids found among lupin species (Table 10.4) with 13-hydroxy lupanine being much less toxic than sparteine (Hatzold et al., 1983).

In a research study, eight generations of pigs were fed with 10–40% lupin in their diets. Lupin was in the starter, grower, and finisher diets. No negative health effect was found (van Barneveld, King, Mullan, & Dunshea, 1995). Rats were fed lupin, soybean, and cowpea for about 2 years. Researchers found that feeding of lupin (*L. angustifolius*) led to no negative effect. However, the long-term feeding of soybean or cowpea caused pancreatic enlargement (Grant, Dorward, Buchan, Armour, & Pusztai, 1995).

TABLE 10.3 Antinutritional Factors in Lupin in Comparison to Soybean (Kyle, 1994)

Botanical Name	L. albus	L. angustifolius	G. max
Total alkaloids (mg/kg)	<100	200.00	nd
Oligosaccharides (%)	6.70	5.20	5.70
Saponins (mg/kg)	nd	573.00	19,000.00
Condensed tannins	0.01	<0.01	<0.01
Lectins	nd	nd	nd
Trypsin inhibitors (mg/kg)	0.13	0.14	17.90
Phytate (%)	0.79	0.58	1.59

TABLE 10.4 Alkaloid Content in Lupin Varieties

Alkaloid	L. albus	L. angustifolius	L. luteus	L. mutabilis
Albine	15			
Lupanine	70	70		46
Multiflorine	3			
3-Hydroxy lupanine				12
13-Hydroxy lupanine	8	12		12
Angustifoline		10		
Lupinine			60	
Sparteine			30	16

Source: Adapted from The Biology of Lupinus L. Australian Government, Office of the Gene Technology Regulator, 2013, http://www.ogtr.gov.au/internet/ogtr/publishing.nsf/Content/biologylupin2013-toc/$FILE/biologylupin2013-2.pdf.

Pilegaard and Gry (2008) have provided a comprehensive review of the studies on alkaloids from lupin. Thus far, there have been seven known cases of human poisoning (four fatal), where an intake of alkaloids was at least 100 times higher than the alkaloid concentration of 200 mg/kg found in modern lupin cultivars. Lupin seed coat cell wall is mainly composed of cellulose and hence dehulling will not reduce the alkaloids (http://www.irwinvalley.com.au/?page_id=37).

Lupin plants can be attacked by a fungus *Diaporthe toxica* during the growth phase. This fungus produces toxic secondary metabolites, phomopsins, which can affect liver function potentially leading to hepatic failure (http://www.dpi.nsw.gov.au/__data/assets/pdf_file/0010/478243/Reducing-the-risk-of-lupinosis-and-the-incidence-of-phomopsis.pdf). Infected lupin seeds can be sorted out on gravity/size-sorting tables. Moreover, the fungus is separated during hulling of the seeds because the fungus grows on the outside of the seed. Although germination can lower the alkaloid content by fermentation, formation of other bioactive compounds such as esters is undesirable. Therefore, germination of lupin seeds for up to 3 days can reduce alkaloid levels and prevent the formation of the quinolizidine alkaloid esters (de Cortes Sanchez et al., 2005).

10.6.1.3 Raffinose Family Oligosaccharides

Lupin seeds are rich in nonstarch polysaccharides (30−40%), oil (5−15%), and protein (Faluyi et al., 2000; Huyghe, 1997; Petterson & Machintosh, 1994). However, one factor that deters people from consuming lupin is flatulence

(Price, Lewis, Wyatt, & Fenwick, 1988). This is caused by α-galactosides or raffinose family of oligosaccharides (RFOs), which are found in the range from 7% to 15% of raw seeds. These RFOs also have a positive effect on health in the bowel function (see Section 10.10).

Extraction processes can remove α-galactosides. When a 50% (v/v) ethanol solution was used to extract α-galactosides, high retention of protein, fat, and polysaccharides were observed in processed seeds. Sucrose and soluble dietary fiber, however, decreased significantly because of processing and retentions ranged from 10% to 60%, depending on the variety studied. In addition, vitamins B1, B2, E, and C were also reduced. Reduction of vitamin E decreased the antioxidant capacity (Torres, Frias, & Vidal-Valverde, 2005). It can be concluded that the lupin with low (extracted) α-galactoside level can be a product of nutritional importance due to their high protein content, dietary fiber and fat contents, as well as acceptable levels of thiamin, riboflavin, and vitamin E.

10.6.2 Off-Tastes

Lupin ingredients are promising alternatives to soybean products due to the presence of similar levels of protein. Lupin also has green and beany flavor similar to other pulses.

A series of unsaturated and saturated aldehydes, ketones, carboxylic acids, alkyl-methoxy pyrazines, and terpenes were identified for the first time as odor-active contributors to the aroma of lupin flour (Bader et al., 2009; Mittermaier, Czerny, Eisner, & Buettner, 2009). These off-notes arise from lipoxygenase activity which breaks down unsaturated fatty acids and is similar to that which occurs in soy (Honig & Rackis, 1975).

10.6.3 Allergenicity

About 1–2% of all adults have a food allergy (http://www.eufic.org/article/en/expid/basics-food-allergy-intolerance/) while a small subsection of this populace are allergic to lupin. Those showing allergic response to lupin also have allergic reaction toward peanuts and soybeans (Smith et al., 2008). A skin prick test with 200 Chilean children found that sensitivity toward lupin was very low, while 20% of the kids were sensitive to either peanuts or soybeans (Gross, 1990).

Most studies for determination of allergic reactions have been conducted on cross-reactions between peanuts and other pulses. Like for other pulses, lupin consumption has a risk for allergic reactions. This risk is comparable with the risk in eating soybeans and pea. In addition, the cross-reactions with peanut for lupin are comparable with soybean and pea (Bahr, Fechner, Kaatz, & Jahreis, 2014). A recent study on allergy to *L. angustifolius* was performed at the Erasmus University (http://www.lupinfood.eu/wp-content/uploads/2015/06/Lupin-allergy.pdf) in the Netherlands. A large group of people with higher sensitivity to peanut, soya, and lupins was tested. Of the 372 people tested, 220 people appeared to be negative, 135 were positive for peanut, 58 were positive for soybeans, and 22 were positive for lupin.

The current list of potential allergenic foods includes lupines. Soybean and peanut were already included (European Commission Directive 2000/13/EC). The inclusion of lupin should be interpreted as a precautionary measure and not as a real limitation, since it simply establishes mandatory labeling of this ingredient in lupin-based foods. Thus, sensitive consumers are alerted to the potential risks, while those who are not affected by lupin can benefit from the protein, minerals, vitamins, and high-fiber content (Duranti et al., 2008).

10.7 USES AND FUNCTIONALITY

There are different functionalities for lupin derivatives (flour, concentrates, and isolates) and their properties of these lupin ingredients are discussed below.

10.7.1 Lupin Flour

Milling of whole lupin without thermal processing provides flour with an intact lipoxygenase (Yoshie-Stark, Bez, Wada, & Wasche, 2004). This enzyme creates a bleaching effect that can be utilized in bread and bread improvers. Lupin flour can bind a lot of water (1.5 times own weight on water) and can aid in extending the keeping quality of bread. A variety of flours were tested for water binding, and lupin had the highest water-binding ability followed by hemp, fava bean, buckwheat, green pea, and wheat having the lowest binding (Raikos, Neacsu, Russel, & Duthie, 2014).

Another functional property of lupin flour is emulsification (Pollard, Stoddard, Popineau, Wrigley, & MacRitchie, 2002). This property is derived when lupin is dehulled, toasted, and milled. The high protein and fiber content provide emulsification to replace eggs, while the yellow color of the flour is an added benefit. In addition, the flour provides water binding, which extends the keeping quality. Use of this toasted flour benefits cakes, waffles, and other specialty-baked items.

10.7.2 Lupin Protein Concentrate

The high protein content (55—60%) of lupin concentrates can form the base for meat alternatives or replacers. In addition, lupin concentrates have good emulsifying properties for use in cakes, while the elasticity and crispiness properties find use in batters. Lupin protein concentrate is especially suitable for use in batters because it is more flexible and elastic than other proteins (https://www.fraunhofer.de/en/press/research-news/2012/december/tasty-and-gluten-free.html).

10.7.3 Lupin Protein Isolate

The Fraunhofer Institute in Germany developed various LPIs and determined their functional properties. Similar to the protein concentrates, the isolates find uses in replacement of animal protein (https://www.fraunhofer.de/en/press/research-news/2011/january/low-fat-lupin-proteins.html). The functional properties of seed storage proteins from indigenous European legume crops (lupin, pea, and broadbean or faba bean) were studied. Emulsions stabilized by these protein isolates obtained by ultrafiltration and isoelectric precipitation showed similar or smaller initial droplet size distribution but ultrafiltered isolates had lower stability throughout the storage time. The addition of salt destabilized these emulsions, by altering the protein structure while xanthan gum enhanced protein absorption and increased the emulsion stability (Makri, Papalamprou, & Doxastakis, 2004). The authors also studied foam formation and stability for the isolates. Foam formation ability for pea protein isolate (PPI) was the best among the studied isolates, followed by fava bean isolate (FPI) and LPI. The foam stability was quite good for PPI and FPI, but appeared to be inferior for LPI. Foams prepared by protein isolates of ultrafiltration had bigger foam volumes and were more stable than the isoelectric precipitated ones. The addition of salt increased the foaming ability, while xanthan gum increased both foaming ability and stability.

Lupin protein products formed gels with the greater fracture properties among all three legumes, for all combinations studied. Conglutin γ has the exceptional characteristic of being a sulfur-rich protein, which contains amino acids that are scarce in other grain legumes.

10.8 APPLICATION/CURRENT PRODUCTS

Lupin can be used in a variety of applications. This is due to the high protein and fiber content, which are significantly higher in comparison with pea, beans, and lentil. In addition, lupin has a superior taste relative to pea, beans, and lentil. Lupin is used to make a variety of foods including sweet and savory. Other factors encouraging use of lupin are that is vegetarian, gluten-free, and genetic modified organism (GMO)-free like other pulses. Lupin hulls can be removed and milled into flour, which is full of fiber suitable to enrich bread and bakery products.

10.8.1 Bakery Applications

Lupin flour finds use as a bread improver. In bread improvers, the concentration of lupin flour is about 80%. In a bread application, the improver constitutes 1—5% of the bread weight. In these applications, native (nonheat-treated) lupin flour is used. The functional properties of lupin including water binding (extending keeping quality of the bread), enzyme activity (bleaching), and emulsification play a role in product application (Kohajdova, Karovicova, & Schmidt, 2011). In baked applications such as special breads, waffles, cookies, and cake, similar levels of bread improver containing toasted lupin flour are used. This flour provides water-binding, emulsification, yellow color, structure, texture, similar to functional properties of eggs as discussed earlier.

10.8.2 Egg Replacement in Baked Goods

Frank Products (http://frankfoodproducts.com/), an ingredient manufacturer in the Netherlands, produces a lupin protein concentrate. The composition of lupin protein is quite similar to egg protein, although the protein quality is lower in comparison with egg protein. To achieve a 100% egg replacement in bakery applications, the addition of other ingredients is needed. A 50% egg replacement can be achieved by combining lupin protein concentrate (20%), whey protein concentrate (3%), and potato starch (7%) with water.

10.8.3 Application of Lupin Protein Concentrate in Batters

The functionalities of adhesion, emulsification, freeze–thaw tolerance, creating a barrier during frying, crispiness, fat uptake, etc., are important for batters. Depending on the type of batter, addition of 5–10% lupin protein in the dry components in the batter premix is recommended. This will help in emulsification (stabilizing the batter), viscosity (increasing water addition while reducing costs), and excellent adhesive properties (forming a stable film around the surface of products). Consequently, there is better freeze–thaw stability; less fat uptake during frying; and better expansion and crispiness of the layer, improving the eating properties.

The Fraunhofer Institute in Germany developed different LPIs with the techniques mentioned earlier, lupin protein type E and type F. Type E LPI is a better emulsifier, while type F is more soluble with better whipping and foaming capabilities. Type E is applied to emulsify in mixed meat products, mayonnaise, dressings, fillings, and ice creams. Type F is applied in whipped products like marshmallow, mousse products, and beverages.

10.9 CURRENT FOOD PRODUCTS

Lupin ingredients are used in numerous products around the globe, especially Europe. Prolupin (http://www.prolupin.com/indexen.html), a lupin food manufacturer, has a new vegan product line based on protein isolates. The brand is called "Made with Luve" with products including ice cream, drinks, desserts, yogurt alternatives, pasta, mayonnaise, and dressings. Lopino (http://www.lopino.com/), another small company in Germany, produces a LPI via a gentle process. LPI contains around 82% protein and has very good emulsification properties. These isolates can replace chicken protein or milk proteins, which are often used for their emulsifying properties. Examples for application include mayonnaise, ice cream, bakery, meat, health products, protein drinks, milk replacements, and pasta products.

Cheese replacements were evaluated using lupin. A lupin paste was prepared by soaking the seeds in tap water for a week, changing the water daily, and then boiled in water for 2 h, cooked and peeled. The peeled seeds were minced, blended to get a very fine paste and kept frozen until use. In matured Egyptian Ras cheese (3 months old) 25%, 50%, 75%, and 100% cheese was replaced with the lupin-based analog. In the mixed cheeses, the meltability, penetration, and fat separation are decreased. All levels of cheese replacement produced acceptable processed cheese analogs, but the most acceptable blend was produced with substituting 25% of cheese base as lupin paste. Feeding rats with the mixed product resulted in improved heat value like blood sugar levels (Awad, Salama, & Farahat, 2014).

In a research study, LPIs were added at 2% (w/w) concentration to meat systems. This resulted in an increase in gel network resistance to compression. Lupin protein tends to adsorb at the fat particle surfaces of the meat systems (Drakos, Doxastakis, & Kiosseoglou, 2007). In salad dressing trials, LPI was added to model salad dressing emulsions. Type E LPI, which contains globulins, was found to best stabilize the emulsion. In comparison, type F LPI did not perform well due to its higher content of albumins (Papalamprou, Doxastakis, & Klosseoglou, 2006). This stabilization ability was attributed to the bridging effect of the globulin aggregates, which strengthen droplet–droplet interactions within the emulsion droplet gel network.

10.9.1 Nutritional Applications

Lupin ingredients are used extensively in application for their nutritional properties and advantages. The main nutritional characteristics are the large amount of good-quality highly digestible proteins. The carbohydrates are present as dietary fiber providing extra health effects. Based on these nutritional qualities, bread containing 50% lupin is available on the market. This bread only contains wheat, lupin, water, and salt with high protein and fiber, is very tasty, and fits a low digestible carbohydrate diet. Consuming lupin improved satiety, stabilized blood sugar level, enhanced bowel health, reduced low-density lipoprotein (LDL) cholesterol levels in the blood, and lowered blood pressure. These are discussed in detail in Section 10.10.

When lupin flour, lupin protein concentrate and LPI were added at 3%, 6%, 9%, and 12% (w/w) of the wheat flour in bread, breads with the highest percentage of added lupin ingredients (12%) had a decreased loaf volume. The addition of the lupin ingredients increased the content of protein, especially the amino acid lysine. This addition also improved in vitro protein digestibility of wheat–lupin bread. *L. albus* showed the greatest potential as a bread additive

(Paraskevopoulou, Provatidou, Tsotsiou, & Kiosseoglou, 2010). The loaf height and crumb structure were not altered when lupin flour was substituted for wheat flour at levels up to 5%. Protein products of *L. albus* showed better emulsification properties, while *L. angustifolius* had better foaming capabilities.

In extruded snacks, where traditionally corn, potato, and wheat were used, pulses and lupin are becoming more popular due to their protein content and dietary fiber. Consequently, starch levels are lowered in the extruded snack. In addition, the popularity of global, ethnic food and the nice savory tastes from pulses can add something new to the extruded snacks (http://www.lupinfoods.com.au/zh/food-applications/).

Pasta is an extruded product, normally produced from durum wheat. Lupin flour can be used to produce gluten-free pasta. Due to the high protein content of lupin flour, lower amounts of flour are used since the high-protein dough will be unable to pass through the extruder (Kohajdova et al., 2011; Mahmoud, Nassef, & Basuny, 2012). In addition, starch is required to enable the dough to pass through the pasta extruder. High-protein pasta is another option to target the products involved in sports nutrition. To achieve this, lupin flour can be added to the wheat and extruded together.

Lupin flours and protein concentrates find use in texturized proteins to produce meat-like products. The company "Meatless" (the Netherlands; http://www.meatless.nl/en/) is producing lupin flour-based meat replacers. These products are based on protein gelation and the semifinished products are shipped to The Vegetarian Butcher (https://www.vegetarianbutcher.com/), a company producing meat alternatives. In addition, Vivera (http://www.wabel.com/c/vivera), yet another Dutch food manufacturer, is developing meat replacers. Vivera uses extrusion technologies to produce chicken muscle-like chunks, sausages, and other meat-like products from lupin flour. The lupin beans required for these products are cultivated around their factory premises.

Lupin can be consumed with minimum processing as whole seeds similar to peanuts. A big disadvantage of lupin in the modern kitchen is the long preparation time. Lupin requires overnight soaking followed by cooking for a soft and edible bean and this process may be time-consuming for a typical household in developed economies. A potential solution for time-strapped households is packages of soaked seed and cooked lupin in a jar. These ready-to-use forms of lupin beans would find consumers in southern Europe, where a typical past-time is consumption of beer with a side of cooked whole white lupin (*L. albus*). In northern Europe, beer is consumed with peanuts. Peanuts and lupin come from the same family and contain a high amount of protein. Peanuts contain a lot of fat, while lupin has a lot of fiber.

Several stores around the Netherlands sell white lupin in jars, including Ekoplaza and other organic food stores. This lupine product was developed by MFH-Pulses (http://www.mfh-pulses.com/en/index.html). To encourage consumers to eat more lupin, Powerpeul (http://powerpeul.nl/en/index.html), based in the Netherlands, produces small packs for consumer (white lupin) with raw harvested white lupin. The company provides recipes like bread filled with lupin paste, lupin spreads, lupin salads, etc. In addition, Powerpeul promotes lupin during fairs and festivals in the Netherlands. Lopino (http://www.lopino.com/products) is a small Italian company that produces hummus di lupino among other lupin ingredients, and products.

Lupin is also consumed as fermented products. De Hobbit (http://www.hobbit.be/Engels/FAQ%20HTML/LUPEH%20ENG.html) is a small Belgian company that makes products out of fermented lupin, called Lupeh; the brother of Tempeh. Lupeh is produced from cooked white lupin fermented with a mold suitable for human consumption. Birra Di Fiemme produces beer from lupin (http://www.birradifiemme.it/home.asp), while a coffee product is available from Caffe di Anterivo (http://www.comune.anterivo.bz.it/system/web/zusatzseite.aspx?menuonr=219763272&detailonr=219798498&sprache=3).

Lupin is popular in Australia. Lupin Foods (http://www.lupinfoods.com.au/) produces lupin flakes in consumer packs. These flakes find use in baked foods, biscuits and cakes, fermented foods, dal, muesli bars, and sauces. The flakes need cooking for 3 min to be consumed. Coorow Seeds (http://www.coorowseeds.com.au/products/lupin-products/) offers Australian sweet lupin products like lupin splits, lupin grits, lupin flour, and lupin bran.

10.10 HEALTH ASPECTS OF LUPIN

Lupin is a remarkable legume containing one of the highest sources of protein (40%) and dietary fiber (37%). They are easily digested, providing high bioavailability of essential nutrients and minerals (calcium, magnesium, and iron). In addition, lupin does not contain cholesterol and is high in essential amino acids. Finally, lupin is very low in lectins, phytates, trypsin inhibitors, and saponins (two known gastric irritants), the latter of which afflicts the soybeans even after extensive baking and processing.

These benefits enable lupin to be an important component of a healthy menu. Consumption of lupin has a beneficial influence on satiety (appetite suppression), energy balance (obesity), and glycemic control (type II diabetes). In addition, lupin is thought to prevent heart and vascular diseases by increasing LDL and reducing blood pressure. Moreover, lupin improves bowel health by prebiotic functionality. Each of these health benefits is explained in the following subsections.

10.10.1 Cholesterol

Several studies have focused on the cholesterol-lowering effect of lupin ingredients (protein, kernel fiber, and whole lupine flour). Lupin protein was found to downregulate genes involved in lipid synthesis, thus reducing LDL cholesterol (Bettzieche et al., 2008). An increase in good HDL cholesterol was observed, though it was not significant. Other lupin ingredients including protein isolate and whole lupin seed reduced accumulation of body fat.

Lupin kernel fiber lowered LDL cholesterol without an effect on HDL cholesterol (Hall, Johnson, Baxter, & Ball, 2005a) and was found to be as efficient as β-glucan or guar gum. The mechanism involved in the lower LDL levels by kernel fiber is thought to be related to the formation of short-chain fatty acids due to the high water-soluble fiber content (Fechner, Kiehntopf, & Jahreis, 2014). Dehulled lupin consists of mainly lupin kernel fiber and lupin proteins, a variety of studies have found a large decline in LDL cholesterol with pure lupin flour, possibly via a decrease in the intestinal absorption of cholesterol (Rahman, Hossain, & Moslehuddin, 1997).

Beside kernel fiber and proteins, phytosterols also play a role in the downregulation of LDL cholesterol. Phytosterols prevent the absorption of cholesterol through the intestine with several mechanisms, as reviewed by Hicks and Moreau (2001). Levels of 1−1.4 g/day of phytosterols may help to lower the LDL cholesterol in 10−15% of the populace. Phytosterols are fat-soluble and are present in the oil fraction. Lupin oil consists of 2.4% phytosterols, levels that are greater than any other known phytosterol-rich oil such as rapeseed (1.2%) and soybean (0.4%). The FDA has approved a health claim for phytosterols in Becel Margarine Plus (http://www.becel.ca/en/), one of the best-known products with added phytosterols.

10.10.2 Bowel Function

In lupin, the α-galactosides (raffinose family oligosaccharides or RFOs) are present in large quantities (5−11%). Depending on the variety and season, RFOs increase during periods of low moisture and provide the seeds with longer storage stability without losing their germination ability. The benefits of oligosaccharides in the diet are dependent on the increase in the *Bifidobacterium* population in the colon, which in turn supports a healthy gut. Bifidobacteria prevent the growth of pathogenic microbes and the excessive growth of detrimental microflora through production of acid, which reduces fecal pH. Bifidobacteria are one of the cultures added to several popular yogurts to improve bowel functioning. Gulewicz et al. (2002) showed that lupin RFOs were an excellent carbon source for Bifidobacteria. However, the bacteria did not metabolize RFOs to gaseous products.

Lupin kernel fiber, with 40% oligosaccharide content, reduced fecal pH during a human dietary intervention study. A similar result was obtained with isolated galactosides in rats (Johnson, Chua, Hall, & Baxter, 2006). Furthermore, it was shown that lupin kernel fiber could improve bowel function and reduce the fecal parameters related to colon cancer risk.

10.10.3 Satiety and Glucose Blood Level

One of the major challenges in weight management is the reduction of daily caloric intake. Due to the mechanization of our lives, the daily energy demand is lowered. On the other hand, the availability of ready-to-eat high-caloric processed foods has increased. This combination has led to a dramatic increase in body mass and obesity in Europe over the last decade. Currently, more than 33% of the European population is overweight or obese according to the World Health Organization (WHO: http://www.euro.who.int/en/health-topics/noncommunicable-diseases/obesity).

Reduction of caloric density (light product) alone does not reduce the daily energy uptake. Although lowering the fat content of a product lowers the energy density, it may also decrease satiety and increase digestibility. Thus, people consuming low-fat products may tend to eat more and feel hungry quickly. There is increasing evidence that consuming a high-protein diet is more satisfying than a high-carbohydrate diet and that high-fiber diets are more satiating than low-fiber diets (Burton-Freeman, 2000; Halton & Hu, 2004). Thus, lupin has the potential to increase satiety and reduce energy intake, due to its high protein and fiber content.

Lupin kernel fiber or flour increased satiety by 20% (Archer, Johnson, Devereux, & Baxter, 2004; Lee et al., 2006). It was found that lupin flour suppressed the hormone ghrelin in the stomach for more than 3 h, leading to reduced appetite. Hence, the total caloric energy uptake after a lupin-rich breakfast was reduced by 20% (Lee et al., 2006). Lower blood glucose levels and glycemic index (GI) were found in a study comparing lupin bread to white bread (Hall, Thomas, & Johnson, 2005b). The increase in satiety was not found to be significant, and a likely reason may be attributed to the lower quantity of lupin flour used. The lower GI indicated that the lupin carbohydrates were digested slower compared to white bread carbohydrates. In addition, fiber present in lupin flour did not cause lower GI, like other dietary fiber present in guar gum. Studies with lupin kernel fiber on the glycemic response did not show any difference with the standard (Johnson et al., 2006). On the other hand, it was found that a lupin protein component (γ-conglutin) is capable of interacting with insulin. Purified γ-conglutin was found to be significant in reducing glycemic levels in rats fed high levels of glucose. The γ-conglutin-lowering effect was comparable to the effect obtained with approximately half a dose of metformin, a well-known hypoglycemic drug (Magni et al., 2004). This result suggests that γ-conglutin may have a pharmacological response (Morazzoni & Duranti, 2008).

10.10.4 Blood Pressure

Hypertension is a well-known risk factor for various cardiovascular complications and is linked to the pathophysiology of type II diabetes (http://www.world-heart-federation.org/cardiovascular-health/cardiovascular-disease-risk-factors/hypertension/). Pilvi et al. (2006) compared the effects of lupin protein diets on blood pressure and vascular function in an animal model with type II diabetes, where the development of hypertension was accelerated by sodium loading. Lupin protein treatments normalized the elevated blood pressure back to the level of the control group. One possible explanation for the positive effect in the lupin group may be the relatively high arginine content of lupin protein (99.3 mg/g protein). L-arginine has been shown to improve vascular function and attenuate blood pressure in other animal models (Laurant, Demolombe, & Berthelot, 1995). The hypocholesterolemic effect of the proteins may be a possible mechanism behind the improved blood pressure. Epidemiological data show that an increased protein intake, and especially plant protein intake, are associated with lower blood pressure and a reduction in blood pressure over time, at least in humans (Appel, 2003). A study by Lee et al. (2009) showed a reduction of 3.5 mmHg pulse pressure by overweight and obese men and women after lupin protein intake. In a large population, this observed difference may be associated with a 10% difference in the prevalence of hypertension, a 4% difference in the risk for coronary artery disease, and a 10% difference in the risk for stroke (Collins & MacMahon, 1994).

10.10.5 Other Health Effects

Australian sweet lupin sprouts are an excellent source of isoflavones, which are often referred to as "phytoestrogens." Isoflavones are natural antioxidants and consuming them may play a role in lowering cardiovascular disease risk. The isoflavones, daidzein and genistein, may improve bone health by conserving calcium, thereby reducing the risk for osteoporosis (http://www.isoflavones.info/osteoporosis.php). Some isoflavones are believed to inhibit the growth of cancerous cells (Sarkar & Li, 2003) and in some studies have slowed prostate cancer growth by killing prostate cancer cells in a similar way to many common cancer drugs (Ahmad et al., 2013).

10.11 CONCLUSION

We are likely to consume less meat in the future, or at least, not the kind we are familiar with today. The way we produce our meat just is not sustainable. According to numerous studies, livestock production takes up 30% of the land surface of the planet and produces more greenhouse gas emissions than all the cars and trucks on the road. "Eating one four-ounce hamburger is equivalent to leaving your bathroom faucet running 24 h a day for a week" (Patrick O. Brown, Impossible Foods). We cannot continue on this path. Only a small percentage of the North American population is vegetarian, but as meat prices climb, consumers will have no choice but to cut back.

Switching diets to new protein sources is another option, including smaller animals like rabbit or edible insects. Our future seafood may come from "mega fish warehouses." Perhaps the meat of the future will actually be made from vegetables. Several companies are making meat alternatives from plants, including Impossible Foods (http://impossiblefoods.com/). These companies want to produce alternatives that even meat lovers will devour. The prairies in Canada/United States are known for their wheat farms but Newman predicts a thriving lentil industry will grow as farmers opt to grow more legumes instead (lentils use less water) (http://www.macleans.ca/society/life/tomorrows-food/). We can eat the pulses without investing in new technology as mentioned above when we have to develop meat alternatives.

Large amounts of soybean are imported by Europe, while a large percent of all soybeans on the market have been genetically modified to resist the herbicide Roundup (http://www.nytimes.com/2010/05/04/business/energy-environment/04weed.html?pagewanted = all). In 2010, 13.5 million tons of soybeans were imported to Europe, whereas only 2146 tons of lupin were imported. In Europe, lupin cultivation is easier in comparison with soy, and lupin can grow in cool climates. For Europe, cultivating lupin for the feed market would enable less dependence on soy. In addition, GMO soy continues to face consumer resistance in much of Europe, with concerns focused on the possible risks to health, biodiversity, and the environment.

Lupin has a number of advantages above all other pulses and can become one of the most important and sustainable protein sources to feed the growing global population. In addition, lupin can fix atmospheric nitrogen, to reduce the demand for fossil-based nitrogenous fertilizers. The nutritional properties of high-protein, nondigestible starch and unsaturated fats make lupin an importance source of nutrition. In addition, with physical properties such as emulsification and foaming, lupin ingredients find use in a variety of food products, including baked goods and meat alternatives. Finally, the health benefits of lowering LDL, blood pressure while boosting satiety are all valuable when faced with exploding health costs of treating chronic diseases. The current world population of seven billion is expected to be more than nine billion by 2050; with climate change, limited sources like land and water, and growing wealth in developing countries food prices will increase enormously. The value adding of lupin and lupin ingredients in addressing global food issues needs to be robustly pursued.

REFERENCES

Ahmad, A., Biersack, B., Li, Y., Bao, B., Kong, D., Ali, S., ... Sarkar, F. H. (2013). Perspectives on the role of isoflavones in prostate cancer. *The AAPS Journal, 15*(4), 991–1000. Available from http://dx.doi.org/10.1208/s12248-013-9507-1.

Appel, L. J. (2003). The effect of protein intake on blood pressure and cardiovascular disease. *Current Opinion in Lipidology, 14*(1), 55–59.

Archer, B. J., Johnson, S. K., Devereux, H. M., & Baxter, A. L. (2004). Effect of fat replacement by inulin or lupin-kernel fibre on sausage patty acceptability, post-meal perceptions of satiety and food intake in men. *British Journal of Nutrition, 91*(4), 591–599.

Awad, R. A., Salama, W. M., & Farahat, A. M. (2014). Effect of lupin as cheese base substitution on technological and nutritional properties of processed cheese analogue. *Technologia Alimentaria, 13*(1), 55–64.

Azo, W. M., Lane, G. P. P., Davis, W. P., & Cannon, N. D. (2012). Bi-cropping white lupins (*Lupinus albus* L.) with cereals for wholecrop forage in organic farming: The effect of seed rate and harvest dates on crop yield and quality. *Biological Agriculture & Horticulture, 28*(2), 86–100.

Bader, S., Czerny, M., Eisner, P., & Buettner, A. (2009). Characterization of odour-active compounds in lupin flour. *Journal of Food and Agricultural Chemistry, 89*(14), 2421–2427.

Bahr, M., Fechner, A., Kaatz, M., & Jahreis, G. (2014). Skin prick test reactivity to lupin in comparison to peanut, pea, and soybean in atopic and non-atopic German subjects: A preliminary cross-sectional study. *Immunity, Inflammation and Disease, 2*(2), 114–120. Available from http://dx.doi.org/10.1002/iid3.24.

Bettzieche, A., Brandsch, C., Weisse, K., Hirche, F., Eder, K., & Stangl, G. I. (2008). Lupin protein influences the expression of hepatic genes involved in fatty acid synthesis and triacylglycerol hydrolysis of adult rats. *British Journal of Nutrition, 99*(5), 952–962.

Brennan, R. F., & Mann, S. S. (2005). Accumulation of cadmium by lupin species as affected by Cd application to acidic yellow sand. *Water, Air and Soil Pollution, 167*(1), 243–258.

Burton-Freeman, B. (2000). Dietary fiber and energy regulation. *Journal of Nutrition, 130*(2), 272S–275S.

Clements, J. C., Buirchell, B. J., Yang, H., Smith, P. M. C., Sweetingham, M. W., & Smith, C. J. (2005). Lupin, Chapter 9. In R. Singh, & P. Jauhar (Eds.), *Genetic resources, chromosome engineering and crop improvement, volume I: Grain legumes*. CRC Press.

Collins, R., & MacMahon, S. (1994). Blood pressure, antihypertensive drug treatment and the risks of stroke and of coronary heart disease. *British Medical Bulletin, 50*, 272–298.

Cowling, W. A., Buirchell, B. J., & Tapia, M. E. (1998). Lupinus *spp. Promoting the conservation and use of underutilised and neglected crops. 23. Institute of Plant Genetics and Crop Plant Resources* (p. 105). Rome: Gatersleben/International Plant Genetic Resources Institute.

de Cortes Sanchez, M., Altares, P., Pedrosa, M. M., Burbano, C., Cuadrado, C., Goyoaga, C., ... Davila-Ortiz, G. (2005). Alkaloid variation during germination in different lupin species. *Food Chemistry, 90*, 347–355.

De Silva, L. C., Trugo, L. C., da Costa Terzi, S., & Couri, S. (2005). Low phytate lupin flour based biomass obtained by fermentation with a mutant of *Aspergillus niger*. *Process Biochemistry, 40*(2), 951–954.

Drakos, A., Doxastakis, G., & Kiosseoglou, V. (2007). Functional effects of lupin proteins in comminuted meat and emulsion gels. *Food Chemistry, 100*(2), 650–655.

Duranti, M., Consonni, A., Magni, C. H., Sessa, F., & Scarafoni, A. (2008). The major proteins of lupin seed: Characterisation and molecular properties for use as functional and nutraceutical ingredients. *Trends in Food Science and Technology, 19*, 624–633.

European Commission Research-Biosociety. (2007). A decade of EU-funded GMO research. <https://ec.europa.eu/research/biosociety/pdf/a_decade_of_eu-funded_gmo_research.pdf>.

Faluyi, M. A., Zhou, X. M., Zhang, F., Leibovitch, S., Migner, P., & Smith, D. L. (2000). Seed quality of sweet white lupin (*Lupinus albus*) and management practice in Eastern Canada. *European Journal of Agronomy*, *13*(1), 27–37.

Fechner, A., Kiehntopf, M., & Jahreis, G. (2014). The formation of short-chain fatty acids is positively associated with the blood lipid-lowering effect of lupin kernel fiber in moderately hypercholesterolemic adults. *Journal of Nutrition*, *144*, 599–607. Available from http://dx.doi.org/10.3945/jn.113.186858.

French, R. J., & Buirchell, B. J. (2005). Lupin, the largest grain legume crop of Western Australia, its adaptation and improvement through plant breeding. *Australian Journal of Agricultural Research*, *56*, 1169–1180.

Gershenzon, J. (1984). Phytochemical adaptations to stress. In: B. N. Timmerman, C. Steelnik, & F. A. Loewus (Eds.), *Recent advances in phytochemistry* (Vol. 18, ix, 334 p.) New York, NY: Plenum Press.

Grant, G., Dorward, P. M., Buchan, W. C., Armour, J. C., & Pusztai, A. (1995). Consumption of diets containing raw soya beans (*Glycine max*), kidney beans (*Phaseolus vulgaris*), cowpeas (*Vigna unguiculata*) or lupin seeds (*Lupinus angustifolius*) by rats for up to 700 days: Effects on body composition and organ weights. *British Journal of Nutrition*, *73*(1), 17–29.

Gross, R. (1990). In: Proceedings of the joint CEC-NRCD workshop. Y. Birk, A. Dourat, M. Waldman, & C. Uzureau (Eds.), 1989. pp. 164–176.

Gulewicz, P., Szymaniec, S., Bubak, B., Frias, J., Vidal-Valverde, C., Trojanowska, J., & Gulewicz, D. (2002). Biological activity of alpha-galactoside preparations from *Lupinus angustifolius* L. and *Pisum sativum* L. seeds. *Journal of Agricultural and Food Chemistry*, *50*(2), 384–389.

Hall, R. S., Johnson, S. K., Baxter, A. L., & Ball, M. J. (2005a). Lupin kernel fibre-enriched foods beneficially modify serum lipids in men. *European Journal of Clinical Nutrition*, *59*, 325–333.

Hall, R. S., Thomas, S. J., & Johnson, S. K. (2005b). Australian sweet lupin flour addition reduces the glycemic index of a white bread breakfast without affecting palatability in healthy human volunteers. *Asia Pacific Journal of Clinical Nutrition*, *14*(1), 91–97.

Halton, T. L., & Hu, F. B. (2004). The effects of high protein diets on thermogenesis, satiety and weight loss: A critical review. *Journal of the American College of Nutrition*, *23*(5), 373–385.

Han, J.-Y., & Khan, K. (1990). Functional properties of pin-milled and air-classified dry edible bean fractions. *American Association of Cereal Chemists—Cereal Chemistry*, *67*(4), 390–394.

Hansen, R. P. (1976). Fatty acid composition of the total lipids from seeds of three cultivars of sweet lupin: *Lupinus albus* cv. 'Neuland' L. albus cv. 'WB2', and L. luteus cv. 'Weiko III'. *New Zealand Journal of Agricultural Research*, *19*(3), 343–345. Available from http://dx.doi.org/10.1080/00288233.1976.10429075.

Hatzold, T., Elmadfa, I., Gross, R., Wink, M., Hartmann, R., & Witte, L. (1983). Quinolizidine alkaloids in seeds of *Lupinus mutabilis*. *Journal of Food and Agricultural Chemistry*, *31*, 934–938.

Hicks, K. B., & Moreau, R. A. (2001). Phytosterols and phytostanols: Functional food cholesterol busters. *Food Technology*, *55*, 63–67.

Hojilla-Evangelista, M. P., Sessa, D. J., & Mohamed, A. (2004). Functional properties of soybean and lupin protein concentrates produced by ultrafiltration-diafiltration. *Journal of the American Oil Chemists Society*, *81*(12), 1153–1157.

Honig, D. H., & Rackis, J. J. (1975). Volatile compounds of maturing soybeans. *Cereal Chemistry*, *52*(3), 396–402.

Hospes, O. (2008). Overcoming barriers to the implementation of the right to food. *European Food and Feed Law Review*, *3*(4), 246–261.

Hung, T. V., Peter, D., Handson, P. D., Amenta, V. C., Kyle, W. S., & Richard, S. T. (1988). Mineral composition and distribution in lupin seeds and in flour, spray dried powder and protein isolate produced from the seeds. *Journal of the Science of Food and Agriculture*, *45*, 145–154.

Huyghe, C. (1997). White lupin (*Lupinus albus* L.). *Field Crops Research*, *53*(1), 147–160.

Johnson, S. K., Chua, V., Hall, R. S., & Baxter, A. L. (2006). Lupin kernel fibre foods improve bowel function and beneficially modify some putative faecal risk factors for colon cancer in men. *British Journal of Nutrition*, *95*(2), 372–378.

Kohajdova, Z., Karovicova, J., & Schmidt, S. (2011). Lupin composition and possible use in bakery—A review. *Czech Journal of Food Science*, *29*(3), 203–211.

Kurlovich, B. S. (2002). Lupins (geography, classification, genetic resources and breeding). (P. 468). St. Petersburg: N.I. Vavilov Institute of Plant Industry.

Kyle, W. S. A. (1994). The current and potential uses of lupins as food. In M. Dracup, & J. Palta (Eds.), *Proceedings of the First Australian Lupin Technical Symposium* (pp. 89–97). South Perth: Department of Agriculture.

Lampert-Szczapa, E., Korczak, J., Nogala-Kalucka, M., & Zawirska-Wojtasiak, R. (2003). Antioxidant properties of lupin seeds products. *Food Chemistry*, *83*, 279–285.

Laurant, P., Demolombe, B., & Berthelot, A. (1995). Dietary L-arginine attenuates blood pressure in mineralocorticoid-salt hypertensive rats. *Clinical and Experimental Hypertension*, *17*(7), 1009–1024.

Lawrence, L. (2007). *Lupin—Australia's role in world markets*. Canberra, Australia: Australian Bureau of Agricultural and Resource Economics (ABARE). available online at: <http://adl.brs.gov.au/data/warehouse/pe_abarebrs99001376/ac_june_07_lupins_article.pdf>.

Lee, Y. P., Mori, T. A., Puddey, I. B., Sipsas, S., Ackland, T. R., Beilin, L. J., & Hodgson, J. M. (2009). Effects of lupin kernel flour-enriched bread on blood pressure: A controlled intervention study. *American Journal of Clinical Nutrition*, *89*(3), 766–772.

Lee, Y. P., Mori, T. A., Sipsas, S., Barden, A., Puddey, I. B., Burke, V., ... Hodgson, J. M. (2006). Lupin-enriched bread increases satiety and reduces energy intake acutely. *American Journal of Clinical Nutrition*, *84*, 975–980.

Luckett, D. J., Cowley, R. B., Richards, M. F., & Roberts, D. M. (2008). Improved methodology for screening for resistance to *Pleiochaeta setosa* root rot in *Lupinus albus*. In J. A. Palta, & J. Berger (Eds.), *12th International Lupin Conference* (pp. 447–450). Fremantle: International Lupin Association.

Magni, C., Sessa, F., Accardo, E., Vanoni, M., Morazzoni, P., Scarafoni, A., & Duranti, M. (2004). Conglutin γ, a lupin seed protein, binds insulin in vitro and reduces plasma glucose levels in hyperglycaemic rats. *Journal of Nutritional Biochemistry, 15*, 646–650.

Mahmoud, E. A. M., Nassef, A. L., & Basuny, A. M. M. (2012). Production of high protein quality noodles using wheat flour fortified with different protein products from lupine. *Annals of Agricultural Sciences, 57*(2), 105–112.

Makri, E., Papalamprou, E., & Doxastakis, G. (2004). Study of functional properties of seed storage proteins from indigenous European legume crops (lupin, pea, broad bean) in admixture with polysaccharides. *Food Hydrocolloids, 19*(3), 583–594.

Martin, W. F., Armstrong, L. E., & Rodriguez, N. R. (2005). Dietary protein intake and renal function. *Nutrition and Metabolism, 2*, 25. Available from http://dx.doi.org/10.1186/1743-7075-2-25.

Martínez-Villaluenga, C., Frías, J., & Vidal-Valverde, C. (2006). Functional lupin seeds (*Lupinus albus* L. and *Lupinus luteus* L.) after extraction of α-galactosides. *Food Chemistry, 98*, 291–299.

Mittermaier, S., Czerny, M., Eisner, P., & Buettner, A. (2009). Characterization of the odour-active compounds in lupin flour. *Journal of the Science of Food and Agriculture, 89*(14), 2421–2427.

Mohamed, A. A., & Rayas-Duarte, P. (1995). Composition of *Lupinus albus*. *Cereal Chemistry, 72*(6), 643–647.

Monteiro, M. R. P., Costa, A. B. P., Campos, M. R., da Silva, C. O., Martino, H. S. D., & Silvestre, M. P. C. (2013). Evaluation of the chemical composition, protein quality and digestibility of lupin (*Lupinus albus* and *Lupinus angustifolius*). *O Mundo da Saude 09/2014, 38*(3), 251–259. Available from http://dx.doi.org/10.15343/0104-7809.20143803251259.

Morazzoni, P., & Duranti, M. (2008). Use of lupin conglutin for the treatment of type II diabetes. US Patent No. 7,323,441.

Papalamprou, E., Doxastakis, G., & Klosseoglou, V. (2006). Model salad dressing emulsion stability as affected by the type of the lupin seed protein isolate. *Journal of the Science of Food and Agriculture, 86*, 1932–1937.

Paraskevopoulou, A., Provatidou, E., Tsotsiou, D., & Kiosseoglou, V. (2010). Dough rheology and baking performance of wheat flour–lupin protein isolate blends. *Food Research International, 43*(4), 1009–1016.

Petterson, D. S., & Mackintosh, J. B. (1994). *The chemical composition of lupin seed grown in Australia*. Perth, Western Australia: Proceedings of the first Australian Lupin Technical Symposium.

Pilegaard, K., & Gry, J. (2008). Alkaloids in edible lupin seeds: A toxicological review and recommendations. <http://www.diva-portal.org/smash/get/diva2:701152/FULLTEXT01.pdf>.

Pilvi, T. K., Jauhiainen, T., Cheng, Z. J., Mervaala, E. M., Vapaatalo, H., & Korpela, R. (2006). Lupin protein attenuates the development of hypertension and normalises the vascular function of NaCl-loaded GotoKakizaki rats. *Journal of Physiology and Pharmacology, 57*, 167–176.

Pollard, N. J., Stoddard, F. L., Popineau, Y., Wrigley, C. M., & MacRitchie, F. (2002). Lupin flours as additives: Dough mixing, breadmaking, Emulsifying and foaming. *Cereal Chemistry, 79*(5), 662–669.

Price, K. R., Lewis, J., Wyatt, G. M., & Fenwick, G. R. (1988). Flatulence—Causes, relation to diet and remedies. *Die Nahrung, 32*(6), 609–626.

Rahman, M. S., Hossain, M. I., & Moslehuddin (1997). Mineral balance of rats fed on diets containing sweet lupin (*Lupinus angustifolius* L.) or its fractions. *Animal Feed Science and Technology, 65*(1–4), 231–248.

Raikos, V., Neacsu, M., Russel, W., & Duthie, G. (2014). Comparative study of the functional properties of lupin, green pea, fava bean, hemp, and buckwheat flours as affected by pH. *Food Science and Nutrition, 2*(6), 802–810.

Ruitenberg, R. (2014).Wheat group seeks 50% yield boost by 2034 to feed the world. <https://olduvaiblog.wordpress.com/tag/food/>.

Sarkar, F. H., & Li, Y. (2003). Soy isoflavones and cancer prevention. *Cancer Investigation, 21*(5), 744–757.

Schoeneberger, H., Gross, R., Cremer, H. D., & Elmadfa, I. (1982). Composition and protein quality of *L. mutabilis*. *Journal of Nutrition, 112*(1), 70–76.

Schulze, J., Temple, G., Temple, S. J., Beschow, H., & Vance, C. P. (2006). Nitrogen fixation by white lupin under phosphorus deficiency. *Annals of Botany, 98*(4), 731–740.

Smith, P. M. C., Goggin, D. E., Mir, G. A., Cameron, E., Colinet, H., Stuckey, M., . . . Loblay, R. H. (2008). Characterization of allergenic proteins in lupin seeds and the relationship between peanuts and lupin allergens. In J. A. Palta, & J. B. Berger (Eds.), *'Lupins for Health and Wealth' Proceedings of the 12th International Lupin Conference*. Fremantle, Western Australia: International Lupin Association, Canterbury, New Zealand. ISBN 0-86476-153-8.

Sujak, A., Kotlarz, A., & Strobel, W. (2006). Compositional and nutritional evaluation of several lupin seeds. *Food Chemistry, 98*(4), 711–719.

Tome, D. (2013). Digestibility issues of vegetable versus animal proteins: Protein and amino acid requirements—Functional aspects. The United Nations University. *Food and Nutrition Bulletin, 34*(2), 272–274.

Torres, A., Frias, J., & Vidal-Valverde, C. (2005). Changes in chemical composition of lupin seeds (*Lupinus angustifolius*) after selective galactoside extraction. *Journal of the Science of Food and Agriculture, 85*(14), 2468–2474.

Tulbek, M.C. (2010). Pulse milling: Wet and dry fractionation applications of peas, lentils and chickpeas in gluten-free foods. In M. C. Tulbek (Ed.), Institute of Food Technologists Annual Meeting, Fargo, ND.

Tyler, R. D., & Panchuk, B. D. (1982). Effect of seed moisture content on the air classification of field peas and faba beans. *Cereal Chemistry, 59*, 31–33.

van Barneveld, R.J., King, R.H., Mullan, B.P., & Dunshea, F.R. (1995). Maximising the efficiency of lupin use in pig diets. <http://livestocklibrary.com.au/handle/1234/19775>.

Viveros, A., Centeno, C., Arija, I., & Brenes, A. (2007). Cholesterol-lowering effects of dietary lupin *(Lupinus albus* var Multolupa) in chicken diets. *Poultry Science, 86*, 2631−2638.

WHO. Technical report series protein and amino acid requirements in Human nutrition.

Yoshie-Stark, Y., Bez, J., Wada, Y., & Wasche, A. (2004). Functional properties, lipoxygenase activity, and health aspects of *Lupinus albus* protein isolates. *Journal of Agricultural and Food Chemistry, 52*, 7681−7689.

Chapter 11

Lentil: Revival of Poor Man's Meat

A. Samaranayaka
POS Bio-Sciences, Saskatoon, SK, Canada

11.1 INTRODUCTION

Lentil is a small legume seed belonging to the *Lens culinaris* species and the Leguminosae (Fabaceae or Papilionaceae) family. It is one of the most ancient food crops that has been grown in the world, and originated from southwestern Asia as early as 7000 BC (Dhuppar, Biyan, Chintapalli, & Rao, 2012). Lentil is classified as a pulse with other legume seeds such as pea, chickpea, and dry beans. Pulses, such as lentil, contain approximately twice the amount of protein as wholegrain cereals like wheat, oats, barley, and rice. About one-third of the calories in lentil come from protein, making it the third-highest level of protein by weight of any legume or nut (http://www.cgiar.org/our-strategy/crop-factsheets/lentil/). In west Asia and the Indian subcontinent, where many people are vegetarians, lentil has become the cheapest protein source to fulfill their nutritional requirements. Lentil protein, like other pulse proteins, is a good source of the essential amino acids, particularly leucine, lysine, threonine, and phenylalanine, but is deficient in the sulfur-containing essential amino acids methionine and cysteine (Table 11.1). Cereal grain proteins on the other hand are rich in methionine, but low in lysine (Table 11.1). Hence, a lentil–rice or lentil–wheat combination provides a complete protein profile of all essential amino acids. Lentil seeds also contain dietary fiber, vitamin B, and minerals such as iron needed for women of child-bearing age, growing children, and vegetarians.

The name "lentil" derives from its typical lens-shaped seeds. Different types/market classes of lentil are available which are different in seed size and seed coat and cotyledon color. Depending on the size, lentil seeds can be classified into two types: Chilean or large-seeded (greater than 50 grams per 1000 seeds) and Persian or small-seeded (45 grams or less per 1000 seeds) (http://saskpulse.com/growing/lentils/varieties/). The two main market classes of lentil are the green and red types. Green lentil is usually marketed as whole seed, while red lentil is marketed as whole seed or in dehulled and split form. The majority of world lentil production and trade is in red lentil. The color of lentil seed coat can range from clear to light green to deep purple, mottled, gray, brown, or black. Lentil seed cotyledon color can be yellow, red, or green (http://www.agriculture.gov.sk.ca/Default.aspx?DN=a88f57f0-242b-40f6-8755-1fc6df4dfa14).

Several popular varieties of lentils include Chilean, Brewer, Spanish brown (pardina); French green (Puy, dark speckled blue-green); Indianhead; Red chief; Beluga lentil; Eston and Milestone (small green); Richlea and Vandage (medium green); Laird, Glamis, Sovereign, and Grandora (large green), Masoor (brown-skinned lentils which are orange inside); Petite Golden; Crimson/red (decorticated masoor lentils); and *Macachiados* (big Mexican yellow lentils); among others (http://www.agrostats.com/fabaceae/table-of-lentil-varieties.html; http://www.ars.usda.gov/is/np/lentils/lentils.htm). The variety CDC Sovereign is the predominant lentil grown in western Canada, but red lentils are also gaining popularity rapidly. According to Canadian Grain Commission analysis (https://www.grainscanada.gc.ca/lentils-lentille/harvest-recolte/2014/hql14-qrl14-en.pdf), the size classes of green lentils include: small seed (3.5–5.0 mm), medium (4.5–6.5 mm) and large (5.0–7.0 mm); while red lentil are in the range of 3.5–5.5 mm.

11.2 SUSTAINABILITY

11.2.1 Land Use

Lentil crop is best adapted to the cooler temperate zones of the world, or the winter season in Mediterranean climates. Typically, seeds begin to germinate about 10 days after sowing, and the plants are ready to harvest in

TABLE 11.1 Amino Acid Composition of Lentil Compared to Pea, Chickpea, Soybean, Egg, Whole Wheat, and Brown Rice

Amino Acid	Lentil	Pea	Chickpea	Soybean	Egg	Whole Wheat	Brown Rice
Alanine	4.2	4.4	4.3	5.2	–	3.7	5.8
Arginine	7.7	8.9	9.4	8.6	6.2	4.9	7.6
Aspartic acid	11.1	11.8	11.8	14.0	11.0	5.5	9.4
Cystine	1.3	1.5	1.3	1.8	2.3	2.1	1.2
Glutamic acid	15.5	17.1	17.5	21.6	12.6	32.8	20.4
Glycine	4.1	4.4	4.2	5.2	4.2	4.3	4.9
Histidine	2.8	2.4	2.8	3.0	2.4	2.7	2.5
Isoleucine	4.3	4.1	4.3	5.4	6.6	3.4	4.2
Leucine	7.3	7.2	7.1	9.1	8.8	6.8	8.3
Lysine	7.0	7.2	6.7	7.4	5.3	2.7	3.8
Methionine	0.9	1.0	1.3	1.5	3.2	1.7	2.3
Phenylalanine	4.9	4.6	5.4	5.8	5.8	5.2	5.2
Proline	4.2	4.1	4.1	6.5	4.2	15.7	4.7
Seine	4.6	4.4	5.0	6.5	6.9	4.7	5.2
Threonine	3.6	3.6	3.7	4.8	5.0	2.8	3.7
Tryptophan	0.9	1.1	1.0	1.6	1.7	1.3	1.3
Tyrosine	2.7	2.9	2.5	4.2	4.2	2.1	3.8
Valine	5.0	4.7	4.2	5.6	7.2	4.3	5.9

Source: USA Dry Pea & Lentil Council Webinar (http://www.pea-lentil.com/core/files/pealentil/uploads/files/Webinar_4a.pdf).

3–4 months (http://www.harvesttotable.com/2009/07/how_to_grow_lentil/). Plants are able to tolerate frosty conditions. In addition, they are able to thrive in a variety of soil types including loamy, alluvial, and even heavy soils. Soil pH levels of 6–8 are better suited for lentil cultivation and the lentil plant does not tolerate water-logging, flooding, or soils with high salinity. Canada, India, Turkey, Australia, the United States, Nepal, China, and Ethiopia are the major players in global lentil production, where Canada is the world's largest exporter of lentil (FAOSTAT, 2013: http://faostat3.fao.org). In 2014, Canada and India produced 1.54 and 1.05 million metric tonnes, respectively (http://www.mapsofworld.com/world-top-ten/lentil-producing-countries.html). This is roughly about 460,000 and 296,000 metric tons of lentil proteins, respectively, mainly for food use.

11.2.2 Water Use

Lentil crop can tolerate extreme environmental conditions such as minimal rainfall and hot temperatures, making them a crop that can thrive in the warming earth. However, such variable weather conditions, especially during flowering and fruit set, can have an effect on the yield. In addition, lentil plants have shallow roots and are able to manage water efficiently (https://www.ag.ndsu.edu/pubs/plantsci/rowcrops/a1636.pdf). Average rainfall and irrigated water supply totaling 20–25 cm will enable a good harvest. In addition, too much moisture or wet climates are detrimental to the plant. Lentil crop is mainly grown in semiarid regions of the world without the need for a proper irrigation system, depending on water conserved in the soil after fall and winter rains. Thus, countries in Asia and sub-Saharan Africa can depend on lentil as a source of protein in the decades to come.

11.2.3 Energy Use

Due to their ability to fix atmospheric nitrogen into usable plant proteins, legumes have always been critical components of the agro-ecosystems throughout the world. Lentil is often grown in rotation with cereals due to several reasons (http://www.ars.usda.gov/is/np/lentils/lentils.htm):

1. Reduction of soil erosion when a lentil crop replaces summer fallow;
2. Less severe disease infestations occur in any following cereal crop because lentil is not an alternative host for certain cereal pathogens;
3. Better control of grassy weeds compared to cropping systems containing only cereals; and
4. Fixation of dinitrogen when effectively nodulated (nodules can contain symbiotic bacteria), therefore reducing the demand for nitrogen fertilizers and the depletion of inorganic nitrogen from soil (http://www.ars.usda.gov/is/np/lentils/lentils.htm).

Various studies of dinitrogen fixation by lentil have indicated values ranging from 35 to 115 kg/ha (31−103 lb/acre). For example, a study conducted by Saxena and Wassimi (1980) pointed out that lentil have the capacity to fix up to 107 kg/ha of nitrogen. Total nitrogen fixation in lentil is also influenced by both crop variety and rhizobial strain (Abi-Ghanem, Carpenter-Boggs, & Smith, 2011; Oplinger, Hardman, Kaminski, Kelling, & Doll, 1990). These findings suggest that nitrogen fixation improvement in lentil may be addressed via breeding crops for greater nitrogen fixation hosting capacity.

11.2.4 Diseases Affecting Lentil Plant

A variety of pathogens affect the lentil plant during various stages of growth (https://www.ag.ndsu.edu/pubs/plantsci/rowcrops/a1636.pdf). Similar to lupin beans, anthracnose (caused by *Colletotrichum truncatum*) affects plant growth, resulting in reduced yields. Other pathogens such as *Ascochyta lentis* cause Ascochyta blight leading to half the actual yield. Moist conditions can promote the growth of pathogens including Botrytis gray mold and *Sclerotinia sclerotiorum*. The gray mold affects all parts of the plant and can cause significant damage to crops and yields, while *Sclerotinia* damages the stems leading to stem rot. Fugicides and proper soil management are required to combat these pathogens for good harvests.

11.3 LENTIL PROTEINS: CHARACTERIZATION AND PROCESSING INTO CONCENTRATES AND ISOLATES

11.3.1 Characterization

Canadian lentil cultivars are reported to contain 26−28% protein on dry weight basis, with no difference between green and red or the market classes based on seed size. Starch content is also in the range of 45.8−48.7% for both green and red lentil. Major proteins found in pulses according to solubility classification are globulins and albumins, which impart functional properties such as water-holding, fat-binding, foaming, and gelation in different food formulations (Boye, Aksay, et al., 2010). Albumins are water-soluble proteins that have molecular weights ranging from 5 to 80 kDa. Globulins are salt-soluble proteins and major types found in legumes are legumin (11S) and vicilin (7S) (Schwenke, 2001). Proteins of prolamin and gluelin classes are also found in pulses, where alkali-soluble glutelins are of nutritional interest because of high levels of methionine and cystine in these proteins. Several research studies have suggested that the development of breeding technologies to produce pulses with higher glutelin content improves the protein quality (Singh & Jambunathan, 1982). Bhatty (1988) showed that albumins and globulins represented 19.6 and 53.9% of the solubilized lentil protein, respectively. The 11S globulin represents the major fraction of lentil proteins (Boye, Aksay, et al., 2010; Swanson, 1990). Gupta and Dhillon (1993) reported that isolated protein fractions were found to be glycosylated, with about 2.8% carbohydrates in the vicillin fraction. Furthermore, the albumin, globulin, legumin, vicilin, glutelin, and prolamin fractions from lentil contained 13, 22, 19, 5, 4, and 10 polypeptides, with molecular masses of 20.2 kDa, 82.2 kDa, 14.6−92.6 kDa, 13.8−92.26 kDa, 20.2−82.2 kDa, 17.0−46.2 kDa, and 16.98−63.8 kDa, respectively (Gupta & Dhillon, 1993).

11.3.2 Processing Into Protein Concentrates or Isolates

During protein concentrate or isolate production, lentil is first preprocessed (postharvest) to remove the hull (seed coat) and milled to appropriate fineness. Both dry and wet fractionation techniques have been tested to make protein products from lentil. Air classification is a dry fractionation technique that allows the fractionation of grains/seeds into high-starch and high-protein flour fractions. Lentil is first milled using an impact milling technique, such as hammer milling or pin milling. The type and extent of milling used for air classification have to be selected to produce a find grind, yet selective enough to break up cells and cell fragments without severely damaging the starch granules (Jones, Taylor, & Senti, 1959). The purities of the coarse (starch) and the fine (protein) fractions obtained by air classification are often lower than the proteins produced through aqueous extraction processes due to the difficulty of complete separation of starch fraction from protein. Protein fractions enriched with ~49–65% protein have been produced from lentil using this dry fractionation technique (Elkowicz & Sosulski, 1982; Tyler, Youngs, & Sosulski, 1981). AGT Foods (Saskatoon, SK, Canada) has developed a lentil protein product with about 50% protein content employing a dry fractionation technique (http://www.agt-foods.com/products/pulse-ingredients.html). VITESSENCE pulse 2550 from Ingredion (http://www.ingredion.us/content/dam/ingredion/us_assets/Pulses_Cereals_FS.pdf) is also a yellow lentil protein product containing 55% protein.

Aqueous alkaline extraction (~pH 8–11) followed by isoelectric precipitation (~pH 4–5) is the most common aqueous processing technique employed for the extraction of legume proteins due to the nature of major proteins present. Salt extraction or micellization can also be used. Acid extraction (pH < 4) is also used depending on the type of proteins to be extracted targeting different product applications (eg, water-soluble protein fractions). Ultrafiltration membranes can also be used instead of isoelectric precipitation to concentrate proteins. Protein isolates with more than 80% purity can be obtained from lentil by employing these wet processing techniques. High processing cost associated with wet processing is the major concern in producing lentil protein isolates by these approaches. Furthermore, protein purity, yield, flavor, and functionality are easily affected by processing conditions used, such as extraction temperature, time, flour: water ratio, condition and protein solubility of the starting material, and type of equipment and process used.

11.4 NUTRITIONAL VALUE, ANTINUTRIENTS, AND ALLERGENICITY

11.4.1 Nutritive Value

Research studies reveal that consumption of pulses provides an array of health benefits such as reduced risk of cardiovascular disease, cancer, diabetes, and reduction of LDL cholesterol (Hu, 2003; Tharanathan & Mahadevamma, 2003). Lentil is a good source of plant protein providing 9 g of protein in ½ cup of cooked lentil, and contains high amounts of iron, phosphorus, potassium, zinc, folate, and niacin (Table 11.1). It is also a good source of soluble fiber that can help reduce blood cholesterol levels. In addition, lentil contains starch that has low glycemic index (55 or less) and can support the maintenance of blood glucose levels.

Lentil flour is gluten-free and legumes like lentil are recommended by dietitians as useful for people with celiac disease. Lentil can also be used in vegetarian diets due to their iron and protein levels. Among the vitamins, lentil is an excellent source of the B vitamin folate which is an essential nutrient. In addition, folate consumption during pregnancy has been shown to reduce the risk of neural tube defects (http://www.cdc.gov/ncbddd/folicacid/recommendations.html). According to the USDA, folate may also provide beneficial effects in reducing heart disease and supporting mental health and a properly functioning nervous system (http://www.nal.usda.gov/fnic/DRI/DRI_Thiamin/196-305_150.pdf). Increasing folate in the diet can also lower the chances of developing colon and cervical cancer, according to researchers at the University of Chicago (http://www.thecco.net/article/view/1858/3044) and the University of Alabama (Piyathilake et al., 2009). Boye, Roufik, Pesta, and Barbana (2010) showed that in vitro tryptic digestion of red lentil protein can produce peptides with angiotensin-I-converting enzyme inhibitory activity.

The nutritional profile of whole red lentil is shown in Table 11.2. Depending on the variety, protein content of lentil from different countries can vary from 22% to 32% (Karakoy et al., 2012; Qayyum, Butt, Anjum, & Nawaz, 2012; Zia-Ul-Haq et al., 2011). The high protein content of lentil seeds makes it a great food source to feed people in developing countries who are unable to afford expensive animal protein products. Lentil is called "poor man's meat" due to its low price compared to meat, and can complement cereal-rich foods in providing a nourishing meal by balancing the amino acid and micronutrient requirements of the diet (Table 11.1). Increased production and utilization of lentil and lentil-derived protein products is therefore in high demand since most of the poor people in the world are dependent on it as a source of protein to meet their nutritional requirements (Abraham, 2015). Moreover, due to the low fat content of lentil (~0.8–2.0%), concentrated or isolated lentil proteins can be a good source of protein suitable for the formulation of various health-promoting foods without the need for supplementary costly industrial operations (eg, solvent extraction) to remove the lipid fraction.

Lentil seeds are mostly used for human consumption and only a small amount, mostly the damaged or defected seeds that are rejected for food use, is diverted to livestock feed. Lentil straw is also a valuable animal feed because

TABLE 11.2 Nutritional Profile of Whole Red Lentil[a]

	Amount	% of Daily Value
Fat	1.0 g	2
Carbohydrates	59.1 g	20
Total fiber	14.2 g	57
Insoluble fiber	12.4 g	
Soluble fiber	1.81 g	
Sucrose	1.79 g	
Protein	28.4 g	
Calcium	97.3 g	10
Iron	7.3 g	41
Potassium	1135 mg	32
Vitamin C	0.73 mg	1
Thiamin	0.34 mg	23
Riboflavin	0.31 mg	18
Niacin	1.73 mg	9
Vitamin B_6	0.28 mg	14
Folate	186 mcg	47

[a]Per 100 g dry seeds.
Source: Pulse Canada publication "Canadian Lentils," Saskatchewan Pulse Growers (http://www.saskpulse.com/).

of the highly palatable nature, high digestibility, and protein, calcium, and phosphorous levels compared to wheat straw (http://www.agriculture.gov.sk.ca/Default.aspx?DN = 5b2ed401-5fd2-483e-bce1-92c8d1687ba4). The leaves and threshed pods are also used for feeding sheep and goats in the Middle East and North Africa (http://www.cgiar.org/our-strategy/crop-factsheets/lentil/).

11.4.2 Phytochemicals

Lentil seeds also contain non-nutritional components including phytochemicals (Rochfort & Panozzo, 2007). These include antioxidant compounds such as triterpinoids, flavonoids, inositol, and steroids (http://www.aicr.org/foods-that-fight-cancer/legumes.html?referrer = https://www.google.com/#intro), phenolic acids, saponins, and tannins (Xu & Chang, 2010). Morton lentil was extracted with acetone and screened for antioxidant activity (Zou, Chang, Gu, & Qian, 2011). Condensed tannins, kaempferol were identified in crude and purified fractions. The study indicated that extracts from Morton phenols may be provided as supplements. Similarly, extracts of red lentil were found to contain phenolics such as quercetin, digallate procyanidin, and catechin (Amarowicz et al., 2009). Much of these antioxidants were found to be present in the seed coat (Hernandez-Salazar et al., 2010). Studies at the University of Illinois' McKinley Health Center found that phytochemicals such as lectins (carbohydrate-binding proteins) may have positive and beneficial effects in preventing and treating several chronic conditions including cancer (De Mejia & Prisecaru, 2005). Multiple mechanisms of action were identified by the authors, including binding to cancer cell membranes or their receptors, causing cytotoxicity, apoptosis, and inhibition of tumor growth. In addition to lentils, lectins are found in many other food sources including wheat, soybean, tomato, peas, and beans.

11.4.3 Protein Quality

Pulse proteins are generally rich in lysine, leucine, aspartic acid, glutamic acid, and arginine, but lack in methionine, cystine, and tryptophan compared to soybean and other protein sources like egg, whole wheat, and rice

TABLE 11.3 Effect of Different Cooking Methods on the Amino Acid Composition of Lentil Seeds[a]

Treatment	Raw	Boiling	Autoclaving	Microwave Cooking
Alanine	4.3	4.0	4.2	3.9
Arginine	7.2	7.0	7.0	7.0
Aspartic acid	11.5	11.4	11.4	11.5
Glutamic acid	15.5	16.6	16.0	16.3
Glycine	4.1	4.5	3.9	4.0
Histidine	3	2.8	2.9	2.9
Isoleucine	4.7	4.6	4.5	4.6
Leucine	7.4	8.0	7.6	7.6
Lysine	7.0	6.8	6.6	6.9
Methionine	1.4	1.2	1.2	1.3
Cystine	1.2	1.1	1.0	1.2
Phenylanine	6.1	5.8	6.0	6.0
Tyrosine	2.3	3.1	2.2	2.3
Proline	4.0	3.7	4.5	4.5
Serine	4.6	4.2	4.5	4.3
Threonine	3.8	4.6	4.8	4.5
Tryptophan	0.7	0.5	0.6	0.6
Valine	5.2	5.1	5.1	5.1

[a]Reported as g/16 g nitrogen.
Source: Hefnawy, T. H. (2011). Effect of processing methods on nutritional composition and antinutritional factors in lentil (Lens culinaris). Annals of Agricultural Sciences 56(2), 57–61.

(Table 11.1; Swanson, 1990). The cooking method employed also has an effect on the amino acid composition of cooked lentil (Table 11.3). Cooking treatments decreased the concentration of lysine (except microwave cooking), tryptophan, and total aromatic and sulfur-containing amino acids, but lysine, isoleucine (except autoclaving), and total aromatic amino acid contents remained high (Hefnawy, 2011). This study suggested that microwave cooking retains the most nutritive value of lentils compared to boiling and autoclaving, and all cooking treatments improved the in vitro protein digestibility and the protein efficiency ratio (PER) (Hefnawy, 2011).

The ratios of albumin:globulin and legumin:vicilin vary markedly for different types of pulses (Bulter, 1982). Gupta and Dhillon (1993) reported albumin:globulin ratios of 1:3, 1:6.3, 1: > 3, and 1:4 for lentil, black gram, French bean, and chickpea, respectively. Similar variations in legumin:vicilin ratio were also reported; 10.5:1, 1:6–9, 1:9, 1–3:1, and 4–6:1 for lentil, French bean, cowpea, pea, and chickpea, respectively (Gupta & Dhillon, 1993).

11.4.4 Antinutritional Factors and Protein Digestibility

Pulse seeds may contain enzyme inhibitors (eg, trypsin and chymotrypsin inhibitors) which could have adverse effects on protein digestibility if not properly inactivated during processing. The activity of antinutritional compounds can be significantly reduced through hydration/soaking followed by cooking. Proteins with higher digestibility are more desirable because they have higher nutritional value. Protein digestibility values reported in the literature for lentil include 95.19 (Monsoor & Yusuf, 2002), 81.76–99.88 (Sulieman et al., 2008), 79.1–79.4 (Han, Swanson, & Baik, 2007), and 73.5 (Melito & Tovar, 1995). According to Elkowicz and Sosulski (1982), lentil possess the lowest level of trypsin inhibitor (TI) activity (5.12 TIU/mg, soy has 41.5 TIU/mg sample). A recent estimation of TI level of Canadian cultivars reported 3.18 mg/g for nondehulled green lentil and 2.25 mg/g of seed coat removed red lentil (http://digitool.library.mcgill.ca/webclient/StreamGate?folder_id=0&dvs=1450216738413~698).

Protein digestibility-corrected amino acid score (PACAAS) values reported for lentil ranges from 52−71% (Sarwar, Paquet, & Peace, 1986). Metabolic utilization of lentil reported as PER is usually low compared to other legumes like pea, faba bean, and lupin, but similar to beans and chickpea (Nestares et al., 1993; Nestares, Barrionuevo, Urbano, & López-Frías, 2001). PER values reported for lentil by several studies include 0.30 (Urbano et al., 1995), 0.64 (Porres et al., 2002), and 0.83 (Hernandez-Infante, Sousa, Montalvo, & Tena, 1998). Low amounts of sulfur-containing amino acids and some essential minerals are partly responsible for low PER for lentil. Research has indicated that the supplementation of methionine or a mineral−vitamin premix significantly improved metabolic utilization of lentil protein (Combe, Achi, & Pion, 1991; Porres et al., 2002; Urbano et al., 1995). As noted previously, consumption of lentil with cereal grains like rice also helps in meeting essential amino acid requirements.

11.4.5 Allergenicity

Although pea, chickpea, bean, and lentil are not classified as major allergens, proteins in these pulse crops have been found to be allergenic. These allergic reactions have been confined mostly to Europe, Asia, and the Mediterranean (Martínez San Ireneo et al., 2000), possibly due to higher consumption of pulses in these populations. Multiple proteins in pulses can induce allergic reactions and these proteins are often heat-stable. Furthermore, pea, lentil, bean, and chickpea allergens have been reported to be cross-reactive (Martínez San Ireneo et al., 2000; Szymkiewicz & Jędrychowski, 1998).

The major allergenic protein reported in lentil is Len c 1, a 12−16-kDa protein that corresponds to γ-vicilin storage protein (Lopez-Torrejon et al., 2003). In addition to this, Len c 2, a 66-kDa protein corresponding to seed-specific biotinylated protein has also been reported (Sanchez-Monge et al., 2000). Both these proteins have been isolated from boiled lentil. Heat treatment of lentil shows drastic changes in the polypeptide profile with a strong increase in low-molecular-weight bands of 12−16 kDa and a decrease in 25−45-kDa bands. In a study by Sanchez-Monge et al. (2000), Len c 1 showed binding to 68% of individual sera of lentil-allergic patients while Len c 2 reacted with 41% of individual sera. In addition, protein isoforms Len c 1.0101, Len c1.0102, Len c 1.03103, and Len c 2.0101 have also been identified.

In a study among the Spanish population, symptomatic hypersensitivity to chickpea was frequently seen associated with lentil allergy and crossreactivity or cosensitivity has been observed among blue vetch (chickling pea), chick pea, and lentil (Pascual et al., 2001). Pea allergy and lentil allergy are frequently associated together. Vicilin and convicilin are the potential major allergens from pea, and they crossreact with the major lentil allergen Len c 1 (Sanchez-Monge et al., 2004). When the epitopes of vicilin allergens Ara h 1 from peanut, Len c 1 from lentil, and Pis s 1 from pea are analyzed, they have similarities which may account for the IgE-binding crossreactivity commonly observed among the vicilin allergens of these legumes (Barre, Borges, & Rougé, 2005).

11.5 APPLICATIONS AND CURRENT PRODUCTS

Lentil, along with pea and beans, are the major source of protein for a majority of the South Asian population (http://indiaphile.info/guide-indian-lentils/). The daily menu contains a variety of lentil−rice combinations, which provide a complete protein profile (http://healthyeating.sfgate.com/benefits-eating-rice-daal-together-11619.html). In fact, batters made from rice−lentil combinations are consumed ubiquitously in India for breakfast, lunch, or dinner. These combinations provide a variety of nutrients including protein (http://www.thehealthsite.com/fitness/health-benefits-of-dosa-k214/). Having high-protein and -fiber contents, and being low in glycemic index, pulses emerge as a unique source of energy to be incorporated into various food products.

Split lentils can be used as a main dish, side dish, or in salads. Lentil flour is used to make soups, stews, purees, and is mixed with cereals to make bread and cakes, and is used as a meat extender and as food for infants (Williams & Singh, 1988). Dehulled and split lentil seeds as well as lentil flour are increasingly used in gluten-free diets to meet protein and mineral requirements. General Mills, Inc., recently introduced a new Cheerios Oats & Honey Cereal which contains lentil proteins with a claim to provide 11 g of proteins per serving with milk.

Aider, Sirois-Gosselin, and Boye (2012) evaluated the incorporation of chickpea, pea, and lentil protein isolates into breads. The supplemented breads showed acceptable loaf volume and hardness at 3% supplemented level, but this decreased as the supplementation level was increased to 6% and 9%. With supplemented bread, the crumb and whites also became darker as the supplementation level was increased and with lentil bread, a greener color appeared at 6 and 9% supplemented levels. This study also suggested that the method of protein extraction could also have an effect on the characteristics of the dough and the baked products. Bamdad, Goli, and Kadivar (2006) showed the ability of using lentil proteins to prepare edible films with comparable mechanical, optical, and barrier properties to other edible protein films. Karaca, Nickerson, and Low (2013) reported that lentil protein isolate-based microcapsule formation was efficient for the entrapment and gastrointestinal delivery of flaxseed oil. In this study, microcapsules prepared by employing lentil and chickpea proteins in combination with maltodextrin exhibited a protective effect against lipid oxidation over 25 days of storage period at room temperature. Other potential applications of lentil proteins include textured vegetable protein products, nutrition bars, sport bars, and protein supplements, as well as pet food and aquaculture feeds.

Product launches in the European Union containing lentil increased in the 5-year period starting 2010 (http://www5.agr.gc.ca/eng/industry-markets-and-trade/statistics-and-market-information/by-region/europe/market-intelligence/new-food-products-with-pulse-ingredients-launched-in-the-european-union/?id = 1420648096758#g). England and France introduced the majority of these products, which ranged from meals, sides, and snacks. Whole red and green lentil were used predominantly, followed by lentil flour. Lentil and their flours are also finding uses in new products in Canada such as stews, soups, and even in chocolates (http://www.foodbusinessnews.net/articles/news_home/Supplier-Innovations/2015/10/Pulses_take_off.aspx?ID = {D72B5D5B-B739-45D4-B1C2-9CC673B64F4A}&page = 2).

Considering positioning lentil in this gaining interest in pulses, "protein level and quality" and uses as "whole grain" are the most important factors; whole lentil and lentil products need to go beyond traditional uses. Work conducted at the Canadian International Grains Institute (https://cigi.ca/pulsemillingproject/) shows that the method of milling (hammer, pin, roller, or stone milling) and extent of milling (fine or coarse flour) has an effect on particle size and functionality of flour due to the degree of starch damage. Milling procedures can therefore have an effect on functionalities such as that required in bakery products, fried foods, and coatings. A recent study by Pathiratne, Shand, Pickard, and Wanasundara (2015) showed that heat treatment in the form of infrared heating above 125°C can cause changes in flour functionality and also reduces the activities of oxidative enzymes, particularly lipoxygenase and peroxidase. As a result, flours with a range of functionalities can be obtained by moisture−heat treatment combinations of lentil seeds; therefore, food applications of lentil flour can be widened. These two are good examples that indicate uses of whole lentil can go beyond the traditional applications, enabling wide use of this important protein source.

11.6 PROTEIN FUNCTIONALITY

Protein functionality is a key factor along with flavor in determining potential product applications of lentil flours, protein concentrates, and isolates. Depending on the target application, properties like solubility, water-binding, fat-binding, emulsification, foaming, gelation, thickening, and/or flavor-binding will be of interest. The amino acid composition, protein structure, and conformation (eg, surface hydrophobicity, hydrophobicity/hydrophilicity ratio), as well as processing conditions involved such as pH, temperature, as well as the interactions that occur between proteins and other food components (eg, salts, fats, carbohydrates, and phenolics) will determine the functionality of proteins in a food system.

As with most pulse proteins, the solubility of lentil proteins is high at low acidic and high alkaline pH conditions, with isoelectric points of albumin and globulin protein fractions around pH 3.7 and pH 4.3, respectively (Torki, Shabana, Attia, & El-Alim, 1987). In a study conducted by Karaca, Nickerson, and Low (2011), lentil protein isolates produced by isoelectric precipitation were reported to possess good emulsifying properties compared to chickpea proteins and comparable emulsifying activity/stability indices and creaming behavior to that of soy protein. Suliman, El Tinay, Elkhalifa, Babiker, and Elkhalil (2006) also reported good emulsifying and foaming properties for protein isolates prepared with two Sudanese lentil cultivars. Ma, Boye, Swallow, Malcolmson, and Simpson (2015) assessed the feasibility of preparing salad dressing emulsions with pea, green lentil, and chickpea flours and obtained promising results.

11.7 HEALTH PROPERTIES

11.7.1 Bioactive Peptides

Lentil, chickpea, and pea contain proteins and peptide fractions that can impart angiotensin-I-converting enzyme (ACE) inhibitory activity upon consumption. ACE inhibitors have been associated with a reduction of hypertension. Use of lentil proteins for the production of bioactive peptides for functional food and nutraceutical applications is also another area of importance. The enzymatic hydrolysis of lentil proteins has resulted in the production of hydrolysates with

ACE-inhibitory activity and bile salts binding activity (Barbana & Boye, 2011; Barbana, Boucher, & Boye, 2011). Savinase, a hydrolytic enzyme, was found to be the most effective among several enzymes in liberating bioactive peptides from lentil (Garcia-Mora, Peñas, Frias, & Martinez-Villaluenga, 2014). Specific peptide fragments from legumin, vicilin, and convicilin have been found to be contributing to the antioxidant and ACE-inhibitory activity of lentil hydrolysates (Garcia-Mora et al., 2014).

11.7.2 Chronic Diseases

Consumption of lentil can reduce the incidence of certain chronic diseases (http://healthyeating.sfgate.com/benefits-eating-lentils-4547.html). In addition to protein, lentil contains resistant starches, fiber, phytochemicals, and antioxidants, which can support a healthy lifestyle while reducing conditions like cancer, diabetes, and cardiovascular disease, as discussed in Sections 11.4.1 and 11.4.2.

11.8 OFF-FLAVORS ASSOCIATED WITH LENTIL FLOUR AND LENTIL PROTEIN INGREDIENTS

The hull or seed coat of lentil is often indigestible and bitter. Removal of the seed coat helps improving palatability and taste, and plays an important role in processing and utilization of lentil (Wang, 2005). Indigestible fiber, polyphenols, tannins, and other antinutritional compounds present in lentil hulls can impart this bitter taste and may also impact physicochemical properties of flour and protein fractions.

There is strong evidence that "beany" aroma and flavor of pulse seeds is mediated by the activity of lipoxygenase (LOX) isozymes (Iassonova, Johnson, Hammond, & Beattie, 2009; Rackis, Sessa, & Honig, 1979). Although contains at $\sim 1\%$ level, lentil lipids are rich in oleic (20.8%,) linoleic (44.3%) and linolenic (14.1%) acids (http://www.pulsecanada.com/uploads/c4/91/c491f652f0cf53390d9a5b86aa63aeea/The-Chemical-Composition-and-Nutritive-Value-of-Canadian-Pulses.pdf), and also contain two lipoxygense isozymes (Hilbers, Kerkhoff, Finazzi-Agro, Veldink, & Vliegenthart, 1995). In soybean and products, the gradual decrease in LOX activity with processing was correlated with a decrease in the level of "beany" aroma compounds (Lv, Song, Li, Wu, & Guo, 2011). Working with whole green lentil (var Eston, small green), Shariati-Ievari (2013) have identified 10 volatile compounds that contribute to the "beany" flavor note and a significant reduction of 2-hexanal and 1-hexanol levels in the volatiles released from the same lentil seeds subjected to heating to 150°C.

According to some of the product development testing work conducted with lentil protein isolates, it is evident that utilization of this protein product at higher concentrations, such as in protein shakes, is challenging due to the beany and earthy flavor notes associated with the protein fraction. Not only the inherent flavor compounds contribute to the characteristic flavors of different lentil varieties and lentil-based flours and protein fractions, but also the processing technique employed has a great impact on the generation of new flavor compounds. Troszyńska et al. (2011) reported that catechin gallate and several types of keampferol glycosides were responsible for the off-odor, bitterness, and astringency of sprouted lentil. Ruiz, Price, Rose, Rhodes, and Fenwick (1996) reported the presence of saponin βg, a bitter-tasting compound, in several lentil varieties. Increased cooking time and soaking in water have been shown to be effective in decreasing bitterness by leaching of saponins and by converting saponin βg into a less bitter compound, saponin Bb (Ruiz et al., 1996). Depending on the targeted final product application, it is therefore important to select appropriate processing steps to either minimize off-flavor generation or to eliminate them. Masking of unwanted flavors associated with lentil protein products by selecting a proper formulation matrix is also another approach to increase utilization of lentil proteins in various food and functional food products.

11.9 CONCLUSION

As outlined in this section, lentil proteins are a great contender to fulfill the ever-increasing demand for sustainable plant-based protein sources. Utilization of lentil flours in various food formulations has increased tremendously during recent years, taking advantage of the whole nutrient package that includes fiber, starch, and micronutrients that comes with lentil protein. The added cost of producing more pure protein concentrates and isolates with bland flavor is one of the challenges at present to finding increased applications for lentil protein products. Nevertheless, several companies are trying to introduce lentil protein ingredients to the marketplace. Research are being carried out to optimize processing conditions and to address flavor concerns in order to produce specific protein fractions with targeted applications and functionality using different lentil varieties.

REFERENCES

Abi-Ghanem, R., Carpenter-Boggs, L., & Smith, J. L. (2011). Cultivar effects on nitrogen fixation in peas and lentils. *Biology and Fertility of Soils*, 47(1), 115–120.

Abraham, R. (2015). Lentil (*Lens culinaris* Medikus) current status and future prospect of production in Ethiopia. *Advances in Plants Agricultural Research*, 2(2), 00040. Available from http://dx.doi.org/10.15406/apar.2015.02.00040.

Aider, M., Sirois-Gosselin, M., & Boye, J. I. (2012). Pea, lentil, and chickpea application in bread making. *Journal of Food Research*, 1, 160–173.

Amarowicz, R., Estrella, I., Hernandez, T., Duenas, M., Troszynska, A., Agneiszka, K., & Pegg, R. B. (2009). Antioxidant activity of a red lentil extract and its fractions. *International Journal of Molecular Sciences*, 10(12), 5513–5527.

Bamdad, F., Goli, A. H., & Kadivar, M. (2006). Preparation and characterization of proteinous film from lentil (*Lens culinaris*). Edible film from lentil (*Lens culinaris*). *Food Research International*, 39, 106–111.

Barbana, C., Boucher, A. C., & Boye, J. I. (2011). In vitro binding of bile salts by lentil flours, lentil protein concentrates and lentil protein hydrolysates. *Food Research International*, 44(1), 174–180.

Barbana, C., & Boye, J. I. (2011). Angiotensin I-converting enzyme inhibitory properties of lentil protein hydrolysates: Determination of the kinetics of inhibition. *Food Chemistry*, 127(1), 94–101.

Barre, A., Borges, J. P., & Rougé, P. (2005). Molecular modelling of the major peanut allergen Ara h 1 and other homotrimeric allergens of the cupin superfamily: A structural basis for their IgE-binding cross-reactivity. *Biochimie*, 87(6), 499–506.

Bhatty, R. S. (1988). Composition and quality of lentil (*Lens culinaris* Medik): A review. *Canadian Institute of Food Science and Technology Journal*, 21, 144–160.

Boye, J. I., Aksay, S., Roufik, S., Ribéreau, S., Mondor, M., Farnworth, E., & Rajamohamed, S. H. (2010). Comparison of the functional properties of pea, chickpea and lentil protein concentrates processed using ultrafiltration and isoelectric precipitation techniques. *Food Research International*, 43, 537–546.

Boye, J. I., Roufik, S., Pesta, N., & Barbana, C. (2010). Angiotensin I-converting enzyme inhibitory properties and SDS-PAGE of red lentil protein hydrolysates. *LWT – Food Science and Technology*, 43(6), 987–991.

Bulter, D. (1982). The composition and nutritional value of legumes in relationship to crop improvement by breeding. In: *Proceedings of nutrition society* (vol. 41, pp. 1–6). Cambridge University Press.

Combe, E., Achi, T., & Pion, R. (1991). Compared metabolic and digestive utilization of faba bean, lentil, and chickpea. *Reproduction Nutrition Development*, 31, 631–646.

De Mejia, E. G., & Prisecaru, V. I. (2005). Lectins as bioactive plant proteins: A potential in cancer treatment. *Critical Reviews in Food Science and Nutrition*, 45, 425–445.

Dhuppar, P., Biyan, S., Chintapalli, B., & Rao, S. (2012). Lentil crop production in the context of climate change: An appraisal. *Indian Research Journal of Extension Education*, 2(Special issue), 33–35.

Elkowicz, K., & Sosulski, F. W. (1982). Antinutritive factors in eleven legumes and their air-classified protein and starch fractions. *Journal of Food Science*, 47, 1301–1304.

FAOSTAT (2013). *Agricultural data on primary crops.* <http://faostat3.fao.org> Accessed 13.10.15.

Garcia-Mora, P., Peñas, E., Frias, J., & Martinez-Villaluenga, C. (2014). Savinase the most suitable enzyme for releasing peptides from lentil (*Lens culinaris* var. Castellana) protein concentrates with multifunctional properties. *Journal of Agricultural and Food Chemistry*, 4166–4174.

Gupta, R., & Dhillon, S. (1993). Characterization of seed storage proteins of Lentil (*Lens culinaris* M.). *Annals of Biology*, 9, 71–78.

Han, I. H., Swanson, B. G., & Baik, B. K. (2007). Protein digestibility of selected legumes treated with ultrasound and high hydrostatic pressure during soaking. *Cereal Chemistry*, 84(5), 518–521.

Hefnawy, T. H. (2011). Effect of processing methods on nutritional composition and antinutritional factors in lentil (*Lens culinaris*). *Annals of Agricultural Sciences*, 56(2), 57–61.

Hernandez-Infante, M., Sousa, V., Montalvo, H., & Tena, E. (1998). Impact of microwave heating on hemagglutinins, trypsin inhibitors and protein quality of selected legume seeds. *Plant Foods for Human Nutrition*, 52, 199–208.

Hernandez-Salazar, M., Osorio-Diaz, P., Loarca-Pina, G., Reynoso-Camacho, R., Tovar, J., & Bello-Perez, L. A. (2010). In vitro fermentability and antioxidant capacity of the indigestible fraction of cooked black beans (*Phaseolus vulgaris* L.), lentils (*Lens culinaris* L.) and chickpeas (*Cicer arietinum* L.). *Journal of the Science of Food and Agriculture*, 90(9), 1417–1422.

Hilbers, M. P., Kerkhoff, B., Finazzi-Agro, A., Veldink, G. A., & Vliegenthart, J. F. G. (1995). Heterogeneity and developmental changes of lipoxygenase in etiolated lentil seedlings. *Plant Science*, 111, 169–180.

Hu, F. B. (2003). Plant-based foods and prevention of cardiovascular disease: An overview. *American Journal of Clinical Nutrition*, 78, 544–551.

Iassonova, D. R., Johnson, L. A., Hammond, E. G., & Beattie, S. E. (2009). Evidence of an enzymatic source of off flavors in "lipoxygenase-null" soybeans. *Journal of the American Oil Chemists' Society*, 86(1), 59–64.

Jones, R. W., Taylor, N. W., & Senti, F. R. (1959). Electrophoresis and fractionation of wheat gluten. *Archives of Biochemistry and Biophysics*, 84, 363–376.

Karaca, A. C., Nickerson, M. T., & Low, N. H. (2011). Lentil and chickpea protein stabilized emulsions: Optimization of emulsion formulation. *Journal of Agricultural and Food Chemistry*, 59(24), 13203–13211.

Karaca, A. C., Nickerson, M. T., & Low, N. H. (2013). Microcapsule production employing chickpea or lentil protein isolates and maltodextrin: Physicochemical properties and oxidative protection of encapsulated flaxseed oil. *Food Chemistry*, 139, 448–457.

Karakoy, T., Erdem, H., Baloch, F. S., Toklu, T., Eker, S., Kilian, B., & Ozkan, H. (2012). Diversity of macro- and micronutrients in the seeds of lentil landraces. *The Scientific World Journal, 2012*. Article ID 710412. http://dx.doi.org/10.1100/2012/710412

Lopez-Torrejon, G., Salcedo, G., Martin-Esteban, M., Diaz-Perales, A., Pascual, C. Y., & Sanchez-Monge, R. (2003). Len c 1, a major allergen and vicilin from lentil seeds: Protein isolation and cDNA cloning. *Journal of Allergy and Clinical Immunology, 112*(6), 1208–1215.

Lv, Y. C., Song, H. L., Li, X., Wu, L., & Guo, S. T. (2011). Influence of blanching and grinding process with hot water on beany and non-beany flavor in soymilk. *Journal of Food Science, 76*(1), S20–S25.

Ma, Z., Boye, J. I., Swallow, K., Malcolmson, L., & Simpson, B. K. (2015). Techno-functional characterization of salad dressing emulsions supplemented with pea, lentil and chickpea flours. *Journal of the Science of Food and Agriculture, 96*(3), 837–847. Available from http://dx.doi.org/10.1002/jsfa.7156.

Martínez San Ireneo, M., Ibañez Sandín, M. D., Fernández-Caldas, E., Marañón Lizana, F., Rosales Fletes, M. J., & Laso Borrego, M. T. (2000). Specific IgE levels to *Cicer arietinum* (chick pea) in tolerant and nontolerant children: Evaluation of boiled and raw extracts. *International Archives of Allergy and Immunology, 12*, 137–143.

Melito, C., & Tovar, J. (1995). Cell walls limit in vitro protein digestibility in processed legume seeds. *Food Chemistry, 53*, 305–307.

Monsoor, M. A., & Yusuf, H. K. M. (2002). In vitro protein digestibility of lathyrus pea (*Lathyrus sativus*), lentil (*Lens culinaris*) and chickpea (*Cicer arietinum*). *International Journal of Food Science and Technology, 37*, 97–99.

Nestares, T., Barrionuevo, M., Lopez-Frias, M., Urbano, G., Diaz, C., Prodanov, M., . . . Vidal-Valverde, C. (1993). Effect of processing on some antinutritive factors of chickpea: Influence on protein digestibility and food intake in rats. *Recent advances of research in antinutritional factors in legume seeds* (pp. 487–491). Wageningen, The Netherlands: Wageningen Pers.

Nestares, T., Barrionuevo, M., Urbano, G., & López-Frías, M. (2001). Nutritional assessment of protein from beans (*Phaseolus vulgaris* L.) processed at different pH values, in growing rats. *Journal of the Science of Food and Agriculture, 81*, 1522–1529.

Oplinger, E. S., Hardman, L. L., Kaminski, A. R., Kelling, K. A., Doll, J. D. (1990). Alternative Field Crops Manual. University of Wisconsin-Extension, University of Minnesota Center for Alternative Plant and Animal Products and the University of Minnesota. Available at: https://www.hort.purdue.edu/newcrop/afcm/lentil.html.

Pascual, C. Y., Fernandez-Crespo, J., Sanchez Pastor, S., Ayuso, R., Garcia Sanchez, G., & Martin-Esteban, M. (2001). Allergy to lentils in Spain. *Pediatric Pulmonology-Supplement, 23*, 41–43.

Pathiratne, S. M., Shand, P. J., Pickard, M., & Wanasundara, J. P. D. (2015). Generating functional property variation in lentil (*Lens culinaris*) flour by seed micronization: Effects of seed moisture level and surface temperature. *Food Research International, 76*, 122–131.

Piyathilake, C. J., Macaluso, M., Alvarez, R. D., Bell, W. C., Heimburger, D. C., & Partridge, E. E. (2009). Lower risk of cervical intraepithelial neoplasia in women with high plasma folate and sufficient vitamin B12 in the post-folic acid fortification era. *Cancer Prevention Research (Phila), 2*(7), 658–664.

Porres, J. M., Urbano, G., Fernandez-Figares, I., Prieto, C., Pere, L., & Aguilera, J. F. (2002). Digestive utilisation of protein and amino acids from raw and heated lentils by growing rats. *Journal of the Science of Food and Agriculture, 82*, 1740–1747.

Qayyum, M. M. N., Butt, M. S., Anjum, F. M., & Nawaz, H. (2012). Composition analysis of some selected legumes for protein isolates recovery. *The Journal of Animal & Plant Sciences, 22*(4), 1156–1162.

Rackis, J. J., Sessa, D. J., & Honig, D. H. (1979). Flavor problems of vegetable food proteins. *Journal of the American Oil Chemists' Society, 56*(3), 262–271.

Rochfort, S., & Panozzo, J. (2007). Phytochemicals for health, the role of pulses. *Journal of Agriculture and Food Chemistry, 55*, 798–7994.

Ruiz, R. G., Price, K. R., Rose, M., Rhodes, M., & Fenwick, R. (1996). A preliminary study on the effect of germination on saponin content and composition of lentils and chickpeas. *Zeitschrift für Lebensmittel-Untersuchung und –Forschung, 203*, 366–369.

Sanchez-Monge, R., Lopez-Torrejon, G., Pascual, C. Y., Varela, J., Martin-Esteban, M., & Salcedo, G. (2004). Vicilin and convicilin are potential major allergens from pea. *Clinical and Experimental Allergy, 34*(11), 1747–1753.

Sanchez-Monge, R., Pascual, C. Y., Diaz-Perales, A., Fernandez-Crespo, J., Martin-Esteban, M., & Salcedo, G. (2000). Isolation and characterization of relevant allergens from boiled lentils. *Journal of Allergy and Clinical Immunology, 106*(5), 955–961.

Sarwar, G., Paquet, A., & Peace, R. W. (1986). Bioavailability of methionine in some limiting amino acids in vegetable proteins fed to rats. *Journal of Nutrition, 116*, 1172.

Saxena, M. C., & Wassimi, N. (1980). Effect of fertilizer application and inoculation on the performance of lentil and subsequent wheat crop. *LENS, 7*, 52–53.

Schwenke, K. D. (2001). Reflections about the functional potential of legume proteins. *Nahrung/Food, 45*, 377–381.

Shariati-Ievari, S. (2013). *Effect of micronization on selected volatiles of chickpea and lentil flours and sensory evaluation of low fat beef burgers extended with these micronized pulse flours.* Master of Science thesis. Canada: Department of Human Nutritional Sciences, University of Manitoba.

Singh, U., & Jambunathan, R. (1982). Distribution of seed protein fractions and amino acids in different anatomical parts of chickpea (*Cicer arietinum* L.) and pigeonpea (*Cajanus cajan* L.). *Plant Foods for Human Nutrition, 31*, 347–354.

Sulieman, M. A., Hassan, A. B., Osman, G. O., El-Tyeb, M. M., El-Khalil, E. A. I., El-Tinay, A. H., et al. (2008). Changes in total protein digestibility, fractions content and structure during cooking of lentil cultivars. *Pakistan Journal of Nutrition, 7*, 801–805.

Suliman, M. A., El Tinay, A. H., Elkhalifa, A. E. O., Babiker, E. E., & Elkhalil, E. A. (2006). Solubility as influenced by pH and NaCl concentration and functional properties of lentil proteins isolate. *Pakistan Journal of Nutrition, 5*(6), 589–593.

Swanson, B. G. (1990). Pea and lentil protein extraction and functionality. *Journal of the American Oil Chemists' Society, 67*, 276–280.

Szymkiewicz, A., & Jędrychowski, L. (1998). Evaluation of immunoreactivity of selected legume seed proteins – Short report. *Polish Journal of Food and Nutrition Sciences, 7/48*(3), 539–544.

Tharanathan, R. N., & Mahadevamma, S. (2003). Grain legumes – A boon to human nutrition. *Trends in Food and Science Technology, 14*, 507–518.

Torki, M. A., Shabana, M. K. S., Attia, N., & El-Alim, I. M. A. (1987). Protein fractionation and characterization of some leguminous seeds. *Annals of Agricultural Science, Moshtohor, 25*, 277–291.

Troszyńska, A., Estrella, I., Lamparski, G., Hernández, T., Amarowicz, R., & Pegg, R. B. (2011). Relationship between the sensory quality of lentil (*Lens culinaris*) sprouts and their phenolic constituents. *Food Research International, 44*, 3195–3201.

Tyler, R. T., Youngs, C. G., & Sosulski, F. W. (1981). Air classification of legumes I – Separation efficiency, yield, and composition of the starch and protein fractions. *Cereal Chemistry, 58*, 144–148.

Urbano, G., Lopez-Jurado, M., Hernandez, J., Fernandez, M., Moreu, M. C., Frias, J., ... Vidal-Valverde, C. (1995). Nutritional assessment of raw, heated and germinated lentils. *Journal of Agricultural and Food Chemistry, 43*(7), 1871–1877.

Wang, N. (2005). Optimization of a laboratory dehulling process for lentils (*Lens culinaris*). *Cereal Chemistry, 82*(6), 671–676.

Williams, P. C., & Singh, U. (1988). Quality screening and evaluation in pulse breeding. In R. J. Summerfield (Ed.), *World crops: Cool season food legumes* (pp. 445–457). Dordrecht, Netherlands: Kluwer Academic Publishers.

Xu, B. J., & Chang, S. K. C. (2010). Phenolic substance characterization and chemical and cell-based antioxidant activities of 11 lentils grown in the Northern United States. *Journal of Agriculture and Food Chemistry, 58*, 1509–1517.

Zia-Ul-Haq, M., Ahmad, S., Aslam Shad, M., Iqbal, S., Qayum, M., Ahmad, A., ... Amarowicz, R. (2011). Compositional studies of some of lentil cultivars commonly consumed in Pakistan. *Pakistan Journal of Botany, 43*(3), 1563–1567.

Zou, Y., Chang, S. K., Gu, Y., & Qian, S. Y. (2011). Antioxidant activity and phenolic compositions of lentil (*Lens culinaris* var. Morton) extract and its fractions. *Journal of Agriculture and Food Chemistry, 59*(6), 2268–2276. Available from http://dx.doi.org/10.1021/jf104640k.

Chapter 12

Underutilized Protein Resources From African Legumes

M. Gulzar and A. Minnaar
University of Pretoria, Hatfield, Pretoria, South Africa

12.1 INTRODUCTION

Getting food resources for the burgeoning population of the world is becoming more and more difficult. In this situation, every country has to best utilize its already-available food resources. However, this is not the case in Africa, where its underutilized crops could have tackled the problems of malnutrition, hunger, and rural poverty. In Africa, a number of legume crops that were previously used as an important source of proteins, edible fats, fiber, minerals, and other nutritional components are on the verge of becoming scarce (NRC, 2006). In fact, some of these crops (marama bean, bambara groundnut, cowpea, pigeon pea, yambean, and lablab) have huge potential in terms of their adaptability to the climate and their richness in nutrition. The nutritional composition of these crops is given in Table 12.1, which shows that these crops have huge potential to become sustainable foods or feed resources for the future. However, due to the lack of agronomic, genetic, and food research on these potentially important crops they are in danger of becoming scarce (NRC, 2006). Keeping in mind their climatic adaptability and richness in nutrition, serious attention is required to move these crops out of obscurity.

Even though there are a number of underutilized legume crops in Africa, this chapter uses the case of two nutritionally important underutilized legume crops: (1) marama beans (*Tylosema esculentum*) and (2) bambara groundnut (*Vigna subterranea*). Marama bean is an underutilized oil seed legume of southern Africa, which due to its high drought tolerance (Jackson et al., 2010) and comparable nutritional profile (Mahesh & Sathe, 2006; Mujoo, Trinh, & Ng, 2003) can be a possible replacement of soybean and peanut. Bambara groundnut is the third most important grain legume crop in Africa after groundnut and cowpea (Bamshaiye et al., 2011; Baryeh, 2001) but is still cultivated by small landholders. Interestingly, it contains the highest oil content (6.5–8.5%) of any other grain legume (Bamshaiye et al., 2011; Baryeh, 2001; Hillocks et al., 2012; NRC, 2006; Steve Ijarotimi & Ruth Esho, 2009). The crop in addition to its high drought tolerance can grow under adverse climatic and soil conditions (Amadou, Bebeli, & Kaltsikes, 2001; Azam-Ali et al., 2001; Bamshaiye et al., 2011; Baryeh, 2001) as well being resistant to diseases and pests (NRC, 2006).

12.2 MARAMA BEANS

12.2.1 Introduction (Land, Water, Sustainability)

In fact, the world relies on essentially just two oilseed legumes for food and feed, soya and peanut. This is a huge potential problem as climate-change starts to adversely affect agriculture as neither are water-efficient crops. Marama bean is an underutilized oilseed legume crop of southern Africa, which could be a valuable alternative to other oilseeds due to its high drought-tolerance (Jackson et al., 2010). Marama belongs to genus *Tylosema* of Fabaceae family and belongs to subfamily Ceasalpinoidae (Coetzer & Ross, 1976; Jackson et al., 2010). Under this genus, it has four species: *T. esculentum*, *T. fassoglense*, *T. argentea*, and *T. humifusa* (Coetzer & Ross, 1976). Marama bean is indigenous to the Kalahari desert of southern Africa (Monaghan & Halloran, 1996) and neighboring sandy areas of Namibia, Botswana, and South Africa (Bower, Hertel, Oh, & Storey, 1988). The crop is grown in northern parts of Namibia and Botswana as well as in the Northern Cape in South Africa. Fig. 12.1 shows marama bean (*T. esculentum*) plant and seeds taken

TABLE 12.1 Nutrient Composition (g/100 g) of Some Underutilized African Legumes Compared With Soybean and Navy Bean

Legumes	Protein	Fats	Carbohydrates	Minerals	References
Marama bean	29–38	32–42	19–27	2.5–3.5	Holse, Husted, and Hansen (2010)
Bambara groundnut	17–25	6.5–8.5	53–69	2.5–3.5	Bamshaiye, Adegbola, and Bamshaiye (2011), Baryeh (2001), Hillocks, Bennett, and Mponda (2012), NRC (2006), and Steve Ijarotimi and Ruth Esho (2009)
Cowpea	23.85	2.07	59.64	2.30	USDA National Nutrient Database (2014)
Pigeon pea	21.70	1.49	62.78	2.10	USDA National Nutrient Database (2014)
Lablab	22.4–31.3	1.5–2.0	54.2–67.2	3.3–3.9	Osman (2007) and Deka and Sarkar (1990)
Yambean	19.2–22.5	1.9–2.5	52.1–62.2	2.7–3.5	Edem, Amugo, and Eka (1990) and Ene-Obong and Carnovale (1992)
Soya bean	36.49	19.94	30.16	3.08	USDA National Nutrient Database (2014)
Navy bean	22.33	1.50	60.75	1.93	USDA National Nutrient Database (2014)

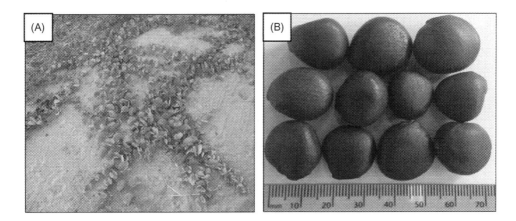

FIGURE 12.1 Marama bean (*Tylosema esculentum*) plant (A) and whole mature beans (B) from southern Africa. *(A) Adapted from Jackson, J. C., Duodu, K. G., Holse, M., Lima de Faria, M. D., Jordaan, D., Chingwaru, W., … Minnaar, A. (2010). Chapter 5 — The morama bean (Tylosema esculentum): A potential crop for Southern Africa, In: Steve, L. T. (Ed.), Advances in food and nutrition research (pp. 187–246). Academic Press.*

from southern Africa. These living cisterns of arid and semiarid regions can thrive in very poor soil and can bear despite severity of climate (drought, high and low temperature) (NRC, 2006; Travlos & Karamanos, 2006).

Marama plant produces brown-colored seeds above ground and highly nutritious tuber below ground. The immature beans are eaten after boiling, while mature beans are roasted and used as a snack (Holse et al., 2010; Jackson et al., 2010). Marama tuber is also highly nutritious, more than yam, potatoes, and sugar beet, as well as being rich in protein content (9%). The tubers are usually large in size (one of the tubers seen in Botswana weighed 277 kg) and are used as a source of energy and water for the plant under severe conditions (NRC, 2006).

As marama has not yet been domesticated and is still in the wild, there is no agronomic research yet to identify the kind of soils needed for the better production of marama beans. However, the characteristics of marama bean-producing soils have been analyzed by Jackson et al. (2010) and Thomas (2004). These authors have observed that in general most of marama bean-growing soils are waterlogged sands containing dolomite and limestone concentrations. However, the marama bean-growing soils in Botswana were characterized as brown sands with the absence of dolomite or limestone.

12.2.2 Composition of Marama Beans

The mature marama beans are yellowish in color and are covered by a hard brown coat. The beans are a rich source of energy in the form of protein, fat, fiber, and minerals, etc. They have high protein (29–38%) and fat (32–42%) content, as well as having 19–27% dietary fiber and 2.5–3.5% mineral salts (Holse et al., 2010). The starch and soluble sugars are less than 1% (Mosele et al., 2011). Marama bean is also a good source of calcium, potassium, magnesium, iron, zinc, phosphate, as well as B vitamins (thiamine, riboflavin, and nicotinic acid) (NRC, 2006; Wehmeyer, Lee, & Whiting, 1969). In terms of protein and fat content the marama beans have a profile almost comparable to soybean (Mujoo et al., 2003) and peanut (Mahesh & Sathe, 2006). However, the protein composition is very much different as compared to soy proteins (Amonsou, Taylor, Beukes, et al., 2012; Maruatona, Duodu, & Minnaar, 2010). Marama beans also possesses high-quality oil, containing approximately 75% unsaturated fatty acids (Bower et al., 1988; Holse, Petersen, Maruatona, & Hansen, 2012).

12.2.3 Composition of Marama Proteins

The composition of legume proteins defines their application in different food products. The composition of marama bean proteins is given in Table 12.2. They contain 23% albumin, 53% globulin, 15.5% prolamins, and 8.3% glutelins (Bower et al., 1988). Marama proteins are unique in the way that their protein composition is different from other common legumes. Amonsou, Taylor, Beukes, et al. (2012) reported that 7S (vicilin) and 11S acidic subunits are absent in marama proteins. They only contains 11S basic subunits (legumin) and some medium (63 kDa) and high (148 kDa) molecular weight protein fractions linked together by covalent bonds other than disulfide bonds. The high tyrosine content in marama proteins (Table 12.3) suggests that the dityrosine bonds may be the binding forces for integrity of these large molecular fractions. The disulfide bonds were also not detected in marama proteins (Amonsou, Taylor, Beukes, et al., 2012). Most of the polypeptides in marama proteome map (as analyzed by two-dimensional electrophoresis) were basic and only one polypeptide matched with those of soybean (Amonsou, Taylor, Beukes, et al., 2012).

12.2.4 Protein Isolation

In spite of being rich in very good-quality proteins there are no commercial protein ingredients of marama beans available in the market. However at the lab scale, defatted marama flour (around 50% protein) and marama protein isolates (around 80% protein) have been prepared and investigated for their functionality by some researchers (Amonsou, Taylor, Beukes, et al., 2012; Amonsou, Taylor, Emmambux, et al., 2012; Amonsou, Taylor, & Minnaar, 2013; Maruatona et al., 2010).

TABLE 12.2 Protein Composition (% Protein) of Marama Bean and Bambara Groundnut Compared With Soybean and Cowpea

Legumes	Protein Content	Albumin	Globulin	Glutelins	Prolamins	References
Marama beans	29–38	23	53	15.5	8.5	Holse, Larsen, Hansen, and Engelsen (2011), Holse et al. (2010), and Bower et al. (1988)
Bambara groundnut	17–25	14–71	6–43	3.3–5.2	1.6–2.2	Hillocks et al. (2012) and Poulter (1981)
Soybean	32–40	10–20	80–90	NR	NR	Amonsou, Taylor, and Minnaar (2011), Amonsou (2010), and Mujoo et al. (2003)
Cowpea	23–28	20–25	49–53	20–24	13–20	Vasconcelos et al. (2010) and Ene-Obong and Carnovale (1992)

NR, Not reported.

TABLE 12.3 The Comparison of Essential Amino Acids Composition (g/100 g Protein) of Marama Bean and Bambara Groundnut Proteins With Soybean Proteins and With FAO/WHO/UNU (2007) Suggested Pattern of Essential Amino Acids Requirement for 1–2-Year Olds

Amino Acids (AA)	Marama Beans	Bambara Groundnut	Soybean	FAO/WHO/UNU Pattern
Lysine	5.70	6.02	6.9	5.2
Isoleucine	4.30	4.04	4.9	3.1
Leucine	7.90	6.59	9.4	6.3
Methionine	1.00	1.40	1.8	2.6
Cysteine	0.10	NR	0.5	
Phenylalanine	3.70	5.01	4.9	4.6
Tyrosine	11.40	7.27	4	
Valine	4.80	5.04	4.9	4.2
Threonine	3.20	4.89	3.9	2.7
Histidine	2.70	2.52	2.7	1.8
Tryptophan	NR	NR	NR	0.7
References	Amonsou, Taylor, Beukes, et al. (2012)	Adebowale, Schwarzenbolz, and Henle (2011)	Amonsou, Taylor, Beukes, et al. (2012)	Joint WHO/FAO/UNU Expert Consultation (2007)

NR, Not reported.

12.2.5 Nutritive Value, Allergenicity, and Antinutritive Factors

The high quantity of proteins (29–38%) in marama beans makes it a nutritionally important food item and potentially important protein-rich food ingredient to be used as a supplement in several other food products. In fact, the protein quality is superior to most legume crops and is comparable with milk and soybean proteins (Bower et al., 1988; Jackson et al., 2010; Powell, 1987). However, marama bean proteins are deficient in sulfur-containing amino acids (cysteine and methionine) as well as in tryptophan (Amonsou, Taylor, Beukes, et al., 2012; Jackson et al., 2010; Maruatona et al., 2010). All the other essential amino acids (lysine, isoleucine, leucine, phenylalanine, tyrosine, valine, and threonine) meet or exceed the minimum level required for a good-quality protein when considered for essential amino acids requirements of growing children (Table 12.3). Unfortunately, there are no data available on the digestibility of marama proteins as well as the impact of processing on their digestibility.

There are very little data available on allergens in marama bean proteins. In a study by Holse et al. (2010), IgE antibodies were used to analyze the allergens in marama proteins. These antibodies react with most of the allergens in peanut and lupin, which are among the most prevalent allergenic foods in the world. However, for marama proteins, the absence of reactivity shows that they may not contain the allergens present in peanut and lupin. However, other allergens need to be tested before ruling out the absence of allergenicity from marama proteins.

Cyanogenic glycosides are toxic compounds present in some plants and legumes. The enzymatic degradation of cyanogenic glycosides by indigenous plant enzymes is called cyanogenesis, which results in the release of cyanide (a respiratory poison). It was shown that the marama proteins do not contain cyanogenic glycosides and the enzymes that cause their degradation (Dubois et al., 1995; Holse et al., 2010).

Raw marama bean proteins have comparatively high trypsin inhibitory activity, which is about 20% of total proteins (Bower et al., 1988), which can be destroyed by heat (Maruatona et al., 2010). Maruatona et al. (2010) have shown that when marama bean flour is dry-heated at 150°C for 20 min around 99% of trypsin inhibitor is inactivated. As while heating in aqueous solution, the rate of chemical reactions is increased due to more water activity, increased protein molecule mobility, and decrease in their denaturation temperature, so a lower temperature/time combination will be required to inactivate the trypsin inhibitor in the aqueous phase. However, this needs to be tested to identify the temperature/time combination required in the aqueous phase.

Phenolic compounds are considered beneficial due to their antioxidant properties. In contrast, these compounds have also been identified as potential antinutritional factors as they make complexes with digestive enzymes, proteins, and minerals, hence decreasing their availability (Bravo, 1998). In marama beans the phenolic compounds are mainly concentrated in seed coat (24.6 mg CE/100 mg) and comparatively lower levels (2.8 mg CE/100 mg) of phenolic compounds are present in cotyledons (Jackson et al., 2010). Marama proteins are also rich in phenolic amino acid, tyrosine (Amonsou, Taylor, Beukes, et al., 2012).

12.2.6 Current and Future Uses and Applications

With the increasing population of the world, we have to find new sources of food to replace a part of the existing foods. The legumes, due to richness in their nutrients, can effectively replace other plant and animal proteins in several food applications. Marama beans are rich in proteins, fats, fiber, and mineral contents (Holse et al., 2010; NRC, 2006; Wehmeyer et al., 1969), so they can effectively be used in several food applications.

Traditionally mature beans are eaten as a snack after roasting (giving cashew nut-like taste) while immature beans are prepared by boiling and are an important part of the diet of the indigenous people (Holse et al., 2010; Jackson et al., 2010). The beans are rich in potent energy, so giving rapid satisfaction. In addition, they can be stored for a long time, giving more value to these beans as a source of food in scarcity, thus providing sustainable food resources.

The defatted marama bean flour is a rich source of protein (around 50%), whereby its amino acid composition is comparable to commercial soybean flour (Maruatona et al., 2010). This makes it a potentially important and economical protein-rich ingredient for supplementation in other food products. In addition, its richness in energy make it a potential food to be effectively used to supplement pregnant and breastfeeding women, elderly people, and babies (Jackson et al., 2010).

Marama bean flour, due to richness in protein and fat contents, has been tested to make marama milk, which has further been reported to be used for making marama yogurt (Jackson et al., 2010). Marama milk contains higher levels of sodium and iron as compared to cow milk but contains lower levels of calcium (Jackson et al., 2010). Like soy milk, marama milk may also possibly be used for making a tofu-like product. Marama bean-based milk and yogurt can provide a very cost-effective source of protein for poor communities.

The adhesive potential of marama proteins is twice as high as soy and five times higher than gluten (Amonsou et al., 2013), so it could potentially be used as a food-grade bioadhesive. In addition, the marama bean proteins have been shown to form highly viscous and extensible doughs, which could be positively exploited in gluten-free products (Amonsou, Taylor, Emmambux, et al., 2012). The other techno-functional properties like foaming, emulsifying, and oil-binding, etc., still need to be explored for further applications in the food industry.

Like other legumes, the amino acid composition of marama bean proteins complements that of cereals so they can effectively be used as a supplement with other cereals in the form of porridges, extrusion products, bakery products, and bread, etc. (Jackson et al., 2010; Kayitesi, de Kock, Minnaar, & Duodu, 2012). In fact, lysine is a limiting essential amino acid in cereals, while the legumes are rich in this amino acid (Jackson et al., 2010; Kayitesi et al., 2012; Maruatona, 2008). Effectively, their mixture can lead to a well-balanced combination of essential amino acids.

As compared to other legumes, marama beans have high trypsin inhibitory activity (Bower et al., 1988; Maruatona et al., 2010). Antinutritional factors in food legumes lose their antinutritional activity on denaturation. However, these denatured proteins have been shown to give tremendous health benefits (Roy, Boye, & Simpson, 2010). They have been shown to control some kinds of cancers as well as have anti-inflammatory properties (Roy et al., 2010). Trypsin and chymotrypsin inhibitors of legumes belong to the Bowman–Birk inhibitor family. These protease inhibitors isolated from pulses have received investigational new drug status by FDA due to their tremendous health benefits (Kennedy, 1995). They have also been suggested to be used as a drug against several diseases like hypertension, neurogenerative disease, human immunodeficiency virus (HIV), as well as several infectious diseases (Roy et al., 2010).

Marama beans have been proposed to be effective in curing and preventing diseases (Jackson et al., 2010). It has also been suggested that they boost the immune system resulting in reduced illness. The use of mashed marama beans in eye infections has also been reported (Jackson et al., 2010). However, further research is required on the bio-active peptides present in marama proteins and their impact on curing different diseases.

12.2.7 Off-Tastes Associated With Marama Beans

There are no data available on off-tastes related to marama bean proteins. However, it has been shown that raw marama beans are bland in taste and have an unpleasant slimy texture. Roasting results in a nutty (cashew nut-like) taste (Mmonatau, 2005), whereby Maillard reaction compounds have been proposed to provide the nutty flavor (Kayitesi et al., 2012). Nyembwe, Minnaar, Duodu, and de Kock (2015) have shown that marama flour has a quite significantly bitter taste, which it has been proposed is due to the presence of saponins, gallic acid, and protocatechuic acid. However, these researchers have worked on selected compounds and further research is needed to find out other phenolic compounds and saponin products (sapogenins) that could also be possibly contributing to the bitter taste.

For commercialization, the bitterness of marama bean flour needs to be addressed. In this regard, marama bean fat has the ability to mask the bitter taste of marama flour. Kayitesi, Duodu, Minnaar, and de Kock (2010) have shown that when full-fat marama flour was used, no bitterness was detected. Blanching and roasting marama beans can also probably be used to improve the taste by removing the bitter components and by giving a nutty flavor (Iwuoha & Umunnakwe, 1997).

The lipoxygenase is an enzyme present in most legumes that causes the oxidation of polyunsaturated fatty acids resulting in the production of off-flavors. It was reported that this enzyme is absent in marama beans (Maruatona, 2008).

12.2.8 Issues and Challenges

Tremendous research is required to move this crop out of obscurity. As marama bean crop has not been domesticated yet and is still the wild, the sufficient and sustainable provision of marama beans for commercial activities is the major challenge of the time to exploit its potential as a crop. In addition, the marama plant takes 18–24 months for maturation (Jackson et al., 2010), therefore intensive agronomic and genetic research is needed to assist the commercial production of this crop.

The commercial utilization of marama proteins as an ingredient requires extensive research on exploration of their intrinsic functionalities as well as the impact of processing parameters on these functionalities. The value addition by improvement or modification of certain techno-functional properties of these proteins via processing will also increase its commercialization. As discussed earlier, marama proteins possess a high level of trypsin inhibitory activity which may decrease its nutritional value (Bower et al., 1988) but will be beneficial in developing specific foods because of the pharmaceutical importance of this activity. Thermal treatment (roasting, dry or wet heating, micronization, etc.) or some physical treatment (pressure) is needed to inactivate this antinutritional factor. However, these treatments can affect the functionality of proteins also. A minimum treatment that completely inactivates the antinutritional factor and least affects the functional properties is needed.

12.3 BAMBARA GROUNDNUT

12.3.1 Introduction (Land, Water, Sustainability)

Bambara groundnut (*V. subterranea*) is the third most important crop in Africa after groundnut and cowpea (Bamshaiye et al., 2011; Baryeh, 2001). It originated in west Africa, however it is now also found in many parts of Asia, South America, and Oceania (Baudoin & Mergeai, 2001; Poulter, 1981). In Africa it is grown across the continent from Senegal to Kenya and from the Sahara to South Africa (Atiku, Aviara, & Haque, 2004). It is a herbaceous, low-growing (0.30–0.35 m height with lateral stems), annual and self-pollinating crop (Amadou et al., 2001; Bamshaiye et al., 2011; NRC, 2006), which belongs to genus *Vigna* of the Fabacae family and subfamily Papilionoideae (Bamshaiye et al., 2011; Baudoin & Mergeai, 2001). There are two main botanical varieties of the crop: *V. subterranea* var. spontanea, and *V. subterranea* var. subterranea, whereby the former includes the wild varieties, while the latter includes the cultivated varieties (Swanevelder, 1998). Bambara groundnut (*V. subterranea*) plant and its seeds are shown in Fig. 12.2. It is classified as a bean, however, like peanut, the bambara seeds are dug from the ground (Bamshaiye et al., 2011). Immature seeds are eaten fresh, while mature seeds are consumed as a pulse or ground to make flour to add to different food dishes (Azam-Ali et al., 2001).

Bambara crop is highly drought-tolerant and can grow under adverse climatic and soil conditions (Amadou et al., 2001; Azam-Ali et al., 2001; Bamshaiye et al., 2011; Baryeh, 2001) as well as being resistant to diseases and pests (NRC, 2006). It can thrive even in areas with average rainfall less than 500 mm (Bamshaiye et al., 2011), however for

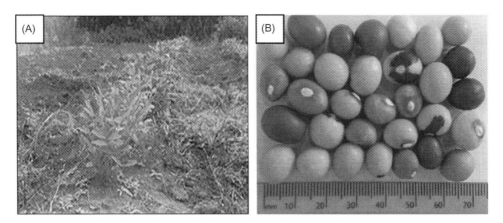

FIGURE 12.2 Bambara groundnut (*Vigna subterranea*) plant (A) and whole mature seeds (B). *(A) Adapted from Wikipedia (https://en.wikipedia.org/wiki/Vigna_subterranea) (accessed September 2015).*

optimum growth rainfall between 750–1000 mm is required (Tweneboah, 2000). It is a low-cost crop as usually fertilizer is not applied to the crop and nodules on the roots of the crop can help in fixing atmospheric nitrogen, hence fulfilling the nitrogen requirements of the crop (NRC, 2006). Due to its nitrogen-fixing ability, it is used for crop rotation (NRC, 2006). The crop also does not require a lot of minerals and is least demanding in minerals.

The crop can be grown in a variety of soils ranging from light loams to sandy loams, as well as in heavier soils, however light sandy loams with pH 5.0–6.5 are highly suitable for its growth (Charles, 2010; Swanevelder, 1998). The crop has a growth period of 110–150 days (Swanevelder, 1998) and performs best on deeply ploughed soil with friable seed bed (Tweneboah, 2000). Soils rich in nitrogen produce excessive vegetation which is not desirable (Tweneboah, 2000).

12.3.2 Composition of Bambara Groundnut

Bambara groundnut is considered as a complete diet as it contains sufficient amounts of proteins, carbohydrates, fats, and minerals. It is composed of 53–69% carbohydrates, 17–25% protein, 6.5–8.5% oil, and 2.5–3.5% mineral salts (Bamshaiye et al., 2011; Baryeh, 2001; Hillocks et al., 2012; NRC, 2006; Steve et al., 2009). The protein content in bambara groundnut is greater than cowpea, pigeon pea, and groundnut (Brough & Azam-Ali, 1992). It also possesses the highest soluble fiber (4–12%) among all other beans (Bamshaiye et al., 2011; NRC, 2006). In addition, it is rich in phosphorous, magnesium, potassium, and calcium (Bamshaiye et al., 2011; Yao et al., 2015).

12.3.3 Composition of Bambara Proteins

Bambara groundnut protein composition is highly variable among different varieties with albumin and globulin being the major storage proteins (Poulter, 1981). The protein composition of bambara groundnut is shown in Table 12.2. It contains 14–71% albumin, 6–43% globulin, 1.6–2.2% prolamins, and 3.3–5.2% glutelins (Hillocks et al., 2012; Poulter, 1981). Some other studies (Adebowale et al., 2011) on brown and white varieties from Nigeria have shown that 7S vicilin (a globulin) is the major storage protein in bambara groundnut. However, more research is required to define the different proteins present in bambara groundnut and the variability in their composition with respect to species, climate, and seasonal variations. It has been shown that disulfide bonds are absent in bambara proteins (Adebowale et al., 2011).

12.3.4 Protein Isolation

The production of protein isolates and concentrates of legume proteins increases their utilization in food applications due to their specific functional properties imparted and impact on the nutritional profile of the final product. Protein isolates and concentrates from legume proteins can effectively be utilized to completely or partially replace other animal proteins.

Even though bambara groundnut is a cheap source of good-quality available proteins there is no commercial production of protein isolates or concentrates from bambara groundnut. Adebowale et al. (2011) prepared bambara groundnut protein isolates at lab scale either by isoelectric precipitation or a micellization process. These authors showed that the isoelectric precipitation gave more yield (56–58%) than micellization (14–16%). However, micellized proteins showed better functional properties (foam capacity and stability, oil binding, emulsification, gelling and water absorption) than isoelectric precipitated protein isolate. The bambara groundnut protein isolates contained higher lysine, arginine, and glutamic acid as compared to soybean (Adebowale et al., 2011).

12.3.5 Nutritive Value, Allergenicity, and Antinutritive Factors

Keeping in view the high protein content (17–25%) in bambara groundnut it can effectively be used in several food applications to improve their nutritional profile. Like most other legumes, bambara groundnut protein is deficient in sulfur-containing amino acids (cysteine and methionine) as well as in tryptophan in terms of essential amino acid requirements for growing children (Table 12.3). However, it has been reported to have higher methionine content (up to 2 g/100 g of protein) than any other beans (Aremu, Olaofe, & Akintayo, 2006; Bamshaiye et al., 2011; NRC, 2006). All other essential amino acids in bambara groundnut proteins meet or exceed the minimum level set by FAO for a good-quality protein for growing children (Adebowale et al., 2011).

There are very few data available on the impact of processing parameters on digestibility of bambara groundnut proteins. Cooking and roasting have been shown to decrease the digestibility of proteins, which has been attributed to protein crosslinking and the presence of bound starch and polyphenols (Yagoub & Abdalla, 2007). Germination has been shown to increase the digestibility of proteins mainly due to a reduction of antinutritional factors and hydrolysis of proteins by proteolytic enzymes of germinating seedlings (Yagoub & Abdalla, 2007). To the best of our knowledge, no information is available on allergenicity of bambara proteins.

Comparatively low levels of antinutritional factors (trypsin inhibitor 6.75–19.08 units/mg) and other compounds like phytic acid (46 mg/100 g), oxalate (3 mg/100 g), and phytin phosphorous (13 mg/100 g) have been reported for bambara groundnut (Bamshaiye et al., 2011; Poulter, 1981; Steve Ijarotimi, & Ruth Esho, 2009). The presence of tannins (0.36–0.94 g/100 g) in bambara groundnut further adds to the list of antinutritional factors (Adegunwa, Adebowale, Bakare, & Kalejaiye, 2014; Bamshaiye et al., 2011; Poulter, 1981). Treatments like soaking, blanching, addition of salts, autoclaving, boiling, cooking, and roasting have been shown to be effective in reducing the antinutritional factors of bambara groundnuts (Adegunwa et al., 2014; Ohene Afoakwa, Simpson Budu, & Bullock Merson, 2007; Yagoub & Abdalla, 2007). In addition, germination has also been shown to decrease phytic acid and other polyphenols (Yagoub & Abdalla, 2007). The toxic compounds like cyanogenic glucoside, alkaloid or phytohalmagglutinin are absent in bambara groundnuts (Bamshaiye et al., 2011).

12.3.6 Current and Future Uses and Applications

Using plant-based foods for a specific application is always a challenge as they are considered as an inferior quality protein source. However, bambara groundnut due to its good-quality protein and other well-balanced nutrients (fats, carbohydrate, and mineral contents) can effectively be used in several food applications.

Immature seeds of bambara groundnut are consumed fresh, boiled, or grilled and eaten alone or mixed with maize or immature groundnut, while mature seeds are boiled, or roasted, and may be pounded into flour and eaten alone or with maize meal as well as added to several traditional dishes (Charles, 2010; NRC, 2006; Swanevelder, 1998). In some areas of Africa, bambara groundnuts are roasted and are used as a salted snack. The boiled seeds are also canned (Baudoin & Mergeai, 2001) and have increasing market value in Africa (NRC, 2006). In countries like Zimbabwe and Ghana, successful commercial canning of bambara groundnuts in gravy have been reported (Mkandawire, 2007). The boiled seeds are also used as a snack and flour is used to make stiff porridge called "nasima" (Mkandawire, 2007). In addition, the roasted seeds are boiled and subsequently crushed and are eaten as a relish called "chipele" (Mkandawire, 2007).

Legumes like bambara groundnut can effectively be used to replace wheat in products like bread, confectionaries, and pasta, etc. (Multari, Stewart, & Russell, 2015). They can also be used partially as a supplement with cereals in products like bread, porridge, bakery, and extrusion products, etc., as the amino acid composition of legume proteins complements the amino acid profile of cereals (Jackson et al., 2010; Kayitesi et al., 2012; Maruatona, 2008). Bread made from blending bambara groundnut flour (up to 50% bambara flour) with wheat flour showed high consumer acceptability, and resulted in high protein contents in the final bread (Alozie, Iyam, Lawal, Udofia, & Ani, 2009).

However, the impact on rheological properties of bread has not been reported. Protein-rich bambara flour is also used for making pancakes, and is used in soups and purees. In Ghana, bambara groundnuts flour paste is fried or steamed to make traditional dishes like "akla" (also called *koose*) and "tubani," respectively (Nti, 2009). It is also used in the form of a bean fritter called "okara" and as a savory pudding called "moin moin." The doughy paste of bambara flour (optionally wrapped in banana leaves) is boiled or steamed to form "okpa" (Barimalaa, Agoha, Oboh, & Kiin-Kabari, 2005; NRC, 2006).

Bambara groundnut is a good source of proteins, calcium, iron, potassium, and fiber; it therefore has huge potential for value-added products (Murevanhema, 2012). Bambara groundnut milk has shown high acceptability in taste and is nutritious (NRC, 2006). It has shown higher acceptability than soybean, pigeon pea, and cowpea milk and its lighter color was much appreciated (Brough, Azam-Ali, & Taylor, 1993). It also contains the lowest content of trypsin inhibitor as compared to other legume milks (Poulter & Caygill, 1980), so it has a better chance of use in various applications. In addition, bambara groundnut milk has shown very good emulsion stability even after pasteurization and curds traditionally prepared from soy milk can be made from bambara milk (Poulter & Caygill, 1980). Probiotic bambara groundnut milk fermented using lactic acid bacteria has shown high consumer acceptability (Murevanhema, 2012). The extruded meat analogs (also called texturized vegetable proteins) made from bambara flour have shown high acceptability and could be an effective cheap protein source to replace some of the meat proteins in the diet (Charles, 2010). This can replace minced meat in several recipes and interestingly contains less fat and sodium as well as providing important quantities of dietary fiber (Charles, 2010). In addition to flour, bambara groundnut protein isolates and concentrates can also be used to make these meat analogs. As bambara groundnuts contain the least quantity of antinutritional factors, it can also be used in baby foods with only slight treatment.

There is an increasing trend of using isolated plant proteins over animal proteins for environmental, economic, and religious reasons (Wong, Pitts, Jayasena, & Johnson, 2013). However, the partial or full substitution of animal proteins by these proteins depends on how these proteins functionally perform in different food applications. Even though bambara groundnut proteins have shown inferior functional properties (foaming, emulsification, and gelling) than soy and egg white proteins (Brough et al., 1993), acetylation and succinylation have been shown to improve foaming, emulsifying, and solubility properties of bambara proteins (Lawal, Adebowale, & Adebowale, 2007). However, further research is needed to substantiate their functional properties using model food systems.

Bambara groundnuts can also possibly replace soybean in animal (fish, rabbit, and dairy cattle, etc.) feed, however studies are also needed to determine up to what level this feed can be tolerated by these farm animals without compromising their performance. As this crop contains the least antinutritional factors, it may be used (with slight treatment) in poultry and pig diets, which are also sensitive to antinutritional factors (Multari et al., 2015).

12.3.7 Off-Tastes Associated With Bambara Groundnut

Unfortunately, there are very few data available on off-tastes related to bambara groundnut proteins. It has been reported that bambara groundnut milk has a beany taste (Brough et al., 1993; Murevanhema, 2012). However, dry frying of presoaked beans before milling has been shown to avoid this beany taste in the resulting milk (Brough et al., 1993). In addition, heat treatment of milk has also been effective in decreasing the beany taste of probiotic bambara groundnut milk (Murevanhema, 2012).

12.3.8 Issues and Challenges

Bambara groundnut is the only legume which is considered as a complete diet due to the sufficient amount of all nutrients available in it (Poulter, 1981). However, the crop is still cultivated at a small scale. In fact, lack of education on crop values, production strategies, optimal conditions for production, pest management, and crop diseases, as well as unavailability of good-quality seed are the major constraints in the development of bambara groundnut as a cash crop (Mkandawire, 2007). In addition, there is no significant access to bambara groundnut in the international market, however, it is playing an important role in the diet of African countries. Tremendous research is required to exploit the potential of this crop.

Even though bambara groundnut has a vast history, it is still cultivated from landraces and no true varieties have been developed for specific agro-ecological conditions (Azam-Ali et al., 2001). In addition, due to the lack of agronomic research data distribution regarding plant optimum growth conditions, farmers are getting 10 times less than the production potential of this crop under optimal conditions (Baudoin & Mergeai, 2001; Brink & Belay, 2006). Due to these reasons, bambara is grown as a subsistence crop rather than a cash crop (Azam-Ali et al., 2001). However, agronomic research and extension programs for farmers could make it an important cash crop.

Like several other legume crops, the seeds are very hard and their cooking time is longer (Tweneboah, 2000), which is one of the major challenges for its processing at a commercial level. In addition to the long cooking time, antinutritional factors and difficult dehulling are also the major challenges for food applications of bambara groundnut (Hillocks et al., 2012). The lack of data on sensory evaluation of bambara groundnut products is also a large challenge to know their acceptability. Despite the fact that bambara groundnut protein isolates and concentrates could potentially be used in several food applications, there is no commercial production. In addition, further research is needed to substantiate their functional potential by testing in model food systems.

12.4 CONCLUSION

The underutilized legume crops of Africa have huge potential for sustainable cultivation due to richness in their nutritional profile and ability to grow in adverse climatic conditions. Marama bean is rich in good-quality protein, oil, and dietary fiber and has the ability to grow in water-deficit conditions, which make it a potential oilseed legume to replace other commercial oilseed legumes (soybean and peanut). The symbiotic nitrogen fixation, drought tolerance, ability to grow in poor soils, and sufficient quantities of all the important nutrients (protein, carbohydrates, fats, and minerals) are important features of bambara groundnut to tackle the agricultural challenges for sustainable crop production. Despite this, there is no commercial production of these crops, therefore serious attention is required to exploit their real potential.

REFERENCES

Adebowale, Y. A., Schwarzenbolz, U., & Henle, T. (2011). Protein isolates from bambara groundnut (*Voandzeia subterranean* L.): Chemical characterization and functional properties. *International Journal of Food Properties*, 14, 758–775.

Adegunwa, M., Adebowale, A., Bakare, H., & Kalejaiye, K. (2014). Effects of treatments on the antinutritional factors and functional properties of bambara groundnut (*Voandzeia subterranea*) flour. *Journal of Food Processing and Preservation*, 38, 1875–1881.

Alozie, Y. E., Iyam, M. A., Lawal, O., Udofia, U., & Ani, I. F. (2009). Utilization of bambara groundnut flour blends in bread production. *Journal of Food Technology*, 7, 111–114.

Amadou, H., Bebeli, P., & Kaltsikes, P. (2001). Genetic diversity in bambara groundnut (*Vigna subterranea* L.) germplasm revealed by RAPD markers. *Genome*, 44, 995–999.

Amonsou, E., Taylor, J., & Minnaar, A. (2011). Microstructure of protein bodies in marama bean species. *Lwt-Food Science and Technology*, 44, 42–47.

Amonsou, E. O. (2010). *Characterisation of marama bean proteins. PhD dissertation*. Pretoria, South Africa: University of Pretoria.

Amonsou, E. O., Taylor, J. R. N., Beukes, M., & Minnaar, A. (2012). Composition of marama bean protein. *Food Chemistry*, 130, 638–643.

Amonsou, E. O., Taylor, J. R. N., Emmambux, M. N., Duodu, K. G., & Minnaar, A. (2012). Highly viscous dough-forming properties of marama protein. *Food Chemistry*, 134, 1519–1526.

Amonsou, E. O., Taylor, J. R. N., & Minnaar, A. (2013). Adhesive potential of marama bean protein. *International Journal of Adhesion and Adhesives*, 41, 171–176.

Aremu, M. O., Olaofe, O., & Akintayo, T. E. (2006). A comparative study on the chemical and amino acid composition of some Nigerian under-utilized legume flours. *Pakistan Journal of Nutrition*, 5, 34–38.

Atiku, A., Aviara, N., & Haque, M. (2004). Performance evaluation of a bambara ground nut sheller. *Agricultural Engineering International: The CIGR Journal of Scientific Research and Development*, Manuscript PM 04 002. Vol. VI

Azam-Ali, S., Sesay, A., Karikari, S., Massawe, F., Aguilar-Manjarrez, J., Bannayan, M., & Hampson, K. (2001). Assessing the potential of an underutilized crop – A case study using bambara groundnut. *Experimental Agriculture*, 37, 433–472.

Bamshaiye, O., Adegbola, J., & Bamshaiye, E. (2011). Bambara groundnut: An under-utilized nut in Africa. *Advances in Agricultural Biotechnology*, 1, 60–72.

Barimalaa, I. S., Agoha, G., Oboh, C. A., & Kiin-Kabari, D. B. (2005). Studies on bambara groundnut flour performance in Okpa preparation. *Journal of the Science of Food and Agriculture*, 85, 413–417.

Baryeh, E. A. (2001). Physical properties of bambara groundnuts. *Journal of Food Engineering*, 47, 321–326.

Baudoin, J., & Mergeai, G. (2001). *Grain legumes in crop production in tropical Africa* (pp. 313–317).

Bower, N., Hertel, K., Oh, J., & Storey, R. (1988). Nutritional evaluation of marama bean (*Tylosema esculentum*, Fabaceae) – Analysis of the seed. *Economic Botany*, 42, 533–540.

Bravo, L. (1998). Polyphenols: Chemistry, dietary sources, metabolism, and nutritional significance. *Nutrition Reviews*, 56, 317–333.

Brink, M., & Belay, G. (2006). *Plant resources of tropical Africa 1. Cereals and pulses* (pp. 213–218). CTA, Wageningen, Netherlands: Prota Foundation. Backhuys Publishers.

Brough, S., & Azam-Ali, S. (1992). The effect of soil moisture on the proximate composition of bambara groundnut (*Vigna subterranea* (L.) Verdc). *Journal of the Science of Food and Agriculture*, 60, 197–203.

Brough, S., Azam-Ali, S., & Taylor, A. (1993). The potential of bambara groundnut (*Vigna subterranea*) in vegetable milk production and basic protein functionality systems. *Food Chemistry, 47*, 277–283.

Charles, O. O. (2010). *Sensory properties of extruded meat analogue from bambara groundnut flour at high moisture contents. Department of Food Science and Technology, College of Food Science and Human Ecology*. Abeokuta: University of Agriculture.

Coetzer, L. A., & Ross, J. H. (1976). Tylosema. *Trees in South Africa, 28*, 77–80.

Deka, R., & Sarkar, C. (1990). Nutrient composition and antinutritional factors of *Dolichos lablab* L. seeds. *Food Chemistry, 38*, 239–246.

Dubois, M., Lognay, G., Baudart, E., Marlier, M., Severin, M., Dardenne, G., & Malaisse, F. (1995). Chemical characterization of *Tylosema fassoglensis* (Kotschy) torre and hillc oilseed. *Journal of the Science of Food and Agriculture, 67*, 163–167.

Edem, D., Amugo, C., & Eka, O. (1990). Chemical composition of yam beans (*Sphenostylis stenocarpa*). *Tropical Science, 30*, 59–63.

Ene-Obong, H. N., & Carnovale, E. (1992). A comparison of the proximate, mineral and amino acid composition of some known and lesser known legumes in Nigeria. *Food Chemistry, 43*, 169–175.

Hillocks, R., Bennett, C., & Mponda, O. (2012). Bambara nut: A review of utilisation, market potential and crop improvement. *African Crop Science Journal, 20*, 1–16.

Holse, M., Husted, S., & Hansen, Å. (2010). Chemical composition of marama bean (*Tylosema esculentum*) – A wild African bean with unexploited potential. *Journal of Food Composition and Analysis, 23*, 648–657.

Holse, M., Larsen, F. H., Hansen, A., & Engelsen, S. B. (2011). Characterization of marama bean (*Tylosema esculentum*) by comparative spectroscopy: NMR, FT-Raman, FT-IR and NIR. *Food Research International, 44*, 373–384.

Holse, M., Petersen, M. A., Maruatona, G. N., & Hansen, Å. (2012). Headspace volatile composition and oxidative storage stability of pressed marama bean (*Tylosema esculentum*) oil. *Food Chemistry, 132*, 1749–1758.

Iwuoha, C. I., & Umunnakwe, K. E. (1997). Chemical, physical and sensory characteristics of soymilk as affected by processing method, temperature and duration of storage. *Food Chemistry, 59*, 373–379.

Jackson, J. C., Duodu, K. G., Holse, M., Lima de Faria, M. D., Jordaan, D., Chingwaru, W., . . . Minnaar, A. (2010). Chapter 5 – The morama bean (*Tylosema esculentum*): A potential crop for Southern Africa. In L. T. Steve (Ed.), *Advances in food and nutrition research* (pp. 187–246). Academic Press.

Joint WHO//FAO/UNU Expert Consultation (2007). *Protein and amino acid requirements in human nutrition*. Geneva: World Health Organization.

Kayitesi, E., de Kock, H. L., Minnaar, A., & Duodu, K. G. (2012). Nutritional quality and antioxidant activity of marama–sorghum composite flours and porridges. *Food Chemistry, 131*, 837–842.

Kayitesi, E., Duodu, K. G., Minnaar, A., & de Kock, H. L. (2010). Sensory quality of marama/sorghum composite porridges. *Journal of the Science of Food and Agriculture, 90*, 2124–2132.

Kennedy, A. R. (1995). The evidence for soybean products as cancer preventive agents. *Journal of Nutrition, 125*, S733–S743.

Lawal, O., Adebowale, K., & Adebowale, Y. (2007). Functional properties of native and chemically modified protein concentrates from bambarra groundnut. *Food Research International, 40*, 1003–1011.

Mahesh, V., & Sathe, S. K. (2006). Chemical composition of selected edible nut seeds. *Journal of Agricultural and Food Chemistry, 54*, 4705–4714.

Maruatona, G. N. (2008). *Physico-chemical, nutritional and functional properties of defatted marama bean flour. MSc dissertation*. Pretoria, South Africa: University of Pretoria.

Maruatona, G. N., Duodu, K. G., & Minnaar, A. (2010). Physicochemical, nutritional and functional properties of marama bean flour. *Food Chemistry, 121*, 400–405.

Mkandawire, C. H. (2007). Review of bambara groundnut (*Vigna subterranea* (L.) Verdc.) production in Sub-Sahara Africa. *Agricultural Journal, 2*, 464–470.

Mmonatau, Y. (2005). *Flour from the marama bean: Composition and sensory properties in Botswana perspective. MSc dissertation*. Stellenbosch, South Africa: Stellenbosch University.

Monaghan, B. G., & Halloran, G. M. (1996). RAPD variation within and between natural populations of morama [*Tylosema esculentum* (Burchell) Schreiber] in southern Africa. *South African Journal of Botany, 62*, 287–291.

Mosele, M. M., Hansen, A. S., Engelsen, S. B., Diaz, J., Sorensen, I., Ulvskov, P., . . . Harholt, J. (2011). Characterisation of the arabinose-rich carbohydrate composition of immature and mature marama beans (*Tylosema esculentum*). *Phytochemistry, 72*, 1466–1472.

Mujoo, R., Trinh, D. T., & Ng, P. K. W. (2003). Characterization of storage proteins in different soybean varieties and their relationship to tofu yield and texture. *Food Chemistry, 82*, 265–273.

Multari, S., Stewart, D., & Russell, W. R. (2015). Potential of fava bean as future protein supply to partially replace meat intake in the human diet. *Comprehensive Reviews in Food Science and Food Safety, 14*, 511–522.

Murevanhema, Y. Y. (2012). *Evaluation of bambara groundnuts (*Vigna subterrenea* (L.) Verdc.) milk fermented with lactic acid bacteria as a probiotic beverage. MSc dissertation*. Cape Peninsula University of Technology.

National Research Council (2006). *Lost crops of Africa. Volume II: Vegetables*. Washington, DC: The National Academies Press.

Nti, C. A. (2009). Effects of bambara groundnut (*Vigna subterranea*) variety and processing on the quality and consumer appeal for its products. *International Journal of Food Science & Technology, 44*, 2234–2242.

Nyembwe, P., Minnaar, A., Duodu, K. G., & de Kock, H. L. (2015). Sensory and physicochemical analyses of roasted marama beans *Tylosema esculentum* (Burchell) A. Schreiber with specific focus on compounds that may contribute to bitterness. *Food Chemistry, 178*, 45–51.

Ohene Afoakwa, E., Simpson Budu, A., & Bullock Merson, A. (2007). Response surface methodology for studying the effect of processing conditions on some nutritional and textural properties of bambara groundnuts (*Voandzei subterranea*) during canning. *International Journal of Food Sciences and Nutrition, 58*, 270–281.

Osman, M. A. (2007). Effect of different processing methods, on nutrient composition, antinutrional factors, and in vitro protein digestibility of *Dolichos lablab* bean [*Lablab purpuresus* (L) sweet]. *Pakistan Journal of Nutrition, 6*, 299–303.

Poulter, N. H. (1981). Properties of some protein fractions from bambara groundnut [*Voandzeia subterranea* (L.) Thouars]. *Journal of the Science of Food and Agriculture, 32*, 44–50.

Poulter, N. H., & Caygill, J. C. (1980). Vegetable milk processing and rehydration characteristics of bambara groundnut [*Voandzeia subterranea* (L.) thouars]. *Journal of the Science of Food and Agriculture, 31*, 1158–1163.

Powell, A. M. (1987). Marama bean (*Tylosema esculentum*, Fabaceae) seed crop in Texas. *Economic Botany, 41*, 216–220.

Roy, F., Boye, J. I., & Simpson, B. K. (2010). Bioactive proteins and peptides in pulse crops: Pea, chickpea and lentil. *Food Research International, 43*, 432–442.

Steve Ijarotimi, O., & Ruth Esho, T. (2009). Comparison of nutritional composition and anti-nutrient status of fermented, germinated and roasted bambara groundnut seeds (*Vigna subterranea*). *British Food Journal, 111*, 376–386.

Swanevelder, C. J. (1998). *Bambara, food for Africa:* Vigna subterranea *(bambara groundnut)*. South Africa: National department of Agriculture. ARC-Grain Crops Institute.

Thomas, T. (2004). *Marama bean (*Tylosema esculentum*), a non-nodulating high protein legume indigenous to the Kalahari sands: Studies of its nutrition. MSc dissertation*. Capetown, South Africa: University of Capetown.

Travlos, I. S., & Karamanos, A. J. (2006). Effects of soil texture on vegetative growth of the tropical legume marama bean (*Tylosema esculentum*). *Journal of Agronomy, 5*, 609–612.

Tweneboah, C. (2000). *Modern agriculture in the tropics, food crops*. Co-Wood Publishers.

USDA National Nutrient Database. *National nutrient database for standard reference release 27*. (2014). Available at <http://ndb.nal.usda.gov> Accessed September 2015.

Vasconcelos, I. M., Maia, F. M. M., Farias, D. F., Campello, C. C., Carvalho, A. F. U., de Azevedo Moreira, R., & de Oliveira, J. T. A. (2010). Protein fractions, amino acid composition and antinutritional constituents of high-yielding cowpea cultivars. *Journal of Food Composition and Analysis, 23*, 54–60.

Wehmeyer, A. S., Lee, R. B., & Whiting, M. (1969). The nutrient composition and dietary importance of some vegetable foods eaten by the Kung Bushmen. *South African Medical Journal (Suid-Afrikaanse tydskrif vir geneeskunde), 43*, 1529–1530.

Wong, A., Pitts, K., Jayasena, V., & Johnson, S. (2013). Isolation and foaming functionality of acid-soluble protein from lupin (*Lupinus angustifolius*) kernels. *Journal of the Science of Food and Agriculture, 93*, 3755–3762.

Yagoub, A., & Abdalla, A. A. (2007). Effect of domestic processing methods on chemical composition, in vitro digestibility of protein and starch and functional properties of bambara groundnut (*Voandzeia subterranea*) seed. *Research Journal of Agriculture and Biological Sciences, 3*, 24–34.

Yao, D. N., Kouassi, K. N., Erba, D., Scazzina, F., Pellegrini, N., & Casiraghi, M. C. (2015). Nutritive evaluation of the bambara groundnut Ci12 landrace [*Vigna subterranea* (L.) Verdc. (Fabaceae)] Produced in Côte d'Ivoire. *International Journal of Molecular Sciences, 16*, 21428–21441.

Chapter 13

Peanut Products as a Protein Source: Production, Nutrition, and Environmental Impact

H.N. Sandefur[1], J.A. McCarty[1], E.C. Boles[2] and M.D. Matlock[3]

[1]*University of Arkansas, Fayetteville, AR, United States,* [2]*Paradigm Sustainability Solutions, Fayetteville, AR, United States,* [3]*University of Arkansas Office for Sustainability, Fayetteville, AR, United States*

13.1 INTRODUCTION

For the past 100 years peanuts have been a plant-based protein source and grocery staple in the American household. Historians believe that the peanut plant originated in South America over 3500 years ago, and was spread to Europe, Africa, and North America during the early 1700s (NPB, 2015). Since it became a widely grown crop for human consumption in the United States, peanuts have been utilized in a number of commercial products, thanks in part to the peanut product development efforts of George Washington Carver. Perhaps the most widely used peanut-based product has been peanut butter, which was included in US rations during World War II, and has since become a common feature of the American pantry and an important protein source for individuals engaging in a vegetarian diet (NPB, 2015).

In spite of the significant increases in meat consumption in the developed world over the past century, a number of lifestyle choices involving alternative diets have emerged since the 1970s. Polling indicates that the current rates of vegetarianism in developed nations range from 3% in the United States to 9% in Germany (Ruby, 2012). In addition, in India, which has the second largest population in the world, approximately 40% of the population identifies as vegetarian (Ruby, 2012). These diets represent a small but not insignificant minority that are seeking alternative, plant-based protein sources (such as peanuts and peanut products) in order to fulfill their daily nutritional requirements.

Given the important role of peanuts in modern food consumption habits, it is important to consider the environmental impact of peanut production, in addition to their nutritional value. The following sections explore the process of cultivating, processing, and preparing peanuts and peanut products, and the environmental impacts associated with these activities. In addition, the nutritional profile and viability of peanuts as a protein alternative is also explored.

13.2 ENVIRONMENTAL IMPACT AND SUSTAINABILITY

In addition to availability and nutritional content, the environmental impacts associated with production are essential considerations when evaluating the sustainability of foodstuffs such as peanuts and peanut products. Agricultural production was responsible for approximately 8% of the greenhouse gas (GHG) emissions produced in the United States in 2011 (EPA, 2013). On a global scale, food production accounts for anywhere from 19% to 29% of the cumulative GHG emissions (McCarty, Sandefur, Matlock, Thoma, & Kim, 2014). Given the potentially significant impacts of crop production on the environment, the following sections review literature documenting the environmental impacts of peanut production, including its impacts on climate change, water use, and land use.

13.2.1 Climate Change Impacts

Life cycle assessment (LCA) methodology has been used to assess the environmental impacts of agricultural products in a number of studies (Kim, Dale, & Jenkins, 2009; McCarty et al., 2014; Thoma, Popp, & Nutter, 2013). During an

LCA, practitioners define a unit of product for which impacts will be assessed. The inputs and outputs associated with the production of the product are then inventoried, and an impact assessment is performed based on the inventory in order to quantify the environmental impacts across the product's life cycle (ISO, 2006). The only cradle-to-grave LCA of the production of peanuts found in existing literature was performed by McCarty et al. (2014) in their assessment of the GHG emissions associated with the production of peanut butter.

In this study, McCarty et al. (2014) inventoried the material inputs and environmental emissions associated with the production of 1 kg of peanut butter in the United States. They adopted a cradle-to-grave approach, which included assessing the impacts associated with activities in the farming, buying point, shelling, processing, retail, and consumer-use phases of the peanut butter life cycle (see Fig. 13.1). McCarty et al. (2014) determined that roughly 2.88 kg of CO_2 equivalents (CO_{2e}) are emitted for each kilogram of peanut butter produced in the United States. While on-farm activities had substantial contributions to the overall GHG footprint, the life cycle stages with the greatest impacts were processing and consumer use. A majority of the CO_{2e} emissions were associated with the consumption of electricity throughout the life cycle, with the processing stage having the most emissions from electricity of any life cycle stage (Fig. 13.2).

A number of other LCAs have been performed for the production of protein sources (Beauchemin, Janzen, Little, McAllister, & McGin, 2010; Boggia, Paolotti, & Castellini, 2010; De Vries & de Boer, 2010; Kim et al., 2013). It is difficult to directly compare the results of different LCA studies, as differences in the underlying assumptions can yield vastly different results. In their review of 52 LCA studies of animal- and plant-based protein sources, Nijdam et al. (2012) found that the carbon footprints for all of the investigated products ranged from 1 to 150 kg CO_{2e} per kg of

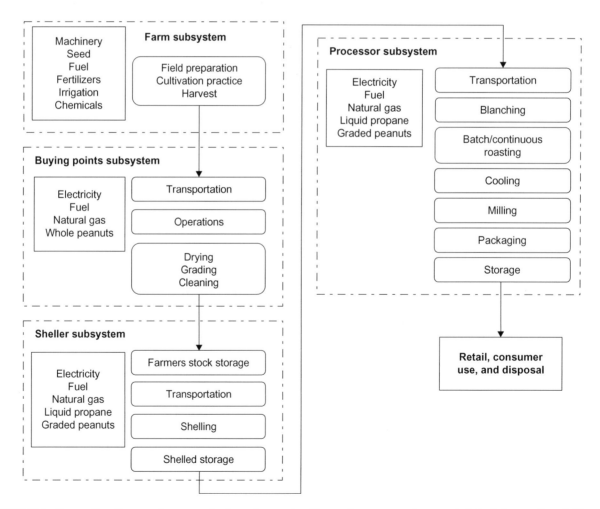

FIGURE 13.1 Process flow diagram of peanut production and processing. The postharvest processing steps include drying, grading, shelling, and endpoint product preparation. *Adopted from McCarty, J.A., Sandefur, H.N., Matlock, M., Thoma, G., & Kim, D. (2014). Life cycle assessment of greenhouse gas emissions associated with production and consumption of peanut butter in the U.S.* Transactions of the ASABE, 57, 1–10.

product (Table 13.1). Results for plant-based protein sources tended to be lower than the results for their meat-based counterparts, and ranged from 1 to 2 kg CO_{2e} per kg. In contrast, values for the carbon footprints of beef, pork, and lamb ranged from 9 to 150 kg CO_{2e} per kg.

13.2.2 Water Use Impacts

The Water Footprint Network (WFN) has developed the concept of the "water footprint," which provides a framework for linking agricultural production with geographically explicit water resources. The water footprint is defined as the total volume of freshwater that is used to produce the goods and services consumed by an individual or a community (Mekonnen & Hoekstra, 2010a). The work of Mekonnen and Hoekstra (2010a) provided the first globally comprehensive assessment of the water footprints of crop and livestock products. In their studies, the WFN reports water consumption values in terms of green, blue, and gray water. The term *green water* refers to the amount of rainwater consumed in the production of the product, while blue water deals with the consumption of freshwater from surface and groundwater sources, such as lakes and aquifers (Mekonnen & Hoekstra, 2010b). Finally, gray water is the amount of water required to assimilate the pollutant loads generated during the production process to ambient water quality conditions (Mekonnen & Hoekstra, 2010b).

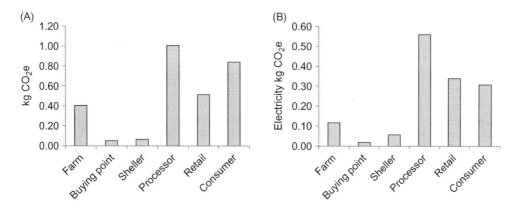

FIGURE 13.2 (A) Global warming impacts for peanut butter production and (B) global warming impacts from electricity consumption for peanut butter production by production stage. Impacts are expressed in terms of carbon dioxide equivalents (CO_{2e}). An overview of the peanut production stages is provided in Fig. 13.1. *Adopted from McCarty, J.A., Sandefur, H.N., Matlock, M., Thoma, G., & Kim, D. (2014). Life cycle assessment of greenhouse gas emissions associated with production and consumption of peanut butter in the U.S. Transactions of the ASABE, 57, 1–10.*

TABLE 13.1 Carbon Footprints per Kilogram of Product for a Variety of Protein Sources

Product	Carbon Footprint (kg CO_{2e}/kg)
Beef (n = 26)	9–129
Pork (n = 11)	4–11
Poultry (n = 5)	2–6
Eggs (n = 5)	2–6
Mutton and lamb (n = 5)	10–150
Milk (n = 14)	1–2
Seafood from fisheries (n = 18)	1–86
Meat substitutes (with egg or milk protein) (n = 2)	3–6
Meat substitutes (100% vegetal) (n = 4)	1–2

The carbon footprint ranges were reported by Nijdam et al. (2012) in their review of 52 life cycle assessment studies of animal- and plant-based protein sources. The value of n refers to the number of analyzed products.
Adapted from Nijdam et al. (2012).

The water footprint findings of Hoekstra (2012) are shown in Table 13.2 for a number of common protein sources, including nuts, eggs, and meat products. Hoekstra shows that the global average blue water consumption within the "nuts" category was actually higher than some of the other protein sources. However, when considering peanuts individually, Mekonnen and Hoekstra (2010b) showed that they have a lower blue water footprint when compared to almonds, walnuts, and pistachios (see Table 13.3).

13.2.3 Land Use Impacts

Land occupation and land use changes are important considerations when assessing the environmental impacts of modern agricultural products. Increasing concern about the related issues of ecosystem and biodiversity loss has gained the attention of the general public. Unfortunately, land use assessments are not as common as studies that quantify water consumption or GHG production in agriculture. However, LCAs of land use have become an area of increasing research interest, and have been performed for some select agricultural products (Borjesson & Tufvesson, 2011; Mattsson, Cederberg, & Blix, 2000; Milài Canals et al., 2014; Thoma, Matlock, Putman, & Burek, 2015).

In 2014, over 326 million acres were planted with crops in the United States (NASS, 2015b). Of the total planted area, approximately 1.35 million acres were planted for the cultivation of peanuts (NASS, 2015a). Unfortunately, there are no detailed LCA studies of the land use impacts and land transformations associated with peanut production that are readily available in the current body of literature. As a result, additional studies will need to be performed in order to better understand the impacts of peanut production on arable land use and transformation.

TABLE 13.2 Green, Blue, and Gray Water Footprints of Various Protein Sources

Product	Global Average Water Footprint (L/kg)				Water Footprint per Unit of Nutritional Value		
	Green	Blue	Gray	Total	Calories (L/kcal)	Protein (L/g)	Fat (L/g)
Nuts	7016	1367	680	9063	3.63	139	47
Eggs	2592	244	429	3265	2.29	29	33
Chicken meat	3545	313	467	4325	3.00	34	43
Pig meat	4907	459	622	5988	2.15	57	23
Bovine meat	14,414	550	451	15,415	10.19	112	153

Results are presented on a per unit weight and per unit of nutritional value basis.
From Hoekstra, A.Y. (2012). The hidden water resource use behind meat and dairy. Animal Frontiers, 2, 3–8.

TABLE 13.3 Green, Blue, and Gray Water Footprints of Various Legumes, Nuts, and Drupes

Product	Global Average Water Footprint (L/kg)			
	Green	Blue	Gray	Total
Peanuts, shelled[a]	3887	236	258	4381
Almonds, shelled	10,212	4206	3323	17,742
Walnuts, shelled	5835	2702	1693	10,229
Pistachios	3412	8380	734	12,526

[a]Values reported for groundnuts, which include peanut varieties.
From Mekonnen, M.M., & Hoekstra, A.Y. (2010b). The green, blue and grey water footprint of crops and derived crop products. UNESCO-IHE Institute for Water Education Research Report Series No. 47.

13.3 PEANUT CULTIVATION AND PRODUCTION

13.3.1 Production Regions

Peanuts are a major agricultural commodity and export product for a number of countries. Worldwide, over 41 million metric tons of peanuts were produced during the cultivation period from 2013 to 2014 (FAS, 2015). The top four peanut-producing countries included China (41% of global production), India (14%), Nigeria (7%), and the United States (5%). In terms of harvested area, global peanut production utilized over 25 million hectares (96,525 square miles) of agricultural land in 2014 (Table 13.4). In the United States, approximately 0.55 million hectares of farmland were cultivated for peanut production in 2014. This corresponded to close to 2.0 million metric tons of peanuts produced in the United States (NASS, 2015a). Combined yields for the four major peanut-producing states made up 79.3% of the total US peanut production, including Georgia (46.5%), Florida (12.8%), Alabama (10.6%), and Texas (9.4%) (NASS, 2015a).

13.3.2 Cultivation Techniques

Peanut cultivation practices include conventional and strip tillage, and can be irrigated or nonirrigated. Conventional tillage practices require both primary and secondary tillage to generate a seedbed that is slightly raised (Clewis, Askew, & Wilcut, 2002). Unlike conventional till, strip tillage operations involve the limited use of tillage equipment and utilize cover crops to prevent soil erosion. The implements that are used in strip tillage result in a relatively narrow seed bed (Monfort, Culbreath, Stevenson, Brenneman, & Perry, 2007). This corresponds to a decrease in the amount of fuel required in the preharvest stages of production (Wright et al., 2009). In addition, the incidence of plant disease is generally lower in crops produced using strip tillage peanut practices. Studies have shown that fungicide applications can be lessened while still obtaining the same yields as conventional tillage operations (Sorensen, Brenneman, & Lamb, 2010). Fertilization, insecticide, and herbicide requirements are generally similar for both methods (Wright et al., 2009).

In the last decade reductions in peanut prices and available labor, along with increases in fuel cost, have led to conversions from conventional intensive tillage to strip tillage. McCarty et al. (2014) reported that approximately 80% of farmers use conventional tillage to cultivate peanuts in Georgia, which is the largest peanut-producing state in the United States. Operations in Georgia with reduced tillage increased from 6% to 22.9% between 1997 and 2003 (Monfort et al., 2007). In addition to tillage, peanut production involves both irrigated and nonirrigated production practices. Irrigated yields are generally higher, but require additional inputs (UGA, 2011). In 2007, irrigated farming operations accounted for 65% of land for cultivated peanuts versus 35% for nonirrigated operations (McCarty et al., 2014).

TABLE 13.4 Country-level Planted Area and Yield Data for Global Peanut Production for the Cultivation Period From 2013 to 2014 (FAS, 2015)

Country/region	Area (Million Hectares)	Production (Million Metric Tons)
World	25.28	41.15
China	4.63	16.97
India	5.4	5.65
Nigeria	2.5	3.00
United States	0.42	1.89
Sudan	2.16	1.77
Burma	0.89	1.38
Indonesia	0.66	1.16
Argentina	0.38	1.00
Senegal	0.77	0.71
Cameroon	0.46	0.64

Results are presented for the top 10 peanut-producing nations.

13.4 PEANUT PROCESSING

Following the successful cultivation and harvest of the peanut plant at the farm, there are a number of postharvest processing stages that peanuts undergo prior to the consumer-use phase. The following sections summarize the steps for processing peanuts after harvest. The postharvest processing stages include drying, grading, shelling, and endpoint product preparation (Fig. 13.1).

13.4.1 Peanut Drying

The peanut drying process begins in the field at the time of harvest. Peanut plants are overturned with a digger so that the top of the plant and leaves are upside down. The peanuts, which were underground, are brought to the surface during this process. The extracted plants are deposited in windrows and left to dry. When first dug, peanuts may have an initial moisture content ranging from 20% to 50% on a wet basis. Depending on environmental conditions, the peanuts are typically left for 2–3 days before the harvesting is complete. Combines are used to separate the peanuts from the plant, after which they are placed in wagons for transport.

The second step of the drying process takes place in the wagons where the harvested peanuts are initially stored. Wagon drying can take place at the farm, but most of the drying during this stage is accomplished at a peanut aggregation facility called the buying point. The buying point takes in all peanuts from a given region over a period of roughly 6 weeks. Fans and heating elements are connected to openings in the wagons where peanuts are dried further to a final moisture content ranging from 7% to 10% (Butts, Davidson, Lamb, Kandala, & Troeger, 2004).

When stored at the proper temperature and moisture content, clean peanuts in hulls can be stored for several years. The lower the temperature and moisture content, the longer peanuts can be stored without risk of spoilage. However, peanuts dried below 7% moisture content result in poor milling quality. Therefore, in order to balance marketability and storage length, the optimum storage conditions involve a target moisture content of 7.5% and target temperature of 10°C. Peanuts stored under these conditions should last for 10 months without a loss in quality (Davidson, Whitaker, & Dickens, 1982).

13.4.2 Grading

If the peanut crop is composed of more than 10% foreign material (FM), an initial precleaning process takes place in order to remove the unwanted materials (Davidson et al., 1982). FM includes everything but in-shell peanuts and loose peanut kernels. Most FM consists of dirt, light trash, rocks, and sticks. The optional precleaning process is then followed by a grading step. Grading is performed by selecting a representative sample of peanuts from each wagon using a 4-inch diameter core sample. During the grading process, a technician looks at the following qualities of the wagon samples in order to make a determination concerning the quality of the harvest peanuts:

- % Foreign material;
- % Loose shelled kernels (LSK);
- % Sound mature kernels (SMK);
- % Sound splits (SS);
- % Total sound mature kernels (TSMK);
- % Damage kernels (DK).

LSK are peanut kernels that are no longer in the hull. LSK are less desirable because they spoil more quickly and are more likely to be contaminated with aflatoxin produced by the *Aspergillus flavus* mold (Dowell, Dorner, Cole, & Davidson, 1990). After the FM and LSK are removed, the sample is shelled. Whole undamaged kernels are referred to as SMK, while undamaged split kernels are SS. The combination of SMK and SS is referred to as the TSMK. Damaged kernels are considered to be any kernels judged inedible because of mold, decay, insect damage, sprouting, freeze damage, discoloration, or freeze damage. The sample is also tested for moisture content and *A. flavus* mold. Samples found to have mold counts above the threshold limit can be cleaned again using screeners to remove FM, LSK, and DK, which in most cases will bring the crop back to within safe levels. Lots that cannot be brought to within threshold values are crushed for oil and their meal is used for nonfood purposes or for animal feed.

13.4.3 Shelling

The peanut shelling operation involves the removal of the hulls from the peanuts. These facilities typically operate year-round, bringing in loads of stored peanuts from the buying points. At the shelling facility the peanuts are cleaned again, separating out soil, vines, stems, and leaves by a series of screens, blowers, and magnets. Peanuts are then sized with screens so that the hulls can be crushed without damaging the kernel. Rollers are then used to crush the hulls with the gap between the rollers being adjusted according to the screened size of the nut to be processed. A horizontal drum with a rotating beater is then used to hull the peanuts. Crushed shells and peanuts are separated by oscillating shaker screens and blown air. Electric eye sorters which detect discoloration are used for grading the final product. Hulls are either land-applied as mulch, used as part of animal bedding, composted, or landfilled. Split kernels are processed for oil. Whole kernels are then stored until ready for final processing (EPA, 1997).

13.4.4 Product Processing

After shelling, the peanut kernels are shipped to a processor for incorporation into a final product. Peanuts are typically roasted and then blanched, which removes the skins, and then roasted using dry or oil-based processes. In dry roasting, ovens at approximately 430°C are used to heat the peanuts to a temperature of 160°C for 40–60 min depending on the desired flavor characteristics. This is done in either a continuous or batch process. In the continuous dry roast process, peanuts may be passed through a gravity-fed operation or moved along a conveyor belt. During this process the peanuts are agitated to ensure uniform roasting. The continuous process has the advantage of reducing labor and ensuring a consistent flow of roasted peanuts. In batch processing, gas-fired revolving drum ovens are used to insure an even roast. Batch processing has the advantage of adjusting for varying moisture content of the peanut lot received (EPA, 1997). Roasting causes a reaction of amino acids and carbohydrates to produce tetrahydrofuran derivatives that give the peanuts their specific flavor profile. Roasting further dries the nut and the heat causes peanut oil to stain the peanut cell wall, darkening the peanut into a roasted look (EPA, 1997). After dry roasting, peanuts are cooled. Cooling occurs in boxes or on conveyors by blown air and stops the roasting from continuing.

When peanuts are oil roasted, blanching takes place first. Coconut oil is preferred; however, peanut and cottonseed oils are also used. Temperatures range from 138°C to 143°C while roasting the nuts for 3–10 min depending on desired peanut characteristics. The roasted peanuts are cooled, by blowing air over them on a conveyor or in a box. Similar to dry roasting, oil roasting can be done in batch or continuous processing. In continuous processing, peanuts are moved on a long conveyor through a tank of heated oil. In batch, peanuts are lowered into a tank of oil for a specified time (EPA, 1997).

Blanching is the process by which skins, dust, mold, and any other material is removed from the nut. The main blanching processes are dry blanching, water blanching, spin blanching, and air impact blanching. Dry blanching is used primarily for peanut butter production because it removes the kernel hearts. Peanuts are heated to 138°C for 25 min to crack and loosen skins. Cooled peanuts are passed through brushes or ribbed rubber to remove skin. Screening is then used to separate the skin and hearts from the peanut halves. In water blanching, conveyors pass peanuts through stationary blades that cut the skins. Pressurized hot water jets loosen the skin, which is removed by oscillating canvas pads on knobbed conveyor belts. Consequently, peanuts must then be dried back to a moisture content of 6–12%. Steaming is used to loosen the skin in spin blanching. Peanuts then move single-file down a grooved conveyor with spinning spindles. The spinning motion unwraps the skin from the peanut. For air impact blanching, peanuts are placed in a horizontal drum and rotated. The drum's inner surface has an abrasive coating and air jets blow air counter to the rotation of the drum (EPA, 1997).

13.5 USES, FUNCTIONALITY, AND CURRENT PRODUCTS

Peanuts have a number of uses and share almost unanimous approval among consumers. Their misnomer status as "top nut" has only recently been challenged (in the late 2000s) by the almond industry. Peanuts are used in daily life as peanut butter, snack nuts, candies, mixes, and bars. Some of the more nontraditional product forms include peanut flour and milk. Peanut butter accounts for roughly half of all the peanuts consumed in the United States. In order to be labeled peanut butter, the product must contain at least 90% peanuts by weight. Peanuts for peanut butter are dry roasted and ground to a fine texture. During the grinding process, additional ingredients are added such as salt, sugar, and oils.

Around 10% of the entire peanut crop in the United States is sold as in-shell peanuts. This means that they bypass the shelling facility and are taken directly to the processor. In-shell peanuts are soaked in salty brine and then lightly roasted. Other salted nuts are shelled first then roasted. This product is used in snacks, as a food garnish, toppings, as well as in baked goods. Peanut candies are available in unlimited variations and the peanut still resides as one of the top ingredients in confections. Candies are available that use whole peanuts to peanut butter and everything in between.

The rise in the use of peanut flour in American homes in recent years has been fueled by an interest in plant-based proteins and gluten-free alternatives. Peanut flour is made from ground peanuts that are pressed to remove the oil. What remains is a flour-like substance that has twice the protein of traditional bread flour. Flours consisting of nuts that are lightly roasted have a mild taste. The longer the roasting, the more peanut taste comes out in the flour. Research has been conducted on the use of peanut flour in protein-fortified cereals, as a flour replacement, and as a supplement in hamburger patties. Peanut flour was found to increase protein levels in cereals to over 21%. Peanut flour used as a flour substitute in baking was found to produce acceptable bread when up to 20% of the bread flour was replaced with peanut flour. The peanut flour gave bread a light texture, uniform brown crust, and acceptable loaf volume. Peanut flour used as a supplement to hamburger patties carried less flavor when compared to soy and these were judged either similar or superior to patties mixed with soy (Ayres & Davenport, 1977).

Peanut milk is a substance that has not gained significant traction yet within the United States. However, there is research underway to offer a viable alternative to the success that almond milk has had as a milk alternative. Peanut milk has been made with full-fat and partially defatted nuts that are typically soaked in water prior to grinding. Standard ratios are one part peanut to six parts water. Much like regular milk, greater stability is achieved by pasteurizing and homogenizing the product. Fermentation of the product into a yogurt or tofu-like substance has the added advantage of removing any potential aflatoxins. Peanut milk has also found success in extending animal milk. Unfortunately, demand for peanut milk still suffers due to consumer sensory profiles and the stability of the product. For a full review of the production of peanut milk and its uses and nutritional profile, see Diarra, Nong, and Jie (2005).

In addition to the peanut kernel, some researchers have suggested that peanut producers use young peanut leaves as a nutritional leafy green. While this application is not common at this time, the greens have been compared to popular collard greens. However, sensory evaluations rank collard greens above peanut greens in appearance and tenderness, but similarly in flavor (Almazan & Begum, 1996).

13.6 NUTRITIONAL VALUE

13.6.1 Calories, Fats, Protein, Carbohydrates

Peanuts can provide a dense source of nutrients, and while the nutritional values associated with peanuts can vary among peanut varieties and processing techniques, the nutritional shifts tend to be minor enough that specific peanut varieties (eg, Runner, Virginia, Spanish, and Valencia) will not be addressed here (Jonnala, Dunford, & Chenault, 2005). Peanut serving sizes tend to vary among the different peanut products; however, 14 g of roasted peanuts (~28 peanuts) or two tablespoons of peanut butter are the most commonly accepted serving sizes. Throughout this section, major nutrients, minerals, vitamins, and amino acids are expressed in units of mass per 100 g of raw peanuts for consistency in comparison. According to the USDA National Nutrient Database for Standard Reference, 100 g of raw peanuts has approximately 567 calories (USDA, 2015). Of the total caloric content, approximately 73% comes from fats, 16% from protein, and 11% from carbohydrates (USDA, 2015). The nutritional composition of peanuts, peanut butter, and roasted peanuts can be found in Table 13.5.

The fats found in raw peanuts are mostly comprised of oleic acid (monounsaturated fatty acid, C18:1) and linoleic acid (polyunsaturated fatty acid C18:2). The high ratio of monounsaturated fats to saturated fats is similar to olive oil, an oil that promotes heart health (American Peanut Council, 2010). Both oil-roasted peanuts and peanut butter have higher overall fat contents than raw peanuts. Oils are added to most peanut butters to achieve the right consistency and oil-roasted nuts absorb some of the heating oil they are cooked in (Holland, Unwin, & Buss, 1992). The fat content in peanuts is high enough that most countries use peanut crops primarily for oil production, however, the US consumes approximately 60% of peanuts as peanut butter, roasted nuts, or other foods (Didzbalis, Ritter, Trail, & Plog, 2004). The carbohydrate composition in most peanut products tends to have a low sugar content with a relatively high dietary fiber content, which results in a low glycemic index (The Peanut Institute, 2008). Consumption of peanuts can also be supportive of a diet high in fiber which has been associated with health and longevity (American Peanut Council, 2010).

TABLE 13.5 Nutritional Composition of Peanuts and Various Peanut Products

Nutrient	Unit	Raw Peanuts	Peanut Butter	Peanuts, Oil-roasted, Salted	Peanuts, dry-roasted, Salted
Proximates					
Water	g	6.5	1.6	1.5	1.8
Ash	g	2.3	3.0	2.8	2.9
Energy	kcal	567.0	588.0	599.0	587.0
Protein	g	25.8	21.9	28.0	24.4
Total lipid (fat)	g	49.2	49.5	52.5	49.7
Fatty acids, total saturated	g	6.3	9.5	8.7	7.7
Fatty acids, total monounsaturated	g	24.4	20.7	26.0	26.2
Fatty acids, total polyunsaturated	g	15.6	11.3	15.3	9.8
Omega-3 fatty acids	g	0.0	0.0	0.0	0.0
Omega-6 fatty acids	g	15.6	11.3	15.1	15.7
Carbohydrate, by difference	g	16.1	24.0	15.3	21.3
Fiber, total dietary	g	8.5	5.7	9.4	8.4
Sugars, total	g	4.7	6.5	4.2	4.9
Vitamins					
Thiamin	mg	0.6	0.0	0.8	0.0
Riboflavin	mg	0.1	0.1	0.1	0.2
Niacin	mg	12.1	0.1	0.1	0.2
Pantothenic acid	mg	1.8	13.2	13.8	14.4
Vitamin B-6	mg	0.3	0.6	0.5	0.5
Folate, total	µg	240.0	35.0	120.0	97.0
Choline, total	mg	52.5	65.7	55.3	64.6
Betaine	mg	0.6	0.4	0.0	0.4
Vitamin E (alpha-tocopherol)	mg	8.3	5.9	6.9	4.9

From USDA. (2015). National nutrient database for standard reference. United States Department of Agriculture. Agricultural Research Service. Release 27.

13.6.2 Amino Acids and Protein

Peanuts have a higher density of protein than all grains, nuts, and most legumes (The Peanut Institute, 2008). As an example, peanuts have more than double the protein content of pinto beans, kidney beans, and chickpeas (USDA, 2015). The quality of peanut protein should be judged by the amino acid composition and presence of antinutritional substances (discussed in subsequent sections) when considering the dietary applications of peanut proteins in humans. As with all plant proteins, peanut protein is an incomplete protein that needs complimentary amino acids from other foods to be effectively used by the human body. The amino acid profile of peanuts can be found in Table 13.6. There are a number of studies indicating that proper processing and use of peanut flour and isolates can enhance the amino acid profile and reduce the presence of toxins. These toxins can include aflatoxin, protease inhibitors, hemagglutinin, goitrogens, saponins, and phytic acid. Aflatoxin is typically removed during the grading process, and others such as goitrogens and saponins, can be removed during blanching (Natarajan, 1980).

TABLE 13.6 Amino Acid Composition of Peanuts and Various Peanut Products

Amino Acid	Unit g/100 g Food Material	Raw Peanuts	Peanut Butter	Peanuts, Oil-roasted, Salted	Peanuts, Dry-roasted, Salted
Tryptophan	g	0.25	0.23	0.23	0.23
Threonine	g	0.88	0.52	0.61	0.81
Isoleucine	g	0.91	0.61	0.98	0.83
Leucine	g	1.67	1.53	1.81	1.54
Lysine	g	0.93	0.67	0.95	0.85
Methionine	g	0.32	0.26	0.29	0.29
Cystine	g	0.33	0.23	0.38	0.30
Phenylalanine	g	1.38	1.19	1.43	1.23
Tyrosine	g	1.05	0.82	1.01	0.96
Valine	g	1.08	0.77	1.15	0.99
Arginine	g	3.09	2.73	3.25	2.83
Histidine	g	0.65	0.55	0.66	0.60
Alanine	g	1.03	0.91	1.09	0.94
Aspartic acid	g	3.15	3.02	3.27	2.89
Glutamic acid	g	5.39	5.03	5.42	4.95
Glycine	g	1.55	1.42	1.62	1.43
Proline	g	1.14	1.39	1.17	1.05
Serine	g	1.27	1.46	1.29	1.17

From USDA. (2015). National nutrient database for standard reference. United States Department of Agriculture. Agricultural Research Service. Release 27.

Products that contain a complete protein source with a well-balanced amino acid composition are rare. It is important to allow proteins to work in concert with others to become well-balanced sources. Therefore, the most important characteristic of a protein is often its ability to supplement the shortcomings of essential amino acids supplied by accompanying foods. When comparing dietary amino acid needs for humans to the amino acid profile of peanuts, peanut proteins are deficient in methionine, lysine, and possibly threonine and tryptophan (FAO, 2002; Natarajan, 1980). Regardless of those shortcomings, peanuts still have a substantially higher level of "true digestibility" when compared to other legumes, whole wheat, and maize (FAO, 2002). For example, Singh and Singh (1991) found peanut flour to have a slightly higher relative nutritive value and protein efficiency ratio than soy protein isolates. The protein digestibility of peanuts is also comparable to that of animal protein, but can be as good or better when paired with other foods that are high in methionine, lysine, and threonine (FAO, 2002).

13.6.3 Micronutrients

Modern American diets tend to be high in energy or calories but low in vitamins, minerals, fiber, and micronutrients. Griel, Eissenstat, Juturu, Hsieh, and Kris-Etherton (2004) evaluated data reported in the Continuing Survey of Food Intake by Individuals and Diet and Health Knowledge Survey to determine the correlation between peanut consumers and their dietary quality. The results demonstrate a correlation between peanut consumption and a higher intake of micronutrients such as vitamin A, vitamin E, folate, calcium, magnesium, zinc, and iron and dietary fiber, along with lower intake of saturated fat and cholesterol (Griel et al., 2004). Individuals with chronic diseases, including heart disease and diabetes, are positively affected by diets containing peanuts and peanut butter (The Peanut Institute, 2008).

Peanuts have a broad range of vitamins and minerals in detectable quantities (Table 13.5). When considering recommended daily nutritional values, minerals such as copper, manganese, calcium, phosphorus, magnesium, zinc, and iron as well as vitamins such as vitamin E, thiamin, niacin, and folate highlight the role of peanuts in a well-balanced diet. Additionally, some of the highest proportions of manganese (a cofactor for enzymes), folate (which helps maintain and produce cells), and niacin (which assists the digestive system, skin, and nerves) are found in peanuts. Other compounds identified in peanuts include arginine, phytosterols, flavonoids, and resveratrol (American Peanut Council, 2010). Resveratrol, found in the skin and cotyledon of peanuts, is touted as a "life-extending" compound (Jang et al., 1997) that can protect against many prominent cardiovascular and neurodegenerative diseases (Das & Das, 2007; Rocha-González, Ambriz-Tututi, & Granados-Soto, 2008).

13.6.4 Taste Profiles and Allergenicity

When using peanuts to enhance the protein content of a particular food, understanding how peanut proteins will transform taste is important. More than 200 compounds have been identified in peanuts that can contribute peculiar flavors to the end product. Some of these include hexanal, octanal, and nonanal, which if not dealt with can contribute a beany flavor to protein-enhanced products. The roasted nut flavor that is commonly associated with peanuts is thought to come from pyrazines (Natarajan, 1980). However, more recent reviews of peanut flavor literature question that premise and suggest that further research must be done to pinpoint the compounds that give peanuts their pleasant roasted flavor (Neta, Sanders, & Drake, 2010). Peanut flavors are affected by genetic, environmental, physiological, and biochemical processes; however, the unique flavor developed during peanut roasting is considered to be the driving force for peanut consumption (Sanders, Vercellotti, Bett, & Greene, 1997). When produced under the proper conditions, peanut protein concentrates and isolates can be off-white in color and bland in flavor, which is necessary when the desire is for little impact to the existing taste and color profile of the product (Natarajan, 1980).

As with any conventional agricultural product, the flavor quality and taste profile can vary from year-to-year, location-to-location, time of harvest, processing techniques, and among various peanut genotypes. Several studies have tried to quantify these taste variations across the spectrum of peanut crop variations (Neta et al., 2010; Ng & Dunford, 2009). There were some common conclusions between the various peanut flavor studies. Immature peanuts and peanuts cured at temperatures around 35–38°C were often characterized as having "off"-flavors with sour and bitter attributes. In addition, premature harvests have resulted in a higher precedence of "off"-flavors (Ng, 2003).

As described in Section 13.6.1, peanuts tend to have a high fat content, with the majority being unsaturated. Unsaturated fats are considered to be healthier than saturated fats, but are more susceptible to lipid oxidation, which can degrade both the nutrition and flavor of the products (Neta et al., 2010). Proper processing and storage and selecting peanuts with high oleic acid contents are two of the best ways to prevent unwanted oxidation. Linoleic acids oxidize about 10 times faster than oleic acids, so shelf-life can be improved with varieties of peanuts containing high oleic acid contents. The preference for monounsaturated lipids (oleic acids) rather than polyunsaturated lipids (linoleic acids) also affects the nutritional and flavor properties of the product; however, the sensory differences between normal and high-oleic peanuts are too minute for the average consumer to differentiate (Neta et al., 2010).

In addition to flavor profiles, the majority of scientific research centered on peanuts and their interactions with consumers is focused on understanding the increasing prevalence of peanut allergies and finding ways to reduce their impacts. There are over 10 allergenic proteins identified in peanuts of which Ara h 1, Ara h 2, and Ara h 3 are the most abundant peanut allergens and cumulatively represent approximately half of the total protein content determined by SDS-PAGE quantitative studies (Kang, Gallo, & Tillman, 2007; Pedreschi, Nørgaard, & Maquet, 2012). There is some evidence to support early exposure to peanuts as a method for reducing the percentage of the populations with peanut allergies, but there is still more research that needs to be done in order to confirm this claim (Du Toit et al., 2008; Fox, Sasieni, du Toit, Syed, & Lack, 2009). All consumers that have a known peanut allergy should create an emergency management plan and have epinephrine and antihistamines readily available at all times (Burks, 2008). At this time, there are many challenges facing food industries when it comes to effectively detecting trace levels of peanut presence in foods (Pedreschi et al., 2012).

13.7 CONCLUSIONS

The versatility of the peanut as a food crop is dramatic; the nutritional value as a plant-based protein alternative alone is impressive, but the nutritional benefits go beyond protein. As the agriculture sector faces an increasing number of global challenges, it is important to consider the environmental impacts of agricultural products in addition to their nutritional contents. While it is difficult to compare the environmental impact results from the different studies that are available in the literature at this time, the emerging knowledge suggests that the climate-change and water-use impacts of peanut production are lower than other plant-based and animal-based protein sources that are currently available in the marketplace. We are in the early stages of quantifying sustainability indicators for agricultural products; additional research will need to be performed across a range of indicators for peanuts and other agricultural commodities in order to better understand the sustainability performance of our food products.

ACKNOWLEDGMENTS

The University of Arkansas' LCA research in peanut production is funded in part by the American Peanut Council.

REFERENCES

Almazan, A. M., & Begum, F. (1996). Nutrients and antinutrients in peanut greens. *Journal of Food Composition and Analysis, 9*(4), 375–383.

American Peanut Council. (2010). Natural Health Food for All. Retrieved from: <http://www.peanutsusa.com/about-peanuts/health-nutrition/56-peanuts-healthy-food-for-all.html>.

Ayres, J. L., & Davenport, B. L. (1977). Peanut protein: A versatile food ingredient. *Journal of the American Oil Chemists' Society, 54*, A109–A111.

Beauchemin, K. A., Janzen, H. H., Little, S. M., McAllister, T. A., & McGin, S. M. (2010). Life cycle assessment of greenhouse gas emissions from beef production in western Canada: A case study. *Agricultural Systems, 103*, 371–379.

Boggia, A., Paolotti, L., & Castellini, C. (2010). Environmental impact evaluation of conventional, organic and organic-plus poultry production systems using life cycle assessment. *World's Poultry Science Journal, 66*, 95–144.

Borjesson, P., & Tufvesson, L. (2011). Agricultural crop-based biofuels—Resource efficiency and environmental performance including direct land use changes. *Journal of Cleaner Production, 19*, 108–120.

Burks, A. W. (2008). Peanut allergy. *Lancet, 371*(9623), 1538–1546.

Butts, C. L., Davidson, J. I., Lamb, M. C., Kandala, C. V., & Troeger, J. M. (2004). Estimating drying time for a stock peanut curing decision support system. *Transactions-American Society of Agricultural Engineers, 47*(3), 925–932.

Clewis, S. B., Askew, S. D., & Wilcut, J. W. (2002). Economic assessment of diclosulam and flumioxazin in strip- and conventional-tillage peanut. *Weed Science, 50*, 378–385.

Das, S., & Das, D. K. (2007). Resveratrol: A therapeutic promise for cardiovascular diseases. *Recent Patents on Cardiovascular Drug Discovery, 2*(2), 133–138.

Davidson, J. I., Jr, Whitaker, T. B., & Dickens, J. W. (1982). *Grading, cleaning, storage, shelling, and marketing of peanuts in the United States* (pp. 571–623). Yoakum, TX: American Peanut Research and Education Society.

De Vries, M., & de Boer, I. J. M. (2010). Comparing environmental impacts for livestock products: A review of life cycle assessments. *Livestock Science, 128*, 1–11.

Diarra, K., Nong, Z. G., & Jie, C. (2005). Peanut milk and peanut milk based products production: A review. *Critical Reviews in Food Science and Nutrition, 45*, 405–423.

Didzbalis, J., Ritter, K. A., Trail, A. C., & Plog, F. J. (2004). Identification of fruity/fermented odorants in high-temperature-cured roasted peanuts. *Journal of Agricultural and Food Chemistry, 52*(15), 4828–4833.

Dowell, F. E., Dorner, J. W., Cole, R. J., & Davidson, J. I., Jr (1990). Aflatoxin reduction by screening farmers stock peanuts. *Peanut Science, 17*(1), 6–8.

Du Toit, G., Katz, Y., Sasieni, P., Mesher, D., Maleki, S. J., Fisher, H. R., & Lack, G. (2008). Early consumption of peanuts in infancy is associated with a low prevalence of peanut allergy. *Journal of Allergy and Clinical Immunology, 122*(5), 984–991.

EPA (1997). *AP 42, Fifth Edition, Compilation of Air Pollutant Emission Factors, Volume 1: Stationary Point and Area Sources. Chapter 9*. Food and Agricultural Industries. Available at: <www.epa.gov/ttnchie1/ap42>. Accessed September 2015.

EPA (2013). *Inventory of U.S. greenhouse gas emissions and sinks: 1990–2011*. Washington, DC: U.S. Environmental Protection Agency.

FAO. (2002). Protein and Amino Acid Requirements in Human Nutrition. Report of a Joint FAO/WHO/UNU Expert Consultation. World Health Org Tech Report No. 935.

FAS (2015). *Production, supply and distribution online. United States Department of Agriculture*. Washington, DC: Foreign Agricultural Service. Retrieved from: <http://apps.fas.usda.gov/psdonline/> Accessed September 2015.

Fox, A. T., Sasieni, P., du Toit, G., Syed, H., & Lack, G. (2009). Household peanut consumption as a risk factor for the development of peanut allergy. *The Journal of Allergy and Clinical Immunology, 123*(2), 417–423.

Griel, A. E., Eissenstat, B., Juturu, V., Hsieh, G., & Kris-Etherton, P. M. (2004). Improved diet quality with peanut consumption. *Journal of the American College of Nutrition, 23*(6), 660–668.

Hoekstra, A. Y. (2012). The hidden water resource use behind meat and dairy. *Animal Frontiers, 2*, 3–8.

Holland, B., Unwin, I. D., & Buss, D. H. (1992). *Fruit and nuts: First supplement to McCance and Widdowson's the composition of food*. Cambridge: RSC/MAFF.

ISO (2006). *ISO 14040: Environmental management—Life cycle assessment—Principles and framework*. Geneva: International Standards Organization.

Jang, M., Cai, L., Udeani, G. O., Slowing, K. V., Thomas, C. F., & Beecher, C. W. (1997). Cancer chemopreventive activity of resveratrol, a natural product derived from grapes. *Science, 275*, 218–220.

Jonnala, R. S., Dunford, N. T., & Chenault, K. (2005). Nutritional composition of genetically modified peanut varieties. *Journal of Food Science, 70*, S254–S256.

Kang, I. H., Gallo, M., & Tillman, B. L. (2007). Distribution of allergen composition in peanut (L.) and wild progenitor () species. *Crop Science, 47*(3), 997–1003.

Kim, D., Thoma, G., Nutter, D., Milani, F., Ulrich, R., & Norris, G. (2013). Life cycle assessment of cheese and whey production in the USA. *The International Journal of Life Cycle Assessment, 18*, 1019–1035.

Kim, S., Dale, B. E., & Jenkins, R. (2009). Life cycle assessment of corn grain and corn stover in the United States. *International Journal of Life Cycle Assessment, 14*, 160–174.

Mattsson, B., Cederberg, C., & Blix, L. (2000). Agricultural land use in life cycle assessment (LCA): Case studies of three vegetable oil crops. *Journal of Cleaner Production, 8*, 283–292.

McCarty, J. A., Sandefur, H. N., Matlock, M., Thoma, G., & Kim, D. (2014). Life cycle assessment of greenhouse gas emissions associated with production and consumption of peanut butter in the U.S. *Transactions of the ASABE, 57*, 1–10.

Mekonnen, M. M., & Hoekstra, A. Y. (2010a). A global and high-resolution assessment of the green, blue and grey water footprint of wheat. *Hydrology and Earth System Sciences, 14*, 1259–1276.

Mekonnen, M. M., & Hoekstra, A. Y. (2010b). *The green, blue and grey water footprint of crops and derived crop products*. UNESCO-IHE Institute for Water Education Research Report Series No. 47.

Milài Canals, L., Michelsen, O., Teixeira, R., Souza, D., Curran, M., & Antón, A. (2014). Building consensus for assessing land use impacts on biodiversity in LCA. In Proceedings of the 9th International Conference on Life Cycle Assessment in the Agri-Food Sector, San Francisco, CA, 8–10 October 2014.

Monfort, W. S., Culbreath, A. K., Stevenson, K. L., Brenneman, T. B., & Perry, C. D. (2007). *Use of resistant peanut cultivars and reduced fungicide inputs for disease management in strip-tillage and conventional tillage systems*. Plant Management Network.

NASS (2015a). *Quick stats. United States Department of Agriculture*. Washington, DC: National Agricultural Statistics Service. Retrieved from: <http://www.nass.usda.gov/Statistics_by_Subject/> Accessed September 2015.

NASS (2015b). *Acreage report, June 2015. United States Department of Agriculture*. Washington, DC: National Agricultural Statistics Service.

Natarajan, K. R. (1980). In Chichester (Ed.), *Advances in food research* (26th volume) New York, NY: Academic Press.

Neta, E. R., Sanders, T., & Drake, M. A. (2010). Understanding peanut flavor: A current review. In Y. H. Hui (Ed.), *Handbook of Fruit and Vegetable Flavors*. NJ, USA: John Wiley and Sons, Inc.

Ng, E. C., & Dunford, N. T. (2009). Flavour characteristics of peanut cultivars developed for southwestern United States. *International journal of food science & technology, 44*(3), 603–609.

Nijdam, D., Rood, T., & Westhoek, H. (2012). The price of protein: Review of land use and carbon footprints from life cycle assessments of animal food products and their substitutes. *Food Policy, 37*(6), 760–770.

NPB (2015). *History of peanuts and peanut butter*. National Peanut Board. Retrieved from: <http://nationalpeanutboard.org/the-facts/history-of-peanuts-peanut-butter/> Accessed September 2015.

Pedreschi, R., Nørgaard, J., & Maquet, A. (2012). Current challenges in detecting food allergens by shotgun and targeted proteomic approaches: A case study on traces of peanut allergens in baked cookies. *Nutrients, 4*, 132–150.

Rocha-González, H. I., Ambriz-Tututi, M., & Granados-Soto, V. (2008). Resveratrol: A natural compound with pharmacological potential in neurodegenerative diseases. *CNS Neuroscience & Therapeutics, 14*(3), 234–247.

Ruby, B. (2012). Vegetarianism. A blossoming field of study. *Appetite, 58*, 141–150.

Sanders, T. H., Vercellotti, J. R., Bett, K. L., & Greene, R. L. (1997). The role of maturation in quality of stackpole—cured peanuts. *Peanut Science, 24*, 25–31.

Singh, B., & Singh, U. (1991). Peanut as a source of protein for human foods. *Plant Foods for Human Nutrition, 41*(2), 165–177.

Sorensen, R. B., Brenneman, T. B., & Lamb, M. C. (2010). Peanut yield response to conservation tillage, winter cover crop, peanut cultivar, and fungicide applications. *Peanut Science., 37*, 44–51.

The Peanut Institute (2008). Super food: Peanuts. *Food for Thought, 12*(1), 65.

Thoma, G., Matlock, M., Putman, B., & Burek, J. (2015). *A life cycle analysis of land use in US pork production: Comprehensive report*. Fayetteville, AR: University of Arkansas Center for Agricultural Sustainability.

Thoma, G., Popp, J., Nutter, D., et al. (2013). Greenhouse gas emissions from milk production and consumption in the United States: A cradle-to-grave life cycle assessment circa 2008. *International Dairy Journal, 31*, S3–S14.

UGA. (2011). 2011 Peanut Update. The University of Georgia Cooperative Extension. <http://www.caes.uga.edu/commodities/fieldcrops/peanuts/2011peanutupdate/index2011.html>.

USDA (2015). *National nutrient database for standard reference*. United States Department of Agriculture. Agricultural Research Service, Release 27.

Wright, D. L., Tillman, B. L., Marois, J. J., Rich, J. R., Sprenkel, R. K., & Ferrell, J. A. (2009). *Conservation tillage peanut production. Agronomy department, Florida cooperative extension service*. Institute of Food and Agricultural Sciences, University of Florida, SS-AGR-185.

Chapter 14

Quinoa as a Sustainable Protein Source: Production, Nutrition, and Processing

L. Scanlin[1] and K.A. Lewis[2]

[1]Colorado State University, Fort Collins, CO, United States, [2]Food Industry Professional Consultant, Littleton, CO, United States

14.1 INTRODUCTION

Quinoa (*Chenopodium quinoa* Willd.) is an emerging world crop and nutritious plant-based source of protein. In either its whole seed form or as a potential protein concentrate or isolate, quinoa offers alternatives to animal-based proteins and may augment the protein needs of a growing world population. Quinoa means "mother grain" in the Quechua and Aymara languages, and has its origins in South America, having been domesticated in the Andean region in 5000 BC (Tapia, 2015). Several million Andean people have grown quinoa on small farms and used it as a staple food for subsistence. Until 1975, cultivation was limited to such "subsistence farms." Today, quinoa has developed into a value-added crop in Bolivia and Peru, and cultivation has expanded outside of its origins due to its favorable nutritional attributes, tolerance to harsh growing conditions, and high biodiversity value.

Quinoa has been consumed for thousands of years as whole seed, boiled or toasted, or ground into flour using a grinding stone called a qhuna (Quiroga et al., 2015). Traditional food uses include soups, stews, pilaf, main dishes, porridges, pastries, and thick or fermented beverages called q'usa or chicha (Rojas, 2011). Quinoa leaves are also consumed as salad and in cooked dishes. There are nonfood uses as well for the plant biomass, such as feed and traditional medicine.

Quinoa has gone from near obscurity at the end of the 20th century to an international crop in a little over a decade. Several noteworthy events laid the foundation for today's global recognition. Early research showed quinoa to be a nutritious Andean crop and digestible source of protein (Posnansky, 1945; White et al., 1955). In 1977, the International Congress on Andean Food Crops was formed under the sponsorship of the International Development Research Centre of Canada and the Inter-American Institute for Cooperation in Agriculture (Cusack, 1984). Cusack was instrumental in collaborating with South and North American scientists on this important initiative to identify, preserve, and study quinoa. One objective was to foster the propagation and promotion of quinoa to facilitate its revival in the Andes. Another objective was to make quinoa a viable alternative crop in other semiarid regions of the world, which led to research trials in Colorado, United States. It was also introduced in Europe in 1978 by Leakey at the University of Cambridge which laid the foundation for subsequent breeding programs of Galwey and Risi (Bazile & Baudron, 2015). Since the 1980s, research trials or small-scale cultivation have spread across all continents.

In the beginning of the 21st century, quinoa was still generally unknown to the world. After the Smithsonian Institute, Washington, DC, described quinoa as "the most nutritious grain in the world," quinoa was soon introduced to European consumers as a "superfood" and an "ancient grain" (FAIR, 2000). Up until 2005, there were sparse articles or recipes on quinoa, yet they were published in well-known newspapers or magazines. Such publications included France-Amérique (Reale, 2003), O, The Oprah Magazine (Neff, 2003), Martha Stewart Living (Clark, 2004), Natural Foods Merchandiser (NFM, 2004), The Wall Street Journal (McLaughlin, 2005), and Prevention (Simmons, 2005). In 2005 on The Oprah Winfrey Show, a television broadcast with a viewing audience in the millions, Oprah discussed quinoa as one of the best grains to eat for good health (Egeland, 2005). In the past decade, over 1400 products containing quinoa have been launched in the United States alone (Innova Database, 2015). In a short period from 2010 to 2013, the number of new products containing quinoa increased nearly 100% in Europe and North America (Frank, 2014). The UN General Assembly and FAO Director-General José Graziano da Silva declared 2013 as the International

Year of Quinoa, to stimulate quinoa development as a worldwide crop and recognize the accumulated knowledge and sustainable practices of Andean smallholder farmers as major producers (FAO, 2013a). Recently, quinoa was named "Whole Grain of the Month" by the Whole Grain Council (WGC, 2015a).

Today, quinoa is recognized by consumers in the United States, Europe, Canada, and Australia, which account for 94% of all exports from Peru and Bolivia, the leading quinoa-producing countries (CAC, 2015). Other countries that import quinoa include: Brazil, Israel, Japan, New Zealand, Russian Federation, Chile, United Arab Emirates, Mexico, South Africa, Argentina, Thailand, India, Malaysia, Uruguay, Ecuador, Venezuela, China, Hong Kong SAR, Costa Rica, China, Ethiopia, Turkey, Lebanon, Columbia, Singapore, and Panama.

A global interest in quinoa has grown quickly due to its protein quality, culinary versatility, gluten-free status, biodiversity, and stress-tolerance. While a third of the world consumes a mostly meat-based diet and two-thirds consumes a plant-based diet, most of the plant protein sources originate from a narrow selection of crops (some for animal feed). New protein resources must be developed from alternative sources and protein-rich crops like quinoa, that produce equitable yields in underutilized growing regions, are of paramount value to feed a growing global population. The superior nutritional quality of quinoa is recognized by numerous countries today. In addition, quinoa protein concentrate (QPC), as a value-added ingredient, may have merit in future food and beverage applications.

14.2 PRODUCTION OF QUINOA

14.2.1 Growing Regions and Yields

Quinoa was domesticated in the Andean region of South America, from Ecuador to southern Chile, especially within the Altiplano highlands of Bolivia and Peru (Tapia, 2015). Quinoa is a remarkably hardy crop, which has been shown to grow in cooler regions of South America, North America, Europe, Africa, Asia, and Australia. Quinoa is above all resilient to the harsh climates and atmospheric conditions of the Andean Altiplano and tolerates temperatures of $-4°C$ to $-8°C$ (CAC, 2015). Quinoa is considered a stress-tolerant species as are other indigenous crops which are grown on local scales around the world (Ruiz et al., 2014). Since quinoa has been cultivated in many different environments from sea level to high elevation within the Andean region, it has a wide genetic diversity (high biodiversity value) with potential to be adapted to other regions of the world. The greatest limitation to quinoa cultivation is heat sensitivity and sustained temperatures above 35°C which may cause plant dormancy or pollen sterility (OMAFRA, 2015).

The main quinoa-producing countries are Bolivia and Peru, which account for over 90% of total world production (CAC, 2015; FAO-FAOSTAT, 2013). A little over a decade ago, world production of quinoa remained under 50,000 metric tonnes (t) per year. By 2011, production increased substantially to 80,000 t, of which Peru, Bolivia, and Ecuador accounted for 51%, 48%, and 1%, respectively. In a short 2-year period, Bolivia alone increased production by 60% to reach 61,182 t in 2013. Since 2013, Peru has doubled its production to 95,000 t (Valdez & Bajak, 2014) and was forecast to reach 108,000 t for the 2015 crop year (USDA-FAS, 2014). Peru and Bolivia have rapidly increased production to meet a new export demand. More than half of quinoa produced in South America is exported, most of which goes to the United States and Europe (CAC, 2015).

Quinoa has achieved global recognition since 1973, and countries with commercial quinoa production of less than 5000 t include Argentina, Australia, Brazil, Canada, Chile, Columbia, Ecuador, France, India, Morocco, England, and the United States (Bazile & Baudron, 2015; CDC, 2010). As dry soil conditions and salinity increase in other areas of the world due to climate change, quinoa's high biodiversity value is of interest. Quinoa is being tested in research trials around the world, including Uruguay, Paraguay, Venezuela, Denmark, Finland, Pakistan, Tanzania, China, Mongolia, New Zealand, Kenya, and Himalayas, and the states of Nevada (USA), Washington (USA).

Within a 30-year period from 1983 to 2013, the average production of quinoa in Bolivia was 0.55 tonne per hectare (t/ha) with a range from 0.43 to 0.68 t/ha (CAC, 2015). From 2007 to 2014, yield efficiencies in Peru have nearly doubled from 0.97 to 1.93 t/ha (USDA-FAS, 2014). Yields of over 3.92 t/ha have been reported in various regions around the world (Jacobsen, 2003). In commercial production, most quinoa producers declare yields reflective of unprocessed quinoa prior to saponin removal. A processing yield loss of 5% to reduce saponin is a commonly accepted value (Quiroga et al., 2015).

Considering an average protein content for processed quinoa is 14.12% (USDA, 2015), total world production of 200,000 t provides 26,828 t of useable plant protein (assumes 5% yield loss). Applying this same rationale, yields of 2–3 t/ha provide 268–402 kg of useable plant protein per hectare.

14.2.2 Land Use

In a 30-year period (from 1983 to 2013), land dedicated to quinoa production in Bolivia increased over fourfold from 32,609 to 131,192 ha (CAC, 2015). In Peru, since 2007, harvested areas have increased from 32,959 to 55,000 ha (CAC, 2015; USDA-FAS, 2014). Intermediate levels of cultivation (500–5000 ha) occur in Ecuador, Chile, and Canada, and small levels of cultivation (<500 ha) occur in Argentina, Australia, Brazil, Colombia, India, Morocco, and United States (Bazile & Baudron, 2015). In 2014, in Europe (Netherlands, France, England, Belgium, and Germany), 1500 ha were dedicated to quinoa, a Wageningen UR bred cultivar (FVU, 2015).

Most of the world's quinoa is produced on smallholder farms (1–2 ha in size) in the Altiplano on arid and semiarid, high-salinity soils at altitudes of 2500–4000 m above sea level (CAC, 2015). The main soil type is sandy, salty, and dry, which is considered severe for today's major world crops such as rice, corn, and wheat. In contrast, major crops are typically produced on premium soils and adapted to specific growing conditions by large agro-industrial farms. Quinoa is considered salt-tolerant. The majority of quinoa produced is grown on saline soils from the Salare of Bolivia to the coastal regions of Chile. Some varieties of quinoa can tolerate the salinity of sea water, which has an electrical conductivity of approximately 50 dS/m (the equivalence of 600 mM NaCl) although yields are higher under moderate saline conditions of 10–20 dS/m (Jacobsen, Mujica, & Jensen, 2003).

14.2.3 Water Use

Quinoa is considered drought-tolerant. A main production zone is in southern Altiplano in Bolivia, where annual rainfall is less than 150 mm (Bazile, Salcedo, & Santivañez, 2015). Water requirements for quinoa are between 254 and 381 mm with combined precipitation and irrigation (green + blue water) (Oelke, 1992). Trials in Peru have shown yields of 6 t/ha when both irrigation and fertilizer systems are implemented (Alejandro, Luz, & Wilfredo, 2015). The water footprint required to produce a gram of protein (L water/g protein), as determined by Mekonnen and Hoekstra (2012), is 21 L for cereal grains, 31 L for animal milk, and 112 L for bovine meat. Likewise, considering water requirements for quinoa of 254–381 mm and yields of 2–3 t/ha that would provide 268–402 kg protein/ha, the water footprint of quinoa would be between 6.3 and 14.2 L/g of protein. Quinoa demands only 30% of the water that rice requires, which is enticing rice producers in Peru to switch to growing quinoa (USDA-FAS, 2014).

14.2.4 Energy Use and Cost

There is no known information in the literature on the amount of energy required to product 1 tonne of quinoa and resulting greenhouse gas emissions. Furthermore, a life cycle analysis of quinoa is unknown. In agriculture, a substantial amount of energy goes toward the production of nitrogen fertilizer and diesel fuel. Fertilizer requirements for quinoa are low, although according to Piva, Brasse, and Mehinagic (2015), there is a direct link between nitrogen intake and yield with maximum yields of 10 t/ha achieved under experimental conditions. Recommendations include a first nitrogen input at the 3–4-leaf stage (30–40 kg N/ha) and a second input at the 8–10-leaf stage. Quinoa crop yields and production costs remain unpredictable. According to USDA-FAS (2014), cost of production for conventional, Peruvian quinoa is $2200 USD/t, and prices at farm gate range between $4000–4500 USD/t (conventional) and $5200 USD/t (organic).

14.3 MORPHOLOGY

Unlike true cereal grains that are part of the Poaceae family of monocotyledonous or single-leaf grasses, quinoa is a pseudocereal belonging to the Amaranthaceae family of dicotyledonous or dual-leaf vegetables. This distinction is important as it pertains to quinoa's seed microstructure, which affects quinoa's nutritional properties.

Quinoa fruits are disc-shaped, ranging in diameter from 1 to 3 mm. As shown in Fig. 14.1A, the major anatomical parts are the pericarp, seed coat, embryo, and perisperm (Lorenz & Nyanzi, 1989; Prego, Maldonado, & Otegui, 1998; Variano-Marston & DeFrancisco, 1984). The embryo surrounding the perisperm is part of the bran fraction of the seed and is high in protein, lipid, ash, fiber, and saponin (Becker & Hanners, 1990; Variano-Marston & DeFrancisco, 1984). Lindeboom (2005) found that the bran fraction (pericarp, seed coat, and embryo) represents 48% of the seed weight and contains 22.9% protein, 8.8% oil, 7.4% saponin on a dry basis (db). Conversely, the perisperm accounts for 52% of the seed weight and contains 77.2% starch (db). The ratio of protein-rich bran to starch-rich perisperm is higher than true cereal grains. The proximate composition of quinoa is shown in Fig. 14.1B.

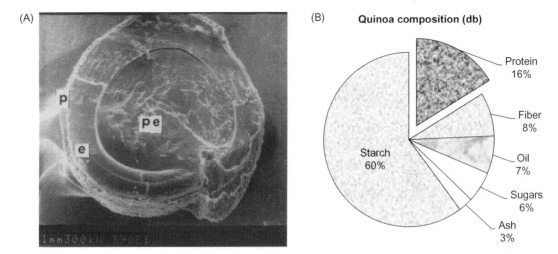

FIGURE 14.1 Quinoa seed structure and composition (A) SEM of gross internal anatomy showing pericarp (p), embryo (e) and perisperm (pe), fracture done parallel to plane of cotyledon and (B) composition of typical quinoa expressed on a dry weight basis. *For (A) with permission from Lorenz and Nyanzi (1989), (B) USDA (2015).*

14.4 NUTRITIONAL QUALITY

Quinoa has gained worldwide recognition for its nutritional properties, primarily the quality of its proteins and essential amino acid (EAA) composition. For some populations, consuming adequate high-quality protein in the diet is an issue, especially for those that limit or avoid intake of animal protein and need to obtain protein from cereals, grains, and legumes. Even when caloric intakes of these foods are sufficient to meet energy requirements; inadequate consumption of EAA may increase the prevalence of malnutrition (FAO, 2013b).

14.4.1 Protein Content

The protein content of quinoa is exceptional as compared to true cereal grains. Relative to the major cereal crops cultivated around the world, quinoa is generally higher in total protein (16.28 g db) than wheat (14.51 g db), corn (10.51 g db), and rice (8.10 g db) (USDA, 2015). The protein-rich embryo comprises 60% of the volume within the pericarp, which accounts for quinoa's higher protein content as compared to cereal grains (Oelke, Putnam, Teynor, & Oplinger, 1992).

As with other crops, studies have shown that the nutrient composition of quinoa varies due to varietal differences, genetic diversity, climatic factors, and growing conditions (FAO, 2013a; Gonzalez, Konishi, Bruno, Valoy, & Prado, 2012; Koziol, 1992). De Bruin (1964) reported protein content ranging from 14.0% to 16.0% (db) in three quinoa genotypes grown in the Netherlands. Koziol (1992) found that the protein content for quinoa seed cultivated in the sierra of Ecuador ranged from 10.8% to 21.9% with an average of 15.7%. More recently, Miranda et al. (2012) studied the nutritional properties of six quinoa ecotypes from three distinctive geographical regions of Chile and found protein ranging from 11.1% to 16.2% (db). The wide ranges in protein content of quinoa are most likely a reflection of differences in the relative ratio of the protein- and fat-rich embryo to perisperm (Taylor & Parker, 2002).

14.4.2 Protein Quality

In addition to total protein, quinoa's EAA composition and bioavailability contribute to its superior protein quality. Quinoa possesses an exceptionally well-balanced composition of EAAs, including lysine, which is the first limiting EAA in most cereal grains (Taylor & Parker, 2002). Table 14.1 shows that the lysine content of quinoa is almost double that of wheat and corn, and 25% higher than rice. Quinoa proteins contain more histidine than wheat and rice proteins, but are comparable to that of corn. While the sulfur and aromatic amino acids in quinoa are adequate to meet the needs of young children and adults, they are present in quantities lower than those of wheat, corn, and rice. According to the WHO/FAO/UNU scoring patterns for young children and adults, quinoa proteins contain sufficient amounts of tryptophan, isoleucine, cysteine, methionine, phenylalanine, tyrosine, and histidine. However,

TABLE 14.1 Amino Acid Composition (mg/g Protein) of the Proteins in Quinoa and Other Cereal Grains in Comparison to the WHO/FAO/UNU Scoring Pattern for Young Children (6 Months to 3 Years) and Older Children, Adolescent, and Adult (3–10 Years)

Amino Acid	Quinoa[a]	Wheat[b]	Corn[c]	Rice[d]	WHO/FAO/UNU Scoring Pattern[e] Young Children	WHO/FAO/UNU Scoring Pattern[e] Older Children, Adolescent, Adult
Tryptophan	12	13	7	12	8.5	6.6
Threonine	30	29	38	36	31	25
Isoleucine	36	36	36	43	32	30
Leucine	59	68	123	83	66	61
Lysine	54	27	28	36	57	48
Sulfur amino acids[f]	36	42	39	44	27	23
Aromatic amino acids[g]	61	78	90	86	52	41
Valine	42	44	51	61	43	40
Histidine	29	23	30	24	20	16
Arginine	77	47	50	83		
Alanine	42	36	75	58		
Aspartic acid	80	51	70	94		
Glutamic acid	132	317	188	195		
Glycine	49	42	41	46		
Proline	55	102	87	47		
Serine	40	46	47	53		

[a]Quinoa, uncooked, No. 20035.
[b]Wheat, hard red winter, No. 20072.
[c]Corn grain, yellow, No. 20014.
[d]Rice, white, long-grain, regular, raw, unenriched, No. 20444.
[e]FAO Expert Consultation (2013).
[f]Cystine + methionine.
[g]Phenylalanine + tyrosine.
[a,b,c,d]Source: USDA National Nutrient Database for Standard Reference Release 28. Retrieved Oct. 16, 2015.

leucine, lysine, threonine, and valine are the limiting amino acids in quinoa for young children, while all of the EAAs, except for leucine, are adequate to meet WHO/FAO/UNU requirements for adults (Table 14.1). Recently, Gonzalez et al. (2012) found that variations in EAAs exist in quinoa, which was influenced by growing region and climate. Lysine, tyrosine, and tryptophan were also found to be limiting amino acids. The high levels of EAAs in its protein allow quinoa to be considered the only plant food that provides all of the EAAs which closely match the human nutrition standards set forth by the FAO, and is considered comparable with casein, the protein in milk (FAO, 2013a).

The major storage proteins of quinoa are primarily albumin and globulin, which account for its high lysine content (Fairbanks, Burgener, Robinson, Andersen, & Ballon, 1990; Koziol, 1992). In contrast, major seed storage proteins of true cereals are of prolamin and glutelin fractions. The main protein group in quinoa is an 11S globulin named chenopodin, comprising 37% of total protein, which is rich in glutamic acid, aspartic acid, arginine, serine, leucine, and glycine (Abugoch James, 2009; Brinegar & Goundan, 1993). The other major quinoa protein is a 2S-type albumin, accounting for 35% of total protein, and is high in cysteine, arginine, histidine, and lysine (Abugoch James, 2009; Brinegar, Sine, & Nwokocha, 1996; Osborne, 1924; Prakash & Pal, 1998). Concentrations of albumins and globulins in quinoa are greater than those found in wheat, maize, or rice (Ríos, Sgarbieri, & Amaya, 1978; Romero, 1981; Scarpati De Briceño & Briceño, 1980), which accounts for its favorable amino acid profile as compared to these grains.

14.4.3 Protein Digestibility

The bioavailability of quinoa protein has long been established using animal and human feeding trials. Though quinoa's digestibility has been studied in many forms (raw, cooked, flour, flakes, extruded), quinoa is most commonly consumed after cooking in water. Several studies found that cooking quinoa improves protein digestibility. Key in vivo studies in which cooked quinoa was fed are summarized below.

14.4.3.1 Animal Feeding Experiments

Mahoney, Lopez, and Hendriks (1975) studied the effects of cooking on the amino acid composition of quinoa and rat response. When fed washed and cooked quinoa, nitrogen efficiency for growth (NEG), weight gain, and protein efficiency ratio (PER) were improved by 40%, 100%, and 29%, respectively. Mixing 20% quinoa and 80% wheat flour improved the NEG by 43%, weight gain by 11%, and PER by 72% as compared to a diet based solely on wheat flour. The protein quality of cooked quinoa was deemed better than casein based on NEG, but comparable to casein based on PER. The improved NEG, weight gain, and PER of the cooked over the uncooked quinoa was not associated with a corresponding change in amino acid composition. These researchers also found that they could match the effects of the 20% quinoa and 80% wheat flour mixture by adding 0.2% lysine to wheat flour. Similar results have been observed when cooked quinoa was used as a protein supplement for pigs (Cardozo & Bateman, 1961), cattle (Martinez, 1946), and chicks (Weber, 1978).

14.4.3.2 Human Feeding Experiments

The suitability of quinoa in infant nutrition was evaluated in two studies of hospitalized Peruvian children recovering from malnutrition. Lopez de Romaña, Creed, and Graham (1978) first studied eight children ranging in age from 4 to 29 months. The children were fed six common Peruvian diets, five of which were based on a potato-wheat noodle supplemented with either milk, fish, egg, beans, or a commercial product. The sixth diet was prepared using equal parts of polished and washed quinoa and oats. Mean nitrogen absorption while on the quinoa-oats diet was significantly lower than when the other five diets were consumed. This was attributed to the lower digestibility of quinoa. Lopez de Romaña, Graham, Rojas, and MacLean (1981) conducted a follow-up study with six hospitalized infants, ages 10–18 months. The children were fed two diets based on whole or milled quinoa and a control diet based on casein protein. Although nitrogen absorption was not significantly different between whole and milled quinoa, both were lower than the casein control. However, the biological values were 43.4% for whole quinoa, 50.7% for milled quinoa, and 45.8% for the casein control. These findings validate the good quality of quinoa protein in a human feeding trial.

Ruales, de Grijalva, Lopez-Jaramillo, and Nair (2002) investigated the effects of a quinoa-based infant food on the nutritional status of 40, low-income boys in Ecuador, ages 50–65 months. The children were selected based on their weight in relation to age, and divided into a reference group of 17 children, a control group of 13 children, and an experimental group of 10 children. Using additional anthropometric measurements, it was determined that there was no acute malnutrition in these children.

The quinoa-based infant food was manufactured by drum drying a precooked slurry of quinoa flour. The infant food was given to the children of the experimental group as a porridge or beverage twice daily for 15 days. Both products contributed 800 calories (about 40% recommended daily allowance) and 30 g protein to the children's daily intakes. Plasma insulin-like growth factor-1 (IGF-1) values, a clinical indicator used to monitor developments in the nutritional status of children, were drawn on the boys in each group at the beginning of the experiment and on days 7, 15, and 30. IGF-1 values increased significantly among the children in the experimental group during the feeding trial and slightly thereafter, while there was no significant change among the control and reference group members. Results indicate that a product with good nutritional quality and acceptability can be made from quinoa for supplemental feeding purposes.

Chemical analysis showed the infant food to be a potential source of valuable nutrients. Animal feeding experiments with rats revealed digestibility of 95 and a 67.7 protein digestibility corrected amino acid score (PDCAAS). The authors attribute the low PDCAAS to the formation of Maillard reaction products during drum drying and damage to lysine during the heat process. Therefore, modifications to the heat treatment of the slurry may further improve protein quality.

14.4.4 Macro- and Micronutrients and Phytochemicals

In addition to its high protein content and superior EAA profile, other important attributes contribute to the quality and unique nutritive value of quinoa.

14.4.4.1 Lipids

Total lipid (fat) content ranges from 1.8% to 9.5% with an average of 5.0−7.2% (Fig. 14.1B) (Bhargava, Shukla, & Ohri, 2006), which is higher than corn (5.29% db) (USDA, 2015). The fatty acid composition is 9.9−12.3% saturated fat with palmitic acid predominant. Monounsaturated fat is 25.0−28.7% total fat and mainly oleic acid. Polyunsaturated fat is 56.20−58.3% total fat and is predominantly two essential fatty acids, linoleic acid (18:2n-6, an omega-6 fatty acid) and α-linolenic acid (an omega-3 fatty acid) (Abugoch James, 2009). The unsaturated fatty acids are well protected from oxidation by a high level of naturally occurring vitamin E present in the forms of tocopherols and tocotrienols (Repo-Carrasco, Espinoza, & Jacobsen, 2003; Ruales & Nair, 1993). Tang et al. (2015) recently revealed that the omega-6/omega-3 ratio is approximately 6/1, which is more favorable than other plant oils regarding potential health benefits.

14.4.4.2 Carbohydrates

Starch is the primary constituent of quinoa carbohydrates, ranging from 32% to 69% (Fig. 14.1B) (Abugoch James, 2009; Atwell, Patrick, Johnson, & Glass, 1983; USDA, 2015), which is lower than that of corn (74.0% db) and rice (88.9% db) (USDA, 2015). Starch granules vary in size from 0.6 to 2.0 μm, which is comparable to amaranth (1−2 μm), but smaller than rice (3−8 μm), and barley (2−3 μm) (Abugoch James, 2009; Atwell et al., 1983). Unlike other small-granule starches such as rice, quinoa starch gelatinizes at relatively low temperatures ranging from 55.5°C to 73°C, which is similar to wheat and potato starches (Koziol, 1992; Repo-Carrasco et al., 2003; Ruales & Nair, 1994). Amylose content of quinoa starch is lower than that of other native starches, ranging from 3% to 20% (Abugoch James, 2009; Atwell et al., 1983). The higher proportion of amylopectin offers unique functional properties, such as excellent freeze−thaw stability and resistance to retrogradation (Ahamed, Singhal, Kulkarni, & Pal, 1996). Maltose, D-ribose, and D-galactose are the main sugars in quinoa, and very low levels of glucose and fructose are present. The small quantities of glucose and fructose indicate that quinoa is a low glycemic food and may improve metabolic control in diabetic individuals (Ogungbenle, 2003; Oshodi, Ogungbenle, & Oladimeji, 1999).

14.4.4.3 Fiber

Total dietary fiber in quinoa seeds ranges from 8.0% to 13.0% (Fig. 14.1B) (Lamothe, Srichuwong, Reuhs, & Hamaker, 2015; Miranda et al., 2012; Ruales & Nair, 1994; Wright, Pike, Fairbanks, & Huber, 2002), up to 30% of which is soluble (Ando et al., 2002). Although both quinoa and long-grain white rice undergo a polishing step to remove the outer layers, the fiber content of quinoa (8.07% db) is notably higher than that of rice (1.47% db) (USDA, 2015). Lamothe et al. (2015) recently conducted a comprehensive investigation of the compositional and structural characteristics of the quinoa seed soluble and insoluble fiber fractions. Approximately 78% was insoluble dietary fiber composed of homogalacturonans, xyloglucans, and cellulose. Quinoa soluble fiber was 22%, as compared to about 15% for wheat and maize, and was composed primarily of homogalacturonans and arabinans. These fiber fractions differ from cereal fibers and more closely resemble those of fruits, vegetables, and leguminous seeds. The dietary fibers from quinoa indicate good potential for favorable function in the colon.

14.4.4.4 Vitamins and Minerals

Quinoa seeds are a rich source of vitamins, including vitamin A precursor β-carotene, thiamin/vitamin B1, riboflavin/vitamin B2, niacin/vitamin B-3, ascorbic acid/vitamin C, folic acid/vitamin B9 and vitamin E B6, and pantothenic acid (Koziol, 1992; Repo-Carrasco et al., 2003; Ruales & Nair, 1993; Tang et al., 2015; USDA, 2015). The mineral (ash) content of quinoa (2.74 g db) (Fig. 14.1B) is higher than that of wheat (1.81 db), corn (1.34 g db), and rice (0.72 g db) (USDA, 2015). Many minerals in quinoa are present in greater quantities than other grains, including phosphorus, magnesium, potassium, calcium, iron, zinc, and copper. The odium content is low (Koziol, 1992; Nascimento et al., 2014; Ruales & Nair, 1993; USDA, 2015). The process of saponin removal decreases vitamin and mineral contents to an extent (Ruales & Nair, 1993).

14.4.4.5 Phytochemicals

There is a growing body of technical information on quinoa's chemical composition, physiologically active compounds, and functional properties, which give quinoa excellent potential in human nutrition (Vega-Gálvez et al., 2010). In recent review articles, Fuentes and Paredes-Gonzalez (2015) and Graf et al. (2015) reported naturally occurring phytochemicals such as phytosterols, betalains, glycine betaine, squalene, phytoecdysteroids, and phenolics, which may have future nutraceutical application. Although the focus of quinoa's health benefits has primarily concentrated on its macro- and micronutrient profiles, quinoa's secondary metabolites may also have a role in the maintenance of human health and wellness.

14.4.5 Antinutritional Factors and Allergenicity

14.4.5.1 Antinutritional Factors

The primary antinutritional factors in quinoa are saponins, a large group of triterpenoid aglycones. Bitterness is associated with quinoa due to saponins present in the pericarp or outer hull of the seed, which is removed prior to consumption. The majority of saponins are removed by polishing. However, since both polarity of the saponins and quality of the polishing procedures vary, some saponin and associated bitterness usually remain in the polished seed. Dependent on quinoa variety, saponin levels can vary considerably from 0.01% to 4.65% in the unpolished seed (Chauhan, Eskin, & Tkachuk, 1992; Galwey, Leakey, Herrera, Price, & Fenwick, 1990; Koziol, 1992; Reichert, Tatarynovich, & Tyler, 1986; Taylor & Parker, 2002; Troisi et al., 2015). Today, most of the commercially grown quinoa has a high level of saponin, although levels may be reduced to less than 0.11% after polishing. Saponins are found in many other plant sources. For example, chickpeas and kidney beans contain 5% and 1.4% saponins, respectively. In addition, quinoa contains 1% phytic acid, 0.5% tannins, but negligible trypsin inhibitors (Taylor & Parker, 2002).

14.4.5.2 Allergenicity

Quinoa is evolutionarily very distant from true cereals of the family Gramineae that contain gluten fractions toxic to those with celiac disease (Berti et al., 2004). Prolamins are present in quinoa in insignificant amounts (Fairbanks et al., 1990; Koziol, 1992). Furthermore, the prolamins of quinoa are unable to agglutinate K562(s) cells (De Vincenzi et al., 1999). De Vincenzi et al. (1999) separated A and B fractions of quinoa prolamins and found fraction A contains protective peptides that interfere with agglutinating activity of toxic peptides found in fraction B. Upon immunochemical and molecular evaluation of quinoa proteins, Berti, Iametti, Porrioni, and Bonomi (2002) and Berti et al. (2004), concluded that quinoa could be a safe choice for the production of gluten-free products. The immunoreactivity of the extracted quinoa proteins was low compared with either commercial antigliadin antibody or serum of a celiac disease subject and was comparable to that of proteins in gluten-free flour. In a recent study evaluating the use of quinoa seeds as a gluten-free alternative to cereal grains, Zevallos et al. (2014) found that gastrointestinal parameters improved in celiac patients on the quinoa diet. It should be noted though that quinoa contains 2S-type albumin, which is of increasing interest in nutritional and clinical studies as it has been reported in seeds of many mono- and dicotyledonous plants as a food allergen (Moreno & Clemente, 2008).

14.5 PROCESSING METHODS

14.5.1 Quinoa Seed From "Farm to Fork"

The majority of quinoa that is consumed is in the whole seed form which is polished (Vega-Gálvez et al., 2010). The seeds originate from the quinoa plant, which has either branched or unbranched stalks with panicles consisting of small flowers. There is one quinoa seed per flower. Although quinoa stalks can be harvested using a combine with a standard- or sorghum-type header (OMAFRA, 2015), harvesting is almost exclusively manual (Winkel et al., 2015). Directly in the field at harvest, quinoa stalks are cut, bundled in sheaves, air-dried, threshed, sifted to separate seeds from chaff, and winnowed to remove lightweight impurities. Quinoa seeds are then transported to a facility where they are cleaned and processed.

With the rise in quinoa's popularity and subsequent production of larger quantities, many advances in industrial processing have been made (Quiroga et al., 2015). Postharvest processing involves a series of steps in order to produce the smooth quinoa seeds. At the processing facility, the steps may include the following: preliminary sorting; sifting to remove impurities; saponin removal (hulling, washing, drying); sorting by size and color; and removal of additional impurities.

One of the most important steps is removal of bitter saponins which are located primarily in the pericarp, the outermost layer that is polished to reveal a smooth seed coat layer. The traditional method to remove saponins involves manually washing with water on an abrasive stone until the outer layer or hull is removed (Quiroga et al., 2015). This method is time-consuming though, requiring 3–6 h to prepare about 11 kg of seed. It is also customary sometimes to toast the seeds prior to washing, which is thought to aid in saponin removal (Andean Naturals, 2015).

As saponins are located mainly in the outermost layers, polishing (also called dry mechanical abrasion) is used to reduce saponin levels by using an abrasive-type dehuller, rice polisher, or modified barley pearler. Newer technology developed by the Sustainable Technologies Promotion Center (CPTS, 2006), includes a revolving rotor equipped with "ribs" inside the drum of the huller which enhances uniform polishing. Dry mechanical abrasion is effective in reducing most of the saponins. However, it can leave behind bitter saponin-laden dust on the seed along with some intact pericarp fragments. Therefore, commercial saponin removal is typically a combination of dry mechanical abrasion followed by washing (soaking, centrifugation, rinsing). The volume of water required is generally > 5 m^3/t and runoff is contaminated with saponins (Quiroga et al., 2015). Saponin removal may be aided with warm, alkaline, or acidic water. In commercial production, a processing yield loss of 5% is commonly accepted, although in research, yield loss up to 14.8% has been reported (Lindeboom, 2005; Reichert et al., 1986; Taylor & Parker, 2002). A rapid test for saponin estimation that is in practice is based on a modified Afrosometric method to measure foam height (Koziol, 1991).

The polished whole seed then is ready to cook and consume or ready for further processing into commercial ingredients. Examples of commercially available quinoa ingredients include: (1) whole seed which may be pasteurized, sprouted, toasted, or boiled and frozen; (2) milled flour which may be pregelatinized or drum-dried; (3) extruded or puffed; and (4) flakes. Methods to prepare these ingredients are beyond the scope of this chapter, and therefore the following section is dedicated to QPC.

14.5.2 QPCs and Isolates

In a recent review by Graf et al. (2015), it was noted that quinoa protein extraction research methods via alkali or enzymatic hydrolysis and precipitation are well documented. Quinoa protein concentrate (QPC) ($\geq 50\%$ protein db) or isolate (QPI) ($\geq 90\%$ protein db) may have application as food ingredients (Scanlin & Stone, 2009), although they are not yet commercially produced. Limitations exist for some research extraction methods. For example, chemicals and/or procedures utilized in the lab are typically not suitable for food manufacturing. Also, research techniques that are focused on protein may degrade other ingredients such as starch, fiber, and oil, which would not be practical for commercial purposes. Certainly, research methods to study protein functionality are valuable, yet lab equipment produces quantities which are too small for evaluation in food prototypes.

Little information exists regarding pilot processing of QPC on industrial equipment. Although QPI has been made in the lab, successful pilot production is unknown. Therefore, the remainder of this section is dedicated to pilot processing of QPC and the knowledge obtained from approximately 30 pilot trial runs. In most cases, conditions change for each run in order to solve a problem previously encountered. Therefore, statistical data are not presented.

Expanding from lab-sized quantities to pilot-sized quantities (a 5000-fold increase) is challenging. In particular, some trials have produced acceptable-tasting QPC with good functional properties, yet some have not done so. However, quantities of QPC up to 25 k per batch have been produced, which allows for evaluation in food prototypes.

In order to prepare for a pilot trial run, some considerations should be taken into account. For example, the amount of protein targeted (such as 50%, 70%, or higher), batch size, extended processing times, food safety parameters, drying procedures, cost of processing, source of quinoa and its form (such as whole seed flour, defatted flour, or mill fraction), and strategies to protect nutritional and functional characteristics of protein and coingredients (starch, fiber, oil). Pilot trials are also batch processing (as opposed to continuous) and monitoring of conditions requires close attention by qualified personnel. The Whole Grains Council recognizes quinoa as a whole grain (WGC, 2015b). During desaponification, the inedible hull is removed, thereby leaving the bran, germ, and endosperm intact. When whole grains are consumed as a single food or as an ingredient in food, these essential fractions and naturally occurring nutrients must be retained in the original proportions in the intact grain. Therefore, quinoa that is processed into QPC would clearly lose its whole grain status. Nevertheless, it should be a consideration that is taken into account.

In order to prepare good-quality QPC, quinoa seeds need to be identified with care as inferior quinoa will yield poor-quality QPC. Raw material should have minimal seed damage and debris, low microbial load, and low saponin ($<0.11\%$). QPC can be produced from either whole seed flour or embryo-rich bran. In the latter case, refined white flour is produced as a coingredient. A flow diagram of a pilot-scale process to make QPC and coingredients is shown in Fig. 14.2.

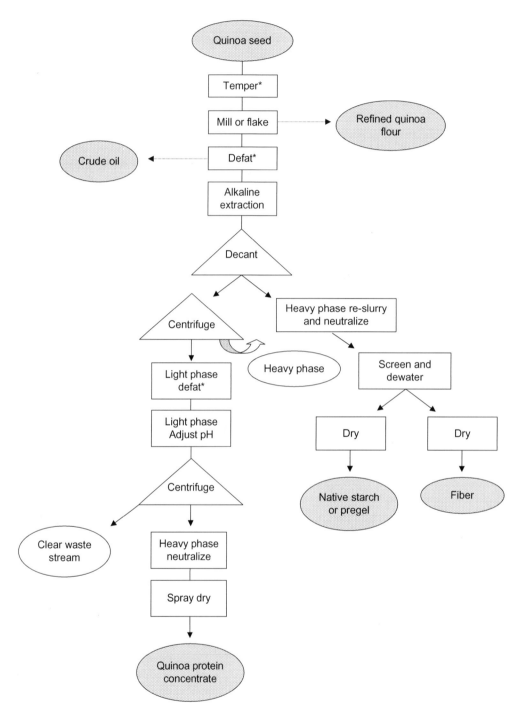

FIGURE 14.2 Flow diagram of a pilot-scale process for quinoa protein concentrate and coingredients (crude oil, starch, fiber, refined white flour); alternate steps are designated by asterisk.

The following examples are suitable starting materials for protein extraction: (1) whole seed flour; (2) defatted flour; (3) protein-rich bran; and (4) defatted, protein-rich bran. On the other hand, a commercially available by-product of popped quinoa, toasted protein-rich bran, is not optimal since the EAA lysine is degraded with Maillard browning.

Whole seed quinoa flour has a typical protein content of 14%. Commercial quinoa flour is made from polished whole seed that is milled using a stone grinder or hammer-type mill. Most commercial flour is too course for protein extraction and fine flour (100% through US Standard Sieve #140 mesh 105 micron opening) is preferred for improved

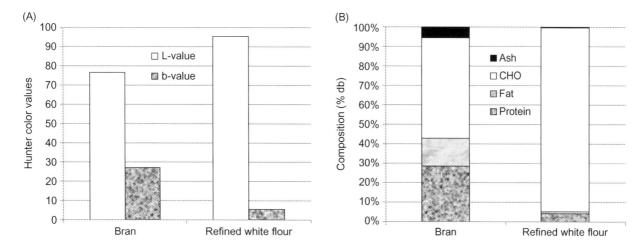

FIGURE 14.3 Quinoa bran (protein-rich) and refined white flour (starch-rich) mill fractions, using Buhler MLU-202 roller mill (A) Hunter color L- and b-values, and (B) ash, carbohydrate (CHO), fat, and protein composition (% db). Averages are presented ($n = 3$).

recoveries. Wet fractionation methods are usually employed to extract and concentrate quinoa protein. If whole seed quinoa flour is used, a substantial amount of starch will need to be dried.

In lieu of using whole seed quinoa flour as the starting material, protein-rich bran can be used which reduces the amount of starch produced. Protein-rich bran and refined white flour (starch-rich) can be prepared using dry fractionation. Dry fractionation methods (such as roller milling, size-classification, air-classification, or electrostatic separation) may be utilized to obtain efficient separation of the tissues or extraction of quinoa protein (FVU, 2015). If protein-rich bran is used to make QPC, bran with small particle size is optimal. For example, protein recovery of 84% was obtained with a bran particle size of 40 μm (Lindeboom, 2005).

In a milling trial, Hunter color values were used to differentiate between bran and refined white flour fractions as shown in Fig. 14.3A (unpublished data provided by the author). The protein-rich bran contained 28% protein (bran to flour ratio of 38:62) as shown in Fig. 14.3B, which is comparable to the results of Föste, Elgeti, Brunner, Jekle, and Becker (2015).

During pilot trials, QPC was prepared from two main types of starting materials; defatted flour (100% through US Standard Sieve #140 mesh 105 micron) and protein-rich bran (90% through US Standard #80 180 micron). As shown in Fig. 14.2, a modified isoelectric precipitation method was used (Mohamed, Wolf, & Spiess, 2000). Batch size was typically 100–200 kg of quinoa starting material with a ratio of 1:10 (w/v) of quinoa to alkaline solution. The quinoa alkaline suspension was continually agitated prior to passing through decanter and disk stack centrifuge. The heavy phase collected from the decanter was resuspended in water and neutralized for starch and fiber separation. The light phase collected from the disk stack centrifuge was pH-adjusted to precipitate the protein and centrifuged again using the disk stack. The second supernatant was discarded as waste stream. The protein pellet collected from the disk stack was resuspended in water, neutralized, and spray-dried to a resulting protein content of approximately 70% (db).

14.6 QUINOA PROTEIN FUNCTIONALITY, OFF-TASTES, AND CHALLENGES

A 70% QPC has functional properties for use in food applications. For instance, it forms stable foams, gels, and retains moisture in food prototypes such as bars and bakery. It is soluble at neutral pH, stable to heat, and has a creamy texture as evaluated in UHT beverages. Abugoch James (2009) prepared a literature review of quinoa protein functionality. QPC has emulsifying, foaming, solubility, bioactive, and water-holding properties. The water-holding capacity was shown to be 3.5–5 mL water per g protein. Minimum solubility of QPC was found to be between 3 and 6 pH. Oshodi et al. (1999) found maximum solubility occurs at pH 10.0. Upon hydrolysis of QPC to produce peptides, foam expansion was shown to increase although foam stability decreased. In addition, solubility and bioactive properties of protein hydrolysate have been shown to increase relative to QPC and may be a potential plant-based alternative to commercially available animal peptides (Aluko & Monu, 2003).

The primary off-tastes associated with QPC made during some of the pilot trials are bitterness and grassiness, likely due to residual saponin and volatile organic compounds (VOCs), respectively. It may seem logical that using a wet fractionation method may remove saponins and VOCs in the waste water. However, because the QPC can be bitter and grassy, there may be interactions between the extracted proteins, saponins, and VOCs. In a study of pea (*Pisum*) saponin and VOCs by Heng (2005), protein–saponin interactions are well documented in literature review. Saponins are found in soy and pea protein isolates. Saponins have been observed to form complexes with protein at low pH during precipitation. In addition, Heng (2005) found that during precipitation, pea protein had increased binding affinities for VOCs. Furthermore, saponins can be removed with aqueous ethanol and heating releases VOCs providing an improved flavor of protein concentrates. Indeed, off-flavors observed in QPC made during some of the pilot trials need to be eliminated or masked and present a challenge in commercial scale-up. Sensory studies of QPC are limited. Added challenges include: (1) high cost of quinoa seed; (2) low protein content and low recovery compared to existing vegetable proteins (soy and pea); (3) variability in the quality of quinoa seed and starting material for protein extraction; and (4) an undeveloped market for coingredients (starch, oil, fiber). The economic viability of QPC is dependent on the marketability of its coingredients.

14.7 CONCLUDING REMARKS AND FUTURE RESEARCH NEEDS

Quinoa as a value-added crop is likely to advance the livelihood for people of the Andes. Moreover, increased consumer demand in the past decade, along with efforts from companies like Andean Naturals, has brought thousands of native quinoa farmers out of poverty. For instance, Bolivia is one of the poorest countries in the western hemisphere and a leading producer of quinoa. More than 45,000 smallholder farmers have been lifted out of poverty by the increased export demand (Núñez de Arco, 2015). Andean Naturals, representing 21 farmers' associations, has played a key role in the dramatic rise in family farm incomes from $35 US$ to over 400 US$ per month between 2007 and 2014 (Andean Naturals, 2015). In addition, Andean Naturals launched a program with industry partners called Andean Family Farmers in 2013. The program is based upon environmental, social, and financial initiatives that enable farmers to develop entrepreneurial skills and maintain sustainable farming practices. Furthermore, industry partners such as Kashi, provide funding to bring solar energy to even the remotest parts of quinoa farmlands (MarketWatch Press Release, 2015).

Yet there are many factors in the sustainability of quinoa as a global food source, especially in growing regions outside of its Andean origins. Ruiz et al. (2014) proposed a cluster, or "quinoa network," for a sustainable productive system in order to preserve the heterogeneous genetic and cultural heritage, yet caution against an exclusive use of select quinoa varieties (such as large, white seeds).

There are several interesting areas that warrant further research on quinoa. Agro-ecological and biogeographical studies conducted on quinoa ecotypes in Chile, Argentina, and Bolivia demonstrate that genetic diversity, environmental factors, and climatic factors affect the nutritional composition of quinoa (Gonzalez et al., 2012; Miranda et al., 2012; Vidueiros et al., 2015). Such findings could offer tools for breeding strategies designed to improve the nutritional attributes and crop adaption in ecotypes in regions where climate and soil conditions are limiting. This may potentially be accomplished through genetic improvement trials and development of high-quality quinoa varieties, particularly in areas of the world where hunger and malnutrition remain unresolved (Miranda et al., 2012; Vidueiros et al., 2015). In addition, heat sensitivity is a limiting factor with quinoa cultivation and research to develop heat-tolerant ecotypes is also needed.

Despite quinoa's nutrition halo, some of today's quinoa ingredients undergo severe processing, such as toasting, that reduce protein quality. Innovation will likely come from improved processing techniques that maintain protein quality and improve digestibility. Further research is needed into the effects of processing on protein yield, functionality, nutrition, and protein digestibility. This type of work is actively being conducted at Wageningen University and Research Centre. For example, in just one of several new studies, Ruiz, Xiao, van Boekel, Stieger, and Minor (2015) found that quinoa protein isolate extracted by alkaline treatment at lower pH (8 and 9) formed semisolid gels upon heating protein suspensions, whereas extractions at higher pH (10 and 11) did not form self-supporting gels.

It is also unknown how certain commercially used processes, such as pasteurization with superheated steam treatment to remove saponins, may affect protein extraction. Saponins are still considered a waste by-product by most quinoa processors. However, in a review by Troisi et al. (2015), the authors critically evaluated the literature and found a substantial body of evidence in support of dietary saponins with positive biological activity such as (1) anti-inflammatory properties; (2) anticarcinogenic traits; (3) antimicrobial activities; and (4) abilities to lower plasma cholesterol. Therefore, future commercial applications for saponins are possible. In addition, bioactive quinoa protein hydrolysate may be a potential plant-based alternative to commercially available animal peptides. In recent reviews on other bioactives, Fuentes and Paredes-Gonzalez (2015) and Graf et al. (2015) reported naturally occurring phytochemicals such as phytosterols, betalains, squalene, phytoecdysteroids, and phenolics, which may have future nutraceutical application. Future studies on quinoa's role in the treatment and prevention of complex human diseases are merited based on the mounting evidence on quinoa's health benefits. In such clinical studies, quinoa products with well-characterized and standardized phytochemical contents must be used in order to link the observed effects to specific constituents (Graf et al., 2015). Further studies on quinoa fiber and their impact on colon health are also warranted based on the previous findings of Lamothe et al. (2015).

Climate change is expected to continue to degrade conditions of major crop production. As a result, dry, salty soils are forecast to increase in most parts of the world. Stress-tolerant and protein-rich plant species like quinoa may play an important role in future agriculture and food security to feed a growing global population.

REFERENCES

Abugoch James, L. E. (2009). Quinoa (*Chenopodium quinoa* Willd.): Composition, chemistry, nutritional and functional properties. *Advances in Food and Nutrition Research*, 58, 1–31.

Ahamed, N. T., Singhal, R. S., Kulkarni, P. R., & Pal, M. (1996). Physicochemical and functional properties of *Chenopodium quinoa* starch. *Carbohydrate Polymers*, 31(1–2), 99–103.

Alejandro, B., Luz, G.-P., & Wilfredo, R. (2015). Quinoa breeding and modern variety development. Chapter 2.5. In D. Bazile, D. Bertero, & C. Nieto (Eds.), *State of the art report of quinoa in the world in 2013* (pp. 172–191). Rome: FAO & CIRAD.

Aluko, R. E., & Monu, E. (2003). Functional and bioactive properties of quinoa seed protein hydrolysates. *Journal of Food Science*, 68(4), 1254–1258.

Andean Naturals. (2015). Retrieved from: <http://www.andeannaturals.com/impact/thechallenge> Accessed October 2015.

Ando, H., Chen, Y., Tang, H., Shimizu, M., Watanabe, K., & Miysunaga, T. (2002). Food components in fractions of quinoa seed. *Food Science and Technology Research*, 8(1), 80–84.

Atwell, W. A., Patrick, B. M., Johnson, L. A., & Glass, R. W. (1983). Characterization of quinoa starch. *Cereal Chemistry*, 60(1), 9–11.

Bazile, D., & Baudron, F. (2015). The dynamics of the global expansion of quinoa growing in view of its high biodiversity. Chapter 1.4. In D. Bazile, D. Bertero, & C. Nieto (Eds.), *State of the art report of quinoa in the world in 2013* (pp. 42–55). Rome: FAO & CIRAD.

Bazile, D., Salcedo, S., & Santivañez, T. (2015). Conclusions: Challenges, opportunities and threats to quinoa in the face of global change. Chapter 7.1. In D. Bazile, D. Bertero, & C. Nieto (Eds.), *State of the art report of quinoa in the world in 2013* (pp. 586–589). Rome: FAO & CIRAD.

Becker, R., & Hanners, G. D. (1990). Compositional and nutritional evaluation of quinoa whole grain flour and mill fractions. *Lebensmittel-Wissenschaft Technologie*, 23(5), 441–444.

Berti, C., Ballabio, C., Restani, P., Porrini, M., Bonomi, F., & Iametti, S. (2004). Immunochemical and molecular properties of proteins in *Chenopodium quinoa*. *Cereal Chemistry*, 81(2), 275–277.

Berti, C., Iametti, M., Porrioni, M., & Bonomi, F. (2002). *Chenopodium quinoa* may represent a viable alternative for gluten-free products. International Workshop on Food Supplementation in Food Allergy and Immunity. Olsztyn, August 30–September 1.

Bhargava, A., Shukla, S., & Ohri, D. (2006). Chenopodium quinoa—An Indian perspective. *Industrial Crops and Products*, 23, 73–87.

Brinegar, C., & Goundan, S. (1993). Isolation and characterization of Chenopodin, the 11S seed storage protein of quinoa (*Chenopodium quinoa*). *Journal of Agricultural and Food Chemistry*, 41(2), 182–185.

Brinegar, C., Sine, B., & Nwokocha, L. (1996). High-cysteine 2S seed storage proteins from quinoa (*Chenopodium quinoa*). *Journal of Agricultural and Food Chemistry*, 44(7), 1621–1623.

CAC (2015). *Project document: Codex standard for quinoa, prepared by Bolivia*. Joint FAO/WHO Food Standards Programme, Codex Alimentarius Commission. 38th Session. Geneva: CICG.

Cardozo, A., & Bateman, J. V. (1961). La quinua en la alimentación animal. *Turrialba*, 11, 72–77.

CDC. (2010). Growth Charts. Centers for Disease Control and Prevention. Retrieved from: <http://www.cdc.gov.growthcharts/cdc_chart.htm> Accessed October 2015.

Chauhan, G. S., Eskin, N. A. M., & Tkachuk, R. (1992). Nutrients and antinutrients in quinoa seed. *Cereal Chemistry*, 69(1), 85–88.

Clark, M. (2004). Fit to eat: The healthiest foods, and how to prepare and enjoy them. *Martha Stewart Living*, October 2004.

CPTS. (2006). Empresa: Andean Valley. Centro de Promoción de Tecnologías Sostenibles. Estudio de Caso PML 29:1–8.

Cusack, D. F. (1984). Quinua: Grain of the Incas. *Ecologist*, 14(1), 21–31.

De Bruin, A. (1964). Investigation of the food value of quinoa and cañihua seed. *Journal of Food Science*, 29, 872–876.

De Vincenzi, M., Silano, M., Luchetti, R., Carratù, B., Boniglia, C., & Pogna, N. E. (1999). Agglutinating activity of alcohol-soluble proteins from quinoa seed flour in celiac disease. *Plant Foods for Human Nutrition*, 54(2), 93–100.

Egeland, T. (2005). Oprah and quinoa! Communication Connection Issue #171, May 6, 2005. Retrieved from: <http://agapps16.agric.gov.ab.ca/$department/newslett.nsf/all/con7272> Accessed June 2005.

FAIR. (2000). Ancient grain becomes biotech snack. Cooperative Research Measures, Anglesey North Wales, UK. FAIR-CT96-9506 July 2000.

Fairbanks, D. J., Burgener, K. W., Robinson, L. R., Andersen, W. R., & Ballon, E. (1990). Electrophoretic characterization of quinoa seed proteins. *Plant Breeding*, 104(3), 190–195.

FAO. (2011). Quinoa: An ancient drop to contribute to world food security. Retrieved from: <www.fao.org/docrep/017/aq287e/aq287e.pdf> Accessed July 2015.

FAO. (2013a). International year of quinoa: A future sown thousands of years ago. Retrieved from: <http://www.fao.org/quinoa-2013/en> Accessed October 2015.

FAO. (2013b). Food and Nutrition Paper 92. Dietary protein quality evaluation in human nutrition. Report of an FAO Expert Consultation March 31-April 2, 2011.

FAO-FAOSTAT. (2013). Retrieved from: <http://faostat3.fao.org/faostat-gateway/g/to/home/E/> Accessed October 2015.

Föste, M., Elgeti, D., Brunner, A.-K., Jekle, M., & Becker, T. (2015). Isolation of quinoa protein by milling fractionation and solvent extraction. *Food and Bioproducts Processing*, *96*, 20–26.

Frank, J. (2014). Ancient grains in depth. Prospector. November 7, 2014. Retrieved from: <http://knowledge.ulprospector.com/1122/fbn-ancient-grains-amaranth-quinoa/> Accessed October 2015.

Fuentes, F., & Paredes-Gonzalez, X. (2015). Nutraceutical perspectives of quinoa: Biological properties and functional applications. Chapter 3.5. In D. Bazile, D. Bertero, & C. Nieto (Eds.), *State of the art report of quinoa in the world in 2013* (pp. 287–299). Rome: FAO & CIRAD.

FVU. (2015). Quinoa beyond the hype. January 7, 2015. Retrieved from: <http://www.foodvalleyupdate.com/news/quinoa-beyond-the-hype/> Accessed October 2015.

Galwey, N. W., Leakey, C. L. A., Herrera, J., Price, K. R., & Fenwick, G. R. (1990). Chemical composition and nutritional characteristics of quinoa (*Chenopodium quinoa* Willd.). *Food Science and Nutrition*, *42*, 245–261.

Gonzalez, J. A., Konishi, Y., Bruno, M., Valoy, M., & Prado, F. E. (2012). Interrelationships among seed yield, total protein and amino acid composition of ten quinoa (*Chenopodium quinoa*) cultivars from two different agroecological regions. *Journal of the Science of Food and Agriculture*, *92*, 1222–1229.

Graf, B. L., Rojas-Silva, P., Rojo, L. E., Delatorre-Herrera, J., Baldeon, M. E., & Raskin, I. (2015). Innovations in health value and functional food development of quinoa (*Chenopodium quinoa* Willd.). *Comprehensive Reviews in Food Science and Food Safety*, *14*, 431–449.

Heng, L. (2005). *Flavour aspects of pea and its protein preparations in relation to novel protein foods (PhD Thesis)*. Wageningen: Wageningen University, ISBN 90-8504-198-8.

Innova Database. (2015). Number of products in United States containing quinoa. Date published between 01/2005 and 12/2014. Retrieved from: <http://www.innovadatabase.com> Accessed June 2015.

Jacobsen, S.-E. (2003). The world potential for quinoa (*Chenopodium quinoa* Willd.). *Food Reviews International*, *19*(1), 167–177.

Jacobsen, S.-E., Mujica, A., & Jensen, C. R. (2003). The resistance of quinoa (*Chenopodium quinoa* Willd.) to adverse abiotic factors. *Food Reviews International*, *19*, 99–109.

Koziol, M. J. (1991). Afrosimetric estimation of threshold saponin concentration for bitterness in quinoa (*Chenopodium quinoa* Willd). *Journal of the Science of Food and Agriculture*, *54*, 211–219.

Koziol, M. J. (1992). Chemical composition and nutritional evaluation of quinoa (*Chenopodium quinoa* Willd.). *Journal of Food Composition and Analysis*, *5*, 35–68.

Lamothe, L. M., Srichuwong, S., Reuhs, B. L., & Hamaker, B. R. (2015). Quinoa (*Chenopodium quinoa* Willd.) and amaranth (*Amaranthus caudatus* L.) provide dietary fibres high in pectic substances and xyloglucans. *Food Chemistry*, *167*, 490–496.

Lindeboom, N. (2005). *Studies on the characterization, biosynthesis and isolation of starch and protein from quinoa* (Chenopodium quinoa *Willd.) (Thesis)*. Saskatoon: Department of Applied Microbiology and Food Science, University of Saskatchewan.

Lopez de Romaña, G., Creed, H. M., & Graham, G. G. (1978). "Alimentos comunes" peruanos. Tolerancia y digestibilidad en infantes desnutridos. *Archivos Latinoamericanos de Nutrición*, *28*, 419–433.

Lopez de Romaña, G., Graham, G. G., Rojas, M., & MacLean, W. C. (1981). Digestibilidad y calidad proteínica de la quinua: Estudio comparativo, en niños, entre semilla y harina de quinua. *Archivos Latinoamericanos de Nutrición*, *31*, 485–497.

Lorenz, K., & Nyanzi, F. (1989). Enzyme activities in quinoa (*Chenopodium quinoa*). *International Journal of Food Science and Technology*, *24*, 543–555.

Mahoney, A. W., Lopez, J. G., & Hendriks, D. G. (1975). An evaluation of the protein quality of quinoa. *Journal of Agricultural and Food Chemistry*, *23*(2), 190–193.

MarketWatch Press Release. (2015). Kashi joins Andean Naturals to help Light-A-Community in rural Bolivia. Published October 7, 2015 8:00 a.m. E.T. Retrieved from: <http://www.marketwatch.com/story/kashi-joins-andean-naturals-to-help-light-a-community-in-rural-bolivia-2015-10-07> Accessed October 2015.

Martinez, C. (1946). *La Quinua. Divulgacion Botanica. Agricola y de Utilizacion Industrial y Culinaria*. Lima: Direccion de Agricultura. Ministerio de Agricultura.

McLaughlin, K. (2005). Eating around: Quinoa.. *The Wall Street Journal*, March 31 2005.

Mekonnen, A. A., & Hoekstra, A. Y. (2012). A global assessment of the water footprint of farm animal products. *Ecosystems*, *15*, 401–415.

Miranda, M., Vega-Galvez, A., Martinez, E., Lopez, J., Rodriguez, M. J., Henriquez, K., & Fuentes, F. (2012). Genetic diversity and comparison of physiochemical and nutritional characteristics of six quinoa *(Chenopodium quinoa* Willd.) genotypes cultivated in Chile. *Ciene Technology Aliment Campinas*, *32*(4), 835–843.

Mohamed, A. M., Wolf, W., & Spiess, W. E. L. (2000). Recovery and characterization of *Balanites aegyptiaca* Del. kernel proteins. Effect of defatting, air classification, wet sieving and aqueous ethanol treatment on solubility, digestibility, amino acid composition and sapogenin content. *Nahrung*, *44*(1), 7–12.

Moreno, F. J., & Clemente, A. (2008). 2S Albumin storage proteins: What makes them food allergens? *The Open Biochemistry Journal, 2,* 16−28.

Nascimento, A. C., Mota, C., Coelho, I., Gueifáo, S., Santos, M., Matos, A. S., ... Castanheira, I. (2014). Characterization of nutrient profile of quinoa (*Chenopodium quinoa*), amaranth (*Amaranthus caudatus*), and purple corn (*Zea mays* L.) consumed in the north of Argentina: Proximates, minerals, and trace elements. *Food Chemistry, 148,* 420−426.

Neff, C. (2003). Carrot quinoa. O, The Oprah Magazine. January 2003. Retrieved from: <http://www.oprah.com/foodhome/food/recipes/food_20021217_quinoa.jhtml> Accessed June 2014.

NFM (2004). *Hot new product trends issue for 2005. The Natural Foods Merchandiser Magazine.* Boulder, CO: New Hope Natural Media, October 2014.

Núñez de Arco, S. (2015). Quinoa's calling. In K. Murphy, & J. Matanguihan (Eds.), *Quinoa: Improvements and sustainable production* (pp. 211−226). Hoboken, NJ: John Wiley & Sons, Inc.

Oelke, E.A., Putnam, D.H., Teynor, T.M., & Oplinger, E.S. (1992). Quinoa. In: Alternative field crops manual. Retrieved from: <http://newcrop.hort.purdue.edu/newcrop/afcm/quinoa.html/> Accessed October 2015.

Ogungbenle, H. (2003). Nutritional evaluation and functional properties of quinoa (*Chenopodium quinoa*) flour. *International Journal of Food Sciences and Nutrition, 54,* 153−158.

OMAFRA (2015). *Specialty cropportunities, a resource for specialty crop growers: Quinoa.* Canada: Ontario Ministry of Agriculture Food and Rural Affairs. Retrieved from: <http://www.omafra.gov.on.ca/CropOp/en/field_grain/spec_grains/quin.html/> Accessed October 2015.

Osborne, T. En (1924). *The vegetable proteins* (2nd ed.). New York, NY: Longmans y Green.

Oshodi, A. A., Ogungbenle, H. N., & Oladimeji, M. O. (1999). Chemical composition, nutritionally valuable and functional properties of benniseed (*Sesamum radiatum*), pearl millet (*Pennisetum typhoides*) and quinoa (*Chenopodium quinoa*) flours. *International Journal of Food Sciences and Nutrition, 50*(5), 325−331.

Piva, G., Brasse, C., & Mehinagic, E. (2015). Quinoa d'Anjou: The beginning of a French quinoa sector. Chapter 6.1.2. In D. Bazile, D. Bertero, & C. Nieto (Eds.), *State of the art report of quinoa in the world in 2013* (pp. 447−453). Rome: FAO & CIRAD.

Posnansky, A. (1945). Kinoa (Quinoa). *Boletin de la sociedad. Geografica de La Paz,* , 98−107.

Prakash, D., & Pal, M. (1998). *Chenopodium*: Seed protein, fractionation and amino acid composition. *International Journal of Food Sciences and Nutrition, 49*(4), 271−275.

Prego, I., Maldonado, S., & Otegui, M. (1998). Seed structure and localization of reserves in *Chenopodium quinoa. Annals of Botany, 82*(4), 481−488.

Quiroga, C., Escalera, R., Aroni, G., Bonifacio, A., González, J. A., Villca, M., ... Ruiz, A. (2015). Traditional processes and technological innovations in quinoa harvesting, processing and industrialization. Chapter 3.1. In D. Bazile, D. Bertero, & C. Nieto (Eds.), *State of the art report of quinoa in the world in 2013* (pp. 218−249). Rome: FAO & CIRAD.

Reale, A., 2003. Art de vivre: Le quinoa, vieux comme les Incas. France-Amerique. October, p. 25.

Reichert, R. D., Tatarynovich, J. T., & Tyler, R. T. (1986). Abrasive dehulling of quinoa (*Chenopodium quinoa*): Effect on saponin content as determined by an adapted hemolytic assay. *Cereal Chemistry, 63*(6), 471−475.

Repo-Carrasco, R., Espinoza, C., & Jacobsen, S.-E. (2003). Nutritional value and use of the Andean crops quinoa (*Chenopodium quinoa* Willd.) and kañiwa (*Chenopodium pallidicaule*). *Food Reviews International, 19,* 179−189.

Ríos, M. L. T., Sgarbieri, V. C., & Amaya, J. (1978). Chemical and biological evaluation of quinoa (*Chenopodium quinoa* Willd.). Effect of extracting the saponins by heat treatment. *Archivos Latinoamericanos de Nutrición, 28,* 253−263.

Rojas, W. (2011). La quinua: Cultivo milenario para contribuir a la seguridad alimentaria mundial. Santiago, FAO, Oficina Regional para America Latina y el Caribe.

Romero, J.A. (1981). Evaluación de las características físicas, químicas y biológicas de ocho variedades de quinua (*Chenopodium quinoa* Willd.). Thesis. Instituto de Nutrición de Centro America y Panamá, Facultad de Ciencias Químicas y Farmacia. Quinoa Universidad de San Carlos de Guatemala, Guatemala.

Ruales, J., de Grijalva, Y., Lopez-Jaramillo, P., & Nair, B. M. (2002). The nutritional quality of an infant food from quinoa and its effect on the plasma level of insulin-like growth factor-1 (IGF-1) in undernourished children. *International Journal of Food Science and Technology, 53,* 143−154.

Ruales, J., & Nair, B. M. (1993). Content of fat, vitamins and minerals in quinoa (*Chenopodium quinoa,* Willd) seeds. *Food Chemistry, 48*(2), 131−136.

Ruales, J., & Nair, B. M. (1994). Effect of processing on in vitro digestibility of protein and starch in quinoa seeds. *International Journal of Food Science and Technology, 29,* 449−456.

Ruiz, G.A., Xiao, W., van Boekel, M., Stieger, M., & Minor, M. (2015). Effect of extraction pH on yield, denaturation properties and functionality of quinoa protein (*Chenopodium quinoa* Willd). Submitted for publication.

Ruiz, K. B., Biondi, S., Oses, R., Acuña-Rodríguez, I. S., Antognoni, F., Martinez-Mosqueira, E. A., ... Molina-Montenegro, M. A. (2014). Quinoa biodiversity and sustainability for food security under climate change: A review. *Agronomy for Sustainable Development, 34,* 349−359.

Scanlin, L., & Stone, M. (2009). Quinoa Protein Concentrate, Production, and Functionality. U.S. Patent No.:7,563,473 B2. Issued July 21, 2009.

Scarpati De Briceño, Z., & Briceño, P. O. (1980). Evaluación de la composición química y nutricional de algunas entradas de quinua (*Chenopodium quinoa,* Willd.) del banco de germoplasma de la Universidad Técnica del Altiplano. *Anales Cientificos, 18,* 125−143.

Simmons, M. (2005). The new carbs: Flavor-packed whole grain recipes banish fat, boost health. *Prevention,* May 2005

Tang, Y., Li, X., Chen, P. X., Zhang, B., Hernandez, M., Zhang, H., ... Tsao, R. (2015). Characterization of fatty acid, carotenoid, tocopherol/tocotrienol compositions and antioxidant activities in seeds of three *Chenopodium quinoa* Willd. genotypes. *Food Chemistry, 174*, 502−508.

Tapia (2015). The long journey of quinoa: Who wrote its history? Foreword. In D. Bazile, D. Bertero, & C. Nieto (Eds.), *State of the art report of quinoa in the world in 2013* (pp. 3−9). Rome: FAO & CIRAD.

Taylor, J., & Parker, M. (2002). Quinoa. In P. S. Belton, & J. Taylor (Eds.), *Pseudocereals and less common cereals* (pp. 93−122). Berlin Heidelberg: Springer-Verlag.

Troisi, J., Di Fiore, R., Pulvento, C., D'andria, R., Vega-Gálvez, A., Miranda, M., ... Lavini, A. (2015). Saponins. Chapter 3.3. In D. Bazile, D. Bertero, & C. Nieto (Eds.), *State of the art report of quinoa in the world in 2013* (pp. 267−277). Rome: FAO & CIRAD.

USDA. (2015). National Nutrient Database for Standard Reference Release 27. Retrieved from: <www.ndb.nal.usda.gov/ndb> Accessed September 2015.

USDA-FAS. (2014). Peru: Quinoa outlook. USDA Foreign Agricultural Service GAIN Report. December 23, 2014.

Valdez, C., & Bajak, F. (2014). Influx of cheap Peruvian quinoa riles Bolivia. Retrieved from: <http://bigstory.ap.org/article/c66b7261e15a484a-b661e14c9d97f17d/influx-cheap-peruvian-quinoa-riles-bolivia> Accessed October 2015.

Varriano-Marston, E., & DeFrancisco, A. (1984). Ultrastructure of quinoa fruit (*Chenopodium quinoa* Willd.). *Food Microstructure, 3*, 165−173.

Vega-Gálvez, A., Miranda, M., Vergara, J., Uribe, E., Puente, L., & Martínez, E. A. (2010). Nutrition facts and functional potential of quinoa (*Chenopodium quinoa* Willd.), an ancient Andean grain: A review. *Journal of the Science of Food and Agriculture, 90*, 2541−2547.

Vidueiros, S. M., Curti, R. N., Dyner, L. M., Binaghi, M. J., Peterson, G., Bertero, H. D., & Pallaro, A. N. (2015). Diversity and interrelationships in nutritional traits cultivated in quinoa (*Chenopodium quinoa* Willd.) from northwest Argentina. *Journal of Cereal Science, 62*, 87−93.

Weber, E. J. (1978). The Inca's ancient answer to food shortage. *Nature, 272*, 486.

WGC. (2015a). Quinoa—March Grain of the Month. Whole Grains Council. Retrieved from: <http://wholegrainscouncil.org/whole-grains-101/quinoa-march-grain-of-the-month> Accessed September 2015.

WGC. (2015b). Whole Grains 101: Definition of Whole Grains. Whole Grains Council. Retrieved from: <http://www.wholegrainscouncil.org/whole-grains-101/definition-of-whole-grains> Accessed September 2015.

White, P. L., Alvistur, E., Días, C., Viñas, E., White, H. S., & Collazos, C. (1955). Nutrient content and protein quality of quinoa and cañihua, edible seed products of the Andes Mountains. *Journal of Agricultural and Food Chemistry, 3*(6), 531−534.

Winkel, T., Álvarez-Flores, R., Bommel, P., Bourliaud, J., Chevarría, L. M., Cortes, G., ... Vieira, P. M. (2015). The southern Altiplano of Bolivia. Chapter 5.1.b. In D. Bazile, D. Bertero, & C. Nieto (Eds.), *State of the art report of quinoa in the world in 2013* (pp. 362−377). Rome: FAO & CIRAD.

Wright, K. H., Pike, O. A., Fairbanks, D. J., & Huber, C. S. (2002). Composition of *Atriplex hortensis*, sweet and bitter *Chenopodium quinoa* seeds. *Journal of Food Science, 67*(4), 1383−1385.

Zevallos, V. F., Herencia, L. I., Chang, F., Donnelly, S., Ellis, H. J., & Ciclitira, P. J. (2014). Gastrointestinal effects of eating quinoa (*Chenopodium quinoa* Willd.) in celiac patients. *The American Journal of Gastroenterology, 109*, 270−278.

Chapter 15

Amaranth Part 1—Sustainable Crop for the 21st Century: Food Properties and Nutraceuticals for Improving Human Health

D. Orona-Tamayo[1] and O. Paredes-López[1,2]

[1]Centro de Investigación y de Estudios Avanzados del IPN, Irapuato, Mexico, [2]Université Pierre et Marie Curie, Paris, France

15.1 INTRODUCTION

The genus *Amaranthus* (L.) belongs to the order of the Caryophyllales and the Amaranthacea family and includes C4 dicotyledonous herbaceous plants (Mlakar, Turinek, Jakop, Bavec, & Bavec, 2010; Sauer, 1967). Amaranth has some agronomic advantages including fast growth and some resistance and tolerance to extreme conditions and poor soils. Amaranth plants have a remarkable ability to adapt to disadvantageous growing conditions such as low-nutrient soil, sand, a wide range of temperature, and irradiation. Its tolerance to different stresses constitutes the potential use of amaranth as a nutritious green crop in semiarid regions (Myers, 1996). Even soils with an excess of inorganic salts as a result of drought and heat (Ebert, 2014) may enable and lead to amaranth adaptability, cultivation, and production. Physiologically, amaranth exhibits a high capacity of osmotic adjustment to ensure different functions in severe drought conditions (Liu & Stützel, 2002); amaranth plants are able to control transpiration water loss by reducing leaf expansion and thereby preventing the dehydration of leaf tissues (Liu & Stützel, 2004). This sustainability of amaranth may derive in production of seeds and young leaves in poor agricultural areas of developing societies, with high contents of proteins, vitamins, and minerals for human consumption (Omamt, Hammes, & Robbertse, 2006; Paredes-López, 1994). The Amaranthacea family is composed by 70 genera and 85 species which are able to grow and produce in wild environments, whose continuous expansion is taking place worldwide (Montoya-Rodríguez, Gómez-Favela, Reyes-Moreno, Milán-Carrillo, & González de Mejía, 2015; Stallknecht & Schulz-Schaeffer, 1993).

Amaranths are widely distributed in temperate and tropical regions of the world but, according to Sauer (1950), the three main amaranth species that produce grain are natives of the New World. *Amaranthus hypochondriacus* is native to the northwestern and central area of Mexico, *Amaranthus caudatus* is native to the Andes, and *Amaranthus cruentus* is from southern Mexico and the central region of Guatemala. However, the cultivable species can be derived from cosmopolitan weeds such as *Amaranthus retroflexus*, *Amaranthus hybridus*, *Amaranthus powellii*, *Amaranthus spinosus*, and *Amaranthus viridis* (Martínez-Cruz, Cabrera-Chávez, & Paredes-López, 2014). It has been hypothesized that three cultivable amaranth species were domesticated directly in different regions and derived from their wild species: *A. hypochondriacus* from *A. powellii*, *A. caudatus* from *Amaranthus quitensis*, and *A. cruentus* from *A. hybridus* (Mallory et al., 2008; Xu & Sun, 2001). In Mexico, the Aztec civilization used *A. hypochondriacus* as one of the basic foods in its diets, and Mayan and Incan civilizations in Peru used *A. cruentus* and *A. caudatus*, respectively, as staple foods (Pavlik, 2011). These civilizations used the amaranth in beverages, sauces mixed with maize flour to prepare tortillas, medicinal treatments, and they also used the plant and grains for religious practices (Mlakar et al., 2010). However, because of the similarity between the Spanish religion (Catholic) and the Native American communion ritual, the Spaniards banned the cultivation and uses of amaranth, ignoring its nutritional and agricultural features (Kauffman, 1992; Mlakar et al., 2010; Rastogi & Shukla, 2013).

The studies on the uses, practice, and nutritional value of amaranth began in the 1970s, when researchers described it as a crop with a promising economic value (Sciences, 1984) and interest grew more when it was found to be a potential source of high-quality proteins and with outstanding nutritious components in the 1980s (Mlakar et al., 2010; Myers, 1996; Paredes-López, 1994; Tucker, 1986). However, in the last 20 years amaranth grain has gained more interest by different types of researches (Martínez-Cruz et al., 2014; Montoya-Rodríguez et al., 2015). Amaranth is considered a pseudocereal with higher protein concentration than the three most important staple cereals, rice, wheat, and maize, which contribute with more than half of the total protein at the global level (Table 15.1; FAO, 2009). In addition, amaranth has a higher amount of lysine, dietary fiber, important content of calcium and iron than these grains (Venskutonis & Kraujalis, 2013). As a result, this plant has become an important crop which is now being cultivated in several regions and countries of the world including South America, Africa, India, China, and the United States (Aguilar et al., 2013).

15.2 NUTRITIONAL COMPONENTS IN AMARANTH

Nowadays, consumers seek and demand foods with important attributes, such as high nutritive value, rich in good-quality proteins, and nutraceutical compounds. Amaranth is considered a multipurpose grain with high nutritional quality (Venskutonis & Kraujalis, 2013). The approximate composition of seed flour from the three main amaranth species is shown in Table 15.2. The amaranth grain contains highly digestible proteins (approximately 90%) with good levels of essential amino acids; its balance being close to the optimum required in the human diet (FAO, 1973, 2011). Depending on the species, the total protein content ranges from 13.2% to 18.4% (Segura-Nieto, Barba De La Rosa, & Paredes-López, 1994). Amaranth proteins are rich in lysine (3.2–13.1 g/100 g protein) and the sulfur amino acids (cysteine and methionine in the ranges of 2.0–3.8 and 0.6–2.4 g/100 g protein, respectively) (Awasthi, Kumar, Singh, & Thakur, 2011; Mlakar et al., 2010; Písaříkováet al., 2005; Saunders & Becker, 1984; Schmidt, 1977; Segura-Nieto et al., 1994). The essential amino acids from different amaranth grains are shown in Table 15.3. Regarding fiber content, amaranth seeds have high fiber values (2.2–5.8%) which may vary depending of the species (Repo-Carrasco-

TABLE 15.1 Proximate Composition of Amaranth and Three Important Cereals

Compound	Amaranth	Corn	Rice	Wheat
Protein (%)	17.9	10.3	8.5	14.0
Fat (%)	7.7	4.5	2.1	2.1
Fiber (%)	2.2	2.3	0.9	2.6
Ash (%)	4.1	1.4	1.4	1.9
Carbohydrates (%)	57.0	67.7	75.4	66.9

Percentage in dry weight basis.
Adapted from Segura-Nieto, M., Barba De La Rosa, A., & Paredes-López, O. (1994). Biochemistry of amaranth proteinsin. In O. Paredes-López (Ed.), Amaranth: Biology, chemistry and technology (pp. 75–106). Boca Raton, FL: CRC Press.

TABLE 15.2 Proximate Composition of the Main Amaranth Seed Species

Compound	A. hypochondriacus	A. cruentus	A. caudatus
Protein (%)	17.9	13.2–18.2	17.6–18.4
Fat (%)	7.7	6.3–8.1	6.9–8.1
Fiber (%)	2.2	3.6–4.4	3.2–5.8
Ash (%)	4.1	2.8–3.9	3.1–4.4

Percentage in dry weight basis.
Adapted from Segura-Nieto, M., Barba De La Rosa, A., & Paredes-López, O. (1994). Biochemistry of amaranth proteinsin. In O. Paredes-López (Ed.), Amaranth: Biology, chemistry and technology (pp. 75–106). Boca Raton, FL: CRC Press.

TABLE 15.3 Amino Acid Composition of Different Amaranth Species

Amino Acid	A. caudatus (g/100 g Protein) (Del Valle et al., 1993)	A. caudatus (g/100 g Protein) (Saunders & Becker, 1984)	A. cruentus (g/100 g Protein) (Schmidt, 1977)	A. cruentus (g/100 g Protein) (Escudero, De Arellano, Luco, Gimenez, & Mucciarelli, 2004)	A. hypochondriacus (g/100 g Protein) (Saunders & Becker, 1984)	A. hypochondriacus (g/100 g Protein) (Písaříková et al., 2005)
Isoleucine	3.6	3.6	3.7	4.8	2.8	3.8
Leucine	5.7	5.9	5.9	9.2	5.0	6.9
Lysine	4.8	5.7	5.8	13.1	3.2	8.0
Sulfure amino acids	4.5			5.7		5.2
Cysteine		2.3	3.8		2.0	2.9
Methionine		2.4	1.6		0.6	2.3
Aromatic amino acids	7.2			10.0		
Phenylalanine		3.4	4.5		3.8	
Tyrosine		2.8	4.0		3.1	
Threonine	3.3	3.8	4.2	4.3	2.6	4.5
Tryptophan	1.1	1.1		2.8	3.1	
Valine	4.5	4.1	4.3	5.1	3.2	5.3
Histidine				4.0		1.7
Arginine				13.2		14.5
Alanine				5.4		6.2
Aspartic acid				11.3		10.7
Glutamic acid				22.8		17.7
Glycine				10.7		15.2
Proline				5.9		3.7
Serine				8.6		9.3
Met + Cys		4.7	5.4		2.6	5.2
Phe + Tyr		6.2	8.5		6.9	

Essential amino acids are in bold.
Adapted from Venskutonis, P. R., & Kraujalis, P. (2013). Nutritional components of amaranth seeds and vegetables: A review on composition, properties, and uses. *Comprehensive Reviews in Food Science and Food Safety, 12,* 381–412.

Valencia, Peña, Kallio, & Salminen, 2009; Segura-Nieto et al., 1994; Singhal & Kulkarni, 1988). The lipid content is reported as between 1.9% and 13% (Alvarez-Jubete, Arendt, & Gallagher, 2010; Caselato-Sousa & Amaya-Farfán, 2012; Segura-Nieto et al., 1994); the main fatty acids found in *Amaranthus* grain species are palmitic (19.1−23.4%), oleic (18.7−38.9%), and linoleic (36.7−55.9%) acids. Linoleic acid is the most abundant and other fatty acids are found in lower concentrations (He, Cai, Sun, & Corke, 2002). Carbohydrates are the principal constituent of amaranth grain and starch is the main compound in this fraction (57−62.0%; Alvarez-Jubete et al., 2010; Paredes-López, Barba De La Rosa, & Cárabez-Trejo, 1990), followed by sucrose as the major sugar, raffinose, glucose, fructose, staquiose, maltose, and inositol are present in low concentrations (Becker et al., 1981). Amaranth starch has been classified as a waxy-type due to its prominent amylopectin content which confers useful and unique applications such as high viscosity and gelatinization at high temperatures (Bello-Pérez & Paredes-López, 2009; López, Bello-Pérez, & Paredes-López, 1994). Other important valuable bioactive compounds in amaranth grains include phenolic acids, flavonoids, anthocyanins, tannins, and phytosterols (Alvarez-Jubete et al., 2010; Pasko, Sajewicz, Gorinstein, & Zachwieja, 2008; Repo-Carrasco-Valencia et al., 2009). Amaranth grains are also a good source of minerals such as Ca, Fe, Mg, Mn, K, P, and Na, and high concentration of B complex vitamins (Alvarez-Jubete et al., 2010; Ferreira & Areas, 2010; Gamel, Linssen, Mesallam, Damir, & Shekib, 2006).

15.3 AMARANTH PROTEINS AND AMINO ACIDS FOR HUMAN NUTRITION

Amaranth grains are a good source of high-quality proteins including an excellent amino acid balance, making it a valuable plant material for human nourishment and the food industry (Venskutonis & Kraujalis, 2013). Amaranth proteins are mainly storage macromolecules with some features of legumin-like proteins (Tovar-Pérez, Guerrero-Legarreta, Farrés-González, & Soriano-Santos, 2009), and according to their solubility (Osborne's method) they are classified as albumins soluble in water, globulins soluble in high-salt concentrations, and prolamins soluble in aqueous alcohol and glutelins soluble in acid or alkaline solutions (Osborne, 1924). Globulins and glutelins are the main protein fractions and comprise over 50% of the total seed proteins, followed by albumins and prolamins (Table 15.4) (Paredes-López, Mora-Escobedo, & Ordorica-Falomir, 1988; Vasco-Méndez & Paredes-López, 1994). Amaranth grains also contain other important proteins involved in important metabolic pathways that derive in mechanisms of seed formation and protection (Montoya-Rodríguez et al., 2015).

Seed proteins generally serve as storage biomolecules providing nutrients during germination and to the growing plant (Fukushima, 1991). For many years, seed albumins were considered as "housekeeping proteins" or enzymes (Vasco-Méndez & Paredes-López, 1994). Albumins are defined by their solubility in water or in low ionic-strength solutions (Silva-Sáchez, González-Castañeda, De León-Rodríguez, & Barba de la Rosa, 2004). Amaranth albumins have low sedimentation patterns and are integrated by two components, one group of 1.4S−2S as the major and 4.6S proteins are the minor component (Oszvald et al., 2009). The main set of albumins sediment between 1.4S and 2S and consists of polypeptides with molecular masses of 4−20 kDa, respectively (Mora-Escobedo, Paredes-López, & Ordorica-Falomir, 1990; Mylne, Hara-Nishimura, & Rosengren, 2014; Segura-Nieto et al., 1994). The 1.7S (1.4−2S) albumins are one of the major groups of polypeptides in the amaranth grain, they are similar to some oil seed albumins (Bashir et al., 1998; Lavine & Ben-Shoshan, 2015; Moreno & Clemente, 2008; Shewry, Casey, & Pandya, 1999). These proteins have high polymorphism, typical of albumin 2S storage proteins, showing a compact structure due to disulfide

TABLE 15.4 Main Storage Protein Fractions of Amaranth Species

Protein Fraction	A. caudatus	A. caudatus	A. cruentus	A. cruentus	A. hypochondriacus	A. hypochondriacus	A. hypochondriacus
Albumin (%)	6.7	8.7	9.7	8.1	8.5	8.2	8.9
Globulin (%)	41.9	39.3	47.5	40.9	38.5	33.3	43.7
Prolamin (%)	8.5	6.9	9.2	8.9	9.1	7.1	7.5
Glutelin (%)	21.1	26.8	26.6	20.5	29.1	22.1	21.5

Percentage in dry weight basis.
Adapted from Bressani, R., & Garcia-Vela, L. A. (1990). Protein fractions in amaranth grain and their chemical characterization. *Journal of Agricultural and Food Chemistry, 38*, 1205−1209.

bonds which confer stability under hard conditions (Moreno & Clemente, 2008). 2S albumins are rich in methionine and are called 2MRP (methionine-rich proteins) with a molecular weight of 18 kDa; amaranth presents a group of 2S polypeptide with 16–18% methionine content (Segura-Nieto et al., 1994).

Globulins constitute the principal protein fraction from the amaranth isolates (Barba de la Rosa, Gueguen, Paredes-López, & Viroben, 1992). Currently, there are two main classes of globulins based on sedimentation coefficient designed globulin 11S and 7S. 11S globulin, also called amarantin (ie, legumin), is a protein with a molecular mass between 300 and 400 kDa and composed of six subunits with molecular masses of 50–60 kDa (Barba de la Rosa, Herrera-Estrella, Utsumi, & Paredes-López, 1996). These subunits are formed by an acidic polypeptide (27–40 kDa) and a basic polypeptide (20–25 kDa) linked together with disulfide bonds (Wright, 1987). Vicilins or 7S globulin are formed by four subunits between 66, 52, 38, and 16 kDa and together compose a polypeptide between 150 and 200 kDa (Quiroga, Martínez, Rogniaux, Geairon, & Añón, 2010; Wright, 1987). Garcia-Gonzalez, Flores-Vazquez, Barba de la Rosa, Vazquez-Martinez, and Ruiz-Garcia (2013) showed that the 7S globulin is characterized by a trimeric organization, consisting of nonidentical subunits, α of 57–68 kDa, α′ of 57–72 kDa, and β of 42–52 kDa; these 7S globulins are N-glycosylated and lack disulfide bridges joining their subunits (Marcone, 1999b; Quiroga et al., 2010). The 11S globulin proteins are found in the seeds of mono- and dicotyledonous plants such as rice, oat, sesame, rape, quinoa, pumpkin, and soybean (Brinegar & Goundan, 1993; Hara-Nishimura, Nishimura, & Akazawa, 1985; Liu et al., 2007; Shotwell, Afonso, Davies, Chesnut, & Larkins, 1988; Tai, Lee, Tsai, Yiu, & Tzen, 2001; Yano, Wong, Cho, & Buchanan, 2001), while 7S proteins are present in legumes (Fukushima, 1991; Shewry & Halford, 2002). In terms of essential amino acids, globulins are relatively rich in lysine (3.7–7.6%), compared to other important cereal and legume globulins (Barba de la Rosa et al., 1992; Bressani & Garcia-Vela, 1990; Gorinstein et al., 2002; Marcone, Kakuda, & Yada, 1998; Peterson, 1978); amaranth globulins show good levels of sulfur amino acids (3.1–7.1%) (Segura-Nieto et al., 1994). In examination of amino acid profiles of the isolated amaranth 7S/11S globulins, 7S globulins showed lower levels of tryptophan and methionine (0.23–0.59% and 0.3–0.7%, respectively), with respect to other important and essential amino acids. Although 7S globulins of amaranth were found substantially low in lysine (3.0–3.7%), histidine (1.3–1.7%), phenylalanine (4.8–5.0%), valine (5.2–5.8%), and isoleucine (5.5–6.8%), the 11S globulins contain more essential amino acids, such as methionine and tryptophan (1.77% and 1.6%, respectively). The 11S globulins of amaranth are also reported to have high levels of lysine (4.25%), histidine (2.62%), phenylalanine (6.78%), and valine (6.3%) and low amounts of isoleucine (5.0%) (Marcone, 1999a). Reported amino acid levels of amaranth are similar to those of 7S and 11S globulins from different plants seeds (Derbyshire, Wright, & Boulter, 1976) and suggest that the 11S globulins may have superior nutritive and nutraceutical value to 7S globulins.

Prolamin fractions occur in low concentration in amaranth grains and have few polypeptides. Depending on the protocol of extraction and the amaranth species, four main components can be detected in the prolamin fraction; two polypeptides with 18 and 22 kDa and another two polypeptides between 10 and 12 kDa (Segura-Nieto et al., 1994). Barba de la Rosa et al. (1992) reported that amaranth grain prolamins with disulfide bonds intact, separate into α (high molecular weight), β (94 kDa), and γ (a doublet having main bands of 67–60 kDa and 94 kDa). Upon reduction of S–S bonds of prolamins with 2-ME, five polypeptides of 67, 38, 35, 26, and 24 kDa can be visualized. Leyva-Lopez, Vasco, de la Rosa, and Paredes-López (1995) support these results, because the pattern of prolamins changes depending on the treatment with organic solvents to defat the amaranth flour and in fact when the hexane is used, the prolamin proteins show high-molecular-weight bands; otherwise, with acetone the prolamins show mainly bands of low molecular weight. In relation to amino acids, prolamins of cereals such as maize and rice are normally deficient of lysine and tryptophan (Rascón-Cruz, Sinagawa-García, Osuna-Castro, Bohorova, & Paredes-López, 2004). Prolamins from amaranth grains show relatively high values of essential amino acids such as leucine (5.5–10.0%) and threonine (3.1–7.2%) but lysine is not as high (6.7%) as the phenylalanine (9.0%) (Barba de la Rosa et al., 1992; Bressani & Garcia-Vela, 1990; Segura-Nieto et al., 1994).

Glutelins are quantitatively the second most important protein fraction in amaranth seeds; these are storage-aggregated proteins and are only soluble in alkaline or acidic solutions (Paredes-López, Mendoza, & Mora, 1993; Tovar-Pérez et al., 2009; Vasco-Méndez & Paredes-López, 1994). Native amaranth glutelins are made up of six main sets of polypeptides, two of them corresponding to 55–67 kDa, two between 35–38 kDa and two corresponding to 22–23 kDa (Barba de la Rosa et al., 1992, 2010; Vasco-Méndez & Paredes-López, 1994). The amino acid composition of glutelins shows high leucine (5.9–10.2%), tyrosine phenylalanine (6.7–10.3%), isoleucine (5.0%), and hisitidine (4.7%) levels. In general, the four principal storage proteins from amaranth grains contain adequate amounts of essential amino acids to fulfill nutritional requirements for the children and adults recommended by FAO/WHO, suggesting that this grain could be used in combination with other cereals to improve the quality of the proteins and increase the nutritive value of foods (Gorinstein et al., 2002; Mlakar et al., 2010).

15.4 BIOACTIVE PEPTIDES RELATED TO ANTIHYPERTENSIVE FUNCTIONS

Dietary proteins constitute the main source of amino acids, a good amount of energy and diverse peptides derived from these proteins, which are needed for maintenance of sustainability of human physiological functions; the importance lies in the fact that many of these physiological functions in all organisms are mediated by peptides. These bioactive components are fragments that are inactive within the sequence parent protein, however when the enzymatic proteolysis occurs during gastrointestinal digestion, amino acids and peptides are released in high amounts and later they can be absorbed and transported by the bloodstream, and finally they can participate in different metabolic functions (Martínez-Maqueda, Miralles, Recio, & Hernández-Ledesma, 2012). Peptides may have different sizes, around 2−20 amino acid residues per molecule with molecular masses between 1 and 6 kDa and based on their physical properties and amino acid composition, peptides possess diverse functional properties (Moure, Domínguez, & Parajó, 2005; Sarmadi & Ismail, 2010). Amaranth seeds can be a potential source of several bioactive peptides with different bioactivity functions with relevance in some important disorders in human health such as cancer, hypertension, antioxidant functions, and diabetes mellitus and other important diseases (Caselato-Sousa & Amaya-Farfán, 2012; Silva-Sánchez et al., 2008). Due to these health-promoting attributes and safety behavior, the peptides may be used to produce food with nutraceutical benefits.

The need to obtain physiological health benefits from functional food sources has led consumers to replace drug therapies against different diseases such as cardiovascular disorders. Bioactive peptides have been evaluated as a new alternative against hypertension (Martínez-Maqueda et al., 2012). Hypertension treatments are based on the inhibition of the angiotensin-converting enzyme (ACE; peptidylpeptidase hydrolase; EC 3.415.1) that plays an important role in the regulation of blood pressure via the renin−angiotensin system. The angiotensinogen is released in response to blood pressure; the reduction in plasma volume increases the production of a deca-peptide angiotensin-I, followed by the cleavage of the dipeptide His-Leu by the ACE enzyme to form the angiotensin-II potent vasoconstrictor (Caselato-Sousa & Amaya-Farfán, 2012; Haulica, Bild, & Serban, 2005; Ondetti & Cushman, 1982).

Amaranth biopeptides are emerging as natural ACE inhibitors and represent a promising alternative with no apparent side-effects (Cao, Zhang, Hong, Ji, & Hao, 2010). Most of the biopeptides from amaranth reported some effects against hypertension (Fig. 15.1; Martínez-Cruz et al., 2014).

Montoya-Rodriguez et al. (2015) performed in silico analysis of the sequence and performed prediction of the bioactive peptides present in amaranth proteins; they showed the potential of biological peptides formed from 11S globulin (Fig. 15.1) using different types of proteases, such as pepsin, trypsin, chymotrypsin, Alcalase, and a combination of serin-proteases; the resulting peptides exhibited ACE inhibition, antioxidant, and hypocholesterolemic activities. However, diverse in vitro and in vivo studies have exhibited the antihypertensive properties of these bioactive peptides from 7S and 11S globulin amaranth seeds with different proteases. Therefore, proteins isolated from amaranth seeds hydrolyzed under gastrointestinal simulation with pancreatin and pepsin showed higher ACE inhibition than the peptides digested with Alcalase (Tiengo, Faria, & Netto, 2009). Amaranth contains different important proteins which are composed of an extensive list of antihypertensive peptides (Table 15.5).

Peptides from the hydrolysis of *Amaranthus mantegazzium* seed flour have been evaluated for in vitro and in vivo hypertension capacity in animal models, and they exhibited ACE-inhibitory activity equal to or higher than the peptides purified from *A. hypochondriacus* protein fractions (Fritz, Vecchi, Rinaldi, & Añón, 2011). In that sense, Tovar-Pérez et al. (2009) evaluated peptides from albumin and globulin fractions from *A. hypochondriacus* seeds with ACE-inhibitory activity; they found that albumin and globulin peptides presented ACE-inhibitory activities of 40% and 35% respectively, after 18 and 15 h of digestion with Alcalase enzyme; this inhibition could be exerted by the peptide's interaction with the ACE enzyme. Peptides from albumin fraction showed a noncompetitive mode of ACE inhibition and globulin peptides had competitive interactions with the ACE enzyme. Most of the ACE inhibitors derived from food-protein hydrolysates belong to the competitive mode and are able to enter the catalytic site in the enzyme and avoid the substrate interaction (Vermeirssen, Camp, & Verstraete, 2004).

The identification of peptides involved in ACE inhibition for treatment of hypertension is a challenge for scientists. Silva-Sánchez et al. (2008) analyzed peptides from globulin and glutelin protein fractions in silico, revealing dipeptides and tripeptides such as Leu-Phe, His-Tyr, Gly-Lys-Pro, and Arg-Phe with strong inhibitory potential against ACE. Similarly, Vecchi and Añon (2009) reported that tetrapeptides from 11S globulin from *A. hypochondriacus* are involved in the ACE-inhibitory activity, demonstrating that these peptides (-ALEP- and -VIKP-) have high occurrence in the 11S globulin sequences. These peptides were validated by in vitro studies, resulting in them having ACE inhibition with IC_{50} values of 6.32 and 175 μM for -ALEP- and -VIKP-, respectively. Additionally, Luna-Suárez, Medina-Godoy, Cruz-Hernández, and Paredes-López (2010) modified the acidic subunit of 11S globulin inserting four -Val-Tyr- peptides in tandem with antihypertensive activity against ACE enzyme; and when the protein was digested the resulting

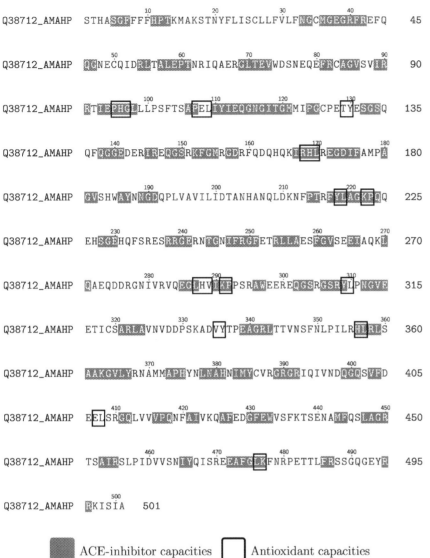

FIGURE 15.1 Bioactive peptide sequences encrypted in the 11S globulin seed protein from *A. hypochondriacus*. Protein sequence was obtained from UniProt (http://www.uniprot.org/uniprot/Q38712); shaded and remarked peptides were taken and modified from Silva-Sánchez et al. (2008) and Montoya-Rodríguez et al. (2015), respectively. Amino acid nomenclature: A, alanine; C, cysteine; D, aspartic acid; E, glutamic acid; F, phenylalanine; G, glycine; H, histidine; I, isoleucine; K, lysine; L, leucine; M, methionine; N, asparagine; P, proline; Q, glutamine; R, arginine; S, serine; T, threonine; V, valine; W, tryptophan; Y, tyrosine; B, either of D or N; Z, either of E or Q.

peptides were confronted with the ACE enzyme and showed high inhibition effect against this enzyme of around eightfold more than the nonmodified globulin. These peptides where overexpressed in different bacterial systems such as *Escherichia coli* strains, and the modified proteins showed high ACE inhibition (Arano-Varela, Dominguez-Dominguez, & Paredes-López, 2012; Castro-Martínez, Luna-Suárez, & Paredes-López, 2012; Morales-Camacho, Dominguez-Dominguez, & Paredes-López, 2013). Later, the same peptides were tested by in vivo studies in spontaneously hypertensive rats, and the inhibitory peptides significantly caused a reduction in the mean arterial pressure, similar to the positive group treated with captopril (Medina-Godoy et al., 2013). On the other hand, Quiroga, Aphalo, Ventureira, Martínez, and Añón (2012) performed in silico studies and showed the presence of the ACE-inhibitory peptides encrypted in 7S proteins and peptides released from these proteins after enzymatic digestion showed a high ACE-inhibitory capacity similar to the 11S globulin peptides.

ACE inhibition promotes a decrease in blood pressure levels (Koike, Ito, Miyamoto, & Nishino, 1980). ACE catalyzes the inactivation of the vasodilator bradykinin, which regulates different biological processes including vascular endothelial nitric oxide (NO) release; NO exerts a strong effect on the vascular smooth muscle cells promoting vascular relaxation (Ju, Venema, Marrero, & Venema, 1998). The identification of the antihypertensive potential and NO production from amaranth peptides supported by bioinformatic studies can be found in other important protein fractions. Barba de la Rosa et al. (2010) found that peptides from a glutelin protein fraction showed strong ACE inhibition comparable to captopril; they also stimulated the endothelial NO production in coronary endothelial cells

TABLE 15.5 Antihypertensive Biopeptides Identified by Sequence Prediction

Protein Fraction	Bioactive Peptides Sequences	References
Albumin	AG, GL, RY, LQ, LA, EV, VE, RW, LY, EG, LG, GH, TE, VG, GG, GS, TG, VF, IF, TF, KG, NG, GK, GV, FG, GY, YG, LN, AH, MF,GT, KF, PR, EA, AA, FR, KR, SG, TQ,AI, EI, IE, RL	Cheung, Wang, Ondetti, Sabo, and Cushman (1980), Bella, Erickson, and Kim (1982), Sentandreu and Toldra (2007), van-Platerink, Janssen, and Haverkamp (2008)
Globulin	SG, GF, HP, PT, NG, MG, GE, EG, GR, FR, QG, GL, TE, EV, AG,GV, RR, IE, PH,HG, AP, IY, GI, TG, GM, IP, PG,GS, GG, KF, FG, GD, HL, IF, AY, FY, LA, GK, PQ, EI, LQ, AW, RY, VE,AR, EA, AA, KG, LY, LN, AH,MY, GQ,VF, VP,AI, AF, EW,MF,RL, IR, IKP, GKP, IEP, ALEP	Cheung et al. (1980), Bella et al. (1982), Sentandreu and Toldra (2007), van-Platerink et al. (2008)
7S Globulin	DA, GK, QG, LQ, RL 2VF, PR, PL, AP, GF, FR, VG, AG, 2GE, MG	Quiroga et al. (2012)
	GK, GD, EG, EA, 2LQ, LN, PQ, EW, HP	
	LVL, HY, FP, PR, 4LF,GPL, 2GP, PL, VK, 2AF, 2LA, KR, VP, 3FR, GL, GH, GR, 2FG, GK, GT, GG, 2EG, NG,2PG, VR, GHF, NY, NF, 2LQ, LN, EK	
	VLP, LNP, 2YL, GPL, PL, AF, AP, 3GA, 3AG, 2FG, GS, 2GV, 2GT,QG, 4SG, GHF, RR, AR, PH, 2VF,GY, AY, AA, VG, GE, QG, EA, NG, NF, YK, EV	
	2LY, LVL, RF,HY, GY, LNP, YL, 2LF,VK, 2AF, AP, 2LA, FR, GA, 3GL, GR, FG, GS, GT, 2SG, 2LG, 2EG, NY, 2SF, KL, LVE, VE, LQ, LN, TQ, EK. KE, PH	
	VLP, RL, PR, LSP, LF, FFL, VP, GF, AG, SY, LN, PQ, TF, EL, FA, LP, VLP, VF, HY, GY, AF, LA, KR, FR, VG, 2NF	
	VF, FP, GF, GL, FG, LN, HY, PR, LF, GP, AF, LA, KR, PG, NF	
Glutelin	AY, FP, FY, GY, HY, IR, IY, LF, LW, LY, MF, MY, PR, RF, RL, RY, VF, VW, VY, YG, YL, YP	Silva-Sánchez et al. (2008)
	AAP, AIP, ALPP, AVP,FNQ, IKP, ILP, IRA, FQP, GGY, GKP, GRP, HIR, LAA, LAMA, LAY, LLP, LNP, LPP, LQP, LQQ, LRP, LSP, LVL, LVR, PLP, PQR, PRY, TAP, VAA, VAP, VAY	
	VLP,VPP, VRP, VSP, VYP, YGGY	
Alpha-amylase inhibitor	IP, KW, GP, DG, GV, YG	Cheung et al. (1980), Byun and Kim (2002)
Trypsin-inhibitor	AR, GK, EW, VG,GE, GY, AA, IE, GF, FR, TG, GV, YP, PR, YG, YPR,	Cheung et al. (1980), Bella et al. (1982), Sentandreu and Toldra (2007)
Prosystemin	KE, EK, KG, GG, GD, IE, TQ, EI, IP, ME, EG, GY, VE, DA, KG, GE, GA, PP, KR	Cheung et al. (1980), van-Platerink et al. (2008)
Cystatin	KF, IF, QG, GS, LG, GG, GL, GA, AA, DA, EI, IE, LA, AR, KE, KA,AG, GT, EA, AI, GK, LY, LQ, TE, EG, GH, AP, PG, GW, EV, VP, AH, VE, HL, KR, HK, LN, MG, RL, IQP	Cheung et al. (1980), Bella et al. (1982), Sentandreu and Toldra (2007), van-Platerink et al. (2008)
Glucosyltransferase	LQ,VF, AY, YG, GH, IP, PT, AR, AA, GV, TQ, AI, IE, EK, KA, HG,GS, IY, TE, EI, IF, NG, GL, KF, VE, LN, RP, PH, MF, VP, PR, GT, TF, EV, KE, FY, YA, GR, RR, RA, AW, IG, GP, KR, GI, EA, KW, FG, MG, IW, PQ, QG, GF, ME, EG, GK, KG, GW, GA, TG,VG, GD,RL, LVR	Cheung et al. (1980), Bella et al. (1982), Sentandreu and Toldra (2007), van-Platerink et al. (2008)
Polyamide oxidase	ME, MG, GS, NG, RP, VE, KE, SG, GM, VF, VG, GA, EV, AP, TG, GG, GL, LG, GD, AA, AR, PR, RW, KR, GV, IF, HP, GI, YG, GP, AG, EA, GE, AY, AI, IY, KG, YP, GY, GR, LQ, YA, IG, GF, IP, EK, IE, EI, LY, KF, HK, TE, HG, EG, MY, FY, FG, GT, RR, LA, TF, PG, IW, RL, VSP	Cheung et al. (1980), Bella et al. (1982), Sentandreu and Toldra (2007), van-Platerink et al. (2008)

See Fig. 15.1 for the amino acid nomenclature used in this table.
Adapted from Silva-Sánchez, C., de la Rosa, A. B., León-Galván, M., De Lumen, B., de Leon-Rodriguez, A., & de Mejía, E. G. (2008). Bioactive peptides in amaranth (Amaranthus hypochondriacus) seed. Journal of Agricultural and Food Chemistry, 56, 1233–1240 and Montoya-Rodríguez, A., Gómez-Favela, M. A., Reyes-Moreno, C., Milán-Carrillo, J., & González de Mejía, E. (2015). Identification of bioactive peptide sequences from amaranth (Amaranthus hypochondriacus) seed proteins and their potential role in the prevention of chronic diseases. Comprehensive Reviews in Food Science and Food Safety, 14, 139–158.

inducing vasodilatation in isolated rat aortic rings. Therefore these studies suggest that glutelin peptides induce endothelial NO production and vasodilatation by ACE-inhibition activity.

Nutraceutical compounds may usually have low capacities as bioactive chemical components, but if they are regularly consumed as a long-term complement in the diet, the physiological effects are perceptible (Espín, García-Conesa, & Tomás-Barberán, 2007). Therefore, globulin and glutelin protein fractions from amaranth seeds are a natural source of antihypertensive peptides and can be used as a natural remedy without undesirable side effects.

15.5 ANTIOXIDANT CAPACITIES OF AMARANTH PEPTIDES

Free radicals are generated by metabolic pathway reactions in the organism (Sarmadi & Ismail, 2010), that is, reactive oxygen species (ROS) such as single oxygen (O_2), hydroperoxyl (HO_2), peroxide (H_2O_2), and hydroxyl (HO) radicals, and reactive nitrogen species (RNS). However, an excessive amount of these ROS can evoke cell damage which may promote the onset of diseases like arthritis, diabetes, cancer, and cardiovascular diseases (Alashi et al., 2014; Paravicini & Touyz, 2008). The human organism has an important antioxidant mechanism to diminish the oxidative damage stress due to ROS. The most important defenses are oxidative enzymes such as catalase and superoxide dismutase and other low-molecular-weight molecules such as vitamin C or E and glutathione that scavenge free radicals. Other important molecules involved in metal chelation are ferritin and transferritin (Noguchi, Watanabe, & Shi, 2000) and recently attention has been given to the antioxidant peptides.

Plant food proteins can act as a natural source of antioxidant peptide and their biological activities have been widely studied (Sarmadi & Ismail, 2010). Antioxidant peptides are simple structures that, in small quantities, are able to retard the oxidation and production of ROS involved in the damage stress of biological structures such as membrane lipids, cellular proteins, enzymes, and DNA (Haque, Chand, & Kapila, 2008; Segura-Campos, Salazar-Vega, Chel-Guerrero, & Betancur-Ancona, 2013). The antioxidant capacity of peptides is related to the protease action and specifically to the extension of the hydrolysis process in their structural characteristics (molecular weight and the amino acidic composition) (Orsini-Delgado, Galleano, Añón, & Tironi, 2015), but the molecular mechanisms of action are not totally known. However, some studies have described that the antioxidant peptides are inhibitors of lipid peroxidation (Peñta-Ramos & Xiong, 2002), scavengers of free radicals (Wu, Chen, & Shiau, 2003), and chelators of metal ions (Durak, Baraniak, Jakubczyk, & Åswieca, 2013; Siow & Gan, 2013). Similar to some other seed proteins (Marambe, Shand, & Wanasundara, 2008), biopeptides from amaranth have attracted interest as natural antioxidants (Table 15.6) because these fragments are unique and in the past decade they were characterized from different natural food sources (Devasagayam et al., 2004).

The physiological effect of amaranth seeds on human health has been demonstrated (Guzmán-Maldonado & Paredes-López, 1998). Some studies have proved the in vitro effect of the antioxidant peptide activities against oxidant reagents. Tironi and Añón (2010) analyzed the presence of peptides with antioxidative capacities and the inhibition of linoleic acid oxidation by *Amaranthus manteggazianus* seed; they demonstrated that peptides from glutelin fraction have the most effective antioxidant capacity, followed by globulin, albumin, and prolamin fractions. Alcalase hydrolysis

TABLE 15.6 Antioxidative Biopeptides Identified by Sequence Prediction

Protein Fraction	Bioactive Peptides	References
Albumin	LK, TY, RW, LH, KP, EL, LHV, LVR	Huang et al. (2010)
Globulin	IR, EL, TY, HL, YL, LH, KP, VY, LK, PHG, PEL, RHL, LHV	Huang et al. (2010)
Glutelin	HH, HL, LH, LHH	Silva-Sánchez et al. (2008)
Prolamin	Due this protein fraction is a minor component, antioxidant capacity did not performed.	Barba de la Rosa et al. (1992), Silva-Sánchez et al. (2008)

See Fig. 15.1 for the amino acid nomenclature used in this table.
Adapted from Silva-Sánchez, C., de la Rosa, A. B., León-Galván, M., De Lumen, B., de Leon-Rodriguez, A., & de Mejía, E. G. (2008). Bioactive peptides in amaranth (Amaranthus hypochondriacus) seed. Journal of Agricultural and Food Chemistry, 56, 1233–1240 and Montoya-Rodríguez, A., Gómez-Favela, M. A., Reyes-Moreno, C., Milán-Carrillo, J., & González de Mejía, E. (2015). Identification of bioactive peptide sequences from amaranth (Amaranthus hypochondriacus) seed proteins and their potential role in the prevention of chronic diseases. Comprehensive Reviews in Food Science and Food Safety, 14, 139–158.

was able to improve the scavenging activities, and prolamin peptides presented the highest antioxidant activity followed by glutelin, albumin, and globulin. Orsini-Delgado, Tironi, and Añón (2011) evaluated the in vitro antioxidant capacity of amaranth peptides and showed that antioxidant peptides that can scavenge radicals better than the ones obtained from digestion with Alcalase alone could be released into the gastrointestinal system alone. Also Orsini-Delgado et al. (2015) showed that amaranth peptides released by gastrointestinal digestion produced a strong increment in the scavenging activity against peroxyl, hydroxyl radicals, and also with peroxynitrites. These peptides could act as metal chelators. The mechanism of action of the antioxidant peptides encrypted in amaranth storage proteins is not clear, however some studies indicate that peptides may inhibit the onset or propagation of free radicals by donating a hydrogen atom (Gordon, 1990; Kong & Xiong, 2006; Orsini-Delgado et al., 2015).

Antioxidative properties of the biopeptides are more related to their physical and chemical properties such as composition, structure, and hydrophobicity (Chen, Muramoto, Yamauchi, Fujimoto, & Nokihara, 1998). Examples of amino acids with antioxidant capacities are Tyr, Trp, Met, Lys, Cys, Phe, and His (Wang, Mejia, & Gonzalez, 2005). In addition, aromatic amino acids lead to antioxidant activities when they donate protons from the phenolic group to electron-deficient radicals improving radical-scavenging properties. In this sense, SH- groups from cysteine interact in a direct manner with the radicals produced. Peptides containing histidine pose antioxidant activity in relation to the ability of the imidazole group for hydrogen-donating, lipid peroxyl radical trapping, and metal ion-chelating ability (Sarmadi & Ismail, 2010).

Amaranth seed proteins contain an extensive profile of bioactive peptides with antioxidant capacities such as Cys, Met, Tyr, Trp, Lys, His, Pro, Gly, Ala, and Thr (Tiengo et al., 2009). In the same line, Silva-Sánchez et al. (2008) identified four peptides rich in His from fragmented 11S globulin related to antioxidant capacities. Montoya-Rodríguez, Mejía, Dia, Reyes-Moreno, and Milán-Carrillo (2014) demonstrated that extruded and unprocessed amaranth hydrolysates contain sulfur and aromatic amino acids with antioxidant capacities, such as Lys, Prol, His, Gly, Ala, and Thr. In this context, Montoya-Rodríguez et al. (2015) determined the bioactive sequence peptides from the 15 most important proteins present in amaranth seeds; these proteins presented high occurrence frequencies of many bioactive peptides with different potential functions that included peptides with high antioxidative activities. They found that amaranth 11S globulin storage protein contains important amounts of dipeptides and tripeptides with antioxidant capacity on the long chain of the protein (see Fig. 15.1). Amaranth antioxidant peptides showed potential to scavenge free radical products from the metabolic pathways in the human body; these peptides can act as a new, cheap, organic alternative and a basic compound of functional foods.

To determine the total antioxidant capacity of food peptides is a challenge, because there is no "ideal" or "best method" to analyze the individual antioxidant potential of each peptide. Diverse antioxidant in vitro assays have been proposed and they are used actually as primary methods for researches; due to their simplicity and fast results, these methods should only be used for preliminary screening purposes (Amorati & Valgimigli, 2015; Gostner, Becker, Ueberall, & Fuchs, 2015). However, if they are tested in combination with other assays such as in vivo, in cell, genetic and enzymatic tests, they may be provide good results that can offer a global overview of the biological potential of the antioxidant peptides (Amorati & Valgimigli, 2015; Orsini-Delgado et al., 2015).

15.6 POTENTIAL USES OF AMARANTH PROTEINS IN THE FOOD INDUSTRY

Amaranth grains have high contents of several nutrients and have attributes not only for direct consumption but for food processing, to be converted into various ingredients and key complements. Its high-protein content converts amaranth into a remarkable complement for some processed foods such as meat foods (Dodok, Modhir, Buchtova, Halasova, & Polaček, 1997). Proteins are commonly used as a food ingredient and formulation due to their nutritional value and their versatile functional performance. It is well known that the high cost of animal proteins for the human population and for the food industry itself leads to vegetable proteins as the most viable alternative for the elaboration of some key food products (Martínez-Cruz et al., 2014).

Previous studies on amaranth proteins have clearly shown that they may be employed as supplement in foods since they display a wide range of functional properties that benefit the foods (Fidantsi & Doxastakis, 2001). However, to increase their functional properties, the proteins may be modified by different physical, enzymatic, and chemical treatments; thus, the availability of food ingredients based on amaranth proteins increases the commercial options to the food industry (Davis & Williams, 1998). The enzymatic modifications are one of the most viable parameters, due to their relatively milder processing, and to fast control of the reaction, with minimal formation of undesirable products (Mannheim & Cheryan, 1992; Panyam & Kilara, 1996).

Protein hydrolysates with high level of hydrolysis are used commonly as food supplements (Clemente, 2000), while protein hydrolysates with a low degree of hydrolysis improve the foaming and emulsifying properties (Rodríguez Patino, Rodríguez Niño, & Carrera Sánchez, 2007). Scilingo, Ortiz, Martínez, and Añón (2002) developed a methodology that optimized the amaranth protein hydrolysis with papain, cucurbita, and thermal treatments; the amaranth hydrolysates keep the solubility under different temperatures, and consequently these hydrolysates are a suitable ingredient in foods considering that they retain high solubility after heating. Thermal treatment in combination with enzymatic hydrolysis improves the functional properties of proteins. In that sense, Condés, Scilingo, and Añón (2009) prepared *A. hypochondriacus* protein hydrolysates using trypsin enzyme and evaluated the structure, solubility, and foaming properties. The results showed that the protein solubility increased with hydrolysis and the foam properties were more dense and stable than those prepared with nondigested proteins.

Another important characteristic of proteins is gelation. The high proportion of 11S globulin in amaranth and their high gelation properties is a desirable blank to form self-supporting gels that could be applied in different gel-like foods (Martínez-Cruz et al., 2014). In that sense, Avanza et al. (2005a) studied the gel-forming properties of amaranth proteins under different thermal conditions and protein concentrations; and reported that elasticity of heated dispersion and gels increased when they increased the protein concentration; this behavior could be related to the great proportion of disulfide bonds formed during protein gelation. In the same way, Avanza et al. (2005b) evaluated the gel color intensity, and water-holding under different temperature conditions. They reported that color gel intensity increased, while the luminosity decreased by increasing the protein concentration and allowed the formation of gel matrices with high water-holding capacity; additionally, the increase in temperature and protein concentration resulted in the formation of more ordered matrix with smaller pores. A rapid denaturation of globulins stabilized by disulfide bonds between protein molecules led to a gelation phenomenon enhanced by protein aggregation (Avanza et al., 2005a, 2005b).

Molecular biology and protein engineering techniques have been used with the aim of improving the functional properties of the amaranth 11S globulin (Martínez-Cruz et al., 2014); and these tools may be used to upgrade the functional characteristics of *A. hypochondriacus* 11S globulin; also termed amarantin protein. In that sense, Carrazco-Peña et al. (2013) modified the primary structure of amaranth 11S globulin. They inserted four continuous Met amino acids in variable region V; solubility and heat-induced gelation were compared with the unmodified native protein. The modified amarantin showed highest hydrophobicity and strongest gel matrices compared with the native amarantin that presented the weakest gels, and the authors concluded that the incorporation of four Met amino acids in this protein increased the hydrophobicity and self-hardness in the gel matrix. These functional properties could be used in the food industry for the development of new products based on amaranth proteins (Carrazco-Peña et al., 2013). Several other successful examples have been developed aiming at food industry considerations, or are under generation by some key groups located in different countries. Thus, the future of amaranth proteins will be surely brighter.

15.7 GENETIC ENGINEERING OF AMARANTH PROTEINS

The FAO estimates that about 70% of the human diet must be comprised of cereals, legumes, fruits, and vegetables (Mandal & Mandal, 2000). Seed storage proteins from grain crops contain the main dietary protein requirements for human. In developing countries the daily diet depends mostly on seed proteins due to the fact that animal proteins are more expensive. Plant proteins are generally deficient in some of the essential nutrients, which can cause malnutrition (Han, Chee, & Cho, 2015), and these must be supplied by complementation and by a diet rich in diverse sources. In addition, genetic manipulation may play an important additional role. Cereals contain proteins usually deficient in lysine and tryptophan (Charalampopoulos, Wang, Pandiella, & Webb, 2002) and legumes are commonly deficient in sulfur amino acids such as methionine and cysteine (Iqbal, Khalil, Ateeq, & Khan, 2006). But their complementation improves substantially the quality of the diet, not only in the protein but also in other important components.

With the advent of the recombinant DNA and new "-omics" technologies, studies have been focused on the isolation, purification, characterization, identification, and development of technologies to offer alternative strategies to address food and nutraceutical challenges. Techniques are being developed to resolve the nutritional seed quality, with the potential to isolate and manipulate gene introduction or reintroduction to produce transgenic crop plants with modified seed genes to improve the nutritional value of food crops and the processed products (Galili & Höfgen, 2002). The isolation and expression of genes to code heterologous proteins with nutraceutical potential may be advantageous to express important seed proteins in different plant species with the objective of producing foods with functional benefits. The 11S globulin or amarantin is the most important seed storage protein in amaranth and several studies have been developed for its molecular characterization and other studies to understand processing and deposition in the amaranth grain. In a pioneering research performed by Barba de la Rosa et al. (1996), amarantin cDNA was isolated and characterized. The authors compared the derived amino acid sequence clones with other species, concluding that amarantin is synthesized as a precursor called preproamarantin, with similar structure to other 11S-like proteins. In this context, Osuna-Castro et al. (2000) overexpressed amarantin in *E. coli*, and after purification found the in vitro refolding of the protein. These studies determined that the recombinant globulin is able to acquire the proper molecular conformation and their physicochemical and biochemical properties (Tandang-Silvas et al., 2012) that are essential to exhibit the expected grain's nutritional functionality.

Amarantin gene is an excellent candidate to be expressed in diverse important crops in order to improve the nutritional value of staple foods. In this sense, Rascón-Cruz et al. (2004) used the 11S globulin cDNA to transform tropical maize plants and their molecular analysis describes the insertion and expression of the amarantin gene in transformed plants. The amarantin protein was accumulated in the seed and its content and amino acid profile increased in particular Lys and Trp compared to nontransformed maize plants. In addition, Germán-Báez et al. (2014) transformed tomato fruit plants with the acidic subunit of amarantin from *A. hypochondriacus*; the amarantin protein accumulation and stability were confirmed with immunoblot assays. They also confirmed an increase in total protein content and higher concentrations of some essential amino acids, such as Val, Tyr, Ile, and Leu, compared to nontransformed plants. Albumin gene, an important protein from *A. hypochondriacus* seed, was used to transform potato tuber plants and an increase in the size and production of tuber in transgenic plants was found, as well as in total protein content and in most of the essential amino acids (Chakraborty, Chakraborty, & Datta, 2000).

However, this alternative to insert important genes and their subsequent expression to improve the nutritional attributes in plant crops has been used to increase the essential amino acids without allergenic side effects (Goodman et al., 2008), an important feature when considering genetically modified food plants (Verma, Kumar, Das, & Dwivedi, 2013). In this context, Sinagawa-García et al. (2004) evaluated in vitro the allergenicity of genetically modified maize with an 11S globulin; they purified the amarantin protein and did not find immunoreactivity against IgE antibody in BALB/c mice. In another study on the expression of albumin protein from amaranth seeds in potato plants, the authors exposed animal models with the albumin proteins and they showed that this protein did not evoke any IgE response (Chakraborty et al., 2000). Both studies reveal that amaranth albumin and globulin proteins do not cause negative effects and allergenicity in humans.

The importance of amaranth seed proteins has led researchers to isolate, modify, and overexpress the protein in different microbial systems, to achieve a high yield of a target protein under controlled conditions. There are some studies related to the expression and production of recombinant protein in bacterial systems. The most commonly employed bacteria is *E. coli*, due to its genetic background, different and available chromosomes or plasmid used for the protein expression and gene manipulation (Martínez-Cruz et al., 2014).

In the last few decades researchers have used these systems to understand the native physicochemical properties of the most important amaranth seed proteins. When 11S globulin was expressed and purified from *E. coli* bacteria, the protein exhibited the same properties as those of the native amarantin seed (Barba de La Rosa et al., 1996; Osuna-Castro et al., 2000). However, other systems improved the potency of purification of the recombinant protein. In that sense, Medina-Godoy et al. (2004) cloned and expressed a modified cDNA of histidine-tagged 11S globulin from *A. hypochondriacus* in *E. coli* strain; the recombinant amarantin was expressed and assembled into trimers inside of the strain, the resulting proamarantin was purified in one step with high yields. Moreover, physicochemical properties have been evaluated in transgenic tobacco plants and multicellular systems, triggering high protein efficiency and quality. Valdez-Ortiz et al. (2005) cloned the amarantin gene in tobacco plants; this gene encoded to a polyhistidine tag, which produced high purification in one step without changes in the biochemical and physicochemical properties of amarantin. Similar studies were performed in *Pichiapastoris* by Medina-Godoy, Valdez-Ortiz, Valverde, and Paredes-López (2006), who used a signal peptide tagged to retrieve the amarantin and overexpress and enhance the protein. The one-step purification expressed in different systems will facilitate further researches of the different storage proteins.

Amarantin gene has been used to modify the protein sequence; in this case the acidic subunit has potential as a functional and nutraceutical protein, and it is structurally an important candidate for modifications since this subunit contains four hypervariable regions of five regions detected in the 11S seed globulin (Tandang-Silvas et al., 2012). Moreover, Luna-Suárez et al. (2008) modified the third variable region of the acidic subunit of a His-tagged 11S globulin, and this subunit was expressed in *E. coli*. Additionally, Arano-Varela et al. (2012) expressed the 11S amaranth protein and studied the parameters to obtain the highest recombinant acidic subunit concentration in a bioreactor and demonstrated that the aeration rate and temperature were the most important variables to increase protein concentration. In the same context, Castro-Martínez et al. (2012) found that the modified amarantin protein increased around threefold in a bioreactor when temperature, agitation speed, and oxygen conditions were optimal for a better protein yield. Later, Morales-Camacho et al. (2013) expressed the acidic subunit of the amarantin manipulating some parameters in a bioreactor in two minimal media with supplementation of an inducer, isopropyl-β-D-thiogalactopyranoside or lactose, and they found high productivity of the recombinant acidic subunit in a short time of around 4–6 h of induction.

However, with the scientific progress, new technologies such as RNA interference and DNA-editing applied in animal models (Cox, Platt, & Zhang, 2015) emerge as new-generation tools to produce genetically edited organisms and their applications in the very short future in functional staple crops improvement is in front us (Kanchiswamy, Sargent, Velasco, Maffei, & Malnoy, 2015; Ricroch&Hénard-Damave, 2015). The future is here.

15.8 CONCLUDING REMARKS

Amaranth grain has been consumed since ancient civilizations, for its beneficial properties for human nutrition and health. Nowadays, our knowledge on this crop has improved. The seed is loaded with a high amount of excellent-quality proteins; its importance is mainly based on the balance of essential amino acids and other key compounds. Globulin and glutelins are the main protein fractions, followed by albumin and prolamins. These proteins have important bioactive peptides which may act as modulators of metabolism and possess other outstanding biological activities, such as antihypertensive and antioxidant properties. Globulin peptides have been extensively studied in vitro and have probed their effectivity for inhibition, which has been clearly supported by in vivo analysis suppressing the inactivation of ACE enzyme. Amaranth peptides contribute strongly for the inactivation of ROS; organic molecules involved in different human disorders. With the modern advances of different molecular tools and expression of key amaranth genes and subsequent production of recombinant proteins in different biological systems, amaranth proteins are the main target of researches addressing their nutritional and nutraceutical potential. Thus, there is a strong basis to consider that their potential will be highly commercially improved in the near future.

ACKNOWLEDGMENTS

We thank Talia Hernandez-Perez for her kind and helpful assistance. This project was partially supported by Consejo Nacional de Ciencia y Tecnologia (CONACyT-Mexico).

REFERENCES

Aguilar, E. G., Peiretti, E. G., Uñates, M. A., Marchevsky, E. J., Escudero, N. L., & Camiña, J. M. (2013). Amaranth seed varieties. A chemometric approach. *Journal of Food Measurement and Characterization, 7*, 199–206.

Alashi, A. M., Blanchard, C. L., Mailer, R. J., Agboola, S. O., Mawson, A. J., He, R., ... Aluko, R. E. (2014). Antioxidant properties of Australian canola meal protein hydrolysates. *Food Chemistry, 146*, 500–506.

Alvarez-Jubete, L., Arendt, E. K., & Gallagher, E. (2010). Nutritive value of pseudocereals and their increasing use as functional gluten-free ingredients. *Trends in Food Science & Technology, 21*, 106–113.

Amorati, R., & Valgimigli, L. (2015). Advantages and limitations of common testing methods for antioxidants. *Free Radical Research, 49*, 633–649.

Arano-Varela, H., Dominguez-Dominguez, J., & Paredes-López, O. (2012). Effect of environmental conditions on the expression levels of a recombinant 11S amaranth globulin in *Escherichia coli*. *Recent Patents in Biotechnology, 6*, 23–31.

Avanza, M., Puppo, M., & Añón, M. (2005a). Rheological characterization of amaranth protein gels. *Food Hydrocolloids, 19*, 889–898.

Avanza, M. V., Puppo, M. C., & Añón, M. C. (2005b). Structural characterization of amaranth protein gels. *Journal of Food Science, 70*, E223–E229.

Awasthi, C., Kumar, A., Singh, N., & Thakur, R. (2011). Biochemical composition of grain amaranth genotypes of Himachal Pradesh. *Indian Journal of Agricultural Biochemistry, 24*, 141–144.

Barba de la Rosa, A. P., Barba Montoya, A., Martínez-Cuevas, P., Hernández-Ledesma, B., León-Galván, M. F., De León-Rodríguez, A., & González, C. (2010). Tryptic amaranth glutelin digests induce endothelial nitric oxide production through inhibition of ACE: Antihypertensive role of amaranth peptides. *Nitric Oxide, 23*, 106–111.

Barba de la Rosa, A. P., Gueguen, J., Paredes-López, O., & Viroben, G. (1992). Fractionation procedures, electrophoretic characterization, and amino acid composition of amaranth seed proteins. *Journal of Agricultural and Food Chemistry, 40*, 931–936.

Barba de la Rosa, A. P., Herrera-Estrella, A., Utsumi, S., & Paredes-López, O. (1996). Molecular characterization, cloning and structural analysis of a cDNA encoding an amaranth globulin. *Journal of Plant Physiology, 149*, 527–532.

Bashir, M., Hubatsch, I., Leinenbach, H. P., Zeppezauer, M., Panzani, R. C., & Hussein, I. H. (1998). Ric c 1 and Ric c 3, the allergenic 2S albumin storage proteins of *Ricinus communis*: Complete primary structures and phylogenetic relationships. *International Archives of Allergy and Immunology, 115*, 73–82.

Becker, R., Wheeler, E., Lorenz, K., Stafford, A., Grosjean, O., Betschart, A., & Saunders, R. (1981). A compositional study of amaranth grain. *Journal of Food Science, 46*, 1175–1180.

Bella, A. M., Erickson, R. H., & Kim, Y. S. (1982). Rat intestinal brush bordermembrane dipeptidyl-aminopeptidase IV: Kinetic properties and substratespecifities of the purified enzyme. *Archives of Biochemistry and Biophysics, 218*, 156–162.

Bello-Pérez, L. A., & Paredes-López, O. (2009). Starches of some food crops, changes during processing and their nutraceutical potential. *Food Engineering Reviews, 1*, 50–65.

Bressani, R., & Garcia-Vela, L. A. (1990). Protein fractions in amaranth grain and their chemical characterization. *Journal of Agricultural and Food Chemistry, 38*, 1205–1209.

Brinegar, C., & Goundan, S. (1993). Isolation and characterization of chenopodin, the 11S seed storage protein of quinoa (*Chenopodium quinoa*). *Journal of Agricultural and Food Chemistry, 41*, 182–185.

Byun, H. G., & Kim, S. K. (2002). Structure and activity of angiotensin I-convertingenzyme inhibitory peptides derived from Alaskan pollack skin. *Journal of Biochemistry and Molecular Biology, 35*, 239–243.

Cao, W., Zhang, C., Hong, P., Ji, H., & Hao, J. (2010). Purification and identification of an ACE inhibitory peptide from the peptic hydrolysate of *Acetes chinensis* and its antihypertensive effects in spontaneously hypertensive rats. *International Journal of Food Science & Technology, 45*, 959–965.

Carrazco-Peña, L., Osuna-Castro, J. A., De León-Rodríguez, A., Maruyama, N., Toro-Vazquez, J. F., Morales-Rueda, J. A., & Barba de la Rosa, A. P. (2013). Modification of solubility and heat-induced gelation of amaranth 11S globulin by protein engineering. *Journal of Agricultural and Food Chemistry, 61*, 3509–3516.

Caselato-Sousa, V. M., & Amaya-Farfán, J. (2012). State of knowledge on amaranth arain: A comprehensive review. *Journal of Food Science, 77*, 93–104.

Castro-Martínez, C., Luna-Suárez, S., & Paredes-López, O. (2012). Overexpression of a modified protein from amaranth seed in *Escherichia coli* and effect of environmental conditions on the protein expression. *Journal of Biotechnology, 158*, 59–67.

Chakraborty, S., Chakraborty, N., & Datta, A. (2000). Increased nutritive value of transgenic potato by expressing a nonallergenic seed albumin gene from *Amaranthus hypochondriacus*. *Proceedings of the National Academy of Sciences, 97*, 3724–3729.

Charalampopoulos, D., Wang, R., Pandiella, S., & Webb, C. (2002). Application of cereals and cereal components in functional foods: A review. *International Journal of Food Microbiology, 79*, 131–141.

Chen, H. M., Muramoto, K., Yamauchi, F., Fujimoto, K., & Nokihara, K. (1998). Antioxidative properties of histidine-containing peptides designed from peptide fragments found in the digests of a soybean protein. *Journal of Agricultural and Food Chemistry, 46*, 49–53.

Cheung, H. S., Wang, F. L., Ondetti, M. A., Sabo, E. F., & Cushman, D. W. (1980). Binding of peptide substrates and inhibitors of angiotensin-converting enzyme. *The Journal of Biological Chemistry, 255*, 401–407.

Clemente, A. (2000). Enzymatic protein hydrolysates in human nutrition. *Trends in Food Science & Technology, 11*, 254–262.

Condés, M. C., Scilingo, A. A., & Añón, M. C. (2009). Characterization of amaranth proteins modified by trypsin proteolysis. Structural and functional changes. *LWT- Food Science and Technology, 42*, 963–970.

Cox, D. B. T., Platt, R. J., & Zhang, F. (2015). Therapeutic genome editing: Prospects and challenges. *Nature Medicine, 21*, 121–131.

Davis, P., & Williams, S. (1998). Protein modification by thermal processing. *Allergy, 53*, 102–105.

Del Valle, F., Escobedo, M., Sanchez-Marroquin, A., Bourges, H., Bock, M., & Biemer, P. (1993). Chemical and nutritional evaluation of two amaranth (*Amaranthus cruentus*)-based infant formulas. *Plant Foods for Human Nutrition, 43*, 145–156.

Derbyshire, E., Wright, D., & Boulter, D. (1976). Legumin and vicilin, storage proteins of legume seeds. *Phytochemistry, 15*, 3–24.

Devasagayam, T., Tilak, J., Boloor, K., Sane, K., Ghaskadbi, S. S., & Lele, R. (2004). Free radicals and antioxidants in human health: Current status and future prospects. *Journal of the Association of Physicians of India, 52*, 794–804.

Dodok, L., Modhir, A., Buchtova, V., Halasova, G., & Polaček, I. (1997). Importance and utilization of amaranth in food industry. Part 2. Composition of amino acids and fatty acids. *Nahrung, 41*, 108–110.

Durak, A., Baraniak, B., Jakubczyk, A., & Åšwieca, M. (2013). Biologically active peptides obtained by enzymatic hydrolysis of Adzuki bean seeds. *Food Chemistry, 141*, 2177–2183.

Ebert, A. W. (2014). Potential of underutilized traditional vegetables and legume crops to contribute to food and nutritional security, income and more sustainable production systems. *Sustainability, 6*, 319–335.

Escudero, N., De Arellano, M., Luco, J., Gimenez, M., & Mucciarelli, S. (2004). Comparison of the chemical composition and nutritional value of *Amaranthus cruentus* flour and its protein concentrate. *Plant Foods for Human Nutrition, 59*, 15–21.

Espín, J. C., García-Conesa, M. T., & Tomás-Barberán, F. A. (2007). Nutraceuticals: Facts and fiction. *Phytochemistry, 68*, 2986–3008.

FAO (1973). *Energy and protein requirements, Nutritional Meeting Report Series*. Rome: Food and Agriculture Organization.

FAO. (2009). FAO and traditional knowledge: The linkages with sustainability, food security and climate change impacts. Rome.

FAO. (2011). Food and nutrition paper. Dietary protein quality evaluation in human nutrition: Report of an FAO expert consultation. Auckland.

Ferreira, T. A., & Areas, J. A. G. (2010). Calcium bioavailability of raw and extruded amaranth grains. *Food Science and Technology, 30*, 532–538.

Fidantsi, A., & Doxastakis, G. (2001). Emulsifying and foaming properties of amaranth seed protein isolates. *Colloids and Surfaces B: Biointerfaces, 21*, 119–124.

Fritz, M., Vecchi, B., Rinaldi, G., & Añón, M. C. (2011). Amaranth seed protein hydrolysates have in vivo and in vitro antihypertensive activity. *Food Chemistry, 126*, 878–884.

Fukushima, D. (1991). Structures of plant storage proteins and their functions. *Food Reviews International, 7*, 353–381.

Galili, G., & Höfgen, R. (2002). Metabolic engineering of amino acids and storage proteins in plants. *Metabolic Engineering, 4*, 3–11.

Gamel, T. H., Linssen, J. P., Mesallam, A. S., Damir, A. A., & Shekib, L. A. (2006). Effect of seed treatments on the chemical composition of two amaranth species: Oil, sugars, fibres, minerals and vitamins. *Journal of the Science of Food and Agriculture, 86*, 82–89.

Garcia-Gonzalez, A., Flores-Vazquez, A. L., Barba de la Rosa, A. P., Vazquez-Martinez, E. A., & Ruiz-Garcia, J. (2013). Amaranth 7S globulin Langmuir films and its interaction with l-α-dipalmitoilphosphatidilcholine at the air−fluid interface. *The Journal of Physical Chemistry B, 117*, 14046–14058.

Germán-Báez, L. J., Cruz-Mendívil, A., Medina-Godoy, S., Milán-Carrillo, J., Reyes-Moreno, C., & Valdez-Ortiz, A. (2014). Expression of an engineered acidic-subunit 11S globulin of amaranth carrying the antihypertensive peptides VY, in transgenic tomato fruits. *Plant Cell, Tissue and Organ Culture, 118*, 305–312.

Goodman, R. E., Vieths, S., Sampson, H. A., Hill, D., Ebisawa, M., Taylor, S. L., & van Ree, R. (2008). Allergenicity assessment of genetically modified crops-what makes sense? *Nature Biotechnology, 26*, 73–81.

Gordon, M. H. (1990). The Mechanism of antioxidant action in vitro. In B. J. F. Hudson (Ed.), *Food antioxidants* (1st ed., pp. 1–18). Dordrecht: Springer.

Gorinstein, S., Pawelzik, E., Delgado-Licon, E., Haruenkit, R., Weisz, M., & Trakhtenberg, S. (2002). Characterisation of pseudocereal and cereal proteins by protein and amino acid analyses. *Journal of the Science of Food and Agriculture, 82*, 886–891.

Gostner, J. M., Becker, K., Ueberall, F., & Fuchs, D. (2015). The good and bad of antioxidant foods: An immunological perspective. *Food and Chemical Toxicology, 80*, 72–79.

Guzmán-Maldonado, S. H., & Paredes-López, O. (1998). Functional products of plants indigenous to Latin America: Amaranth, quinoa, common beans, and botanicals. In G. Mazza (Ed.), *Functional foods: Biochemical and processing aspects* (pp. 293–328). Lancaster, PA: Technomic Publishing Company.

Han, S.-W., Chee, K.-M., & Cho, S.-J. (2015). Nutritional quality of rice bran protein in comparison to animal and vegetable protein. *Food Chemistry, 172*, 766–769.

Haque, E., Chand, R., & Kapila, S. (2008). Biofunctional properties of bioactive peptides of milk origin. *Food Reviews International, 25*, 28–43.

Hara-Nishimura, I., Nishimura, M., & Akazawa, T. (1985). Biosynthesis and intracellular transport of 11S globulin in developing pumpkin cotyledons. *Plant Physiology, 77*, 747–752.

Haulica, I., Bild, W., & Serban, D. N. (2005). Review: Angiotensin peptides and their pleiotropic actions. *Journal of the Renin-Angiotensin-Aldosterone System, 6*, 121–131.

He, H.-P., Cai, Y., Sun, M., & Corke, H. (2002). Extraction and purification of squalene from Amaranthus grain. *Journal of Agricultural and Food Chemistry, 50*, 368–372.

Huang, W. Y., Majumder, K., & Wu, J. (2010). Oxygen radical absorbance capacity of peptides from egg white protein ovotransferrin and their interactions with phytochemicals. *Food Chemistry, 123*, 635–641.

Iqbal, A., Khalil, I. A., Ateeq, N., & Khan, M. S. (2006). Nutritional quality of important food legumes. *Food Chemistry, 97*, 331–335.

Ju, H., Venema, V. J., Marrero, M. B., & Venema, R. C. (1998). Inhibitory interactions of the bradykinin B2 receptor with endothelial nitric-oxide synthase. *The Journal of Biological Chemistry, 273*, 24025–24029.

Kanchiswamy, C. N., Sargent, D. J., Velasco, R., Maffei, M. E., & Malnoy, M. (2015). Looking forward to genetically edited fruit crops. *Trends in Biotechnology, 33*, 62–64.

Kauffman, C. S. (1992). Realizing the potential of grain amaranth. *Food Review International, 8*, 5–21.

Koike, H., Ito, K., Miyamoto, M., & Nishino, H. (1980). Effects of long-term blockade of angiotensin converting enzyme with captopril (SQ14,225) on hemodynamics and circulating blood volume in SHR. *Hypertension, 2*, 299–303.

Kong, B., & Xiong, Y. L. (2006). Antioxidant activity of zein hydrolysates in a liposome system and the possible mode of action. *Journal of Agricultural and Food Chemistry, 54*, 6059–6068.

Lavine, E., & Ben-Shoshan, M. (2015). Allergy to sunflower seed and sunflower butter as proposed vehicle for sensitization. *Allergy, Asthma & Clinical Immunology, 11*, 1–3. Available from http://dx.doi.org/10.1186/s13223-014-0065-6.

Leyva-Lopez, N., Vasco, N., de la Rosa, A. B., & Paredes-López, O. (1995). Amaranth seed proteins: Effect of defatting on extraction yield and on electrophoretic patterns. *Plant Foods for Human Nutrition, 47*, 49–53.

Liu, C., Wang, H., Cui, Z., He, X., Wang, X., Zeng, X., & Ma, H. (2007). Optimization of extraction and isolation for 11S and 7S globulins of soybean seed storage protein. *Food Chemistry, 102*, 1310–1316.

Liu, F., & Stützel, H. (2002). Leaf water relations of vegetable amaranth (*Amaranthus* spp.) in response to soil drying. *European Journal of Agronomy, 16*, 137–150.

Liu, F., & Stützel, H. (2004). Biomass partitioning, specific leaf area, and water use efficiency of vegetable amaranth (*Amaranthus* spp.) in response to drought stress. *Scientia Horticulturae, 102*, 15–27.

López, G. M., Bello-Pérez, A., & Paredes-López, O. (1994). Amaranth carbohydrates. In O. Paredes-López (Ed.), *Amaranth: Biology, chemistry and technology* (pp. 107–130). Boca Raton, FL: CRC Press.

Luna-Suárez, S., Medina-Godoy, S., Cruz-Hernández, A., & Paredes-López, O. (2010). Modification of the amaranth 11S globulin storage protein to produce an inhibitory peptide of the angiotensin I converting enzyme, and its expression in *Escherichia coli*. *Journal of Biotechnology, 148*, 240–247.

Luna-Suárez, S., Medina-Godoy, S., Cruz-Hernández, A., & Paredes-López, O. (2008). Expression and characterization of the acidic subunit from 11S amaranth seed protein. *Biotechnology journal, 3*, 209–219.

Mallory, M. A., Hall, R. V., McNabb, A. R., Pratt, D. B., Jellen, E. N., & Maughan, P. J. (2008). Development and characterization of microsatellite markers for the grain amaranths. *Crop Science, 48*, 1098–1106.

Mandal, S., & Mandal, R. (2000). Seed storage proteins and approaches for improvement of their nutritional quality by genetic engineering. *Current Science, 79*, 576–589.

Mannheim, A., & Cheryan, M. (1992). Enzyme-modified proteins from corn gluten meal: Preparation and functional properties. *Journal of the American Oil Chemists' Society, 69*, 1163–1169.

Marambe, P. W. M. L. H. K., Shand, P. J., & Wanasundara, J. P. D. (2008). An in-vitro investigation of selected biological activities of hydrolysed flaxseed (*Linum usitatissimum* L.) Proteins. *Journal of the American Oil Chemists' Society, 85*, 1155–1164.

Marcone, M. (1999a). Possible nutritional implications of varietal influence on the 7S/11S seed globulin ratios in amaranth. *Plant Foods for Human Nutrition, 54*, 375–380.

Marcone, M. F. (1999b). Biochemical and biophysical properties of plant storage proteins: A current understanding with emphasis on 11S seed globulins. *Food Research International, 32*, 79–92.

Marcone, M. F., Kakuda, Y., & Yada, R. Y. (1998). Salt-soluble seed globulins of various dicotyledonous and monocotyledonous plants-I. Isolation/purification and characterization. *Food Chemistry, 62*, 27–47.

Martínez-Cruz, O., Cabrera-Chávez, F., & Paredes-López, O. (2014). Biochemical characteristics, and nutraceutical and technological uses of amaranth globulins. In S. D. Milford (Ed.), *Globulins: Biochemistry, production and role in immunity* (pp. 41–70). New York, NY: Nova Science Publishers.

Martínez-Maqueda, D., Miralles, B., Recio, I., & Hernández-Ledesma, B. (2012). Antihypertensive peptides from food proteins: A review. *Food Function, 3*, 350–361.

Medina-Godoy, S., Rodriguez-Yanez, S. K., Bobadilla, N. A., Perez-Villalva, R., Valdez-Ortiz, R., Hong, E., ... Valdez-Ortiz, A. (2013). Antihypertensive activity of AMC3, an engineered 11S amaranth globulin expressed in *Escherichia coli*, in spontaneously hypertensive rats. *Journal of Functional Foods, 5*, 1441–1449.

Medina-Godoy, S., Valdez-Ortiz, A., Valverde, M. E., & Paredes-López, O. (2006). Endoplasmic reticulum-retention C-terminal sequence enhances production of an 11S seed globulin from *Amaranthus hypochondriacus* in *Pichia pastoris*. *Biotechnology Journal, 1*, 1085–1092.

Medina-Godoy, S., Nielsen, N. C., & Paredes-López, O. (2004). Expression and Characterization of a His-Tagged 11S Seed Globulin from *Amaranthus hypochondriacus* in *Escherichia coli*. *Biotechnology progress, 20*, 1749–1756.

Mlakar, S. G., Turinek, M., Jakop, M., Bavec, M., & Bavec, F. (2010). Grain amaranth as an alternative and perspective crop in temperate climate. *Journal for Geography, 5*, 135–145.

Montoya-Rodríguez, A., Gómez-Favela, M. A., Reyes-Moreno, C., Milán-Carrillo, J., & González de Mejía, E. (2015). Identification of bioactive peptide sequences from amaranth (*Amaranthus hypochondriacus*) seed proteins and their potential role in the prevention of chronic diseases. *Comprehensive Reviews in Food Science and Food Safety, 14*, 139–158.

Montoya-Rodríguez, A., Mejía, E. G., Dia, V. P., Reyes-Moreno, C., & Milán-Carrillo, J. (2014). Extrusion improved the anti-inflammatory effect of amaranth (*Amaranthus hypochondriacus*) hydrolysates in LPS-induced human THP-1 macrophage-like and mouse RAW 264.7 macrophages by preventing activation of NF-κB signaling. *Molecular Nutrition & Food Research, 58*, 1028–1041.

Mora-Escobedo, R., Paredes-López, O., & Ordorica-Falomir, C. (1990). Characterization of albumins and globulins from amaranth. *LWT-Food Science and Technology, 23*, 484–487.

Morales-Camacho, J., Dominguez-Dominguez, J., & Paredes-López, O. (2013). Overexpression of a modified amaranth protein in *Escherichia coli* with minimal media and lactose as inducer. *Recent Patents on Biotechnology, 7*, 61–70.

Moreno, F. J., & Clemente, A. (2008). Albumin storage proteins: What makes them food allergens? *The Open Biochemistry Journal, 2*, 16–28.

Moure, A., Domínguez, H., & Parajó, J. C. (2005). Fractionation and enzymatic hydrolysis of soluble protein present in waste liquors from soy processing. *Journal of Agricultural and Food Chemistry, 53*, 7600–7608.

Myers, R. L. (1996). Amaranth: New crop opportunity. In J. Janick (Ed.), *Progress in new crops* (pp. 207–220). Alexandria, VA: ASHS Press.

Mylne, J. S., Hara-Nishimura, I., & Rosengren, K. J. (2014). Seed storage albumins: Biosynthesis, trafficking and structures. *Functional Plant Biology, 41*, 671–677.

Noguchi, N., Watanabe, A., & Shi, H. (2000). Diverse functions of antioxidants. *Free Radical Research, 33*, 809–817.

Omamt, E., Hammes, P., & Robbertse, P. (2006). Differences in salinity tolerance for growth and water-use efficiency in some amaranth (*Amaranthus* spp.) genotypes. *New Zealand Journal of Crop and Horticultural Science, 34*, 11–22.

Ondetti, M., & Cushman, D. (1982). Enzymes of the renin-angiotensin system and their inhibitors. *Annual Review of Biochemistry, 51*, 283–308.

Orsini-Delgado, M. C., Tironi, V. A., & Añón, M. C. (2011). Antioxidant activity of amaranth protein or their hydrolysates under simulated gastrointestinal digestion. *LWT-Food Science and Technology, 44*, 1752–1760.

Orsini-Delgado, M. C. O., Galleano, M., Añón, M. C., & Tironi, V. A. (2015). Amaranth peptides from simulated gastrointestinal digestion: Antioxidant activity against reactive species. *Plant Foods for Human Nutrition, 70*, 27–34.

Osborne, T. B. (1924). *The vegetable proteins, monographs in biochemistry* (2nd ed., p. 25). London: Longmans Green and Co.

Osuna-Castro, J. A., Rascón-Cruz, Q., Napier, J., Fido, R. J., Shewry, P. R., & Paredes-López, O. (2000). Overexpression, purification, and in vitro refolding of the 11S globulin from amaranth seed in *Escherichia coli*. *Journal of Agricultural and Food Chemistry, 48*, 5249–5255.

Oszvald, M., Tamás, C., Rakszegi, M., Tömösközi, S., Békés, F., & Tamás, L. (2009). Effects of incorporated amaranth albumins on the functional properties of wheat dough. *Journal of the Science of Food and Agriculture, 89*, 882–889.

Panyam, D., & Kilara, A. (1996). Enhancing the functionality of food proteins by enzymatic modification. *Trends in Food Science & Technology, 7*, 120–125.

Paravicini, T. M., & Touyz, R. M. (2008). NADPH oxidases, reactive oxygen species, and hypertension clinical implications and therapeutic possibilities. *Diabetes Care*, *31*, S170–S180.

Paredes-López, O. (1994). *Amaranth: Biology, chemistry and technology* (1st ed.). Boca Raton, FL: CRC Press.

Paredes-López, O., Barba De La Rosa, A. P., & Cárabez-Trejo, A. (1990). Enzymatic production of high-protein amaranth flour and carbohydrate rich fraction. *Journal of Food Science*, *55*, 1157–1161.

Paredes-López, O., Mendoza, V., & Mora, R. (1993). Isolation of amaranth flour proteins by fractionation procedures and sonication. *Plant Foods for Human Nutrition*, *43*, 37–43.

Paredes-López, O., Mora-Escobedo, R., & Ordorica-Falomir, C. (1988). Isolation of amaranth proteins. *LWT-Food Science Technology*, *21*, 59–61.

Pasko, P., Sajewicz, M., Gorinstein, S., & Zachwieja, Z. (2008). Analysis of selected phenolic acids and flavonoids in *Amaranthus cruentus* and *Chenopodium quinoa* seeds and sprouts by HPLC. *Acta Chromatographica*, *20*, 661–672.

Pavlik, V. (2011). The revival of amaranth as a third-millennium food. *Neuroendocrinology Letters*, *33*, 3–4.

Peñta-Ramos, E., & Xiong, Y. (2002). Antioxidant activity of soy protein hydrolysates in a liposomal system. *Journal of Food Science*, *67*, 2952–2956.

Peterson, D. M. (1978). Subunit structure and composition of oat seed globulin. *Plant Physiology*, *62*, 506–509.

Písaříková, B., Kráčmar, S., & Herzig, I. (2005). Amino acid contents and biological value of protein in various amaranth species. *Czech Journal of Animal Science*, *50*, 568–573.

Quiroga, A., Martínez, E. N., Rogniaux, H., Geairon, A., & Añón, M. C. (2010). Amaranth (*Amaranthus hypochondriacus*) vicilin subunit structure. *Journal of Agricultural and Food Chemistry*, *58*, 12957–12963.

Quiroga, A. V., Aphalo, P., Ventureira, J. L., Martínez, E. N., & Añón, M. C. (2012). Physicochemical, functional and angiotensin converting enzyme inhibitory properties of amaranth (*Amaranthus hypochondriacus*) 7S globulin. *Journal of the Science of Food and Agriculture*, *92*, 397–403.

Rascón-Cruz, Q., Sinagawa-García, S., Osuna-Castro, J., Bohorova, N., & Paredes-López, O. (2004). Accumulation, assembly, and digestibility of amarantin expressed in transgenic tropical maize. *Theoretical and Applied Genetics*, *108*, 335–342.

Rastogi, A., & Shukla, S. (2013). Amaranth: A new millennium crop of nutraceutical values. *Critical Reviews in Food Science and Nutrition*, *53*, 109–125.

Repo-Carrasco-Valencia, R., Peña, J., Kallio, H., & Salminen, S. (2009). Dietary fiber and other functional components in two varieties of crude and extruded kiwicha (*Amaranthus caudatus*). *Journal of Cereal Science*, *49*, 219–224.

Ricroch, A. E., & Hénard-Damave, M.-C. (2015). Next biotech plants: New traits, crops, developers and technologies for addressing global challenges. *Critical Reviews in Biotechnology*, *36*(4) 1–16.

Rodríguez Patino, J. M., Rodríguez Niño, M. R., & Carrera Sánchez, C. (2007). Physico-chemical properties of surfactant and protein films. *Current Opinion in Colloid & Interface Science*, *12*, 187–195.

Sarmadi, B., & Ismail, A. (2010). Antioxidative peptides from food proteins: A review. *Peptides*, *31*, 1949–1956.

Sauer, J. D. (1950). The grain amaranths: A survey of their history and classification. *Annals of the Missouri Botanical Garden*, *37*, 561–632.

Sauer, J. D. (1967). The grain amaranths and their relatives: A revised taxonomic and geographic survey. *Annals of the Missouri Botanical Garden*, *54*, 103–137.

Saunders, R., & Becker, R. (1984). Amaranthus: A potential food and feed resource. In Y. Pomeranz (Ed.), *Advances in cereal science and technology* (pp. 357–397). St. Paul, MN: American Association of Cereal Chemist.

Schmidt, D. (1977). *Grain amaranth: A look at some potentials, Proceedings of the First Amaranth Conference* (pp. 121–129). Maxatawny, PA: Rodale Press.

Sciences, N. A. (1984). *Amaranth: Modern prospects for an ancient crop* (pp. 55–85). Washington, DC: National. Academic Science Press.

Scilingo, A. A., Ortiz, S. E. M., Martínez, E. N., & Añón, M. C. (2002). Amaranth protein isolates modified by hydrolytic and thermal treatments. Relationship between structure and solubility. *Food Research International*, *35*, 855–862.

Segura-Campos, M. R., Salazar-Vega, I. M., Chel-Guerrero, L. A., & Betancur-Ancona, D. A. (2013). Biological potential of chia (*Salvia hispanica* L.) protein hydrolysates and their incorporation into functional foods. *LWT-Food Science and Technology*, *50*, 723–731.

Segura-Nieto, M., Barba De La Rosa, A., & Paredes-López, O. (1994). Biochemistry of amaranth proteins. In O. Paredes-López (Ed.), *Amaranth: Biology, chemistry and technology* (pp. 75–106). Boca Raton, FL: CRC Press.

Sentandreu, M. A., & Toldra, F. (2007). Evaluation of ACE inhibitory activity of dipeptides generated by the action of porcine muscle dipeptidyl peptidases. *Food Chemistry*, *101*, 1629–1633.

Shewry, P., Casey, R., & Pandya, M. (1999). *The 2S albumin storage proteins, seed proteins* (pp. 563–586). Dordrecht: Springer.

Shewry, P. R., & Halford, N. G. (2002). Cereal seed storage proteins: Structures, properties and role in grain utilization. *Journal of Experimental Botany*, *53*, 947–958.

Shotwell, M. A., Afonso, C., Davies, E., Chesnut, R. S., & Larkins, B. A. (1988). Molecular characterization of oat seed globulins. *Plant Physiology*, *87*, 698–704.

Silva-Sáchez, C., González-Castañeda, J., De León-Rodríguez, A., & Barba de la Rosa, A. P. (2004). Functional and rheological properties of amaranth albumins extracted from two Mexican varieties. *Plant Foodsfor Human Nutrition*, *59*, 169–174.

Silva-Sánchez, C., de la Rosa, A. B., León-Galván, M., De Lumen, B., de Leon-Rodriguez, A., & de Mejía, E. G. (2008). Bioactive peptides in amaranth (*Amaranthus hypochondriacus*) seed. *Journal of Agricultural and Food Chemistry*, *56*, 1233–1240.

Sinagawa-García, S. R., Rascón-Cruz, Q., Valdez-Ortiz, A., Medina-Godoy, S., Escobar-Gutiérrez, A., & Paredes-López, O. (2004). Safety assessment by in vitro digestibility and allergenicity of genetically modified maize with an amaranth 11S globulin. *Journal of Agricultural and Food Chemistry*, *52*, 2709–2714.

Singhal, R. S., & Kulkarni, P. R. (1988). Composition of the seeds of some Amaranthus species. *Journal of the Science of Food and Agriculture, 42*, 325−331.

Siow, H.-L., & Gan, C.-Y. (2013). Extraction of antioxidative and antihypertensive bioactive peptides from *Parkia speciosa* seeds. *Food Chemistry, 141*, 3435−3442.

Stallknecht, G., & Schulz-Schaeffer, J. (1993). Amaranth rediscovered. In J. Janick, & J. E. Simon (Eds.), *New crops* (pp. 211−218). New York, NY: Wiley.

Tai, S. S. K., Lee, T. T. T., Tsai, C. C. Y., Yiu, T.-J., & Tzen, J. T. C. (2001). Expression pattern and deposition of three storage proteins, 11S globulin, 2S albumin and 7S globulin in maturing sesame seeds. *Plant Physiology and Biochemistry, 39*, 981−992.

Tandang-Silvas, M. R., Cabanos, C. S., Carrazco Peña, L. D., Barba de la Rosa, A. P., Osuna-Castro, J. A., Utsumi, S., . . . Maruyama, N. (2012). Crystal structure of a major seed storage protein, 11S proglobulin, from *Amaranthus hypochondriacus*: Insight into its physico-chemical properties. *Food Chemistry, 135*, 819−826.

Tiengo, A., Faria, M., & Netto, F. (2009). Characterization and ACE-inhibitory activity of amaranth proteins. *Journal of Food Science, 74*, 121−126.

Tironi, V. A., & Añón, M. C. (2010). Amaranth proteins as a source of antioxidant peptides: Effect of proteolysis. *Food Research International, 43*, 315−322.

Tovar-Pérez, E., Guerrero-Legarreta, I., Farrés-González, A., & Soriano-Santos, J. (2009). Angiotensin I-converting enzyme-inhibitory peptide fractions from albumin 1 and globulin as obtained of amaranth grain. *Food Chemistry, 116*, 437−444.

Tucker, J. B. (1986). Amaranth: The once and future crop. *BioScience, 36*, 9−13.

Valdez-Ortiz, A., Rascón-Cruz, Q., Medina-Godoy, S., Sinagawa-García, S. R., Valverde-González, M. E., & Paredes-López, O. (2005). One-step purification and structural characterization of a recombinant His-tag 11S globulin expressed in transgenic tobacco. *Journal of Biotechnology, 115*, 413−423.

van-Platerink, C. J., Janssen, H. G. M., & Haverkamp, J. (2008). Application of at-line two-dimensional liquid chromatography-mass spectrometry for identification of small hydrophilic angiotensin I-inhibiting peptides in milk hydrolysates. *Analytical and Bioanalytical Chemistry, 391*, 299−307.

Vasco-Méndez, N. L., & Paredes-López, O. (1994). Antigenic homology between amaranth glutelins and other storage proteins. *Journal of Food Biochemistry, 18*, 227−238.

Vecchi, B., & Añon, M. (2009). ACE inhibitory tetrapeptides from *Amaranthus hypochondriacus* 11S globulin. *Phytochemistry, 70*, 864−870.

Venskutonis, P. R., & Kraujalis, P. (2013). Nutritional components of amaranth seeds and vegetables: Are view on composition, properties, and uses. *Comprehensive Reviews in Food Science and Food Safety, 12*, 381−412.

Verma, A. K., Kumar, S., Das, M., & Dwivedi, P. D. (2013). A comprehensive review of legume allergy. *Clinical Reviews in Allergy & Immunology, 45*, 30−46.

Vermeirssen, V., Camp, J. V., & Verstraete, W. (2004). Bioavailability of angiotensin I converting enzyme inhibitory peptides. *British Journal of Nutrition, 92*, 357−366.

Wang, W., Mejia, D., & Gonzalez, E. (2005). A new frontier in soy bioactive peptides that may prevent age-related chronic diseases. *Comprehensive Reviews in Food Science and Food Safety, 4*, 63−78.

Wright, D. J. (1987). The seed globulins. In B. J. F. Hudson (Ed.), *Developments in food proteins* (p. 81). London: Elsevier Applied Science.

Wu, H.-C., Chen, H.-M., & Shiau, C.-Y. (2003). Free amino acids and peptides as related to antioxidant properties in protein hydrolysates of mackerel (*Scomber austriasicus*). *Food Research International, 36*, 949−957.

Xu, F., & Sun, M. (2001). Comparative analysis of phylogenetic relationships of grain amaranths and their wild relatives (*Amaranthus*; Amaranthaceae) using internal transcribed spacer, amplified fragment length polymorphism, and double-primer fluorescent intersimple sequence repeat markers. *Molecular Phylogenetics and Evolution, 21*, 372−387.

Yano, H., Wong, J. H., Cho, M.-J., & Buchanan, B. B. (2001). Redox changes accompanying the degradation of seed storage proteins in germinating rice. *Plant Cell Physiology, 42*, 879−883.

Chapter 16

Amaranth Part 2—Sustainability, Processing, and Applications of Amaranth

D.K. Santra[1] and R. Schoenlechner[2]

[1]University of Nebraska-Lincoln, Scottsbluff, NE, United States, [2]University of Natural Resources and Life Sciences, Vienna, Austria

16.1 SUSTAINABILITY OF AMARANTH PRODUCTION

16.1.1 Origin and Distribution

Amaranths are broad-leaved plants, one of the few nongrasses that produce significant amounts of edible small-seeded grain, also often called pseudocereals. It was reported to have originated both in Central and Latin America (Sauer, 1967, 1993; Stallknecht & Schulz-Schaeffer, 1993; Sumar, 1983). Among the three grain-type species of amaranth, *Amaranthus cruentus* was reported to be cultivated 6000 years ago in Central America, *Amaranthus hypochondriacus* was cultivated in Mexico at least approximately 1500 years, and the third grain type *Amaranthus caudatus* was reported to be grown in Andean mountain valleys of south America (Sauer, 1993). Presently, *A. cruentus* production is limited to Andean mountains because of its adaptability to higher elevation. *Amaranthus hypochondriacus* is the most common grain amaranth since it is more adapted to lower elevation, which is represented by the worlds' major production regions (Myers, 1996). Grain amaranth was a major food in Aztecs, Mayan, and Incan diets and cultures until the 1500s when the Spanish conquered (Graham, 2010; NRC, 1989; Sooby et al., 1998). By the 1700s it was spread from Latin America and grown in Eastern Europe and Russia as a herb and ornamental (NRC, 1984). Grain amaranth was presumably introduced from these points of origin to the northern Indian subcontinent, the mountain valleys of Nepal, and part of Africa in the late 1800s (Joshi and Rana, 1991; Sauer, 1967, 1993). During the 20th century, its production was reported in Asia, Africa, Europe, and North and South America (Sooby et al., 1998). It was largely ignored in the United States until the 1970s, when amaranth grain protein was reported as high quality and could be used as a food ingredient in the American diet (Breene, 1991; Senft, 1980).

16.1.2 Production and Yield

Although traditionally cultivated within 30° latitude of the equator, amaranth can be grown in higher latitudes using varieties requiring longer day length than that of the tropics (NRC, 1989; Weber, 1987). Most grain amaranth cultivation was concentrated in highland valleys, such as those in the Sierra Madre, Andes, and Himalayas. By the middle of the 20th century, cultivation of grain amaranth had declined to the point where it was grown only in small plots in Mexico, the Andean highlands, and in the Himalayan foothills of India and Nepal (Kauffman & Weber, 1990; Myers, 1996; Weber, 1987). Cultivation of grain amaranth is now in the process of expanding in a number of countries (Mexico, Guatemala, Peru, Venezuela, Kenya, Uganda, Nigeria, India, China, Thailand, United States, and Canada) (Graham, 2010). As of the mid-1990s, South Asia was the world's only region where grain amaranth production was increasing (Brenner et al., 2000).

Amaranth production was slowly started and increased in the United States during the 1980s and 1990s, primarily because of an initiative by the Rodale Research Center, Pennsylvania (Weber, 1987). The United States has been the leading commercial producer of grain amaranth during this period, although production has been less than 2000 ha annually (Myers, 1996; Weber, 1987). Most of the United States production has been in the upper Midwest and Great Plains (Nebraska, South Dakota, North Dakota, Missouri, Minnesota, Kansas, and Iowa) and with widely scattered fields in other parts of the country (Montana, California, Maryland, and Kentucky) (Myers, 1996; Sooby et al., 1998; Weber, 1987). Production in none of these states is on a large scale, which possibly will not change in the near future based on the limited market. In 1988, approximately 1200 ha of grain amaranth were planted in the Great Plains of the United States. According to the 2002 US Census of Agriculture, 10 farms grew amaranth on 939 acres. Although the United States has been the leading producer of grain amaranth for retail food products, the largest production area in the last decade is believed to have been in China (Sooby et al., 1998). The main Chinese use of amaranth is reportedly to feed the forage to hogs, rather than harvesting the grain (Myers, 1996).

In North America (United States and Canada), optimal planting time is between mid-May to mid-June when soil temperature is at or above 65–70°F (Myers, 1996; Weber, 1987). Yield was decreased substantially when planting time was delayed to July. Grain amaranth was usually harvested either after natural senescence (such as Missouri, Texas) or after first frost (northern Great Plains and upper mid-west) in September–October (Myers, 1996; Weber, 1987). Yields of grain amaranth, like any new crop, are highly variable. One of the most important factors of grain loss is seed loss due to shattering before harvest from wind or during harvest (Myers, 1996; Weber, 1987). Seed yield of grain amaranths is very comparable to the yields of most other cereals when yield loss due to shattering was minimal. Hand-harvested yield has been as high as 4000 kg/ha in Montana (Cramer, 1988) and 6000 kg/ha in Peru (Sumar, 1983). When harvested mechanically, 1000 kg/ha is considered to be a good yield, which has often been achieved in research plots in a number of states throughout the United States (Myers, 1994). However, potential yields could be several-fold more than this base level depending on location and condition of the trials. In Pennsylvania, test plots yielded 1800 kg/ha, whereas in California the yield was ~3000 kg/ha (Myers, 1994). In the sub-Himalayan region in India (Himachal Pradesh and Uttar Pradesh) selected landraces yielded 3000 kg/ha in a research plot (Joshi, 1985, 1986). Grain yield of up to 5000 kg/ha has been reported in Uganda (Stallknecht & Schulz-Schaeffer, 1993). Grain amaranth breeding programs in Latin America have achieved yields of 7200 kg/ha and 4600 kg/ha for certain varieties in Peru and Mexico, respectively (Brenner et al., 2000).

16.1.3 Land, Water, and Energy Uses

Conventional cereals (eg, corn, wheat, rice) require high levels of water and nitrogen fertilizer, which is chemically produced through energy-intensive chemical processes. Therefore, such modern food grain crops are very energy-intensive for production of protein-rich human diet. In contrast, pseudocereal crops like grain amaranth are low energy-requiring crops because of the low requirement for water and fertilizer.

The grain amaranths exhibit C4 photosynthesis, grow rapidly, tolerate a variety of unfavorable abiotic conditions, including high salinity, acidity, or alkalinity, making them highly suited for production under subsistence agricultural practices that are inhospitable to conventional cereal crops (Myers, 1996; Sooby et al., 1998; Weber, 1987). Therefore, by implication, the grain amaranth has the potential for a significant impact on malnutrition (Emokaro & Ekunwe, 2007). Historically, people have cultivated amaranths in environments ranging from the true tropics to semiarid lands and from sea level to some of the highest farms in the world.

Amaranth has evolved so that it can produce grain under moisture stress. Grain amaranth has the ability to produce good seed yield even under severe drought conditions when most modern grain crops fail. The grain amaranth field in western Nebraska during 2012, an historic drought year in the United States, is a perfect example (Fig. 16.1). Little is known about actual water requirements of grain amaranth. Amaranths require well-moistened soil for germination and root establishment but once seedlings are established, it does well with limited water, making it especially valuable in areas with limited water resources such as Sub-Sahara Africa and the west-central Great Plains of the United States (Chaudhari, Patel, & Desai, 2009; Johnson & Henderson, 2002; Joshi & Rana, 1991; Mng'omba, Kwapata, & Bokosi, 2003; Piha, 1995; Sooby et al., 1998). In fact, they grow best under dry, warm conditions. Grain amaranths have been grown in dry-land agriculture in areas receiving as little as 200 mm of annual precipitation (Putnam, 1990).

Observations in many test plots and farmers' fields suggest that grain amaranth is drought-tolerant at later stages of growth. Amaranth has the ability to grow back to full vigor if rain occurs within a few days of wilting. Researchers in China have reported that the water requirement for growing grain amaranth is 42–47% that of wheat, 51–62% that of maize, and 79% that of cotton (Kauffman & Weber, 1990). Kenyan farmers in regions with marginal rainfall plant amaranth rather than maize because they believe there is less risk of a crop failure with amaranth (Gupta & Thimba, 1992). Observations indicate that amaranth in the coastal desert of Peru requires half the irrigation required by corn (Sumar, 1983). In the United States, total water use by grain amaranth ranged from 27–32 cm on an average year in eastern North Dakota (Henderson, Schneiter, & Johnson, 1993). A farmer in western Nebraska uses 30 cm water for irrigated grain amaranth production, which is about 50% of irrigated corn production (Sooby et al., 1998).

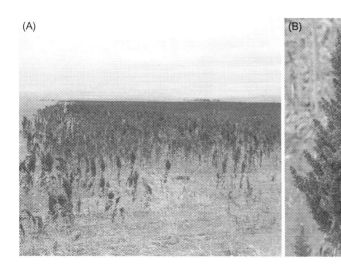

FIGURE 16.1 Grain amaranth production field (A) with large and healthy head (B) in Garden Co. in western Nebraska during 2012 when most of the dryland crops in the area failed due to severe drought. *Photos were taken by Mr. Gary L. Stone, Extension Educator, Panhandle Research and Extension Center, University of Nebraska-Lincoln.*

Limited information is available on the fertility requirements of amaranth. In general, amaranth's fertility requirement, especially for nitrogen (N), in not high. Under dry-land production conditions in western Nebraska typically 22–45 kg N/ha is applied and the rate is 45–90 kg/ha under irrigation (Sooby et al., 1998). More N application above this level increases vegetative growth, which induces more lodging (Elbehri, Putnam, & Schmitt, 1993l; Myers, 1998). Typical phosphorus (P) requirement in western Nebraska is 22 kg/ha (Sooby et al., 1998). With respect to energy requirement, grain amaranth is environmentally friendly and a sustainable source of high-quality protein for healthy human diet. Therefore, grain amaranth is an excellent plant protein source for economically poor people living in the area where water resources are limited, farmers are not able to apply chemical fertilizer, and farmland is poor quality, all of which make the area impossible for the production of conventional crops such as corn, rice, wheat, and soybean.

16.1.4 Harvesting

When it comes to harvesting grain amaranth, "Amaranth is easy to grow but hard to harvest" is a common phrase among the United States grain amaranth farmers, especially in the region with short growing season. The main problem is grain shattering before harvesting and during combine. Although amaranth is a widely adapted plant and can be grown anywhere in the United States, harvesting is more difficult in warm and moist regions. Harvesting time depends on the regional climate. For short growing-season in the northern High Plains and upper mid-west of the United States, harvesting should be done as soon as possible after frost-mediated drying in October (Putnam, 1990; Sooby et al., 1998). It usually takes 2 weeks after the frost to dry enough for combining since plants are full of moisture at first frost. In regions with a longer growing-season (eg, Missouri, Maryland) natural senescence followed by drying usually occurs in September through mid-October before the first frost. In such areas, harvesting is usually done when amaranth heads turn brown (Myers, 1996; Sooby et al., 1998). Windrowing is not desirable in amaranth since soil particles are usually picked up at the time of threshing and particle size is similar to amaranth seed, which makes it difficult to clean later on. Many a time farmers harvest amaranth at higher moisture to minimize seed loss due to shattering and dry the grains later. A standard small-grain combine is usually used to harvest with special precautions to minimize loss of tinny amaranth grain during combining (Myers, 1996; Putnam, 1990; Weber, 1987). Combine setting is similar to wheat but with reduced cylinder speed as much as possible. A canvas or draper type of header may be used to catch the seed and most of these come with a bat reel with no fingers, but a pick-up reel is better for lifting heads that have fallen over (Sooby et al., 1998).

16.1.5 Postharvest Processing (Cleaning and Storage)

Postharvest processing (drying and cleaning) is very important for maintaining high-quality grain. Problems with grain drying will vary from year to year depending on weather conditions. Grain moisture of 10–12% is optimum for storage without further drying. It is important to harvest the grain when the plants are as dry as possible. The longer the plants stay in the field after the first frost, the higher the likelihood that the quality of the grain will be reduced by wet weather. Grain maturity will vary even on a single head because amaranth is an indeterminate type, that is, it is a plant that continues to produce new flower and form seed throughout the season. Therefore, harvested seed will be a mixture of optimally matured (solid "opaque" white or tan appearance) and less matured grain with more moisture (glossy or translucent appearance) (Sooby et al., 1998). Translucent-looking seeds will be lighter and poorer quality than matured seeds and, therefore, should be cleaned to maintain high food quality grain (Myers, 1996). Amaranth grain will mold quickly and become unfit for human consumption if stored when it has a moisture content that is too high. The moisture content of grain amaranth is usually monitored before harvest and accordingly arrangements for drying should be made in advance. It is important to remove as much vegetative material as possible from the harvested grain before drying to reduce the potential sources for the introduction of mold and undesirable flavors. Small quantities of grain can be dried by moving ambient air over a pile of grain with occasional stirring of the grain if possible. In the case of a large pile of grain, forced air is run through a perforated pipe under the pile. Due to the small size of amaranth, conventional grain dryers need to be adapted (eg, fine-mesh nylon cloth over the perforated pipe) for drying amaranth.

It is necessary to pay close attention to cleaning the grain for high-quality food-grade grain amaranth (free from soil dirt, small stem pieces, black seed, mold, and other contamination). Preliminary cleaning of bulk of trash by scalping always minimizes the cost of cleaning since specialized equipment is needed to adequately clean amaranth (Sooby et al., 1998). Many local grain cleaners can do the final cleaning. Specialized cleaning usually involves auguring through a rotary screen to remove large stems and sticks. Then the grain is passed through screens and run over a gravity table to remove smaller foreign materials and dry but immature amaranth seed with lower bulk density. Optical sorters are usually used to remove black-seeded pigweed seed or discolored amaranth seed. Such sophisticated cleaning process finally produces very high-quality grain amaranth with uniform color and without any foreign material. Dried, cleaned grain should be placed in rodent-proof storage with adequate ventilation to prevent a build-up of condensation. Good storage conditions are needed to maintain grain quality at high level. Often heavy-duty paper bags with poly liners are used to store completely dried grain amaranth (Sooby et al., 1998; Weber, 1987). The producers possibly will adapt different strategies for harvesting and postharvest processing depending on resources. However, it should be remembered that suboptimal processing usually makes for inferior quality grain and potentially would make for a lower price or the grain being rejected in the market.

16.1.6 Production Cost

The cost of amaranth is not very high when compared with major crops like corn and soybean. This is due to its ability to grow in marginal land with a low level of input cost associated with fertilizers, water, herbicides (no herbicides are approved for amaranth), and nonsignificant insects and diseases. The only significant insect that may cause yield loss is the Lygus bug. Tarnished leaf bug (*Lygus lineolaris* P. Beauv.) is considered the greatest pest of amaranth globally, damaging plants through its sucking action on meristematic tissue, developing floral buds, blossoms, and embryos (Brenner et al., 2000; Joshi & Rana, 1991; Myers, 1996). Production costs for amaranth are estimated at $247 per hectare, with additional harvest and marketing costs varying from $50 to $500 per hectare, according to the market channel selected. Total expenses per hectare, including both variable and fixed, would come to approximately $570—1000. Presuming gross returns of $790—1600 per hectare, returns to land, capital, and management could range from $247 to $620 per hectare (Grain Amaranth, University of Kentucky, https://www.uky.edu/Ag/CCD/introsheets/amaranth.pdf; AMRC, 2011).

16.2 PROCESSING OF AMARANTH

Processing of amaranth is majorly influenced by the morphology of the seed, particularly as the embryo surrounds the starch-rich perisperm, and by its small seed size, which ranges from 0.8 g to 1.6 g per 1000 seeds (Sooby et al., 1998; Fig. 16.2). Both morphological features pose challenges to many existing food processes that were originally established for cereals, mainly wheat. These existing food processes cannot be simply transferred to amaranth processing. They require several adaptations like choosing the appropriate equipment or modifying the processing parameters. Sometimes rather unconventional and innovative approaches may have to be considered.

16.2.1 Milling and Fractionation

Most cereal food products do not utilize whole seed kernels, thus requiring the preparation of (wholemeal) flour or defined flour fractions. Milling and fractionation of starchy seeds is therefore an important step that influences further product development. Milling is a high shear process, which generates heat and thus causes an increase in the

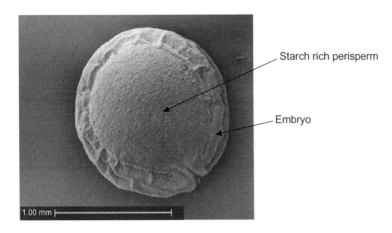

FIGURE 16.2 Scanning electron microscopy (SEM) picture of a single amaranth grain. Embryo and surrounding starch-rich perisperm are indicated by arrows.

temperature of the flour, which has to be considered, as it may affect the properties of the obtained byproducts. Milling can be performed either by dry or wet milling schemes. The aim of dry milling is mainly to produce wholemeal flour or to separate the grain by physical fractionation techniques (eg, grinding, sifting, sieving) into its anatomical parts, that is, separation of the starch-rich endosperm (perisperm in amaranth) from the outer layers (bran and embryo). Wet milling is applied to separate the kernels into its chemical components, that is, starch, protein (concentrates, isolates), dietary fibers, or oil.

The production of wholemeal flour from amaranth is well established and does not have specific problems, so all known processes may be applied. Care has to be taken for the moisture content of the seeds, so tempering (ie, addition of water and resting period) or preconditioning (addition of water and heat treatment) of the seeds is often required to achieve an optimal seed moisture content for easier grinding (Tosi, Ré, Lucero, & Masciarelli, 2000). The production of flour fractions with different chemical composition and physical properties by dry fractionation techniques from amaranth is extremely challenging. Specifically, its small seed size and tightly bound protein and starch cause excess friction on milling equipment designed to handle larger or softer cereal grains. Various milling and fractionation techniques (pilot scale) to produce starch-rich and protein-rich flour fractions from amaranth have been investigated by several researchers, for example, roller mill and plansifter by Berghofer and Schoenlechner (2002) or differential milling process, sieving, and pneumatic separation by Tosi et al. (2000). Abrasive milling seems to have potential for such small seeds. In earlier studies barley pearlers were studied (eg, Betschart, Wood, Shepherd, & Saunders, 1981) and in more recent studies, Roa, Santagapita, Buera, and Tolaba (2014) applied a combination of abrasive milling and planetary ball milling, and found that milling energy influenced the rheological and thermal behavior of amaranth flour (Roa, Baeza, & Tolaba, 2015).

16.2.2 Wet Milling for Production of Starch-Rich, Fiber-Rich, or Protein-Rich Fractions (Protein Concentrates and Isolates)

Wet milling is mainly applied to isolate starch, but other coproducts that are interesting for food applications are the protein-rich and fiber-rich fractions. Typical wet milling includes the following steps:

1. Cleaning of the grain;
2. Soaking in an aqueous solution (often including alkali);
3. Several milling steps to pulverize the particles;
4. Filtration through a series of screens with decreasing mesh sizes (mainly to remove germ and fiber);
5. Separation of starch and protein by centrifugation (mainly for lab scale) or table method (for industrial scale).

The protein fraction (lighter fraction) is then concentrated and dehydrated. The starch suspension is washed and concentrated. The two mentioned separation techniques are based on density differences between starch and protein. For amaranth seeds these separation methods cause problems due to the already mentioned tight starch−protein bonds and small seed size (Middlewood & Carson, 2012a; Wilhelm, Themeier, & Lindhauer, 1998). Thus, screening, microfiltration, or tangential flow filtration (pressure-driven separation process) is more feasible (Middlewood & Carson, 2012a, 2012b).

Wet milling of amaranth has been investigated on a laboratory scale and many methods have been developed, more or less similar to corn wet milling (eg, Calzetta Resio, Aguerre, & Suarez, 2003, 2006; Calzetta Resio, Tolaba, & Suarez, 2009). However, the efficiency of the process has not yet reached a level that may be applied on an industrial scale. There is no commercial wet milling process for amaranth yet. Alkaline soaking has been proposed for amaranth wet milling, in order for easier removal of the protein, but it has to be considered that starch granules might be damaged or lost (decreasing yield) (Perez, Bahnassey, & Breene, 1993). Acid wet milling (Loubes, Calzetta Resio, Tolaba, & Suarez, 2012), use of enzymes (Radosavljevic, Jane, & Johnson, 1998), or sodium metabisulfite (Calzetta Resio et al., 2009) might eventually be alternatives.

If the specific aim of separation is to produce protein concentrates or isolates, the process is performed analogous to the described wet milling methods. This commonly applies alkaline steeping of defatted flour, in order to increase the yield and purity of isolated or concentrated protein. Optimal pH for this alkaline extraction is pH 11 and usually the glutelin, albumin, and globulin proteins are isolated (Martinez & Anon, 1996). On a laboratory scale, Condés, Añón, and Mauri (2015) used alkaline steeping at pH of 11 (using NaOH) and achieved a yield of 2 g isolate/100 g defatted flour with a purity of approximately 90%. Bejarano-Luján and Netto (2010) found that modification of the standard wet milling process of amaranth, by including an acid washing or heating step during alkaline extraction, changed the composition and functionality of the isolated protein fraction. Consequently, this modified the structure and rheological properties of gels obtained from this protein. Pilot-scale or even industrial-scale processing to obtain protein isolates or concentrates has not been investigated much. Castel, Andrich, Netto, Santiago, and Carrara (2012) performed a pilot-scale study to isolate protein from amaranth (*Amaranthus mantegazzianus*). They compared the application of alkaline extraction or acid pretreatment in combination with isoelectric precipitation or ultrafiltration processes on protein yield, protein concentration, and physicochemical characteristics of the protein concentrates. Protein yield was higher after alkaline extraction in comparison to acid pretreatment, but protein concentration was lower. Acid pretreatment, and in particular ultrafiltration, improved protein concentration and its nutritional quality (an improved amino acid composition).

For full exploitation of dry and wet milling processes to obtain defined fractions, isolates, or concentrates of amaranth components, research has to be intensified, in particular for subsequent scaling-up to an industrial level. With respect to nutritional and physicochemical properties, amaranth and its constituents present a valuable alternative to other sources like meat, dairy, or soy.

16.3 FOOD APPLICATIONS

Amaranth can be used in many food applications like cooking, popping, extrusion, fermentation, bread baking, or pasta. Whole seeds can be consumed directly after cooking in threefold water or they can be popped by short and dry heat (without fat addition). These two processes present the oldest forms of consumption that have been traditionally applied. Popping of amaranth is a very interesting alternative use of amaranth because popped amaranth presents a nutty flavor, and thus, may enhance the palatability of food products. In particular, popped amaranth offers a nutty compliment to sweet products such as cakes, cookies, mueslis, or granolas. Popped amaranth grains are quite soft in texture and are ready to be eaten as is or to be incorporated (after milling) into existing or new food formulations. During popping, the embryo stays intact and a partial gelatinization of the starch granules occurs (in the perisperm) and due to the short processing time of only seconds, the nutritional profile of the grain is more or less maintained.

For amaranth processing, the absence of gluten should be considered, therefore, it has no dough-forming properties. A strategy to use amaranth is to blend it with other (gluten-containing) cereals in existing products in order to enhance their nutritional value. Up to 20% amaranth addition does not really ask for intensive adaptation of preparation processes. This has been investigated for different products (eg, bread, pasta, cookies, biscuits, beverages) by several researchers. The main aim of adding amaranth to such cereal products is usually their nutritional enhancement.

Alternatively, the absence of gluten makes amaranth suitable for the production of gluten-free products. The production of gluten-free bread and bakery products or pasta using amaranth flour is of great interest now, since the need for gluten-free products is increasing due to an increased prevalence of celiac disease and gluten-sensitivity. Summarizing all affected persons together, the market can be estimated to be around 8–10% of the global population. Besides being gluten-free, the challenge of gluten-free food is to offer an adequate nutritional balance. As amaranth, as well as other pseudocereals, is nutritionally superior to many gluten-free raw materials, its use is a logical consequence. In fact, the growing gluten-free market can be seen as one of the main driving forces for the increased production and use of amaranth. Production of gluten-free products in general, and including amaranth in particular, is a great challenge and cannot be carried out without addition of further ingredients or without specific adaptation of relevant processing steps.

Gluten-free products like bread and pasta with amaranth have been studied by some researchers (Calderon de la Barca, 2010; Schoenlechner, Drausinger, Ottenschlaeger, Jurackova, & Berghofer, 2010), but still remain under-researched compared to major crops.

In addition to its nutritional advantages, amaranth and isolated fractions or components thereof offer unique properties and technological functionality in food applications that have not been exploited to a large extent. Amaranth proteins, concentrates, or isolates are characterized by excellent solubility, as well as foaming, emulsifying, and stabilizing properties (Bejosano & Corke, 1998; Fidantsi & Doxastakis, 2001) and thus have a high potential for functional foods, in particular where gel formation is desired. Amaranth starch is characterized by the small size of granules, low amylose content, high water-binding capacity, good freeze−thaw stability, resistance to mechanical shear, and excellent gelling and thickening properties (Wilhelm, Aberle, Burchard, & Landers, 2002; Zhao & Whistler, 1994). These functional properties offer a wide range of uses in food applications.

REFERENCES

AMRC (Agricultural Marketing Resource Center). (2011). *Amaranth*: <http://www.agmrc.org/commodities__products/specialty_crops/amaranth.cfm/>.

Bejarano-Luján, D. L., & Netto, F. M. (2010). Effect of alternative processes on the yield and physicochemical characterization of protein concentrates from *Amaranthus cruentus*. *LWT − Food Science and Technology, 5*, 736−743.

Bejosano, F. P., & Corke, H. (1998). Protein quality evaluation of *Amaranthus* wholemeal flours and protein concentrates. *Journal of the Science of Food and Agriculture, 76*, 100−106.

Berghofer, E., & Schoenlechner, R. (2002). Chapter 7: Grain amaranth. In P. S. Belton, & J. R. N. Taylor (Eds.), *Pseudocereals and less common cereals. Grain properties and utilization potential* (pp. 219−253). Berlin Heidelberg: Springer-Verlag.

Betschart, A. A., Wood, I. D., Shepherd, A. D., & Saunders, R. M. (1981). *Amaranthus cruentus*: Milling characteristics, distribution of nutrients within seed components, and the effects of temperature on nutritional quality. *Journal of Food Science, 46*, 1181−1187.

Breene, W. M. (1991). Food uses of grain amaranth. *Cereal Foods World, 36*, 426−430.

Brenner, D. M., Baltensperger, D. D., Kulakow, P. A., Lehmann, J. W., Myers, R. L., Slabbert, M. M., & Sleugh, B. B. (2000). Genetic resources and breeding of *Amaranthus*. *Plant Breeding Reviews, 19*, 227−285.

Calderon de la Barca, A. M., Rojas-Martinez, M. E., Islas-Rubio, A. R., & Cabrera-Chavez, F. (2010). Gluten-free breads and cookies of raw and popped amaranth flours with attractive technological and nutritional qualities. *Plant Foods for Human Nutrition, 65*, 241−246.

Calzetta Resio, A. N., Aguerre, R. J., & Suarez, C. (2003). Study of some factors affecting water absorption by amaranth grain during soaking. *Journal of Food Engineering, 60*, 391−396.

Calzetta Resio, A. N., Aguerre, R. J., & Suarez, C. (2006). Hydration kinetics of amaranth grain. *Journal of Food Engineering, 72*, 247−253.

Calzetta Resio, A. N., Tolaba, M. P., & Suarez, C. (2009). Correlations between wet-milling characteristics of amaranth grain. *Journal of Food Engineering, 92*, 275−279.

Castel, V., Andrich, O., Netto, F. M., Santiago, L. G., & Carrara, C. R. (2012). Comparison between isoelectric precipitation and ultrafiltration processes to obtain *Amaranthus mantegazzianus* protein concentrates at pilot plant scale. *Journal of Food Engineering, 112*, 288−295.

Chaudhari, P. P., Patel, P. T., & Desai, L. J. (2009). Effect of nitrogen management on yield, water use, and nutrient uptake on grain amaranth (*Amaranthus hypochondriacus*) under moisture stress. *Indian Journal of Agronomy, 54*(1), 69−73.

Condés, M. C., Añón, M. C., & Mauri, A. N. (2015). Amaranth protein films prepared with high-pressure treated proteins. *Journal of Food Engineering, 166*, 38−44.

Cramer, C. (Ed.). (1988). Montana releases new amaranth line. *Amaranth Today, 4*(2−3), 6.

Elbehri, A., Putnam, D. H., & Schmitt, M. (1993). Nitrogen fertilizer and cultivar effects on yield and nitrogen-use efficiency of grain amaranth. *Agronomy Journal, 85*, 120−128.

Emokaro, C. O., & Ekunwe, P. A. (2007). Efficiency of resource-use and marginal productivities in dry season amaranth production in Edo South, Nigeria. *Journal of Applied Sciences, 7*, 2500−2504.

Fidantsi, A., & Doxastakis, G. (2001). Emulsifying and foaming properties of amaranth seed protein isolates. *Colloids and Surfaces B: Biointerfaces, 21*, 119−124.

Graham, M. W. (2010). *Grain amaranth production and effects of soil amendments in Uganda. Ph.D. thesis*. Iowa State University. <http://lib.dr.iastate.edu/cgi/viewcontent.cgi?article=2462&context=etd/>.

Gupta, V. K. (1986). *Grain amaranths in Kenya. Proceedings of the third amaranth conference*. Emmaus, PA: Rodale Press, Inc.

Gupta, V. K., & Thimba, D. (1992). Grain amaranth: A promising crop for marginal areas of Kenya. *Food Reviews International, 8*(1), 51−69.

Henderson, T. L., Schneiter, A. A., & Johnson, B. L. (1993). *Production of amaranth in the northern Great Plains. Alternative crop research: A progress report* (pp. 22−30). Fargo: North Dakota State University.

Johnson, B. L., & Henderson, T. L. (2002). Water use patterns of grain amaranth in the northern Great Plains. *Agronomy Journal, 94*, 1437−1443.

Joshi, B. D. (1985). Annapurna, a new variety of grain amaranth. *Indian Farming*, 29−31.

Joshi, B. D. (1986). Genetic variability in grain amaranth, *Amaranthus hypochondriacus* Linn. *Indian Journal of Agricultural Science, 56*, 574−576.

Joshi, J. D., & Rana, R. S. (1991). *Grain amaranths: The future food crop*. India: National Bureau of Plant Genetic Resources.

Kauffman, C. S., & Weber, L. E. (1990). Grain amaranth. In J. Janick, & J. E. Simon (Eds.), *Advances in new crops* (pp. 127–139). Portland, OR: Timber Press.

Loubes, M. A., Calzetta Resio, A. N., Tolaba, M. P., & Suarez, C. (2012). Mechanical and thermal characteristics of amaranth starch isolated by acid wet-milling procedure. *LWT — Food Science and Technology, 46*, 519–524.

Martinez, E. N., & Anon, M. C. (1996). Composition and structural characterisation of amaranth protein isolates. An electrophoretic and calorimetric study. *Journal of Agricultural and Food Chemistry, 44*, 2523–2530.

Middlewood, P. G., & Carson, J. K. (2012a). Extraction of amaranth starch from an aqueous medium using microfiltration: Membrane characterization. *Journal of Membrane Science, 405–406*, 284–290.

Middlewood, P. G., & Carson, J. K. (2012b). Extraction of amaranth starch from an aqueous medium using microfiltration: Membrane fouling and cleaning. *Journal of Membrane Science, 411–412*, 22–29.

Mng'omba, S. A., Kwapata, M. B., & Bokosi, J. M. (2003). Performance of grain amaranth varieties under drought stressed conditions in two contrasting agro-ecological areas in Malawi. *Acta Horticulturae, 618*, 313–319.

Myers, R. L. (1994). Regional amaranth variety test. *Legacy, 7*, 5–8.

Myers, R. L. (1996). Amaranth: New crop opportunity. In J. Janick (Ed.), *Progress in new crops* (pp. 207–220). Alexandria, VA: ASHS Press.

Myers, R. L. (1998). Nitrogen fertilizer effect on grain amaranth. *Agronomy Journal, 90*(5), 597–602.

National Research Council (NRC) (1984). *Amaranth: Modern prospects for an ancient crop*. Washington, DC: National Academy Press.

National Research Council (NRC) (1989). *Lost crops of the Incas. Little known plants from the Andes with promise for worldwide cultivation*. Washington, DC: National Academy Press.

Perez, E., Bahnassey, Y. A., & Breene, W. M. (1993). A simple laboratory scale method for isolation of amaranth starch. *Starch/Stärke, 45*, 211–214.

Piha, M. I. (1995). Yield potential, fertility requirements and drought tolerance of grain amaranth compared with maize under Zimbabwean conditions. *Tropical Agriculture, 72*(1), 7–12.

Putnam, D. H. (1990). *Agronomic practices for grain amaranth. Proceedings of the fourth national amaranth symposium: Perspectives on production, processing and marketing* (pp. 151–159). Minneapolis, Minnesota: American Amaranth Institute; Minnesota Extension Service.

Radosavljevic, M., Jane, J., & Johnson, L. A. (1998). Isolation of amaranth starch by diluted alkaline-protease treatment. *Cereal Chemistry, 75*, 571–577.

Roa, D. F., Baeza, R. I., & Tolaba, M. P. (2015). Effect of ball milling energy on rheological and thermal properties of amaranth flour. *Journal of Food Science and Technology, 52*, 8389–8394.

Roa, D. F., Santagapita, P. R., Buera, M. P., & Tolaba, M. P. (2014). Amaranth milling strategies and fraction characterization by FTIR. *Food and Bioprocess Technology, 7*, 711–718.

Sauer, J. D. (1967). The grain amaranths and their relatives: A revised taxonomic and geographic survey. *Annals of the Missouri Botanical Garden, 54*, 103–137.

Sauer, J. D. (1993). *Historical geography of crop plants: A select roster*. Boca Raton, FL: CRC Press.

Schoenlechner, R., Drausinger, J., Ottenschlaeger, V., Jurackova, K., & Berghofer, E. (2010). Functional properties of gluten-free pasta produced from amaranth, quinoa and buckwheat. *Plant Food Human Nutrition, 65*, 339–349.

Senft, J. P. (1980). *Protein quality of amaranth grain. Proceedings of the Second Amaranth Conference* (pp. 43–47). Emmaus, PA: Rodale Press, Inc.

Sooby, J., Myers, R., Baltensperger, D., Brenner, D., Wilson, R., & Block, C. (1998). *Amaranth production manual for the central United States*. University of Nebraska Cooperative Extension, EC 98-151-S.

Stallknecht, G. F., & Schulz-Schaeffer, J. R. (1993). Amaranth rediscovered. In J. Janick, & J. E. Simon (Eds.), *New crops* (pp. 211–218). New York: Wiley.

Sumar, L. (1983). *Amaranthus caudatus, el pequeño gigante*. Lima: UNICEF.

Tosi, E. A., Ré, E., Lucero, H., & Masciarelli, R. (2000). Amaranth (*Amaranthus* spp.) grain conditioning to obtain hyperproteic flour by differential milling. *Food Science and Technology International, 6*, 433–438.

Weber, E. (1987). *Amaranth grain production guide 1987*. Rodale Research Center Rodale Press, Inc, Copyright 1987 Rodale Press, Inc.

Wilhelm, E., Aberle, T., Burchard, W., & Landers, R. (2002). Peculiarities of aqueous amaranth starch suspensions. *Biomacromolecules, 3*, 17–26.

Wilhelm, E., Themeier, H. W., & Lindhauer, M. G. (1998). Small granule starches and hydrophilic polymers as components for novel biodegradable two-phase compounds for special applications. Part 1: Separation and refinement techniques for small granule starches from amaranth and quinoa. *Starch/Stärke, 50*, 7–13.

Zhao, J., & Whistler, R. L. (1994). Isolation and characterization of starch from amaranth flour. *Cereal Chemistry, 71*, 392–393.

Chapter 17

Chia—The New Golden Seed for the 21st Century: Nutraceutical Properties and Technological Uses

D. Orona-Tamayo[1], M.E. Valverde[1] and O. Paredes-López[1,2]
[1]Centro de Investigación y de Estudios Avanzados del IPN, Irapuato, Guanajuato, Mexico, [2]Université Pierre et Marie Curie, Paris, France

17.1 INTRODUCTION

The *Salvia* genus has around 900 species and some of them are cultivated widely for their taste and used as folk medicines. These plants belong to the Kingdom Plantae, division as vascular plants and family Lamiaceae. The plant is known as "chia" (*Salvia hispanica* L.) and is an annual herb that can grow up to 1 m tall and has oppositely arranged leaves with small white or purple hermaphrodite flowers (3–4 mm; Fig. 17.1). The seeds are oval, smooth, and shiny, and their color varies from black, gray, and black spotted to white (Fig. 17.1); and size ranges from 1 mm to 2 mm (Ayerza & Coates, 2005; Lu & Foo, 2002; Mohd Ali et al., 2012).

Chia is native to central Mexico up to northern Guatemala, and began to be used in human food c.3500 BC (http://www.getnativ.com/chia-seeds-history-health-benefits/). Between 1500 and 900 BC, Aztecs, Mayas, and Incas used the seeds for the preparation of various medicines, foods, and paintings. In addition, chia seeds are also a source of energy vigor. Chia seeds were one of the main crops of pre-Columbian societies, and the Aztecs received them as annual tributes. They were also used as an offering to the gods in religious ceremonies. The Spanish conquest suppressed this traditional crop due to its religious beliefs (http://equinexia.jimdo.com/chia_seed_history.php). The plant has emerged as a super-food in view of its nutraceutical potential (Ayerza & Coates, 2005; Cahill, 2003; Jamboonsri, Phillips, Geneve, Cahill, & Hildebrand, 2012; Muñoz, Cobos, Diaz, & Aguilera, 2013).

17.2 SUSTAINABILITY OF CHIA

17.2.1 Production

The commercial production of chia was only concentrated in specific areas such as Bolivia and Paraguay. However in the last decade, other countries such as Mexico, Australia, and Argentina have good experience in cultivating chia plants. In 2014, speculation and dramatic price increases triggered rapid production growth of chia in several countries, with trading prices that reached US$8000–12,000 per ton (t) in 2013. Chia prices fluctuate according to quality, demand, and production volume. However it lacks the continuous price feedback of a stock market commodity such as coffee or cacao (Peperkamp, 2014). Bolivia ranks among the top country producers of chia, with high exportation of this seed (Table 17.1); the cultivation area increased in recent years from 50,000 ha with a production of 18,000 t to 80,000 ha cultivated with a production of 30,000 t (Peperkamp, 2014).

The optimal yield per hectare depends on different situations, such as genetic health of seeds, climatic regions, cultivation techniques, and harvest equipment. In low-input conditions, the average yield of commercial seeds is around 500–600 kg/ha. However, some growers have obtained up to 1200 kg/ha (Cahill, 2003; Coates, 2011). In optimal agronomic conditions a yield of 2500 kg/ha has also been reported (Cahill, 2003; Coates, 2011; Ullah et al., 2015). Bolivia was able to improve its yield from 350 kg/ha in 2013 to 650 kg/ha in 2014, lower than Argentina and Paraguay

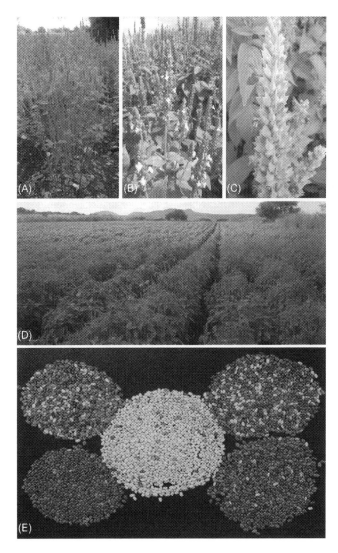

FIGURE 17.1 Chia plants, flowers and seeds. Commercial chia plantations (A); purple (gray in print versions) and white flowers (B); a close-up of purple (gray in print versions) flowers (C); commercial chia plants in Guanajuato, Mexico, with tight-rows to avoid weed growth (D); chia seeds from different commercial cultivars.

that can reach 800–900 kg/ha in optimal circumstances (Peperkamp, 2014). In some regions of Mexico, yields reached 470 kg/ha in 2013 and were improved to 600 kg/ha in 2014 (SAGARPA, 2014).

17.2.2 Land Use

Agronomically, chia plants require different environmental conditions for optimal development and seed production. The temperature for growth development ranges from 11°C to 36°C, with optimal levels between 16–26°C and the plant is very sensitive to low temperatures (Bochicchio et al., 2015). Chia plants do best in sandy and well-drained soils with optimal pH of 6.0–8.5 and are adapted to low-nutrient concentrations (Yeboah et al., 2013). The plant has low resistance to salt concentration and plants that are grown in saline soils can significantly reduce the seed oil content (Heuer, Yaniv, & Ravina, 2002).

17.2.3 Water Use

The chia crop is able to grow in acidic (Muñoz et al., 2013) and semiarid soils that make chia cultivation a good alternative crop (Bochicchio et al., 2015). Chia leaves are rich in metabolites such as phenolic compounds (Amato et al., 2015),

TABLE 17.1 World Production of Chia Seed

Country	2013		2014	
	Acreage (Ha)	Production (tons)	Acreage (Ha)	Production (tons)
Bolivia	50,000	18,000	80,000	30,000
Paraguay	30,000	25,000	100,000	30,000
Argentina	40,000	<10,000	120,000	40,000
Mexico	18,000	8400	50,000	25,000
Australia	ND	<10,000	ND	<10,000
Central America	15,000	10,000	17,000	11,500
Peru	ND	ND	ND	<5000
Ecuador	ND	ND	ND	<1000
Colombia	ND	ND	ND	<100

ND, Not determined.
Source: Data were modified from Peperkamp, M. (2014). Chia from Bolivia: A modern super seed in a classic pork cycle. In: *CBI marked intelligence* (pp. 1–15). Netherlands: Ministry of Foreign Affairs. <www.cbi.eu/market-information/grains-pulses/chia/>.

polyunsaturated fatty acids (PUFAs), and crude protein (Peiretti & Gai, 2009). Due to the high foliage of chia plants, they should be planted between narrow rows to cover the soil completely (Fig. 17.1), which inhibits weed seed germination deriving the soil nutrient competence (Thelen, 2006).

17.2.4 Energy Use

Chia leaves bear a high amount of essential oils, with some components with a repellent effect against herbivorous insects; thus, this crop can be grown without the use of insecticides (Muñoz et al., 2013). These beneficial traits make chia cultivation very sustainable; at present it is cultivated in different regions of Argentina, Australia, Bolivia, Colombia, Ecuador, Guatemala, Mexico, and Peru among others.

17.3 CONSUMPTION OF CHIA

Chia is promoted as a health food product, and is used as a supplement and an ingredient in different proportions. Health aspects and nutritional value are the main reasons for consumers purchasing chia seeds (Peperkamp, 2014; Reyes-Caudillo, Tecante, & Valdivia-López, 2008) and mostly used in food. For example, at the market there are different presentations of packaged chia seeds for consumption, and the recommended use is around 15–25 g/day. The benefits of daily consumption are claimed to be the lowering of cholesterol and blood pressure, weight loss, less joint pain, endurance enhancement, and antioxidant effects. There are different experimental trials where researches found beneficial effects of the daily intake of 35–37 g of ground chia can exert a blood pressure reduction (Toscano et al., 2014; Vuksan et al., 2007). For the athletes that require endurance, the consumption of chia seeds provides ω-3 fatty acids (Illian, Casey, & Bishop, 2011). It has been hypothesized that dietary fiber and ω-3 fatty acids are involved in losing weight; chia mucilage can absorb a high amount of water, forming a large bolus that passes into the stomach evoking great satiety which may reduce consumption of more food. However, while it is considered safe in the short term, there are limited data to suggest safe use in the long term (Egras, Hamilton, Lenz, & Monaghan, 2011; Nieman et al., 2009). Dietary consumption of ground chia, oil, and proteins has long-term health benefits due to its antioxidant properties and the protection of cells against free radicals which may induce different degenerative diseases (Marineli, Lenquiste, Moraes, & Maróstica, 2015; Orona-Tamayo, Valverde, Nieto-Rendón, & Paredes-López, 2015).

Different preparations of chia may be found in the market. These include raw seeds, oil capsules as supplements, seed flour, and ingredients for foods. Raw chia seeds and seed flour are very popular and may be added to muesli, breakfast cereals, crisps, peanut butter, fruit, nut and different seed mixes, drinks, shakes, desserts, or homemade bakery products, such as bread and bread mixes. Cosmetic products that use chia are related to skin cleaners, watery eye essence, and skin creams. Animal foods formulated with chia are prepared mainly for horses and birds (Ayerza & Coates, 2005; Peperkamp, 2014).

17.4 NUTRITIONAL VALUE

In 2009, chia was approved as a novel food by the European Parliament and the European Council (Mohd Ali et al., 2012). Chia seed is approximately 15–24% protein, 26–41% carbohydrates, and 25–40% fat. It has been studied principally due to its oil quality content, possesses almost 55–60% linolenic acid (ω-3), 18–20% linoleic acid (ω-6), 6% monounsaturated ω-9, and 10% saturated fat. On the other hand, the seed has highly soluble and insoluble dietary fiber, over 35% of the total weight, and it is a rich source of the B vitamins and minerals. It also contains 6 times more calcium, 11 times more phosphorus, and 4 times more potassium than 100 g of milk, besides possessing magnesium, iron, zinc, and copper (Ayerza & Coates, 2009). In addition, it has a high amount of natural antioxidants, such as phenolic compounds, which protect against some adverse conditions. Another important characteristic of this seed is that it does not contain gluten and can be consumed by persons with celiac disease (Martínez-Cruz & Paredes-López, 2014; Mohd Ali et al., 2012; Reyes-Caudillo et al., 2008; Ullah et al., 2015).

17.4.1 Fiber

Dietary fiber is an important component in the daily diet due to its beneficial effect on health. Some of these effects are the reduction of cholesterol, modification of the glycemic and insulin responses, changes in intestinal function, decrease of the risk for coronary heart disease, diabetes mellitus type II, and several types of cancer; and also antioxidant activity. The consumption of dietary fiber has been associated with an increase in postmeal satiety, decreasing subsequent hunger (Borderías, Sánchez-Alonso, & Pérez-Mateos, 2005; Esposito et al., 2005; Muñoz et al., 2013).

Chia mucilage has approximately 48% total sugar content, 4% protein, 8% ash, and 1% fat. The fiber is a polysaccharide with a high molecular weight, and its basic structure is a tetrasaccharide with 4-O-methyl-a-D-glucoronopyranosyl residues that branch b-D-xylopyranosyl on the main chain structure. The monosaccharide composition is 16% D-xylose + D-mannose, 2% D-arabinose, 6% D-glucose, 3% galacturonic acid, and 12% glucuronic acid. Chia seeds produce between 35 and 40 g of dietary fiber per 100 g, equivalent to 100% of the daily recommendations for the adult population (Capitani, Spotorno, Nolasco, & Tomás, 2012; Kaczmarczyk, Miller, & Freund, 2012; Vázquez-Ovando et al., 2009).

17.4.2 Lipids

The most important characteristic of chia is its high content of PUFAs. The seed has around 25–40% that comprises 55–60% linolenic acid (ω-3) and 18–20% linoleic acid (ω-6). The human body requires these essential fatty acids for good health (Ayerza & Coates, 2011; Jamboonsri et al., 2012; Martínez-Maqueda et al., 2012; Mohd Ali et al., 2012). Chia contains the highest percentage of any plant source of α-linolenic acid. This fatty acid is the precursor for the long-chain PUFAs considered as essential fatty acids because the human body cannot produce them. Chia seeds contain high concentrations of PUFAs that provide potent lipid antioxidants (Ayerza & Coates, 2011; Marineli et al., 2015).

17.4.3 Phenolic Compounds

Chia seeds are rich in phenolic compounds and have a high antioxidant capacity. Polyphenols responsible for antioxidant activity are most commonly flavonoids and cinnamic acid derivatives. The amounts of phenolic compounds in chia are around 0.88–1.6 mg GAE/g (Table 17.2). The seed contains significant concentrations of gallic, caffeic, chlorogenic, ferulic, and rosmarinic acids. In addition, they also contain myricetin, quercetin, and kaempferol. The most important phenolic compounds present in chia are tocopherols, which are found in a concentration of 238–427 mg/kg; similar to that in peanut oil. Additionally, seeds contain some isoflavones such as daidzin, glycitin, genistin, glycitein, and genistein (Ayerza & Coates, 2001; Reyes-Caudillo et al., 2008; Martínez-Cruz & Paredes-López, 2014; Muñoz et al., 2013; Taga, Miller, & Pratt, 1984).

TABLE 17.2 Concentration of Phenolic Compounds in Chia Seeds

Compound	mg/g Seed
Phenolic Acids	
Galic[b]	0.0115
Caffeic[a,b,c]	0.027–0.086
Chlorogenic[a,b,c]	0.013–0.074
Ferullic[b]	t
Rosmarinic[b]	0.9267
Esters	
Protocatechuic Ethyl Ester[b]	0.7471
Isoflavones	
Daidzin[b]	0.0066
Glycitin[b]	0.0014
Genistin[b]	0.0034
Glycitein[b]	0.0005
Genistein[b]	0.0051
Flavanols	
Quercetin[a,c]	0.0181–0.209
Kaempferol[a,c]	0.0057–0.0435
Myricetin[a]	0.0095

[a]Capitani et al. (2012).
[b]Martínez-Crúz and Paredes-López (2014).
[c]Reyes-Caudillo et al. (2008).
t, trace.

17.4.4 Protein Content and Amino Acids

Chia is a nutrient-dense food with high potential as a functional food (Sandoval-Oliveros & Paredes-López, 2013). Although it is not a well-known global food source, its commercial popularity has grown in Mexico, and South and North America (Ayerza & Coates, 2005; Marineli et al., 2014), due to its exceptional biochemical compounds. One of these components is protein, which makes chia seed an important nutraceutical food providing potential benefits for human health.

The protein content of chia seeds is around 15–24% (Ayerza, 2009; Ayerza & Coates, 2004; Olivos-Lugo, Valdivia-López, & Tecante, 2010; Sandoval-Oliveros & Paredes-López, 2013), thus chia is an important source of great-quality proteins composed in their backbone by essential amino acids (Sandoval-Oliveros & Paredes-López, 2013). Several important storage protein fractions have been found within chia seeds. Globulins are the main protein fraction and comprise around 52–54% of the total storage proteins, followed by 17.3–18.6% albumins, 13.6% glutelin, and 17.9% prolamin (Table 17.3; Orona-Tamayo et al., 2015; Sandoval-Oliveros & Paredes-López, 2013).

Biochemical studies on chia seed protein fraction are limited. However, two recent studies show the molecular biochemistry of its protein fractions (Orona-Tamayo et al., 2015; Sandoval-Oliveros & Paredes-López, 2013). Denaturing electrophoretic patterns show that the proteins are composed of different polypeptides (Fig. 17.2). Albumin fraction represents low-intensity bands with molecular masses between 10–250 kDa, but with apparently intensive bands that range approximately 12, 25, 28, 35, 60, and 68 kDa; globulins show eight intensity protein bands with molecular weights of approximately 10, 15, 18, 24, 28, 33, 50, and 60 kDa. Prolamins showed a different electrophoretic pattern with only three sharp bands between 12–25 kDa; and finally, chia glutelins show main bands with molecular sizes of 25, 28, 35, 60, and 68 kDa with similarity to the main bands of albumins.

TABLE 17.3 Main Storage Protein Fractions of Chia Seeds

	Salvia hispanica L. (%)		
Protein Fraction	Olivos-Lugo et al. (2010)	Sandoval-Oliveros and Paredes-Lopez (2013)	Orona-Tamayo et al. (2015)
Albumin	3.9	17.3	18.6
Globulin	7.0	52.0	54.0
Prolamin	53.8	12.7	7.2
Glutelin	23.0	14.5	6.4

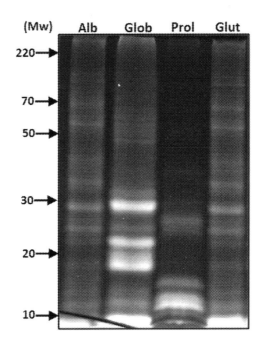

FIGURE 17.2 SDS-PAGE of chia seed storage proteins. *Alb*, albumins; *Glob*, globulins; *Prol*, prolamins; *Glut*, glutelins;. *Mw*, Molecular weight marker. Proteins were separated by a 14% gel concentration and stained with flamingo stain.

17.4.4.1 Chia Globulins

Globulins are widely distributed in nature; they are particularly common as main storage proteins in dicotyledon seeds such as pea, soybean, and bean (Shewry, 1995). Chia seeds fit in this distribution. Sandoval-Oliveros and Paredes-López (2013) determined the sedimentation coefficient of chia globulin and found that 11S globulin is the principal component, followed by 7S-like proteins; however, other minor components such as 6S and 19S, with unusual sedimentation coefficients, can be formed as intermediates derived from 11S globulins. This result is supported by two-dimensional gel electrophoresis for globulin fraction in a broad pH range (3–10; Fig. 17.3). The protein map shows a denaturing globulin profile that confirms a high heterogeneity with molecular masses ranging from 11 kDa to 70 kDa and focused over the range of pI 4–9. In this proteomic map, a chain of six abundant proteins was present at approximately 29–35 kDa with a range of pI between 4.5 and 7.0. This globulin shows acid pH tendencies due to the presence of the acid 11S subunit. The 11S globulin consists of a single band of 383 kDa, comprising a hexameric conformation of about 50–60 kDa; however, under reducing conditions these monomers are resolved into acidic (approximately 30 kDa) and basic (approximately 20 kDa) subunits. Protein identification confirmed the presence of peptides belonging to the 11S protein with less proportion of 7S protein peptides (Sandoval-Oliveros & Paredes-López, 2013) confirming the abundant presence of 11S subunit containing disulfide bonds in its structure.

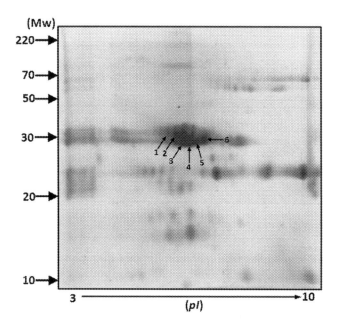

FIGURE 17.3 Two-dimensional gel electrophoresis of chia seed globulins. Arrows indicate the possible subunits of 11S globulin. *Mw*, molecular weight marker; *pI*, isoelectric point. The protein was separated by a 13% gel concentration and stained with flamingo stain.

It is important to study the amino acid composition of chia proteins due to its high quality for human health. The protein composition of chia seed flour is an excellent source of sulfur amino acids (cysteine and methionine), arginine, aspartic, and glutamic amino acids (Table 17.4; Olivos-Lugo et al., 2010; Sandoval-Oliveros & Paredes-López, 2013; Vázquez-Ovando, Rosado-Rubio, Chel-Guerrero, & Betancur-Ancona, 2010). Globulin, the highest protein fraction, also has significant amounts of aromatic and sulfur amino acids, glutamic and aspartic acids, as well as threonine and histidine. Hence, the flour and the isolated globulins from chia seeds contain the essential amino acids for human nutrition, which are histidine, isoleucine, leucine, lysine, methionine, phenylalanine, threonine, tryptophan, and valine (Table 17.4).

The amino acids in chia seeds are important for human metabolic activities, that is, glutamic acid has the potential to stimulate the central nervous system, involved in its immunologic performance and to enhance athletic endurance (Brosnan & Brosnan, 2013; McCormack et al., 2015; Paredes-López, 1991), aspartic acid stimulates the hormonal regulation for the proper functionality of the nervous system (Brosnan & Brosnan, 2013), while other amino acids like arginine apparently protect against cardiovascular diseases (Böger, 2007), and sulfur amino acids may be involved in the functionality of the tertiary and also quaternary structures of the proteins (Sandoval-Oliveros & Paredes-López, 2013). These results suggest that the quality of chia proteins and their amino acids is similar or higher than other important cereals and oilseeds. The presence of these biomolecules in chia seeds represents an important nutraceutical contribution to the daily diet (Sandoval-Oliveros & Paredes-López, 2013).

17.4.4.2 Peptides With Possible Antihypertensive Effects

Peptides are encrypted in the primary structure of the protein, but when proteins are hydrolyzed they can release peptide sequences with functional properties (Fig. 17.4), including those that characteristically contribute to the prevention or treatment of cardiovascular diseases and providing antioxidant properties (Aluko, 2015) with the potential to replace drug therapies (Udenigwe & Aluko, 2012).

Chia seeds provide diverse health benefits due to the high amounts of phytochemicals and proteins that provide a high concentration of biologically active peptides with antihypertensive and other important functions. Literature data on chia proteins and their antihypertensive effects are limited. However, some researchers have isolated globulin, the rich-protein fraction, and obtained peptides by using enzymatic hydrolysis to evaluate antihypertensive peptides as natural inhibitors of angiotensin I-converting enzyme (ACE). Salazar-Vega, Segura-Campos, Chel-Guerrero, and Betancur-Ancona (2012) and Segura-Campos, Salazar-Vega, Chel-Guerrero, and Betancur-Ancona (2013) have hydrolyzed chia seed flour proteins with Alcalase and Flavourzyme at 30, 60, 90, 120, and 150 min and showed that

TABLE 17.4 Amino Acid Composition of Flour and Isolated Globulin From Chia Seeds

	Salvia hispanica L. (g/100 g Protein)					
	Olivos-Lugo et al. (2010)		Vázquez-Ovando et al. (2010)		Sandoval-Oliveros and Paredes-López (2013)	
	Seed Flour	Globulin	Seed Flour	Globulin	Seed Flour	Globulin
Alanine	4.3	3.9	5.1	5.0	2.6	3.9
Arginine	8.9	11.1	10.2	10.6	4.2	9.4
Aspartic acid	7.6	6.0	10.2	9.3	4.7	7.2
Cysteine	1.4	0.1	1.9	2.4		
Glutamic Acid	12.4	12.0	19.9	19.2	7.0	24.3
Glycine	4.2	3.2	5.9	4.9	2.2	7.3
Hystidine	2.5	2.2	2.5	2.7	1.3	4.0
Isoleucine	3.2	3.6	3.3	3.2	2.4	3.0
Leucine	5.8	5.5	7.2	6.9	4.1	4.4
Lysine	4.4	3.7	5.0	5.0	2.9	1.5
Methionine	0.3	2.5	1.3	3.1		
Phenylalanine	4.7	4.0	5.1	5.0		
Proline	4.4	3.0	4.0	4.0	1.9	10.6
Serine	4.8	3.6	6.4	6.3	2.6	6.9
Tyrosine	2.7	2.7	2.3	2.9		
Threonine	3.4	2.9	3.9	3.9	1.8	6.2
Tryptophan			0.9	0.8		
Valine	5.1	4.8	4.6	4.6	2.8	3.5
Met + Cys					2.7	5.7
Phe + Tyr					3.8	10.9

Essential amino acids are in bold.

the resulting peptides exhibit different ACE-inhibitory effects. The highest inhibition was found at 150 min of hydrolysis than those produced at 120 and 90 min or shorter hydrolysis times. The authors concluded that more effective ACE-inhibitory peptides were released from chia seed flour due to extensive hydrolysis. In order to produce peptides with a short size, between 2–20 amino acids and molecular weights around 1–6 kDa, requires extensive hydrolysis and can be achieved by a combination of more than one protease (Orona-Tamayo et al., 2015; Udenigwe & Aluko, 2012). Such peptides may exert different physiological benefits to human health (Moure, Domínguez, & Parajó, 2005; Sarmadi & Ismail, 2010). Di- or tripeptides with antihypertensive functions consist of 2–9 amino acids. Short peptides have more biological activities and are also resistant to the endopeptidase action of the digestive tract (Kitts & Weiler, 2003; Segura-Campos et al., 2013). Segura-Campos et al. (2013) isolated and digested the protein-rich fraction from chia seed flour and found that ACE-inhibitory activity has a relationship with the molecular weight of the peptides in the fractions obtained from ultrafiltration. The peptide fraction with very low-molecular-weight peptides (<1 kDa) had 69.3% of ACE inhibition than the fraction (53.8% of ACE inhibition) containing high-molecular-weight peptides (>10 kDa).

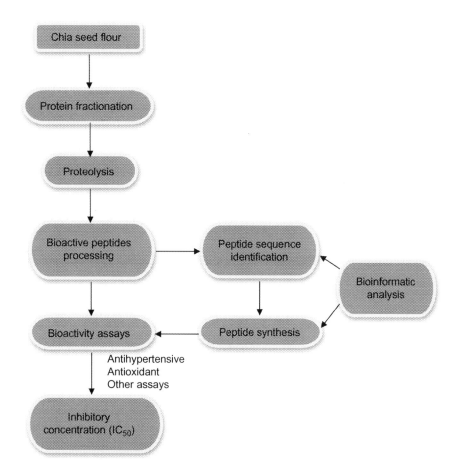

FIGURE 17.4 Classical approach to obtain bioactive peptides from chia seeds. Storage proteins are subjected to hydrolysis with different peptidases to produce the bioactive peptides. Bioactive peptides are processed by different purification methodologies and assayed to identify their specific functional properties. Peptide sequences are identified by mass spectrometry and peptides can be chemically designed and assayed directly to obtain the IC_{50}.

The biological activity of chia protein hydrolysates regarding ACE inhibition is related to the amino acid sequence of the peptides and their high hydrophobicity (Alemán, Giménez, Pérez-Santin, Gómez-Guillén, & Montero, 2011). In di- and tripeptides showing ACE inhibition, the activity is strongly influenced by the C-terminal amino acid and hydrophobicity of the peptide (Murray & FitzGerald, 2007). Chia seeds contain a high concentration of hydrophobic amino acids that include proline, leucine, phenylalanine, and isoleucine and generate peptides with high ACE-inhibitory activity (see Table 17.4; Segura-Campos, Peralta González, Chel Guerrero, & Betancur Ancona, 2013).

Chia is a good source of peptides which can play an important role in the regulation of blood pressure. Orona-Tamayo et al. (2015) isolated and hydrolyzed albumin, globulin, prolamin, and glutelin protein fractions with different peptidases (pepsin, trypsin, and chymotrypsin) and tested for inhibition of ACE. They found that peptides from albumin and globulin protein fractions exhibited the highest ACE-inhibitory activity, with IC_{50} values of 377 and 339 μg/mL, respectively, followed by bioactive peptides from chia seed flour (IC_{50} = 516 μg/mL) and lastly the peptides from prolamin and glutelins with IC_{50} values of 636 and 700 μg/mL, respectively. These results indicate that peptides from albumin and globulin protein fractions as well as unfractionated chia flour are better inhibitors against ACE than the prolamin and glutelin protein fractions.

Alternative antihypertensive drugs are being researched because of the high cost, side effects, and safety issues of existing drugs. Evidence suggests that edible foods such as milk, egg, plants, and grains contain peptides involved in the prevention and reduction of high blood pressure (Hernández-Ledesma, del Mar Contreras, & Recio, 2011; Montoya-Rodríguez, Gómez-Favela, Reyes-Moreno, Milán-Carrillo, & González de Mejía, 2015; Rosales-Mendoza, Paz-Maldonado, Govea-Alonso, & Korban, 2013). The ACE-inhibitory peptides derived from specific protein fractions of chia seeds can be a natural treatment for hypertensive individuals when they consume chia as a supplement.

Some studies also show the positive effects of the intake of whole or ground chia seeds on the blood pressure levels in humans. In this context, Vuksan et al. (2007) evaluated diabetic individuals with cardiovascular risk to determine the effect of the addition of 37 g/day of ground chia seeds as supplement. These patients showed reduced blood pressure by 12 weeks compared to patients with placebo. Compared to the control patients, the chia supplementation reduced systolic blood pressure around 6.3 mmHg and they concluded that the long-term consumption of the seeds can decrease the cardiovascular risk factor. Toscano et al. (2014) studied the effects of chia seed supplementation on the blood pressure in treated and untreated hypertensive individuals. Hypertensive subjects supplemented with 35 g/day of chia seed flour or placebo for 12 weeks, showed a reduction of 5.2 mmHg in blood pressure, while the placebo group showed no change. They concluded that chia flour consumption is able to decrease blood pressure in hypertensive patients. However, when Nieman et al. (2009) evaluated an intake of 50 g/day of whole or ground chia seeds in male and female patients for 12 weeks in terms of hypotensive features, no differences were found for changes in blood pressure in either gender compared with the control groups. Similar results were found by Nieman et al. (2012) when they supplemented 25 g/day of whole or ground chia seeds in overweight women for 10 weeks. They concluded that the ingestion of 25 or 50 g/day of ground or whole chia seeds did not influence the cardiovascular risk factors. Hence, these results can be contradictory and controversial, because the inhibitory capacity of the food peptides on ACE is not always related to their antihypertensive activities; and peptides show high inhibitory effects against ACE in vitro but not in vivo blood pressure-lowering effects (Li, Le, Shi, & Shrestha, 2004). The hypotensive action may also depend on the physiological status of the individual and the period of supplementation as well as the proper absorption of the bioactive peptides (Gostner, Becker, Ueberall, & Fuchs, 2015; Vermeirssen, Camp, & Verstraete, 2004).

The main chemical composition of *S. hispanica* seeds includes not only proteins but also α-linolenic acid and dietary fiber, which are in high concentrations and can exert high antihypertensive effects. Therefore, the chia components such as fatty acids, fiber, and peptides must be separately tested in animal or human models with antihypertensive risk factors in order to analyze their inhibitory effects on blood pressure.

17.4.5 Polyphenols, Oil, and Peptides With Antioxidant Capacity

Biomolecules of chia seed can act as antioxidant compounds, in particular secondary metabolites are the most important components, followed by oil and peptides. The consumption of natural sources with high levels of antioxidant compounds (polyphenols, tocopherols, carotenoids, vitamins, oil, and antioxidant peptides) (Marineli et al., 2015) can prevent DNA and cell damage, thus the onset of degenerative disorders, that is, arthritis, diabetes, cancer, and cardiovascular diseases can be suppressed (Martínez-Cruz & Paredes-López, 2014; Muñoz et al., 2013; Orona-Tamayo et al., 2015). It is important to note that the antioxidant capacity of the phytochemicals isolated from chia seeds has only been evaluated in vitro. A pioneering study by Taga et al. (1984) assessed the antioxidant activities of hydrolyzed and nonhydrolyzed chia seed extracts; techniques based on the bleaching of β-carotene coupled oxidation and linolenic acid in the presence of added antioxidants. They found that flavonol glycosides, chlorogenic and caffeic acids caused the main antioxidant activities in nonhydrolyzed extracts, in contrast, the major antioxidants in the hydrolyzed extracts were kaempferol, quercetin, myricetin, and caffeic acid. In a similar study performed by Reyes-Caudillo et al. (2008) in chia seeds grown in the states of Sinaloa and Jalisco (Mexico), quercetin and kaempferol were identified in the crude and hydrolyzed extracts, while caffeic, chlorogenic acids were present in lower concentrations. The antioxidant capacities of the cultivars from Jalisco state showed a higher antioxidant activity than those from Sinaloa. Vázquez-Ovando et al. (2009) evaluated the antioxidant capacity of a fiber-rich fraction obtained by dry processing of defatted chia seed flour. They found that chia flour antioxidant activity was higher than wheat and sorghum grains and similar to wine, coffee, tea, and orange juice. These antioxidant effects are due to the presence of caffeic and chlorogenic acids, as well as to other phenolic compounds. Martínez-Cruz and Paredes-López (2014) analyzed methanolic extracts of chia seeds and identified and quantified phenolic and isoflavone compounds with high antioxidant activity by ultrahigh-performance liquid chromatography. The total phenolic concentration was 1.8-fold higher than previous reports (Reyes-Caudillo et al., 2008) and the main compounds identified were daidzin, protocatehuic ethyl ester, rosmarinic, ferulic, and gallic acids; additionally, glycitin, genistin, glycitein, and genistein were also detected. The antioxidant activity against DPPH (2,2-diphenyl-1-picrylhydrazyl) radical was higher (68.83% inhibition) than the values reported previously for other *Salvia* species (Tepe, Sokmen, Akpulat, & Sokmen, 2006). Marineli et al. (2014) identified chlorogenic acid, quercetin, kaempferol, myricetin, and decarboxymethylelenolic acid linked to hydroxytyrosol (3,4-DHPEA-EDA) in the ethanolic extracts of chia seeds by direct mass spectrometry using the ambient sonic-spray ionization technique. The authors identified the same phenolic compounds except kaempferol in chia oils. Based on in vitro studies, it can be concluded that chia extracts and oil comprise important antioxidants.

In vivo analyses on the antioxidant potential of chia are limited. Marineli et al. (2015) evaluated the effects of consumption of chia seed and oil for 6 and 12 weeks by obese rats and quantified important biomarkers reduced glutathione (GHS), catalase (CAT), glutathione peroxidase (GPx), and glutathione reductase (GRd) in plasma and liver to establish oxidative stress status. The authors found that a high-fructose (HFF) diet induced lipid peroxidation and oxidative stress in these organs. In contrast, the animals consuming chia seed or oil showed an increase in the activity of GHS, CAT, GPx, and liver GRd. Plasma and hepatic antioxidant capacity increased in chia seed- and oil-consuming groups showing similar antioxidant capacity of around 35% and 47%, respectively, compared to HFF groups.

The high antioxidant capacity of phenolic compounds and oil from chia seeds is of great impact to food research. However, in recent years seed peptides, especially antioxidative peptides, have drawn the attention of researchers due to their simple characteristics such as their low-molecular-weight, easy absorption (Xie, Huang, Xu, & Jin, 2008), capacity of inhibiting lipid peroxidation and scavenging free radicals and chelators of transition metal ions (Sarmadi & Ismail, 2010). These features have focused the attention on peptides as new biomolecules that may act together with phenolic compounds and oil to reduce the oxidative stress more effectively than a single antioxidant compound. Besides, peptides released from proteins isolated from chia seeds have also been evaluated by their antioxidant activities against oxidants chemicals. Orona-Tamayo et al. (2015) reported that peptides of albumin and globulin fractions of chia seeds show high antiradical effects against ABTS (2,2'-azino-bis(3 ethylbenzothiazoline-6-sulfonic acid)). The scavenging activity of ABTS by peptides of albumin and globulin showed the lowest IC_{50} values of 89.3 and 92 μg/mL, respectively, whereas peptides from prolamin and glutelin were higher (161.5 and 184.7 μg/mL, respectively). The authors evaluated the same peptides against DPPH radicals and presented similar results. Peptides from albumin and globulin fractions showed a high antiradical capacity with IC_{50} values of 124.4 and 74.7 μg/mL, respectively. Prolamin and glutelin peptides gave IC_{50} values of 242.8 and 238.4 μg/mL, respectively. The antioxidant capacity of chia peptides against DPPH and ABTS could be derived from extensive protein hydrolysis which results in the formation of shorter peptides. Such peptides may delay their availability as an electron donor. Hydrophobic and acidic amino acids are present in high proportions in chia protein fractions, which may consist of the peptides derived from these fraction (Orona-Tamayo et al., 2015; Sandoval-Oliveros & Paredes-López, 2013; Siow & Gan, 2013).

Transition metal ions, such as iron (Fe^{2+}) and cupper (Cu^{2+}), can catalyze Fenton and Haber−Weiss reactions to produce hydroxyl radicals that trigger the oxidative (Lehmann et al., 2015) reactions generating cell lipid peroxidation and DNA damage in cells as well as in food systems (Durak, Baraniak, Jakubczyk, & Świeca, 2013). Reports indicate that the progression of hydroxyl radical generation by metal ions is effectively inhibited by antioxidant peptides via metal ion chelation (Guo et al., 2014; Xie et al., 2008; Zhou, Chen, Wang, Ye, & Chen, 2012). In this context, Orona-Tamayo et al. (2015) identified that the peptides from prolamin fractions have the highest ability to chelate Fe^{2+} ion with an IC_{50} value of 0.94 mg/mL, followed by globulin and glutelin peptides with similar magnitude of chelation (1.1 and 1.2 mg/mL, respectively), whereas chia seed flour peptides showed an IC_{50} value of 1.6 mg/mL. These results indicate that prolamin and globulin peptides from chia seeds are the most powerful chelating components in chia seeds (Orona-Tamayo et al., 2015).

In general, these seeds are loaded with a high amount of antioxidative molecules, mainly phenolic compounds (Martínez-Cruz & Paredes-López, 2014) accompanied by new sources of antioxidants such as oil with a high proportion of similar components (Marineli et al., 2015); and bioactive peptides with antioxidant and chelating activities derived from protein fractions (Orona-Tamayo et al., 2015).

17.5 CHIA COMPOUNDS SIGNIFICANT TO THE FOOD INDUSTRY

The intake of chia seeds can be important for human health due to the high concentration of nutrients with important functional properties (Mohd Ali et al., 2012). The popularity of these seeds and the different commercial presentations are slowly growing up in the food and cosmetic industries; producers and manufacturers are looking for the best seed constituents that can be incorporated into new products or merely replace ingredients in commercial products. Interestingly, chia seed coat mucilage is composed mainly of polysaccharides, which can absorb 27 times their weight in water (Muñoz, Cobos, Diaz, & Aguilera, 2012). This mucilaginous gel is considered a valuable ingredient in the food industry, due to its good physical properties. This includes working as a foam-stabilizing agent in products such as mayonnaises, sauces, and yogurts (Bochicchio et al., 2015; de la Paz Salgado-Cruz et al., 2013). In addition, the gel is also a suspending agent, emulsifier, adhesive, or binder with water-holding capacity (Vazquez-Ovando, Rosado-Rubio, Chel-Guerrero, & Betancur-Ancona, 2009). In this sense, Steffolani, Martinez, León, and Gómez (2015) mentioned that mucilage from chia seeds can potentially be used in bakery food products as a good and healthy replacement for egg and oil, as well as a solution to decrease fats and sugars in flour bakery (Borneo, Aguirre, & León, 2010).

The hydrocolloids of the mucilage of chia seeds have been used as novel edible films since mucilage exhibits excellent absorption of ultraviolet light and thermal stability; it can be used as an edible film or coating (Dick et al., 2015) for the industry, as a new alternative for edible and biodegradable films to partly or totally substitute packing polymers to resolve environmental problems. Chia contains high concentrations of insoluble and soluble fiber (Reyes-Caudillo et al., 2008) and its addition bring positive changes to some properties of foods such as texture. It can also act as a stabilizing agent, and improves fat-binding and water retention in cooked meat products (Capitani et al., 2012; Raghavendra et al., 2006). Chia mucilage could be a suitable material to reduce the use of fat in processed foods.

17.5.1 Antioxidant Properties

The high antioxidant capacity of chia oil can be used to protect against oxidative reactions in meat and seafood products of mass consumption (Martínez et al., 2015). Emulsions prepared with chia oil and hydrotyrosol have high antioxidant stability in healthy lipid-containing cooked meats, providing long shelf-life of the meat product (Cofrades et al., 2014). In this context, Julio et al. (2015) evaluated the incorporation of chia oil into functional oil–water emulsions with sodium alginate and lactose under different homogenizer pressure levels. Chia emulsions showed low levels of primary and secondary oxidation products during the storage period that followed, suggesting that the oil–water emulsions are a potential alternative against lipid peroxidation and can be incorporated in diverse functional foods (Julio et al., 2015).

Some researchers have investigated the role of chia oil supplementation in marine diets to increase the ω-3 fatty acid contents in the fish muscle tissue that are for human consumption. Montanher et al. (2015) analyzed the effect of chia oil in a diet of tilapia fish regarding antioxidant capacity, and the effect on ω-3 fatty acid content in muscle fillets. The inclusion of this oil produced a significant increase in ω-3 levels and antioxidant capacity; thus chia oil can contribute in the improvement of nutritional quality of tilapia in terms of ω-3 and antioxidant capacity.

17.5.2 Health Benefits

Important benefits can be found with the use of chia oil in skin applications because ω-3 and ω-6 fatty acids can inhibit melanin hyperpigmentation by means of a good epidermal barrier function (Ando, Ryu, Hashimoto, Oka, & Ichihashi, 1998; Rawlings, 2003). Chia seeds are an excellent source of this type of healthy fats. When the effect of chia seed oil extract rich in ω-3/-6 against melanogenesis was examined, inhibition of melanin biosynthesis in Melan-a cells was observed (Ayerza, 1995). The possible mechanism of action was revealed as that the chia seed oil was downregulating the expression of melanogenesis-related genes that encoded key melanogenic enzymes (Diwakar et al., 2014). These results may benefit cosmetic and pharmaceutical industries. Chia seed phenolic compounds have considerable interest in relation to their antioxidant properties acting against oxidants that can promote cell damage and derive in neurodegenerative diseases such as alzheimer and parkinson (Uttara et al., 2009). Chia is a good source of phenolic and isoflavone compounds that represent a novel source of antioxidants without side effects. These compounds could be incorporated as natural additives into processed foods with high oxidants to preserve the quality of the food product. Synthetic antioxidants present different toxicological problems and they are widely used by the food industry (Balasundram, Sundram, & Samman, 2006); antioxidant compounds from chia can be used to replace them.

17.5.3 Functional Benefits

In order to test the suitability of chia seed components as natural antioxidants for the stabilization of polyunsaturated fats and oils, Azeem, Nadeem, and Ahmad (2015) investigated the antioxidant activity of chia extract for the stabilization and preservation of cotton oil under ambient temperature during 90 days of storage. The addition of chia seed extract in cotton oil significantly inhibited the auto-oxidation compared with the control samples. This antioxidative ability could be related to the phenolics of chia seed. Antioxidants contained in chia significantly inhibit the oxidative breakdown of oils and fats with a high degree of unsaturation (Azeem et al., 2015).

The oxidation reactions occurring in fruits and vegetables during handling, harvesting, transportation, and storage have an important impact on browning. These reactions catalyzed by peroxidases (POD) involve phenolic compound polymerization leading to changes in quality (Tomás-Barberán & Espin, 2001). Inhibition of POD using natural antioxidants is a good alternative to avoid enzymatic browning in fruits. Coehlo and Salas-Mellado (2014) demonstrated that phenolic compounds from chia seed extracts can exert POD activity inhibition, which is related to the browning reaction in potato tuber extracts. The authors also found that chia seed phenolic extracts showed their effectiveness in the later times of reaction, while at the beginning it showed the same level of oxidation inhibition as control. The cell damage in fruits leads to decompartmentalization, and activates polyphenol oxidase as well as POD. Both enzymes are responsible for the loss of quality in fruits (Tomás-Barberán & Espin, 2001) and chia phenolic compounds may be used for inhibiting these enzymes.

Protein isolates from vegetal sources are becoming of great interest due to their use as ingredients with functional properties that can improve the nutritive quality of foods (Sandoval-Oliveros & Paredes-López, 2013). Proteins of chia seeds provide a rich source of essential amino acids with high potential as functional ingredients to be used by the food industry. The storage proteins comprise 23% (Sandoval-Oliveros & Paredes-López, 2013) with globulins being the main fraction (Orona-Tamayo et al., 2015) which potentially can be used as functional ingredients in foods. The functional properties of proteins are greatly influenced by their conformation, providing different functional properties such as gelation, foaming, and thermal capacities that may improve the sensory quality of foods.

To date, few studies have evaluated the functional properties of isolated proteins from chia seeds. In that sense, Olivos-Lugo et al. (2010) evaluated different functional properties of chia globulin and glutelin proteins. They reported that these proteins have good gelling capacities and formed a stable gel matrix, with low foaming capacities and presented high water- and oil-holding properties. Similarly, Sandoval-Oliveros and Paredes-López (2013) showed the thermal properties of individual chia seed storage proteins, and found that albumins and globulins had closer denaturation temperatures, 103°C and 105°C, respectively, followed by glutelin and prolamins at 91°C and 85°C, respectively. These functional features of chia seed proteins could potentially be used as nutraceutical ingredients in different food systems.

17.6 THE FUTURE OF CHIA SEEDS: MOLECULAR ENGINEERING AND GENE EDITING

Since chia crop's revival, diverse studies of the seed quality have emerged to exploit the nutraceutical properties to human health benefits. These studies were mainly focused on knowing the chia seed oil composition and its amount of ω-3/-6 fatty acid content (Ayerza & Coates, 2011; Bochicchio et al., 2015; Jamboonsri et al., 2012; Porras-Loaiza, Jiménez-Munguía, Sosa-Morales, Palou, & López-Malo, 2014), phenolic compounds (Marineli et al., 2014; Martínez-Cruz & Paredes-López, 2014), proteins (Sandoval-Oliveros & Paredes-López, 2013), and peptides (Orona-Tamayo et al., 2015). Each of these biomolecules could be genetically manipulated with recombinant DNA and through genome technologies as part of a new revolution in food and biological research (Hsu, Lander, & Zhang, 2014).

Eukaryotic genomes contain a high amount of DNA base pairs, which increases difficulties for manipulation. However, one of the breakthroughs in genome engineering to alleviate the large-size genomes is manipulation by gene targeting or gene editing. This technique integrates artificial nucleases producing double-stranded breaks in genome, and subsequently these breaks can be repaired by endogenous cell repair systems, allowing the precise insertion of specific genes for modification/replacement at its desired genomic location without any foreign DNA source. The absence of strange DNA can help to increase consumer acceptance of novel genetically modified plants (Hsu et al., 2014; Kanchiswamy, Sargent, Velasco, Maffei, & Malnoy, 2015). This advanced tool has been successfully demonstrated in different plants with agronomic importance such as tobacco, rice, sorghum, and soybean (Jiang et al., 2013; Kanchiswamy et al., 2015; Li et al., 2015).

Chia is a diploid plant with only 12 chromosomes ($n = 6$) (Estilai, Hashemi, & Truman, 1990), a small genome, which will facilitate the rapid genetic improvement and consequent plant breeding (Araki & Ishii, 2015; Jamboonsri et al., 2012) by genome-editing modification. Gene editing will facilitate agronomic traits such as abiotic and biotic adaptation, yield components, plant architecture, vigor, seed maturation, and flowering time to facilitate the crosses for plant breeding (Hu & Lübberstedt, 2015; Jamboonsri et al., 2012). Incidentally, reported work on basic molecular techniques, such as plant mutagenesis, to overexpress genes involved in the biosynthetic pathways to overproduce metabolites and recombinant proteins with nutraceutical properties are scarce in chia plants. Genomic information is important since the gene editing technique needs the information and characterization of specific genes that provides insights into the specific functions. High-throughput de novo sequencing approaches, such as whole-genome (Sablok et al., 2015) and next-generation transcriptome sequencing, are necessary for "nonmodel" species without a reference genome. These molecular tools provide information to generate physical maps and facilitate mapping with agronomic traits (Hu & Lübberstedt, 2015) in crop improvement programs.

Genetic and genomic information on chia plants is missing, therefore, there is an opportunity to use advanced molecular tools to identify and reveal important genes involved in polymorphisms associated with beneficial traits that link to important metabolic networks. For example, the high polyunsaturated fatty acids content of chia seeds makes this crop very attractive as a food, for health uses, and for some industrial purposes. From a commercial perspective, it is desirable that seeds must contain high levels of triacylglycerols enriched with beneficial fatty acids (Brown et al., 2012).

In the last two decades, researchers have focused attention on understanding genes encoding the most important enzymes involved in fatty acid and triacylglycerol biosynthesis (Ruiz-Lopez, Usher, Sayanova, Napier, & Haslam, 2015). In that sense, Sreedhar, Kumari, Rupwate, Rajasekharan, and Srinivasan (2015) presented an analysis of a global transcriptome profile for developing chia seeds with special reference to genes involved in lipid metabolism. They analyzed transcripts from five different seed developmental stages and identified and validated through RT-PCR the genes involved in fatty acid and oil accumulation into chia seeds. This genomic information related to lipid metabolism may be useful to improve the quality and quantity of chia seed oil (Sreedhar et al., 2015). With the fast progress in genomics, transcriptomics analysis, proteomics, chemical genomics, metabolomics, lipidomics, and in the new emergent and exciting technologies, such as mutagenesis and gene editing, this could be the beginning of more research on this crop and will promote the development of new cultivars with better nutraceutical attributes.

17.7 CONCLUDING REMARKS

Chia seeds provide several nutrients that have great potential as nutraceutical compounds, which benefit human health. The most important compounds of the seeds include soluble and insoluble fiber, oil with high amounts of ω-3 and -6 fatty acids, proteins with a high level of essential amino acids, minerals, vitamins, and phytochemicals with high antioxidant activities including phenolics and isoflavones. The main components of the seed have been isolated and evaluated to understand their functional properties and nutrition and health benefits for human use. Over the last decade, chia seeds have been the focus of researchers, due to the presence of these active compounds for identification and improving their properties, especially their antihypertensive and antioxidant potentials. Advances in new molecular technologies, such as DNA editing and novel-omic technologies, can be used in chia plants to develop new cultivars with better nutraceutical attributes and intelligent and rational uses in the food industry. Thus chia may become the golden seed of this century.

ACKNOWLEDGMENTS

This project was partially supported by ConsejoNacional de Ciencia y Tecnologia (CONACyT-Mexico).

REFERENCES

Alemán, A., Giménez, B., Pérez-Santin, E., Gómez-Guillén, M. C., & Montero, P. (2011). Contribution of Leu and Hyp residues to antioxidant and ACE-inhibitory activities of peptide sequences isolated from squid gelatin hydrolysate. *Food Chemistry*, 125, 334–341.

Aluko, R. E. (2015). Antihypertensive peptides from food proteins. *Annual Reviews of Food Science and Technology*, 6, 235–262.

Amato, M., Caruso, M. C., Guzzo, F., Galgano, F., Commisso, M., Bochicchio, R., ... Favati, F. (2015). Nutritional quality of seeds and leaf metabolites of chia (*Salvia hispanica* L.) from southern Italy. *European Food Research and Technology*, 241, 615–625.

Ando, H., Ryu, A., Hashimoto, A., Oka, M., & Ichihashi, M. (1998). Linoleic acid and α-linolenic acid lightens ultraviolet-induced hyperpigmentation of the skin. *Archives of Dermatological Research*, 290, 375–381.

Araki, M., & Ishii, T. (2015). Towards social acceptance of plant breeding by genome editing. *Trends in Plant Science*, 20, 145–149.

Ayerza, R. (1995). Oil content and fatty acid composition of chia (*Salvia hispanica* L.) from five northwestern locations in Argentina. *Journal of the American Chemical Society*, 72, 1079–1081.

Ayerza, R. (2009). The seed's protein and oil content, fatty acid composition, and growing cycle length of a single genotype of chia (*Salvia hispanica* L.) as affected by environmental factors. *Journal of Oleo Science*, 58, 347–354.

Ayerza, R., & Coates, W. (2001). Omega-3 enriched eggs: the influence of dietary α-linolenic fatty acid source on egg production and composition. *Canadian Journal of Animal Science*, 81, 355–362.

Ayerza, R., & Coates, W. (2004). Composition of chia (*Salvia hispanica*) grown in six tropical and subtropical ecosystems of South America. *Tropical Science*, 44, 131–135.

Ayerza, R., & Coates, W. (2005). Ground chia seed and chia oil effects on plasma lipids and fatty acids in the rat. *Nutrition Research*, 25, 995–1003.

Ayerza, R., & Coates, W. (2009). Some quality components of four chia (*Salvia hispanica* L.) genotypes grown under tropical coastal desert ecosystem conditions. *Asian Journal of Plant Sciences*, 8, 301.

Ayerza, R., & Coates, W. (2011). Protein content, oil content and fatty acid profiles as potential criteria to determine the origin of commercially grown chia (*Salvia hispanica* L.). *Industrial Crops and Products*, 34, 1366–1371.

Azeem, W., Nadeem, M., & Ahmad, S. (2015). Stabilization of winterized cottonseed oil with chia (*Salvia hispanica* L.) seed extract at ambient temperature. *Journal of Food Science and Technology*, 52(11). Available from http://dx.doi.org/10.1007/s13197-015-1823-2.

Balasundram, N., Sundram, K., & Samman, S. (2006). Phenolic compounds in plants and agri-industrial by-products: Antioxidant activity, occurrence, and potential uses. *Food Chemistry*, 99, 191–203.

Bochicchio, R., Philips, T. D., Lovelli, S., Labella, R., Galgano, F., Di Marisco, A., ... Amato, M. (2015). Innovative crop productions for healthy food: The case of chia (*Salvia hispanica* L.). In A. Vastola (Ed.), *The sustainability of agro-food and natural resource systems in the Mediterranean Basin* (pp. 29–45). Springer International Publishing.

Böger, R. H. (2007). The pharmacodynamics of L-arginine. *Journal of Nutrition, 137*, 1650S–1655S.

Borderías, A. J., Sánchez-Alonso, I., & Pérez-Mateos, M. (2005). New applications of fibres in foods: Addition to fishery products. *Trends in Food Science & Technology, 16*, 458–465.

Borneo, R., Aguirre, A., & León, A. E. (2010). Chia (*Salvia hispanica* L) gel can be used as egg or oil replacer in cake formulations. *Journal of the American Dietetic Association, 110*, 946–949.

Brosnan, J. T., & Brosnan, M. E. (2013). Glutamate: A truly functional amino acid. *Amino Acids, 45*, 413–418.

Brown, A. P., Kroon, J., Swarbreck, D., Febrer, M., Larson, T. R., Graham, I. A., ... Slabas, A. R. (2012). Tissue-specific whole transcriptome sequencing in castor, directed at understanding triacylglycerol lipid biosynthetic pathways. *PLoS ONE, 7*, e30100.

Cahill, J. P. (2003). Ethnobotany of chia, *Salvia hispanica* L. (Lamiaceae). *Economic Botany, 57*, 604–618.

Capitani, M., Spotorno, V., Nolasco, S., & Tomás, M. (2012). Physicochemical and functional characterization of by-products from chia (*Salvia hispanica* L.) seeds of Argentina. *LWT – Food Science and Technology, 45*, 94–102.

Coates, W. (2011). Whole and ground chia (*Salvia hispanica* L.) seeds, chia oil-effects on plasma lipids and fatty acids. In V. Patel, R. Preedy, & V. Watson (Eds.), *Nuts and seeds in health and disease prevention* (pp. 309–314). San Diego: Academic.

Coelho, M. S., & Salas-Mellado, M. D. I. M. (2014). Chemical characterization of chia (*Salvia hispanica* L.) for use in food products. *Journal of Food and Nutrition Research, 2*, 263–269.

Cofrades, S., Santos-Lopez, J., Freire, M., Benedí, J., Sanchez-Muniz, F., & Jiménez-Colmenero, F. (2014). Oxidative stability of meat systems made with W1/O/W 2 emulsions prepared with hydroxytyrosol and chia oil as lipid phase. *LWT – Food Science and Technology, 59*, 941–947.

de la Paz Salgado-Cruz, M., Calderón-Domínguez, G., Chanona-Pérez, J., Farrera-Rebollo, R. R., Méndez-Méndez, J. V., & Díaz-Ramírez, M. (2013). Chia (*Salvia hispanica* L.) seed mucilage release characterisation. A microstructural and image analysis study. *Industrial Crops and Products, 51*, 453–462.

Dick, M., Costa, T. M. H., Gomaa, A., Subirade, M., Rios, A. D. O., & Flôres, S. H. (2015). Edible film production from chia seed mucilage: Effect of glycerol concentration on its physicochemical and mechanical properties. *Carbohydrate Polymers, 130*, 198–205.

Diwakar, G., Rana, J., Saito, L., Vredeveld, D., Zemaitis, D., & Scholten, J. (2014). Inhibitory effect of a novel combination of *Salvia hispanica* (chia) seed and *Punica granatum* (pomegranate) fruit extracts on melanin production. *Fitoterapia, 97*, 164–171.

Durak, A., Baraniak, B., Jakubczyk, A., & Świeca, M. (2013). Biologically active peptides obtained by enzymatic hydrolysis of Adzuki bean seeds. *Food Chemistry, 141*, 2177–2183.

Egras, A. M., Hamilton, W. R., Lenz, T. L., & Monaghan, M. S. (2011). An evidence-based review of fat modifying supplemental weight loss products. *Journal of Obesity, 2011*. Article ID 297315. <http://dx.doi.org/10.1155/2011/297315/>

Esposito, F., Arlotti, G., Bonifati, A. M., Napolitano, A., Vitale, D., & Fogliano, V. (2005). Antioxidant activity and dietary fibre in durum wheat bran by-products. *Food Research International, 38*, 1167–1173.

Estilai, A., Hashemi, A., & Truman, K. (1990). Chromosome number and meiotic behavior of cultivated chia, *Salvia hispanica* (Lamiaceae). *HortScience, 25*, 1646–1647.

Gostner, J. M., Becker, K., Ueberall, F., & Fuchs, D. (2015). The good and bad of antioxidant foods: An immunological perspective. *Food and Chemical Toxicology, 80*, 72–79.

Guo, L., Harnedy, P. A., Li, B., Hou, H., Zhang, Z., Zhao, X., & FitzGerald, R. J. (2014). Food protein-derived chelating peptides: Biofunctional ingredients for dietary mineral bioavailability enhancement. *Trends in Food Science & Technology, 37*, 92–105.

Hernández-Ledesma, B., del Mar Contreras, M., & Recio, I. (2011). Antihypertensive peptides: Production, bioavailability and incorporation into foods. *Advances in Colloid and Interface Science, 165*, 23–35.

Heuer, B., Yaniv, Z., & Ravina, I. (2002). Effect of late salinization of chia (*Salvia hispanica*), stock (*Matthiola tricuspidata*) and evening primrose (*Oenothera biennis*) on their oil content and quality. *Industrial Crops and Products, 15*, 163–167.

Hsu, P. D., Lander, E. S., & Zhang, F. (2014). Development and applications of CRISPR-Cas9 for genome engineering. *Cell, 157*, 1262–1278.

Hu, S., & Lübberstedt, T. (2015). Getting the 'MOST' out of crop improvement. *Trends in Plant Science, 20*, 372–379.

Illian, T. G., Casey, J. C., & Bishop, P. A. (2011). Omega 3 chia seed loading as a means of carbohydrate loading. *The Journal of Strength & Conditioning Research, 25*, 61–65.

Jamboonsri, W., Phillips, T. D., Geneve, R. L., Cahill, J. P., & Hildebrand, D. F. (2012). Extending the range of an ancient crop, *Salvia hispanica* L.—A new ω3 source. *Genetic Resources and Crop Evolution, 59*, 171–178.

Jiang, W., Zhou, H., Bi, H., Fromm, M., Yang, B., & Weeks, D. P. (2013). Demonstration of CRISPR/Cas9/sgRNA-mediated targeted gene modification in Arabidopsis, tobacco, sorghum and rice. *Nucleic Acids Research, 41*, e188 . <http://dx.doi.org/10.1093/nar/gkt780/>

Julio, L. M., Ixtaina, V. Y., Fernández, M. A., Sánchez, R. M. T., Wagner, J. R., Nolasco, S. M., & Tomás, M. C. (2015). Chia seed oil-in-water emulsions as potential delivery systems of ω-3 fatty acids. *Journal of Food Engineering, 162*, 48–55.

Kaczmarczyk, M. M., Miller, M. J., & Freund, G. G. (2012). The health benefits of dietary fiber: Beyond the usual suspects of type 2 diabetes mellitus, cardiovascular disease and colon cancer. *Metabolism, 61*, 1058–1066.

Kanchiswamy, C. N., Sargent, D. J., Velasco, R., Maffei, M. E., & Malnoy, M. (2015). Looking forward to genetically edited fruit crops. *Trends in Biotechnology, 33*, 62–64.

Kitts, D. D., & Weiler, K. (2003). Bioactive proteins and peptides from food sources. Applications of bioprocesses used in isolation and recovery. *Current Pharmaceutical Design*, *9*, 1309–1323.

Lehmann, C., Islam, S., Jarosch, S., Zhou, J., Hoskin, D., Greenshields, A., ... Kelly, M. (2015). The utility of iron chelators in the management of inflammatory disorders. *Mediators of Inflammation*, *2015*. ID 516740. http://dx.doi.org/10.1155/2015/516740

Li, G.-H., Le, G.-W., Shi, Y.-H., & Shrestha, S. (2004). Angiotensin I–converting enzyme inhibitory peptides derived from food proteins and their physiological and pharmacological effects. *Nutrition Research*, *24*, 469–486.

Li, Z., Liu, Z.-B., Xing, A., Moon, B. P., Koellhoffer, J. P., Huang, L., ... Cigan, A. M. (2015). Cas9-guide RNA directed genome editing in soybean. *Plant Physiology*, *169*(2), 960–970. Available from http://dx.doi.org/10.1104/pp.15.00783.

Lu, Y., & Foo, L. Y. (2002). Polyphenolics of Salvia – A review. *Phytochemistry*, *59*, 117–140.

Marineli, R. S., Lenquiste, S. A., Moraes, É. A., & Maróstica, M. R. (2015). Antioxidant potential of dietary chia seed and oil (*Salvia hispanica* L.) in diet-induced obese rats. *Food Research International*, *76*, 666–674.

Marineli, R. S., Moraes, É. A., Lenquiste, S. A., Godoy, A. T., Eberlin, M. N., & Maróstica, M. R., Jr. (2014). Chemical characterization and antioxidant potential of Chilean chia seeds and oil (*Salvia hispanica* L.). *LWT – Food Science and Technology*, *59*, 1304–1310.

Martínez, M. L., Curti, M. I., Roccia, P., Llabot, J. M., Penci, M. C., Bodoira, R. M., & Ribotta, P. D. (2015). Oxidative stability of walnut (*Juglans regia* L.) and chia (*Salvia hispanica* L.) oils microencapsulated by spray drying. *Powder Technology*, *270*, 271–277.

Martínez-Cruz, O., & Paredes-López, O. (2014). Phytochemical profile and nutraceutical potential of chia seeds (*Salvia hispanica* L.) by ultrahigh performance liquid chromatography. *Journal of Chromatography A*, *1346*, 43–48.

Martínez-Maqueda, D., Miralles, B., Recio, I., & Hernández-Ledesma, B. (2012). Antihypertensive peptides from food proteins: a review. *Food & function*, *3*, 350–361.

McCormack, W. P., Hoffman, J. R., Pruna, G. J., Jajtner, A. R., Townsend, J. R., Stout, J. R., ... Fukuda, D. H. (2015). Effects of L-alanyl-L-glutamine ingestion on one-hour run performance. *Journal of the American College of Nutrition*, *34*(6), 488–496. Available from http://dx.doi.org/10.1080/07315724.2015.1009193.

Mohd Ali, N., Yeap, S. K., Ho, W. Y., Beh, B. K., Tan, S. W., & Tan, S. G. (2012). The promising future of chia, *Salvia hispanica* L. *Bio Med Research International*, 9. Article ID 171956.

Montanher, P. F., Costa e Silva, B., Guntendorfer Bonafé, E., Carbonera, F., dos Santos, H. M. C., de Lima Figueiredo, I., ... Visentainer, J. Vl (2015). Effects of diet supplementation with chia (*Salvia hispanica* L.) oil and natural antioxidant extract on the omega-3 content and antioxidant capacity of Nile Tilapia fillets. *European Journal of Lipid Science and Technology*. Available from http://dx.doi.org/10.1002/ejlt.201400334.

Montoya-Rodríguez, A., Gómez-Favela, M. A., Reyes-Moreno, C., Milán-Carrillo, J., & González de Mejía, E. (2015). Identification of bioactive peptide sequences from amaranth (*Amaranthus hypochondriacus*) seed proteins and their potential role in the prevention of chronic diseases. *Comprehensive Reviews in Food Science and Food Safety*, *14*, 139–158.

Moure, A., Domínguez, H., & Parajó, J. C. (2005). Fractionation and enzymatic hydrolysis of soluble protein present in waste liquors from soy processing. *Journal of Agricultural and Food Chemistry*, *53*, 7600–7608.

Muñoz, L. A., Cobos, A., Diaz, O., & Aguilera, J. M. (2012). Chia seeds: Microstructure, mucilage extraction and hydration. *Journal of Food Engineering*, *108*, 216–224.

Muñoz, L. A., Cobos, A., Diaz, O., & Aguilera, J. M. (2013). Chia seed (*Salvia hispanica*): An ancient grain and a new functional food. *Food Reviews International*, *29*, 394–408.

Murray, B., & FitzGerald, R. (2007). Angiotensin converting enzyme inhibitory peptides derived from food proteins: Biochemistry, bioactivity and production. *Current Pharmaceutical Design*, *13*, 773–791.

Nieman, D. C., Cayea, E. J., Austin, M. D., Henson, D. A., McAnulty, S. R., & Jin, F. (2009). Chia seed does not promote weight loss or alter disease risk factors in overweight adults. *Nutrition Research*, *29*, 414–418.

Nieman, D. C., Gillitt, N., Jin, F., Henson, D. A., Kennerly, K., Shanely, R. A., ... Schwartz, S. (2012). Chia seed supplementation and disease risk factors in overweight women: A metabolomics investigation. *Journal of Alternative and Complementary Medicine*, *18*, 700–708.

Olivos-Lugo, B., Valdivia-López, M., & Tecante, A. (2010). Thermal and physicochemical properties and nutritional value of the protein fraction of Mexican chia seed (*Salvia hispanica* L.). *Food Science and Technology International*, *1*, 1–8.

Orona-Tamayo, D., Valverde, M. E., Nieto-Rendón, B., & Paredes-López, O. (2015). Inhibitory activity of chia (*Salvia hispanica* L.) protein fractions against angiotensin I-converting enzyme and antioxidant capacity. *LWT – Food Science and Technology*, *64*, 236–242.

Paredes-López, O. (1991). Safflower proteins for food use. In B. J. F. Hudson (Ed.), *Development in food proteins* (7 ed., pp. 1–33). London, UK: Elsevier.

Peiretti, P., & Gai, F. (2009). Fatty acid and nutritive quality of chia (*Salvia hispanica* L.) seeds and plant during growth. *Animal Feed Science and Technology*, *148*, 267–275.

Peperkamp, M. (2014). *Chia from Bolivia: A modern super seed in a classic pork cycle. CBI Marked Intelligence* (pp. 1–15). Netherland: Ministry of Foreign Affairs. <www.cbi.eu/market-information/grains-pulses/chia/>.

Porras-Loaiza, P., Jiménez-Munguía, M. T., Sosa-Morales, M. E., Palou, E., & López-Malo, A. (2014). Physical properties, chemical characterization and fatty acid composition of Mexican chia (*Salvia hispanica* L.) seeds. *International Journal of Food Science & Technology*, *46*, 571–577.

Raghavendra, S., Swamy, S. R., Rastogi, N., Raghavarao, K., Kumar, S., & Tharanathan, R. (2006). Grinding characteristics and hydration properties of coconut residue: A source of dietary fiber. *Journal of Food Engineering*, *72*, 281–286.

Rawlings, A. V. (2003). Trends in stratum corneum research and the management of dry skin conditions. *International Journal of Cosmetic Science*, *25*, 63–95.

Reyes-Caudillo, E., Tecante, A., & Valdivia-López, M. (2008). Dietary fibre content and antioxidant activity of phenolic compounds present in Mexican chia (*Salvia hispanica* L.) seeds. *Food Chemistry*, *107*, 656–663.

Rosales-Mendoza, S., Paz-Maldonado, L. M. T., Govea-Alonso, D. O., & Korban, S. S. (2013). Engineering production of antihypertensive peptides in plants. *Plant Cell, Tissue and Organ Culture, 112*, 159–169.

Ruiz-Lopez, N., Usher, S., Sayanova, O. V., Napier, J. A., & Haslam, R. P. (2015). Modifying the lipid content and composition of plant seeds: Engineering the production of LC-PUFA. *Applied Microbiology and Biotechnology, 99*, 143–154.

Sablok, G., Kumar, S., Ueno, S., Kuo, J., Varotto, C., Terauchi, R., ... Kamoun, S. (2015). Whole genome sequencing to identify genes and QTL in rice. In G. Sablok, S. Kumar, S. Ueno, & C. Varotto (Eds.), *Advances in the understanding of biological sciences using next generation sequencing (NGS) approaches* (pp. 33–42). Switzerland: Springer International Publishing.

SAGARPA (2014). Cierre de la produccion agricola por cultivo. In: *Servicio de Informacion Agroalimentaria y Pesquera*. <http://www.siap.gob.mx/cierre-de-la-produccion-agricola-por-cultivo/>.

Salazar-Vega, I. M., Segura-Campos, M. R., Chel-Guerrero, L., & Betancur-Ancona, D. (2012). Antihypertensive and antioxidant effects of functional foods containing chia (*Salvia hispanica*) protein hydrolysates. In B. Valdez (Ed.), *Agricultural and Biological Sciences Scientific, Health and Social Aspects of the Food Industry* (pp. 381–398). InTech.

Sandoval-Oliveros, M. R., & Paredes-López, O. (2013). Isolation and characterization of proteins from chia seeds (*Salvia hispanica* L.). *Journal of Agricultural and Food Chemistry, 61*, 193–201.

Sarmadi, B., & Ismail, A. (2010). Antioxidative peptides from food proteins: A review. *Peptides, 31*, 1949–1956.

Segura-Campos, M. R., Peralta González, F., Chel Guerrero, L., & Betancur Ancona, D. (2013). Angiotensin I-converting enzyme inhibitory peptides of chia (*Salvia hispanica*) produced by enzymatic hydrolysis. *International Journal of Food Science, 8*, Article ID 158482

Segura-Campos, M. R., Salazar-Vega, I. M., Chel-Guerrero, L. A., & Betancur-Ancona, D. A. (2013). Biological potential of chia (*Salvia hispanica* L.) protein hydrolysates and their incorporation into functional foods. *LWT – Food Science and Technology, 50*, 723–731.

Shewry, P. (1995). Plant storage proteins. *Biological Reviews, 70*, 375–426.

Siow, H.-L., & Gan, C.-Y. (2013). Extraction of antioxidative and antihypertensive bioactive peptides from *Parkia speciosa* seeds. *Food Chemistry, 141*, 3435–3442.

Sreedhar, R., Kumari, P., Rupwate, S. D., Rajasekharan, R., & Srinivasan, M. (2015). Exploring triacylglycerol biosynthetic pathway in developing seeds of chia (*Salvia hispanica* L.): A transcriptomic approach. *PLoS ONE, 10*, e0123580.

Steffolani, E., Martinez, M. M., León, A. E., & Gómez, M. (2015). Effect of pre-hydration of chia (*Salvia hispanica* L.), seeds and flour on the quality of wheat flour breads. *LWT – Food Science and Technology, 61*, 401–406.

Taga, M. S., Miller, E., & Pratt, D. (1984). Chia seeds as a source of natural lipid antioxidants. *Journal of the American Oil Chemists' Society, 61*, 928–931.

Tepe, B., Sokmen, M., Akpulat, H. A., & Sokmen, A. (2006). Screening of the antioxidant potentials of six Salvia species from Turkey. *Food Chemistry, 95*, 200–204.

Thelen, K. D. (2006). Interaction between row spacing and yield: Why it works. *Crop Management, 5*. Available from http://dx.doi.org/10.1094/CM-2006-0227-03-RV.

Tomás-Barberán, F. A., & Espin, J. C. (2001). Phenolic compounds and related enzymes as determinants of quality in fruits and vegetables. *Journal of the Science of Food and Agriculture, 81*, 853–876.

Toscano, L. T., da Silva, C. S. O., Toscano, L. T., de Almeida, A. E. M., da Cruz Santos, A., & Silva, A. S. (2014). Chia flour supplementation reduces blood pressure in hypertensive subjects. *Plant Foods for Human Nutrition, 69*, 392–398.

Udenigwe, C. C., & Aluko, R. E. (2012). Food protein-derived bioactive peptides: Production, processing, and potential health benefits. *Journal of Food Science, 77*, R11–R24.

Ullah, R., Nadeem, M., Khalique, A., Imran, M., Mehmood, S., Javid, A., & Hussain, J. (2015). Nutritional and therapeutic perspectives of chia (*Salvia hispanica* L.): A review. *Journal of Food Science and Technology*, 1–9. Available from http://dx.doi.org/10.1007/s13197-015-1967-0.

Uttara, B., Singh, A. V., Zamboni, P., & Mahajan, R. T. (2009). Oxidative stress and neurodegenerative diseases: a review of upstream and downstream antioxidant therapeutic options. *Current neuropharmacology, 7*, 65–74.

Vazquez-Ovando, A., Rosado-Rubio, G., Chel-Guerrero, L., & Betancur-Ancona, D. (2009). Physicochemical properties of a fibrous fraction from chia (*Salvia hispanica* L.). *LWT – Food Science and Technology, 42*, 168–173.

Vázquez-Ovando, J., Rosado-Rubio, J., Chel-Guerrero, L., & Betancur-Ancona, D. (2010). Dry processing of chia (*Salvia hispanica* L.) flour: Chemical characterization of fiber and protein. *CyTA – Journal of Food, 8*, 117–127.

Vermeirssen, V., Camp, J. V., & Verstraete, W. (2004). Bioavailability of angiotensin I converting enzyme inhibitory peptides. *British Journal of Nutrition, 92*, 357–366.

Vuksan, V., Whitham, D., Sievenpiper, J. L., Jenkins, A. L., Rogovik, A. L., Bazinet, R. P., ... Hanna, A. (2007). Supplementation of conventional therapy with the novel grain Salba (*Salvia hispanica* L.) improves major and emerging cardiovascular risk factors in type 2 diabetes: Results of a randomized controlled trial. *Diabetes Care, 30*, 2804–2810.

Xie, Z., Huang, J., Xu, X., & Jin, Z. (2008). Antioxidant activity of peptides isolated from alfalfa leaf protein hydrolysate. *Food Chemistry, 111*, 370–376.

Yeboah, S., OwusuDanquah, E., Lamptey, J., Mochiah, M., Lamptey, S., Oteng-Darko, P., ... Agyeman, K. (2013). Influence of planting methods and density on performance of chia (*Salvia hispanica*) and its suitability as an oilseed plant. *Agricultural Science, 2*, 14–26.

Zhou, H., Chen, X., Wang, C., Ye, J., & Chen, H. (2012). Purification and characterization of a novel ~18 kDa antioxidant protein from *Ginkgo biloba* seeds. *Molecules, 17*, 14778–14794.

Part II

Upcoming Sources of Proteins

Chapter 18

Proteins From Canola/Rapeseed: Current Status

J.P.D. Wanasundara[1], S. Tan[2], A.M. Alashi[3], F. Pudel[4] and C. Blanchard[2]

[1]*Agriculture and Agri-Food Canada, Saskatoon, SK, Canada,* [2]*ARC ITTC for Functional Grains, Charles Sturt University, Wagga Wagga, NSW, Australia,* [3]*University of Manitoba, Winnipeg, MB, Canada,* [4]*Pilot Pflanzenöltechnologie Magdeburg e.V., Magdeburg, Germany*

18.1 INTRODUCTION

Rapeseed or canola plant belongs to the Brassicaceae (Cruciferae) family. Prehistoric and archeological evidence, religious texts and teachings, and traditional ethnomedical practices suggest rape was one of the first plants domesticated by humans (Röbeelen, Downey, & Ashri, 1989; Wanasundara, 2011; Zohary & Hopf, 2000). Rape or colza is the term primarily used in Europe to identify oil-bearing seeds of *Brassica napus* and *Brassica rapa*. The term canola has been adopted since 1978 and is derived from "**Can**ada" and "**o**il **l**ow **a**cid" for the oilseed that fits into the international standard for an edible oil and suitable for commercial production. The international standard for "canola quality" oil is worded as the "seeds of the genus *Brassica* (*B. napus*, *B. rapa*, or *Brassica juncea*) from which the oil shall contain less than 2% erucic acid in its fatty acid (FA) profile and the solid component shall contain less than 30 micromoles of any one or any mixture of 3-butenyl glucosinolate, 4-pentenyl glucosinolate, 2-hydroxy-3 butenyl glucosinolate, and 2-hydroxy-4-pentenyl glucosinolate per gram of air-dry, oil-free solid" (CCC, 2015). Both Canada and Australia use this definition, however, European countries, China, and India use the terminology of rapeseed or double-low rapeseed, which refers to more or less the same parameters for oil composition and meal glucosinolate levels. In the international oilseed trade, the terms canola and rapeseed are used interchangeably and it is common to see canola and rapeseed data combined and presented as rapeseed. Canola/rapeseed (C/RS) occupies a significant place in the world oilseed industry; second place (~13.6%) in global oilseed production after soybean (~55%) and third place (for last 25 years) in the global vegetable oil consumption after palm and soybean oil. Among the protein meal and cake products, globally, C/RS meal is the second-largest feed protein source (FEDIOL, 2015).

18.2 PRODUCTION OF C/RS

C/RS grows in a wide range of environments and thrives in cooler temperate zones. Commercial canola production is primarily in the northern hemisphere except for Australia. In 2013, a total of 72.67 million tonnes (mil t) of rapeseed was produced by 63 countries around the world. The top five C/RS producing countries in 2013 were Canada (17.80 mil t), China (14.46 mil t), India (7.83 mil t), Germany (5.78 mil t), and France (4.37 mil t) and together these countries constituted 69.2% of world production (FAOSTAT, 2015). Indian C/RS production occurs in the northern areas of the country where mustard (mainly *B. juncea*) production also occurs. Canola production in Australia has increased significantly since 1995 and contributed 3.8 mil t to global production in 2013 (Agricultural Commodities Australia, 2013) and is the major oilseed cultivated in that country. Yield values reported for C/RS vary depending on the country. In the 2013–14 crop year, an average yield of 3.24 tonne/hectare (t/ha) was reported for European Union (EU) countries in which Germany obtained an average yield of 4.46 t/ha and France obtained an average yield of 3.66 t/ha (AGCanada, 2015). The average yield of canola grown in Canada is 2.24 t/ha (AAFC, 2015) and for Australia it is 1.3 t/ha (ABS, 2015).

C/RS crops generate both oil and protein. Considering the average protein content of C/RS is 20% by weight, in 2013 world canola production resulted in ~14.5 mil t of plant proteins being produced by this crop. At present, the primary use of C/RS protein is in feed rations for dairy cattle, poultry, and swine with a minor amount directed to aquaculture (CCC, 2015).

18.2.1 Land Use

Written records of "rape" cultivation for oil production date back to approximately 4000 years ago. The modern C/RS germplasm is a result of intensive human selection for better agronomic performance. C/RS is adapted to a wide range of soil types and can grow in relatively high-saline and also acidic soils but the yields are comparatively low. C/RS is cultivated as a rotation or break crop after cereals or pulses and can be grown as a spring or winter crop (CCC, 2015; UK Agriculture, 2015). European countries generally obtain higher yields compared to other countries due to superior soil fertility and climatic factors. In 2014, the acreage of rapeseed in EU was 6.70 million hectares (mil ha), while Canada harvested canola from 8.07 mil ha. In 2012–13, the Australian canola cultivation area reached 3.27 mil ha (Agricultural Commodities Australia, 2013).

18.2.2 Water Use

The majority of global C/RS production is under rainfed cultivation and an estimation of the extent of the crop under irrigation is not available. Water usage for C/RS production varies between the geographical regions that the crop is produced. For example, due to the climate differences that exist between European countries, rapeseed shows higher water demand in southern Europe (230 mm) compared to the northern regions (160 mm). The water use efficiency ranges from 582 to 830 kg water/kg DM when rapeseed is grown in European countries. However, rapeseed is predominantly produced in central Europe, where water scarcity is not an issue and the total water use is relatively low. According to Ludwig et al. (2011), rapeseed production in Europe is unlikely to cause unsustainable water use due to the abundance of water in canola-growing areas. In the Canadian prairies, where the majority of the world canola production occurs, 100–125 mm (4–5 in) water is needed to take the crop from germination to the reproductive growth stage to produce seeds. The Canadian canola-growing season is May to mid-September and, in total, 400–480 mm of water is needed. Water use efficiency reported as bushels of yield per inch water is 2.6–3.6 across different soil types in the Canadian prairie cultivation (CCC, 2015).

18.2.3 Energy Use

Under Canadian canola production systems, the estimated amount of energy required to produce 1 t of dry canola in the province of Manitoba is 4630 MJ and the net amount of greenhouse gas emission as a result of producing 1 t of canola is 548 kg CO_2e. According to the breakdown of energy use by input type under the production system practiced in Manitoba, Canada, 70% of the total energy requirement is for the production of nitrogen fertilizer (55% for anhydrous ammonia, 11% for ammonium sulfate, and 4% for monoammonium phosphate), diesel fuel production and use makes up 21% of total energy use, 3% for phosphate fertilizer production, 3% for herbicide production, and 1% each for the production of canola seed and fungicides (LCA Manitoba, 2015).

18.3 PROTEINS OF C/RS

18.3.1 Chemical Composition of the Seed

The chemical composition of C/RS seeds has the unique characteristics of the Brassicaceae family including oil, protein, carbohydrates (cellulose, polysaccharides, free sugars), glucosinolates (GSL), sinapic acid choline esters (sinapine), phenolic compounds, and phytic acid (Table 18.1). Details of the components considered as antinutritional factors (GSL, phenolics, phytic acid, and fiber) are discussed in Section 18.6. Historically, oil (35–38% of seed dwt) is the primary product of C/RS and protein (21–23% seed dwt) can be recovered from the oil-extracted meal, which contains all seed constituents other than oil and oil-soluble compounds. Oil of C/RS is generally used worldwide for human consumption and a small fraction is used as feedstock for biodiesel production in Europe and Canada. C/RS oil has a characteristic FA composition consisting of very low levels of saturated FA (~7%), relatively high levels of monounsaturated FA (61%), and intermediate levels of polyunsaturated FA (32%) with a good balance between omega-

TABLE 18.1 Average Values Reported for Chemical Composition of Canadian Canola Meal

Major Chemical Components and Nutrients		Minerals and Vitamins	
Component	Average Content	Component	Average Content
Proximates (%):[a]		**Minerals (mg/kg):**[b]	
Crude protein (N × 6.25)	34.0–40.0	K	12,000
Oil	2.0–3.8	P	10,600
Ash	6.1–10.1	S	830
Crude fiber	9.7–12.8	Ca	620
Acid detergent fiber	16.4–21.9	Mg	530
Neutral detergent fiber	20.7–35.1	Na	1000
		Cl	1000
		Fe	162
		Zn	57
		Mn	51
		Cu	5.7
		Mo	1.4
Carbohydrates (%):[b]		**Vitamins (mg/kg):**[b]	
Oligosaccharides	2.3	Choline[b]	6500
Free sugars	6.7	Niacin	156
Sucrose	6.9	Vitamin E	13
Fructose + glucose	0.5	Pantothenic acid	9.3
Nonstarch polysaccharides	15.7	Pyridoxine	7.0
Soluble	1.4	Riboflavin	5.7
Insoluble	14.4	Thiamin	5.1
Total dietary fiber	32.3	Biotin	0.96
		Folic acid	0.80
Others:[b]			
Tannins (%)	1.5		
Sinapine (%)	1.5–3.0		
Phytic acid	3.3		
Glucosinolates, μmoles/g (total)	7.2		

[a]Range of values reported from different sources, on "as received basis."
[b]Values reported for Canadian canola meal, and on 12% moisture basis.
Source: Adapted from Bell (1993), CCC. Canola Council of Canada. (2015). <www.canolacouncil.org>.

6 (21%) and omega-3 (one-third of total polyunsaturates) FA. This composition is consistent with nutrition recommendations targeting reduced saturated fat intake and is an important reason for the widespread adoption of C/RS oil by the food industry (CCC, 2015). In addition, the development of high-oleic acid-containing canola oils that are stable and do not require hydrogenation or modification for extended shelf-life has provided food processors with a tangible solution for an oil low in saturated FA which is free of trans-fat.

Simple sugars found in C/RS seed are primarily sucrose, glucose, and fructose, which constitute 5–6% of meal by weight (Table 18.1). Complex carbohydrates of seed coat, endosperm, and cotyledon cell walls contribute to the seed dietary fiber (DF) fraction. Information on micronutrients of C/RS meal or seed is limited. Among the minerals, high potassium and phosphorus levels are reported for C/RS meal (Table 18.1). Phosphorus exists mostly as phytate bound similar to many other seeds and vegetables and only 30–50% of total phosphorus is estimated to be bioavailable. Among the other minerals of the meal, S, Ca, Mg, Fe, Mg, Zn, Mn, Cu, and Se, are found in decreasing order of abundance. Choline, which is a water-soluble component of vitamin B complex is abundant in C/RS. It is usually known that in many of the crucifer oilseeds including C/RS choline exists as sinapic acid ester. Biotin, folic acid, niacin, pantothenic acid, pyridoxine, riboflavin, thiamin, and vitamin E are also found in C/RS (Table 18.1). The meal of C/R is depleted of lipid-soluble vitamins such as tocopherols of vitamin E complex during oil extraction as they are partitioned into oil fraction.

18.3.2 Protein Types of C/RS

Approximately 90% of the proteins found in C/RS are storage proteins. The major seed storage proteins of crucifers are 11S cruciferin of cupin superfamily and 2S napin of prolamin superfamily. Other minor proteins, the oil body proteins (OBP), and lipid transfer proteins (LTP) have also been reported.

18.3.2.1 Cruciferin

According to Malabat, Atterby, Chaudhry, Renard, and Guéguen (2003) double-low rapeseed cultivars produced in France contained cruciferin in the range of 32–53% of total proteins. However, based on expressed protein analysis, at maturity, the *B. napus* seed protein complement consisted of 60% cruciferin (Crouch & Sussex, 1981). Cruciferin is structurally similar to other 11/12S seed storage proteins of eudicots, and has well-organized primary, secondary, tertiary, and quaternary structure levels. Cruciferin subunits of *B. napus* are encoded by 9–12 genes (Breen & Crouch, 1992; Simon, Tenbarge, Scofield, Finkelstein, & Crouch, 1985). (Five cruciferin subunit or protomer isoforms CRU1_BRANA (P33523; cruciferin BnC1 precursor; gene BnC1), CRU2_BRANA (P33524; cruciferin BnC2 precursor; gene BnC2), CRU3_BRANA (P33525; cruciferin CRU1 precursor; gene CRU1), CRU4_BRANA (P33522; cruciferin CRU 4 precursor, gene CRU4), and CRUA_BRANA (P11090; cruciferin precursor, gene CRUA syn CRU2/3) are reported for *B. napus* with polypeptide chain ranges from 465 to 509 amino acid (AA) residues depending on the gene involved in expression (UniProtKB/Swiss-Prot and UniProtKB/TrEMBL database).) Cruciferin primary structure consists of a heavy α-(acidic, ∼30 kDa, 254–296 amino acids) and a light β-(basic, ∼20 kDa, 189–191 amino acids) chain that are linked by one interchain disulfide bond (Dalgalarrondo, Robin, & Azanza, 1986). The secondary structure of the cruciferin contains 27 beta strands and seven helices that are folded into two β-barrel (jelly-roll) domains and two extended helix domains each containing two helices (Adachi, Takenaka, Gidamis, Mikami, & Utsumi, 2001). The mature cruciferin subunit has 48–56 kDa molecular mass (Dalgalarrondo et al., 1986; Robin, Inquello, Mimouni, & Azanza, 1991) and an isoelectric point of 7.25 (Schwenke, Schultz, Linow, Gast, & Zirwer, 1980). Cruciferin may be phosphorylated (Wan, Ross, Yang, Hegedus, & Kermode, 2007) then glycosylated (Schwenke, Raab, Plietz, & Damaschun, 1983). The 3-D structure of *B. napus* cruciferin shows a hexameric quaternary structure made of two trimers composed of cruciferin subunits which are associated with noncovalent interactions. The exact or predominant combination(s) of the protomers composing the mature trimer or hexamer has not been established. The hexameric structure of cruciferin shows reversible association and dissociation due to pH and ionic strength changes (Schwenke et al., 1983).

18.3.2.2 Napin

Napin of crucifers are 2S albumin proteins that belong to the prolamin protein superfamily (Shewry, Napler, & Tatham, 1995). European rapeseed cultivars contain 25–45% of total seed protein as 2S albumin (Malabat et al., 2003). In *B. napus*, napin is encoded by 10–16 genes (Josefsson, Lenman, Ericson, & Rask, 1987; Scofield & Crouch, 1987). At least 14 full-length "napin" sequences can be found under *B. napus* in the databases (UniProt, 2015). The primary structure of napin is composed of 111–180 amino acid residues while the secondary structure is predominantly helical and consists of four helices. Two subunits (short or small ∼4.5 kDa and long or large ∼10 kDa) linked by two disulfide bonds compose napin (Gehrig, Krzyzaniak, Barciszewski, & Biemann, 1998). Brassica napins are hydrophilic proteins (Jyothi, Singh, & Appu Rao, 2007) and remain stable at temperatures as high as 75°C (Jyothi, Sinha, Singh, Surolia, & Appu Rao, 2007). Napin contains a high level of basic and S-amino acids (Müntz, 1998).

18.3.2.3 Minor Proteins

Similar to many other oil- and protein-containing seeds, C/RS oil bodies (oleosomes) are surrounded by OBP, primarily the oleosins (75−80% of total OBP) and to a lesser extent caleosins (Jolivet, Boulad, Bellamy, Larre, & Barre, 2009) prevent coalescence of oil bodies in the cellular structure of the seed through steric hindrance and electrostatic repulsions. OBP retain in oil-expressed meal. Oleosins are ~18-kDa proteins, contain a hydrophobic core, and show good oil−water interface stabilization ability (Wijesundera et al., 2013). The identified rapeseed trypsin inhibitory proteins (RTI, ~19 kDa) are quite distinct from Kunitz- or Bowman−Birk-types and include thermolabile RTI-I and RTI-II specific for trypsin (Visentin, Iori, Valdicelli, & Palmieri, 1992) and thermostable RTI-III (6.5 kDa) that inactivate both trypsin and chymotrypsin (Ceciliani et al., 1994).

18.4 PROCESSES OF PROTEIN PRODUCT PREPARATION

18.4.1 Significant Considerations

The array of chemical compounds found in C/RS (described under antinutritional components) makes the incorporation of C/RS meal directly into human food unsuitable. Several studies have reported the negative nutritional and organoleptic attributes of C/RS meal when it is directly fed to animals or incorporated in food product formulations. The array of nonprotein chemical compounds found in C/RS and their reactive chemical entities (described under antinutritional components) pose negative impact on direct incorporation of C/RS meal into human foods and also affect protein recovery from the seed meal. The unresolved understanding of the chemical and physical interassociations of these components in the seed further complicates processing conditions and the quality of final protein products. Different protein production methods have been described for C/RS (Fig. 18.1) and all of them involve recovering protein via aqueous extraction of oil-free meal. Depending on the conditions and additives employed in protein extraction and recovery from extracts, largely different protein yields and compositions can be expected.

The quality of the starting meal is important in the yield and final quality of protein products recovered from them. A good example is the protein recovery yield of commercial C/RS meal; at an industrial level, C/RS crushing focuses on maximizing oil yields and the processing conditions employed in oil extraction result in decreased protein extractability, therefore protein recovery yield is very low compared to laboratory-prepared nontoasted meal (Newkirk, Classen, & Edney, 2003; Tan, Mailer, Blanchard, & Agboola, 2011a). The protein dispersibility index (PDI) of C/RS is significantly low compared to soy due to inherent differences in the protein composition. (The American Oil Chemists'

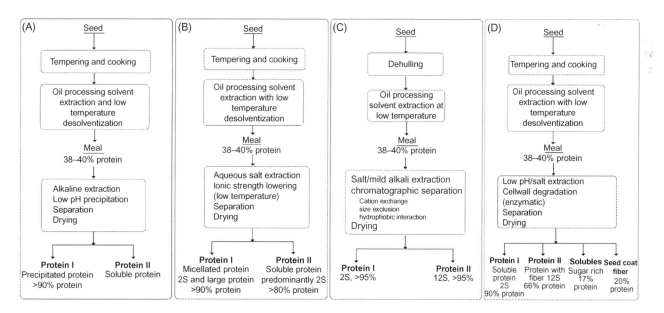

FIGURE 18.1 Flow charts summarizing important processing steps and products for four different methods described and employed to obtain protein products from canola/rapeseed. Processes depicted here are either reported as scaled up to pilot level or patented. (A) Alkali extraction of protein and recovery at low pH (Diosady et al., 2005; Newkirk et al., 2009); (B) protein micelle formation method (Murray, 1999; Schwizer & Greene, 2005); (C) chromatographic separation (Berot et al., 2005); and (D) meal component fractionation method developed by Wanasundara and McIntosh (2013).

Society methods Ba 10a-05 and 09 were developed for PDI of soybean protein products. Modified PDI uses consequent extraction with distilled water, a 0.5 M sodium chloride, and NaOH solution to achieve pH 9.) Pudel, Tressel, and Düring (2015) using modified PDI showed that the commercial hot pressing (19.2) or solvent extraction (27.6) of C/RS meal yields a lesser amount of extractable protein than dehulled cold pressed (84.2) or fluidized bed dried meal. Pressing operation and the desolventizing step (~107°C for more than 1 h) of commercial C/RS processing exert excess thermal stress on seed constituents causing protein denaturation and nonreversible interactions with other components of the seed resulting in very low PDI. Therefore, all the protein recovery processes (Fig. 18.1) described and also scaled-up to commercial level, utilize nontoasted C/RS meal or the white flakes. The fluidized bed desolventizer (Leidt, Mörl, Pudel, Weigel, & Zettl, 2009) which operates ~80°C for about 25 min (superheated hexane is fed from the bottom and distributed by a perforated plate and leaves the separation chamber on top where the meal slurry is fed and fluidized) or desolventizing under vacuum (Newkirk et al., 2003) can bring residual hexane content of the meal to <300 ppm while maintaining protein solubility at similar values to those observed before the desolventizing step.

Inactivation of myrosinase enzyme is also important in the C/RS meal preparation stage as the glucosinolate breakdown products (GBPs; isothiocyanates, nitriles, thiourea, and oxazolidinethione) can be coextracted with protein and makes GBP removal difficult (Fenwick, 1982; Wallig, Belyea, & Tumbleson, 2002). Inactivation of seed myrosinase during the "cooking" step (in the commercial oil extraction process, moisture-adjusted C/RS is heated up to 85°C for ~1 h) ensures GBPs are not generated under the aqueous conditions of protein product preparation. The polymeric phenolic compounds of C/RS seed coat are another consideration because under extreme alkaline pH conditions used in protein solubilization, protein–phenolic interactions result in the generation of dark color compounds.

The industry standards for protein concentrates and protein isolates are generally benchmarked against soy protein industry standards and are also adapted in scientific reporting and when describing nonsoy protein products. The followings methods have been described for C/RS protein product preparation and Fig. 18.1 provides summarized flowcharts for the methods that are either patented or have been developed up to proof-of-concept stage.

18.4.2 Involving Aqueous Alkaline Conditions

Alkaline extraction of proteins followed by precipitation with dilute acid is the widely reported procedure to prepare protein isolates from C/RS (Tan, Mailer, Blanchard, & Agboola, 2011b). Usually, highly alkaline or pH values of 11–12 achieved with NaOH are necessary to obtain high-protein extraction yields and extraction efficiencies from C/RS meal (Mieth, Bruckner, Kroll, & Pohl,1983; Sosulski & Bakal, 1969). Additives such as NaCl (Alireza-Sadeghi, Rao, & Bhagya, 2006) and CaO (Maenz, Newkirk, Classen, & Tyler, 2004) have resulted in improved protein extraction. Recovery of protein is by adjusting the pH of the extract to a value the minimum solubility is observed (sometimes referred to as isoelectric point or pI). Usually, dilute acid solutions, such as HCl or acetic, are used in a laboratory setting to recover proteins, however, alternative acids compatible with extraction equipment are needed in industrial applications. The pH values of 3.5 (Diosady, Xu, & Chen, 2005; Klockeman, Toledo, & Sims, 1997), 4.0 (Aluko & McIntosh, 2001), and 4.5–5.5 (Ghodsvali, Khodaparast, Vosoughi, & Diosady, 2005) or two pH levels in a step-wise manner; first pH 5 then pH 3.5 (Pedroche et al., 2004) or first pH 3.6 then 6.0 (El Nockrashy, Mukherjee, & Mangold, 1977) have been reported to recover the maximum amount of protein from alkaline extracts of C/RS. All C/RS proteins soluble at alkali pH cannot be recovered at the minimum solubility pH. The soluble N content at pH 3–4 is relatively high in canola and is rich in Cys-containing polypeptides (Kodagoda, Nakai, & Powrie, 1973), which are primarily napins (Wanasundara, Abeysekara, McIntosh, & Falk, 2012). Heat shocking of canola protein solution recovers protein in a concentrated curd form (Newkirk, Maenz, & Classen, 2009) but the technological functionalities of the proteins may be compromised. Membrane separation (ultrafiltration, 10 kDa) is an alternative to pH adjustments to recover proteins from alkaline meal extracts and also removes low-molecular-weight phytates, glucosionolates, and polyphenolic compounds (Xu & Diosady, 2000) and the salts used in assisting protein extraction. Isolexx (60–65% globulin and 30–35% albumin; TeuTexx Protein, 2015) is an example of a canola protein product that is produced by extraction at near neutral pH and then concentrated using membrane technology and drying.

Alkali extraction of C/RS results in dark brown to gray color protein products due to oxidation of phenolic compounds and protein–phenolic interactions. Additives such as sodium hexametaphosphate (SHMP) at 1–2% (Mahajan & Dua, 1994; Thompson, Allum-Poon, & Procope, 1976), sodium bisulfite (Blaicher, Elstner, Stein, & Mukherjee, 1983), or sodium sulfite (10% w/w; Tzeng, Diosady, & Rubin, 1990) in the alkaline extraction medium or mixing the meal with insoluble polyvinyl pyrrolidine before extraction (Blaicher et al., 1983) produces lighter, ivory color protein extracts by preventing protein–phenolic interactions.

Phytates of C/RS (3–4% in the seed) usually coextract with the protein. A low-phytate-containing canola protein isolate can be obtained by adding $CaCl_2$ (0.05–0.15 M) (Diosady, Rubin, & Tzeng, 1989; Tzeng et al., 1990) prior to the pH adjustment for isoelectric point precipitation. Phytase enzyme can also be added to the extract to reduce the phytate level of canola protein products (Newkirk et al., 2009), especially when it is for feed applications.

Protein content of isolates prepared by alkaline extraction and acid precipitation have generally been reported in the range of 60–90%. Normally, these protein isolates reported poor solubility characteristics primarily due to the dramatic pH change during extraction that results in changes to native protein conformation (Tan et al., 2011b). The posttreatment of protein isolates using chemicals (acyl derivatives; Guéguen, Bollecker, Schwenke, & Raab, 1990) or enzymes (alcalase, chymotrypsin, pepsin, trypsin, and pancreatin) can improve the solubility of these proteins (Alashi, Blanchard, Mailer, & Agboola, 2013).

18.4.3 Processes Targeting Specific Seed Protein Types/Fractions

To maximize biological, chemical, and technological functionalities of seed protein extracts, fractionation of protein molecules during recovery is necessary and less emphasis on exhaustive recovery of total seed proteins is required. Protein products that contain certain molecular types or compositions are more useful in certain applications as the proteins exhibit particular functionalities that are associated with protein types rather than mixtures of few proteins (eg, 2S and 11S proteins of C/RS) with different properties.

18.4.3.1 Protein Micelle Mass Formation

The micellation process described by Murray, Maurice, Barker, and Myers (1980) is a noncovalent approach that uses salting-in and hydrophobic aggregation properties of canola seed proteins. Protein solubilized in salt (NaCl) solution with appropriate concentration (usually 0.15 M) is concentrated to achieve a desirable dry matter level and later the salt concentration is changed to favor protein aggregation through a hydrophobic interaction. The aggregated, gelatinous protein mass is subsequently recovered as Protein micelle mass (PMM), while some protein remains in solution without micellation. Technological developments of this protein recovery process for canola are covered by several patents (Murray, 1999, 2005; Murray, Myers, & Barker, 1981; Schweizer & Green, 2005). The products of the process are PMM as cruciferin-rich Puratein and the proteins that do not form micelle are napin-rich Supertein proteins (Burcon, 2015). In this process, some degree of protein-type separation occurs.

18.4.3.2 Chromatographic Separation

Cruciferin and napin of C/RS meal that becomes soluble at pH 8.5 and in 50 mM Tri-HCl buffer containing 750 mM NaCl, 5 mM EDTA, and 0.3% $NaHSO_3$ can be separated to a high purity level (>95% protein) by chromatographic means (Bérot, Compoint, Larré, Malabat, & Guéguen, 2005). The first step is to concentrate proteins by removing salts and small molecules, such as phenolics, by using a 1-kDa membrane. Concentrated protein is then subjected to cation exchange chromatography (CEC; alkaline pH) to obtain cruciferin as unbound protein and napin and LTP as proteins eluting with 35% (w/v) NaCl. Further purification of cruciferin is by size exclusion chromatography (SEC) and napin by CEC (pH 5.3) followed by hydrophobic interaction chromatography (HIC; pH 8.5). The LTP fraction is obtained from the napin separation step of the CEC at acidic pH. Bérot et al. (2005) have scaled-up this process to obtain gram quantities of cruciferin, napin, and LTP.

Pudel et al. (2015) describe use of expanded bed adsorption (EBA)-ion exchange chromatography (IEC) for isolation of napin from an aqueous RS protein extract after precipitating cruciferin. The EBA-IEC has the ability to be scaled up to industrial level. This chromatographic separation process results in high-purity napin (>98%) and cruciferin (>95%). Protein products with mixed composition (56–57% napin and 43–44% cruciferin) can also be obtained by modifying some process conditions.

18.4.3.3 Solubility-Based Separation

Bhatty, MacKenzie, and Finlayson (1968) were the first to adapt globulin protein fractionation (Osborne, 1897) of globulins of double-low rapeseed meal by using 10% (w/v) NaCl, followed by protein precipitation via dialysis of excess salt and then further purification by chromatography. Betschart, Fong, and Saunders (1977) adopted the classical procedure of Osborne and Mendel (1914) with some modifications. This involves: (1) obtaining water-soluble albumins by extracting with water (water to meal ratio, 10:1, v-w, 3 extractions) and dialyzing (cellulose acetate membrane against 10 volumes of water); (2) further recovery of "solubles" by consequently extracting the insoluble residue resulting from step 1 with 5% (w/v) NaCl, then with 60% (v/v) ethanol, and finally with 0.4% (w/v) NaOH to obtain globulin, prolamin, and glutelin protein fractions, respectively. Recently, Manamperi, Chang, and Pryor (2012) and Tan et al. (2011a) also adopted similar solubility-based fractionation to recover proteins from canola produced in the United States and Australia, respectively, because of the resulting high cumulative protein yield. Subtle differences were seen in the types of proteins found in these four fractions, interestingly, the glutelin fraction contained similar protein types as the isolates obtained by aqueous alkali extraction (Tan et al., 2011a). Adoption of this sequential protein fractionation has limitations due to multiple solvent compositions and extraction steps, which requires modifications to develop an economically viable process for C/RS.

The differences of molecular size, structure, and amino acid composition of cruciferin and napin result in differences in valuable technological functionalities (Wanasundara, 2011). According to Wanasundara et al. (2012), nearly 20–35% of proteins remain soluble in the pH ranges that the *Brassica* spp. meal proteins exhibit minimum solubility. The napins are soluble at pH levels as low as 3, and addition of neutral salts such as $CaCl_2$ or NaCl increases their solubility while keeping cruciferin insoluble. Wanasundara and McIntosh (2013) describe a process to obtain *Brassica* seed protein products using this opportunity. First, napin is extracted using low pH and salt conditions and further purified through membrane separation (5 MWCO) to remove low-molecular-weight components and achieve >90% protein purity. The cruciferins retained in the residue are recovered either by solubilizing at alkali pH followed by concentrating using membrane filtration (85% protein purity), or by removing cell wall and seed coat fiber by enzyme degradation and a separation step to concentrate cruciferin (65% protein purity). This process is scaled-up successfully and separates canola seed protein types, seed coat, and soluble fiber of cell walls allowing utilization of these various seed components while improving the economics and sustainability of C/RS and commercial viability of the technique.

18.4.4 Combination of Chemical and Physical Methods

The dark, tannin-filled seed coat of C/RS is an impediment to obtaining low-fiber as well as light-color protein products, therefore separation of cotyledon and hulls facilitates obtaining suitable material for protein extraction. Air classification of meal to separate seed coat particles is a possibility when combined with deoiling, and requires a liquid cyclone operating with an organic solvent suitable for oil extraction (Eapen, Tape, & Sims, 1968, 1969; Jones & Holme, 1979). The protein content of the products of this process was between 50% and 69%. Carre, Quinsac, Citeau, and Fine (2015) re-examined the technical feasibility and economic viability of C/RS dehulling in large-scale commercial operations and concluded that dehulling is an economically viable option when C/RS protein products become more valuable than oil.

Cold-pressed oil has become a popular niche C/RS oil product particularly for markets such as organic and nongenetically modified organisms (non-GMO) edible oils. The patented process of Teutoburger–Oelmuehle (2015) produces cold-pressed hull-free cotyledon flour very low in antinutrients (38.8% protein) and can be a carrier, filler, and flavoring substance in foods such as sauces, spice mixes, baked products, sausages, and marinades. Press cakes are high in residual oil content compared to prepress-solvent extracted meal; 10–20% versus <1% (Newkirk, 2009). A more environmentally friendly, solvent-free process involving dehulling, cold pressing, and/or enzyme-catalyzed cell wall degradation, ultrafiltration of the soluble fraction, and flash chromatography to separate proteins was described by Bagger, Sørensen, and Sørensen (1998) and Kvist, Carlsson, Lawther, and Basile de Castro (2003). The final products of the process are oil (no degumming required), protein-enriched (40–55%, w/w) meal, lipophilic proteins complexed with amphiphilic lipids, hydrophilic and amphiphilic compounds, GSL (biocide precursors), and seed coat rich in DF. This process recovers most of the seed components and fits well with the biorefining model that accompanies sustainable production of C/RS proteins.

18.5 NUTRITIONAL VALUE

18.5.1 Amino Acid Composition

The proteins of C/RS are significant in human nutrition because of the high levels of essential amino acids (>400 mg/g protein), and S-containing amino acids (3.0–4.0%, 40–49 mg/g protein), which is closer to the reference protein pattern established by FAO/UNU/WHO requirements for humans than any other vegetable (including legume) protein (Bos et al., 2007). Table 18.2 provides reported amino acid composition for the meal of currently cultivated canola varieties and the protein products derived from various isolation methods. Lysine is the only essential amino acid (EAA) found in the protein isolate in significantly lower levels than those measured in the starting material (Klockeman et al., 1997).

TABLE 18.2 Amino Acid Composition of Canola Meal and Protein Products Derived From Canola by Different Methods

Amino Acid	Canola/Rapeseed Meal % of CP[a]	Alkali Extracted and Acid Precipitated Protein Isolate[b]	PMM[c]		Specific Fractions[d]	
			Supertein g/100 g Protein	Puratein g/100 g Protein	2S Isolate g/100 g Protein	11S Concentrate g/100 g Protein
Essential						
Cysteine	2.39	0.39	4.5	1.6	8.1	1.4
Histidine	3.39	3.17	3.6	2.5	3.5	1.7
Isoleucine	4.33	5.18	3.0	4.4	6.0	6.1
Leucine	7.06	9.26	6.0	8.2	6.8	6.6
Lysine	5.56	5.62	7.4	4.0	3.4	4.6
Methionine	2.06	2.60	2.4	1.9	2.7	2.2
Phenylalanine	3.83	5.13	2.6	4.9	4.3	4.0
Threonine	4.39	5.30	3.2	3.7	4.5	4.3
Tryptophan	1.33	-	1.4	2.0	1.3	1.2
Tyrosine	3.22	3.93	1.4	4.1	3.4	2.5
Valine	5.47	5.85	4.3	5.5	5.1	4.6
Conditionally Essential						
Arginine	5.78	7.66	5.8	7.2	5.4	5.3
Glutamine + glutamate	18.14	17.27	24.6	19.8	14.2	19.8
Glycine	4.92	5.05	4.3	5.4	6.5	6.8
Proline	5.97	4.32	9.2	5.8	4.7	6.8
Nonessential						
Alanine	4.36	5.14	4.0	4.2	5.2	5.3
Aspartic acid + aspartate	7.25	9.41	2.6	9.3	11.4	10.5
Serine	4.00	4.74	3.3	4.1	5.2	5.5

[a]Newkirk (2009).
[b]Tzeng et al. (1988).
[c]GRAS Notice 327 (2010).
[d]Wanasundara and McIntosh (2013), Wanasundara, unpublished data.
Direct comparison of amino acids may not be valid since the different starting canola materials were used for obtaining protein products and most of the time meal amino acid composition is not provided.

Lysine is also the most affected amino acid in C/RS meal during commercial oil extraction process. The available- or reactive-lysine content of expeller press cake or the desolventized toasted meal is always lower (9–10%) than the seed due to the impact of an increase in temperature during oil extraction—most likely due to Maillard-type reactions (Newkirk et al., 2003).

18.5.2 Digestibility in Human and Animal Models and the Processing Effects

Several animal-model studies show that C/RS protein digestibility can be significantly compromised by the presence of other constituents such as phytic acid and phenolic compounds which may interact with proteins, however only a few studies differentiate the effect of protein types on digestibility. Among the protein digestibility studies, only a handful of studies describe C/RS protein digestibility in humans.

Nutritional assessment in C/RS protein in rats gave similar results as beef and even higher values than casein (Friedman, 1996; Sarwar, 1987). Seed coat lignin and polyphenols contribute to low digestibility values of meal, however RS meal even without seed coat exhibited lower digestibility values than soy protein (Grala et al., 1998). The method of protein processing also affects C/RS protein digestibility. Water solubilization and ammonium sulfate precipitation improved digestibility values of RS protein from 81% to 87% while the digestibility of C/RS protein concentrate was found to be 52%, compared to 87% and 89% for 2S and 12S fractions, respectively (Delisle et al., 1984).

Feeding healthy volunteers with a meal prepared with ^{15}N-labeled RS protein product (37.8% globulin, 41% napin, and 2.7% LTP) as the sole source of protein, Bos et al. (2007) showed that *B. napus* protein exhibits comparatively low (84%) real ileal digestibility values indicating low bioavailability. However, the low digestibility of RS protein was compensated by the high postprandial retention of released amino acids (70.5%) compared to the other plant proteins, such as wheat (66%), pea (71%), or lupin (74%), therefore exhibited excellent postprandial biological value (84%). The high cysteine and methionine levels (80% higher than the limiting value for S-AA) and the 1:1 ratio of these two AA (comparable with egg protein) places RS protein at a high biological value (Bos et al., 2007).

Combining digestibility data and AA profile, the calculated protein digestibility corrected amino acid scores (PDCASS; according to WHO/FAO 1989 standards) of napin-rich Supertein and cruciferin-rich Puratein were 0.61 (61%) and 0.64 (64%), respectively. Improved values of 0.83 and 0.71, for Supertein and Puratein, respectively, can be obtained when calculated according to updated FAO/WHO/UNU guidelines in 2002 (WHO/FAO/UNU, 2007). (The difference is in the reference amounts of specific AA and the requirements by age groups of children 1−2 years and 3−10 years.) The limiting AA of these two C/RS protein products are phenylalanine for Supertein and tyrosine and lysine for Puratein (GRAS Notice 327, 2010).

When assessed for subchronic dietary toxicity in a 13-week healthy rat model at 5, 10, and 20% (w/w) dietary admix levels, Puratein showed no negative effect on body weight gain, food consumption, blood parameters, motor activity, ophthalmic, or clinical pathology observed for at all levels (Mejia, Korgaonkar, Schweizer, Chengelis, Marit et al., 2009). For the same assessment, Supertein at the 20% level lowered bodyweight (BW) gain and reduced food intake, particularly at the beginning of the feeding trial. Both males and females showed an increase in thyroid/parathyroid weight at this 20% feeding level but not at a level that exerted any adverse effects (Mejia, Korgaonkar, Schweizer, Chengelis, Novilla et al., 2009). The phytates of the protein product did not affect the plasma Zn levels of test animals, indicating no interference on mineral availability. The recommended levels of these protein suggested to use with no-observed-adverse-effect-level (NOAEL) were 11.24 g/kg BW/day for males and 14.11 g/kg BW/day for females for cruciferin-rich Puratein (Mejia, Korgaonkar, Schweizer, Chengelis, Marit et al., 2009) and 12.46 g/kg BW/day for males and 14.95 g/kg BW/day for females for napin-rich Supertein (Mejia, Korgaonkar, Schweizer, Chengelis, Novilla et al., 2009). Neither of these C/RS protein products showed any significant trend towards genotoxicity (GRAS Notice 327, 2010).

Safety assessment of the C/RS product Isolexx by the European Food Safety Authority (EFSA) reported that the PDCAAS value for this product is similar to soy protein products, with low concentrations of antinutrional factors, an absence of toxicologically relevant effects in subchronic studies with rats, making the protein a suitable candidate for the novel food ingredient category (EFSA, 2013). Allergenic potential of C/RS protein products is a factor that cannot be excluded. It was estimated that "heavy" adult consumer intake (mean +2SD) of Isolexx would be 2.2 g/kg BW per day, 4−6-year-old group mean intake of 3 g/kg BW per day and the 95th percentile intake of 4.73 g/kg BW per day.

18.6 ANTINUTRITIONAL FACTORS OF C/RS

Antinutritional components such as GSL, phenolics (sinapine and tannins), phytates, and fiber, which are listed under chemical composition, are retained in the oil-free C/RS meal. In order to obtain protein products suitable for human food application, many of these components have to be removed or depleted to an acceptable level.

18.6.1 Glucosinolates

GSL levels (along with FA composition) were manipulated during the development of food-grade *B. napus* for C/RS. The aliphatic GSL, 3-butenyl, 4-pentenyl, 2-hydroxy-3butenyl, and 2-hydroxy-4-pentenyl are present in C/RS at low levels (<30 μmol/g of dry defatted meal). Hydrolysis of GSL catalyzed by myrosinase enzyme releases glucose and a range of potentially toxic chemicals such as isothiocyanates (ITC), nitriles, epithioalkanes, oxazolidinethions,

5-vinyloxazolidine-2-thione (VOT), thiocyanate ions, and sometimes organic thiocyanates. Intestinal tract microflora can also metabolize GSL and produce similar chemical entities when ingested, even though seed myrosinase is inactivated (Krul et al., 2002; Li, Huller, Beresford, & Lampe, 2011). The toxic effects of GSL breakdown products on test animals are listed as reduced feed intake, growth depression, impaired thyroid function, enlargement of the kidney, liver or thyroid glands, and decreased egg production in birds (Mawson, Heaney, Zdunczyk, & Kozlowska, 1995). In humans, higher levels of GSL breakdown products may be associated with reduced iodine uptake by the thyroid gland (Fenwick, Heaney, & Mullin, 1983). The total intact GSL level in cruciferin-rich Puratein and napin-rich Supertein, varied from 1.09 to 2.53 and 0.39 to 1.02 μmol/g, respectively, and ITC or nitriles were not detected (GRAS Notice 327, 2010). The Isolexx product contained GSL levels below 0.1 μmol/g (EFSA, 2013). The napin isolate and cruciferin concentrate produced according to Wanasundara and McIntosh (2013) contained no intact GSL normally associated with C/RS. The levels of GSL found in all these protein products are lower than the exposure levels originating from crucifer vegetables consumed by humans.

18.6.2 Phytates

Similar to many other seeds C/RS contains phytates (salts of Ca, Mg, and K of *myo*-inositol 1,2,3,4,5,6-hexakis-dihydrogen phosphate or phytic acid) primarily in the form of *myo*-inositol hexakisphosphate (IP_6) and *myo*-inositol pentakisphosphate (IP_5), which are in the ranges of 15–21 mg/g and 1–2 mg/g, respectively, for commercial oil meal (Matthäus, Lösing, & Fiebig, 1995). Phytates are accumulated as insoluble crystals in the PSV (Raboy, 2003), and are therefore inevitably associated with C/RS proteins and partitioned depending on the pH employed in the protein extraction. At low pHs, phytic–protein complexing is at its maximum between both cruciferin and napin and zero complexing may occur at pH values corresponding to the isoelectric region of both proteins (Schwenke, Mothes, Marzilger, Borowska, & Koslowska, 1987). Protein complexes with phytic acid directly or through mediation by mineral ions, which may alter the protein structure leading to decreased solubility, functionality, and digestibility of the proteins (Sarwar, 1987; Tan et al., 2011b). Phytate levels of 0.12–0.32% and 3.35–3.84% were reported for Puratein and Supertein, respectively (GRAS Notice 327, 2010), whereas 1.45% phytate level was reported for cruciferin concentrate and undetected phytate levels were found in the napin isolate of Wanasundara and McIntosh (2013) process. The phytic acid level of Isolexx is in the range of 0.44–1.1% (EFSA, 2013).

18.6.3 Phenolics

Phenolic compounds found in C/RS are free and esterified phenolic acids and condensed tannins (proanthocyanidins). The total extractable content of phenolics ranges from 1.59 to 1.84 g/100 g of defatted canola meal and 0.62 to 1.28 g/100 g of RS flour (Dabrowski & Sosulski, 1984; Naczk, Amarowicz, Sullivan, & Shahidi, 1998). Phenolics of C/RS are hydroxylated and/or methoxylated derivatives of benzoic and cinnamic acids as esters of glucose, sucrose, malic acid (in the DF fraction), and choline. Sinapic acid (3,5-dimethoxy-4-hydroxy cinnamic acid) is the abundant phenolic acid in C/RS and comprises >73% of free and 99% of esterified phenolic acids (Dabrowski & Sosulski,1984). Sinapine, the choline ester of sinapic acid, is the most prominent; 6.8–10 mg/g seed in European cultivars (Matthäus, 1998), 6–18 mg/g defatted meal for Canadian canola (Newkirk, 2009), and 13–15 mg/g defatted meal for Australian cultivars (Mailer, McFadden, Ayton, & Redden, 2008) are reported. The total phenolic acid content in Puratein was 0.40% and Supertein was 0.26%, in which 93–96% was sinapic acid. Phenolic compounds of C/RS can be effective antioxidants; C/RS is an effective antioxidant in polyunsaturated FA-rich systems (Thiyam, Stöckmann, Zum Felde, & Schwarz, 2006; Wanasundara, Amarowicz, & Shahidi, 1996).

18.6.4 Carbohydrates and Fiber

The DF content of C/RS meal is high compared to soy, and the cotyledon DF has a higher negative effect on digestibility of proteins than DF isolated from seed coat (Bjergegaard, Eggum, Jensen & Sorensen, 1991). Cellulose and lignins are primarily found in the insoluble dietary fiber (IDF) fraction and pectins, hemicellulose, mixed β-glucans, gums, and mucilage are in the soluble dietary fiber (SDF) fraction. The levels of 27.5–33.0% IDF and 3.1–5.2% SDF are reported for spring- and winter-type RS grown in Europe (Ochodzki, Rakowska, Bjergegaard, & Sørensen, 1995). Protein associated with fiber (2.4–6.7% for SDF and 11.8–14.0% for IDF) are not susceptible to pepsin-pancreatin digestion.

18.7 ALLERGENICITY OF C/RS PROTEINS

The 2S albumin is one of the three major groups of allergenic proteins of prolamin superfamily and found in Brassicaceae seeds including C/RS. Most of the studies and reported immune responses are for certain napin proteins of mustard (*B. juncea* and *Sinapis alba*), such as induction of celiac disease and baker's asthma (Monsalve, Villalba, & Rodríguez, 2001) not for C/RS because of the differences in using whole seed in human food. Recently, 2S protein of RS has also been reported to contain allergenic proteins (Poikonen et al., 2008; Puumalainen et al., 2006, 2015). Napin is a gastrointestinal allergen, however, fatal anaphylactic reactions to mustard seeds is rare (Monreal, Botey, Pena, Martin & Eseverri, 1992). Among the several isoforms of napin found in mature C/RS or mustard seed, only certain napin isoforms are capable of eliciting immunogenic response. (An isoform is a protein that has same function, encoded by a different gene but may have small differences in the primary sequence, it could be a domain, a motif usually that is located on the surface.) A study carried out in children with IgE-mediated food allergy and reacted to *B. napus* and *B. rapa* seed extracts in skin prick tests showed Bra n 1 (Napin BnIII, napin nIII or napin 3; P80208, 2SS3_BRANA) and Bra r 1(Q42473, BRACM; UniProtKB/Swiss-Prot entry) as the allergenic proteins of *B. napus* and *B. rapa*, respectively (Poikonen et al., 2008; Puumalainen et al., 2006). Allergenic 2S albumins have four S—S bonds that allow tight packing, forming a compact structure and provide special resistance to proteolytic enzyme access and thermal unfolding, thus protein can reach the gut immune system intact (Mills, Madsen, Shewry, & Wichers, 2003). Currently, no information is available on the effect of processing on C/RS napin allergenic potential. Considering the recognition of mustard as an allergen in EU countries and Canada, it is recommended that C/RS protein-containing foods need to be appropriately labeled to indicate for potential allergenicity (GRAS Notice 327, 2010).

18.8 FUNCTIONAL PROPERTIES OF PROTEIN PRODUCTS

Numerous studies on C/RS protein product preparation, and product functionalites in various model systems and prototype products have been reported since the 1970s. The protein products used in those studies differ in protein composition, processing history, associated component particle size, etc. and as these factors influence the functionalities of protein ingredient in a given system it is difficult to generalize on the key functionalities. As mentioned earlier, the two major proteins of *B. napus* differ in many ways including AA composition, molecular structure, and physicochemical properties. Therfore, the functionalities discussed under this section have been limited to protein products with somewhat defined protein composition.

18.8.1 Solubility

Solubility is a key functional requirement of food-based protein systems. Proteins have to be in soluble or soluble aggregate forms to be active in the air—water and oil—water interfaces and for heat-induced gel formation. The processing history of protein products has a strong influence on the solubility characteristics of the final product. Alkali-extracted and acid-precipitated canola proteins showed depressed solubility around the pH that was employed in protein recovery, for example, pH 3, 4, or 5 depending on the process. Hydrolysis of such protein products with Alcalase 2.4 L (*Bacillus licheniformis* protease with endopeptidase activity from Novozyme) improved solubility over a wide pH range (70% at pH 2, 90% at pH 5, 100% at >pH 6; Vioque et al., 1999). Supertein is soluble in a wide pH range. Wanasundara and McIntosh (2013) also reported that the 2S protein of canola exhibits >90% solubility values in the pH range of 2—10, which is a unique characteristic for a plant (seed) protein. Cruciferin-rich protein products show depressed solubility compared to napin-rich protein products in this pH range compared to the alkaline pH range. The effect of additives such as NaCl, sucrose, and lipids that are common in food product development has not been reported for these protein products.

18.8.2 Emulsifying Properties

The C/RS protein isolates prepared by alkali extraction and acid precipitation generally have limited emulsifying ability and are comparable to soy protein isolates. Limited hydrolysis (3.1—7.7% degree of hydrolysis (DH)) of mixed protein-containing RS protein isolate catalyzed by Alcalase 2.4 L showed improvement in emulsifying capacity (EC) and emulsion stability (ES) in which the 3.1% DH exhibited the maximum values (50% EC and 65% ES) (Vioque, Sánchez-Vioque, Clemente, Pedroche, & Millán, 2000). Studies have shown that the globulin fractions of canola protein isolate exhibit higher emulsion capacity (emulsion activity index (EAI)) than the canola albumin fraction or soy protein isolates (Tan, Mailer, Blanchard, & Agboola, 2014). Using cruciferin and napin separated by chromatography, Wu and Muir (2008), Cheung, Wanasundara, and Nickerson (2014), and Cheung, Wanasundara, and Nickerson (2015) showed that cruciferin exhibited better EC, EAI, and emulsion stabilities than napin. Napin isolate of Wanasundara and McIntosh (2013) process also showed poor emulsification capacity and emulsion stability compared to commercial whey protein isolate (Davisco, USA) or soy protein concentrate (ADM, Co., USA) (Wanasundara & McIntosh, 2015). The hydrophilic nature and the lower flexibility due to internal S−S bonds may contribute to the inefficiency of napin as an oil−water interface active molecule. Emulsifying properties of canola PMM (cruciferin-rich) can be improved when hydrocolloids such as guar gum and κ-carrageenan are present in the media at high pHs (Uruapka & Arntfield, 2005).

18.8.3 Heat-Induced Gel Formation Ability

The ability to form gels has not been a strong functional aspect of C/RS protein isolates as their gelling properties are affected by the phenolic compounds present in protein products (Rubino, Arntfield, Nadon, & Bernatsky, 1996). Cruciferin and napin have opposing properties that contribute to heat-induced gel formation. Compared to cruciferin, napin requires higher temperature to form gels (72°C versus 95°C at pH 7) and forms weak gels with intensive syneresis. Cruciferin has the strongest tendency to form heat-induced gels than napin (Schwenke, Dahme, & Wolter, 1998). Heat-induced gels of albumin and CPI (cruciferin and napin mixes) showed weak gel strength profiles, while globulin fraction (predominately cruciferin) showed a strong gel strength profile at both pH 7 and 9 (Tan, Mailer, Blanchard, Agboola, & Day, 2014). High-pressure processing (400 MPa) can form C/RS mixed protein gels at low concentration (7% vs 11% at 100°C) with improved texture (He, He, Chao, Ju, & Aluko, 2014) and crosslinking of canola PMM (cruciferin-rich) induced by transglutaminase enzymes can improve heat-set gelation and gel properties (Pinterits & Arntfield, 2008).

18.8.4 Foaming Properties

Among the two major storage proteins of C/RS, the 2S proteins have exceptional ability to stabilize air−water interfaces (Krause, 2002). This was further confirmed by Wanasundara and McIntosh (2015) when a napin isolate from scaled up meal fractionation was compared with whey protein isolate and cruciferin-rich protein concentrate for foaming capacity and foam stability. Napin isolate (0.5−5% w/v) was capable of providing >100% foam-forming ability over a pH range of 3−10 which showed nearly 90% stability over a 30-min period and was comparable with whey protein isolate. Supertein has also been reported to be an effective foam former (Burcon, 2015), which indicates that protein-type-based C/RS processing may provide protein products with distinct functionalities.

18.9 APPLICATIONS AND CURRENT PRODUCTS

18.9.1 Potential Food Applications as Protein Supplements or Bulk Proteins

The functional properties mentioned above highlight the potential use of C/RS protein products in food applications. Pinterits and Arntfield (2008) reported the possibility of using rapeseed protein concentrate in German sausages, however, the proteins were shown to have poor gelling properties, most likely due to the high thermal stability of constituent proteins of the isolate. In the preparation of mayonnaise, using hydrolyzed proteins of canola meal, up to 50% (w/w) of the egg yolk could be replaced while the unhydrolyzed canola meal could not exceed 15% replacement before emulsion breakage (Aluko & McIntosh, 2005). Supertein, which has been reported to have unique functional attributes, with excellent foaming properties, allows its use in a wide range of applications including beverages, confectionaries, and baked goods (Burcon, 2015). Both Supertein and Puratein have generally recognized as safe (GRAS) status and US Food and Drug Administration (FDA) approval for food use (GRAS Notice 327, 2010). The proposed food categories that cruciferin-rich and napin-rich protein products can be used in are listed in Table 18.3. In addition, Isolexx which is a C/RS protein product of TeuTexx Proteins has EFSA approval under the novel food category. Furthermore, a range of products including processed meats (Olymel Co., and Lafleur Co., Canada), cheeses (Olymel Co., Canada), pizza, (Casa di Mama, Dr. Oetker Co., Canada), stuffing ingredients (Grissol Co., Canada), Oxo base cooking ingredients (Oxo, Unilever, Canada), lemon pepper seasoning blend (Hy's of Canada), and partially prepared turkey main dish dinners (Maple Leaf, Canada) has been identified that contain hydrolyzed canola protein (GRAS Notice 327, 2010).

TABLE 18.3 Proposed Food Categories and the Usage Level of Protein Product Rich in Cruciferin or Napin

Category of Food	Proposed Level of Cruciferin- or Napin-Rich Protein Product (% as is)[a]
Protein supplement	95
Powdered egg/egg substitute	60
Meal replacement/nutrition bars	50
Fruit and vegetable juices/beverages	10
Dairy products	5
Processed meats	2
Grain products	2
Salad dressings	2

[a]Inclusion levels are estimated based on US population 1999–2004 National Health and Nutrition examination survey (NHANES) databases. Children below 3 years of age were excluded because intended use of canola protein products is not inclusive of infant foods or infant formula.
Source: Adapted from GRAS Notice 327. GRAS notification for cruciferin-rich and napin-rich protein isolates derived from canola/rapeseed (Puratein® and Supertein™). (2010). <www.fda.gov/Food/FoodIngredientsPackaging/GenerallyRecognizedasSafeGRAS/GRASListings/default.htm>.

18.10 POTENTIAL NEW USES, ISSUES, AND CHALLENGES

18.10.1 New Uses

New and potential uses of C/RS proteins have been reported as applications other than their nutritional and functional applications in food products. Most of these proposed uses are based on the biochemical functions related to the structural features of the constituent proteins. Both cruciferin and napin contain amino acid sequence fragments that match with peptide sequences with proven bioactivities (Wanasundara, 2011).

18.10.1.1 Bioactive Peptides

An emphasis on blood pressure-regulating activities is prominent among the bioactivities reported for C/RS. These reports were mostly on angiotensin I-converting enzyme (ACE) inhibition (Pedroche et al., 2004; Wu, Aluko, & Muir, 2008; Aachary & Thiyam, 2011) by the peptides of hydrolyzed seed proteins of *B. napus*. Hydrolysis of *B. napus* seed protein (extracted with 1 M NaCl and extensively dialyzed) assisted by subtilisin (enzyme Carlsberg-type III from *B. licheniformis*) has generated hydrolysates containing peptides of IY, RIY, VW, and VWIS sequences that are highly active towards inhibiting ACE (Marczak et al., 2003). Among these peptides the RIY sequence exhibited high potency as an antihypertensive peptide in spontaneously hypertensive rat models (Marczak et al., 2003). The peptide of the same sequence was capable of blocking cholecystokinin-1 (CCK-1) receptor antagonist lorglumide and decreasing gastric emptying rate by blocking lorglumide when fed to fasting ddY male mice, further resulting in anorexic effects (Marczak, Ohinata, Lipkowski, & Yoshikawa, 2006). The peptide RIY showed no affinity towards the receptor but was found to decrease food intake and gastric emptying by stimulating CCK release indirectly. The RIY peptide sequence is exclusive to napin among the storage proteins of *B. napus* (Wanasundara, 2011). Hydrolysis of C/RS meal proteins catalyzed by Alcalase generates ACEI peptides (Pedroche et al., 2004) and among the active peptides, VSV and FL sequences were found to be significant (Wu et al., 2008). Several sequences that are involved in the reduction of high blood pressure levels through the renin–angiotensin pathway and ACE inhibition have been purified (He, Malomo et al., 2013; Marczak et al., 2003; Wu et al., 2008).

According to Yust et al. (2004) Alcalase-assisted hydrolysis of alkali-extracted and acid-precipitated *B. napus* protein produces peptides capable of inhibiting human immunodeficiency virus (HIV) protease. The ethanol-soluble peptides of RS meal protein possess antioxidant activities. C/RS protein-derived peptides exhibit the ability to intervene in tissue oxidative status. The ethanol-soluble peptides of RS meal protein possess antioxidant activities manifested as reducing power, hydroxyl, and DPPH radical scavenging activity, ferrous-induced phosphatidyl choline oxidation inhibition, and antithrombotic activity (Zhang, Wang, & Xu, 2008). The antioxidant activities of C/RS protein hydrolysates, peptides, and ultrafiltered fractions revealed the ability to scavenge free radicals and thus the ability to attenuate oxidative reactions (Alashi et al., 2014; He, Girgih, Malomo, Ju, & Aluko, 2013). Both napin and cruciferin protein contain amino acid sequence fragments that match with peptide sequences with proven bioactivities (Wanasundara, 2011). The size, charge, and hydrophobic conformation depend on the AA sequences they are composed of and provide the basis for developing therapeutic and/or pharmaceutical compounds from C/RS proteins.

The possibility of generating nanoparticles from cruciferin to deliver bioactive molecules (β carotene as the model) was reported by Akabari and Wu (2015). Cruciferin nanoparticles produced using cold gelation and combination with chitosan showed stability under in vitro gastric digestion conditions but were able to release carrying molecules under intestinal conditions.

18.10.2 Issues and Challenges

The issues and challenges in developing protein products from C/RS can be categorized as those that are inherent to seed composition and current germplasm, and the ones that arise from seed processing for oil. Among the compositional attributes that are inherent to C/RS are the antinutritional factors including phytates, phenolics, GSL, and their breakdown products (Section 18.6) and the allergenic proteins (Section 18.7). Coextraction of these components can be minimized with proper understanding of their interassociation with protein and chemical changes that occur under the conditions of protein extraction. However, all these remedies cannot be included in developing a technically sound and commercially feasible protein product recovery process(es). Therefore some of the negative properties such as slightly colored products may be typical for C/RS products. The presence of allergenic proteins in C/RS is another challenge, however the mainstream plant proteins such as soy and animal proteins, egg, dairy, fish, and meat all are in the list of priority allergens for several world jurisdictions, where proper allergen risk mitigation mechanisms are in place. Inclusion of C/RS protein products into mainstream foods can be done in a similar way to other protein sources that are under the same guidelines. Proper labeling to provide the correct information for consumers, the use of specific tests approved for detection, and the generation of more scientific evidence-based information on C/RS allergenicity prevalence and the effect of processing on allergenic proteins and their activity are needed.

The other concern is consumer perception of genetically modified (GM) food. The majority of canola produced in Canada is genetically modified and an increasing amount of canola produced in Australia is also genetically modified. As the agronomic advantages of GM canola begin to outweigh any advantage of growing nonGM canola, it will become difficult to source non-GM sources of canola. However, there are some states in Australia where the cultivation of GM crops is not allowed, so in the short term, non-GM sources may be available. Contract, close-loop production of non-GM canola destined for niche markets occurs in Canada. However, as GM technology develops and consumer perceptions change, more canola varieties will be developed using GM technology and as has been the case in the corn and soybean industries canola production worldwide will become predominantly based on cultivation of GM varieties.

Among the challenges that arise from processing is the impact of oil extraction on the meal protein extractability and nutritional quality as described in Section 18.5. Most of the commercial-scale C/RS oil extraction (prepress and solvent) is of very large scale and produces desolventizer-toasted meal which is not suitable for protein extraction. C/RS protein meal is primarily directed to animal feed for milk, eggs, and meat production. The inability to use commercial C/RS meal in protein product preparation is one of the primary reasons that integration of protein recovery processes with commercial oil extraction has not occurred. Although low-temperature desolventization or vacuum desolventization can be employed to generate a gently processed meal, to date it has not been considered by the C/RS crushing industry because of the readily accessible feed market. In the soy industry, <4% of total meal production goes for food uses (FAO, 2006). Taking soy as an example, it can be expected that only a minor fraction of C/RS crushing will be diverted to food-grade protein production when appropriate technologies, product applications, and market demand align. Use of press C/RS cake (no solvent extraction) for protein extraction is also challenging because of the high level of retained oil which alters protein extractability. Research in C/RS protein recognizes the importance of press cake, work towards deriving multiple products that may enhance the sustainability of organic (nonsolvent oil) C/RS sectors.

18.11 OFF-TASTES ASSOCIATED WITH USING OILSEED PROTEINS

The phenolic compounds in the cotyledons and seed coat which are easily extractable with proteins under alkaline conditions (pH 7.5–12.5) are the major contributors to the dark color and bitter, astringent taste of the meal. The dark-color protein−phenol complexes can change physicochemical and functional properties of the protein (Schwenke & Dabrowski, 1990; Spencer et al., 1988). Phenolics interact with proteins predominantly via ionic bonding (>50% of extractable phenolics) and hydrophobic interactions while the H-bound or covalently bound portion of phenolics represent <10% of the extractable material (Xu & Diosady, 2000). Binding of free sinapic acid to 11S canola globulins is high when pH is 4.5 and no NaCl is present (Rubino et al., 1996).

Proteins are known to bind small molecules that are flavor- and taste-active. Canola PMM (rich in cruciferin) showed that similar to wheat or pea proteins, canola protein favors binding of C8 (octanal) aldehydes compared to C7 (heptanal) or C6 (hexanal) aldehydes (Wang & Arntfield, 2014).

18.12 CONCLUDING REMARKS

Canola or rapeseed is a food-grade oil-producing crop that has become a major oilseed in the last 40 years. It produces a considerable amount of protein that can be utilized as a plant protein source in human food. As C/RS is a major oilseed crop, utilizing its protein directly in human food will be a model for the production of sustainable sources of food grain protein. There have been numerous studies on C/RS protein properties and nutritional significance. Using oil-free canola meal directly in food is not an option because of its inherent constituents that are of non-nutritional value. Suitable processing regimens that can isolate proteins appropriate for human food application are necessary and the products needs to fit within the regulatory limits required of novel protein sources. Currently, the technologies are available, however, they need to be economically competitive to generate protein products that are affordable when incorporated into food products.

REFERENCES

Aachary, A. A., & Thiyam, U. (2011). A pursuit of the functional nutritional and bioactive properties of canola proteins and peptides. *Critical Reviews in Food Science and Nutrition, 52*, 965−979.

Adachi, M., Takenaka, Y., Gidamis, A. B., Mikami, B., & Utsumi, S. (2001). Crystal structure of soybean proglycinin A1aB1b homotrimer. *Journal of Molecular Biology, 305*, 291−305.

Akabari, A., & Wu, J. (2015). Canola protein nanoparticles: A promising delivery system for encapsulation of bioactive compounds. In: *Proceedings of 14th international rapeseed congress, Abstract 80, July 05−08, 2015, Saskatoon, Canada.*

Alashi, A. M., Blanchard, C. L., Mailer, R. J., & Agboola, S. O. (2013). Technological and functional properties of canola meal proteins and hydrolystes. *Food Reviews International, 29*(3).

Alashi, A. M., Blanchard, C. L., Mailer, R. J., Agboola, S. O., Mawson, A. J., He, R., ... Aluko, R. E. (2014). Antioxidant properties of Australian canola meal protein hydrolysates. *Food Chemistry, 146*, 500−506.

Alireza-Sadeghi, M., Rao, A. G. A., & Bhagya, S. (2006). Evaluation of mustard (*Brassica juncea*) protein isolate prepared by steam injection heating for reduction of antinutritional factors. *Lebensmittel Wissenschaft und Technologie, 39*, 911−917.

Aluko, R. E., & McIntosh, T. (2001). Polypeptide profile and functional properties of defatted meals and protein isolates of canola seeds. *Journal of Science Food and Agriculture, 81*, 391−396.

Aluko, R. E., & McIntosh, T. (2005). Limited enzymatic proteolysis increases the level of incorporation of canola proteins into mayonnaise. *Innovative Food Science & Emerging Technologies, 6*, 195−202.

Bagger, C. L., Sørensen, H., & Sørensen, J. C. (1998). High-quality oils, proteins and bioactive products for food and non-food purposes based on biorefining of cruciferous oilseed crops. In J. Gueguen, & Y. Popineau (Eds.), *Plant proteins from European crops: Food and non-food applications* (pp. 272−291). Berlin: Springer-Verlag.

Bell, J. M. (1993). Factors affecting the nutritional value of canola meal: A review. *Canadian Journal of Animal Science, 73*, 679−697.

Bérot, S., Compoint, J. P., Larré, C., Malabat, C., & Guéguen, J. (2005). Large scale purification of rapeseed proteins (*Brassica napus* L.). *Journal of Chromatography B, 818*, 35−42.

Betschart, A. A., Fong, R. Y., & Saunders, R. M. (1977). Rice by-products: Comparative extraction and precipitation of nitrogen from U.S. and Spanish bran and germ. *Journal of Food Science, 42*, 1088−1093.

Bhatty, R. L., MacKenzie, S. L., & Finlayson, A. J. (1968). The proteins of rapeseed (*Brassica napus*, L.) soluble in salt solutions. *Canadian Journal of Biochemistry, 46*, 1191−1197.

Bjergegaard, C., Eggum, B. O., Jensen, S. K, & Sørensen, H. (1991). Dietary fibres in oilseed rape: Physiological and antinutritional effects in rats of IDF and SDF added to a standard diet. *Journal of Animal Physiology and Animal Nutrition, 66*, 69−79.

Blaicher, F. M., Elstner, F., Stein, W., & Mukherjee, K. D. (1983). Rapeseed protein isolates: Effect of processing on yield and composition of protein. *Journal of Agricultural and Food Chemistry, 31*, 358−362.

Bos, C., Airinei, G., Mariotti, F., Benamouzig, R., Bérot, S., & Evrard, J. (2007). The poor digestibility of rapeseed protein is balanced by its very high metabolic utilization in humans. *Journal of Nutrition, 137*, 594−600.

Breen, J. P., & Crouch, M. L. (1992). Molecular analysis of a cruciferin storage protein gene family of *Brassica napus*. *Plant Molecular Biology, 20*, 1049–1055.

Carre, P., Quinsac, A., Citeau, M., & Fine, F. (2015). A re-examination of the technical feasibility and economic viability of rapeseed dehulling. *OCL, 22*, D304.

Ceciliani, F., Bortolotti, F., Menegatti, E., Ronchi, S., Ascenzi, P., & Palmieri, S. (1994). Purification, inhibitory properties, amino acid sequence and identification of the reactive site of a new serine proteinase from oil-rape (*Brassica napus*) seeds. *FEBS Letters, 342*, 221–224.

Cheung, L., Wanasundara, J. P. D., & Nickerson, M. T. (2014). The effect of pH and NaCl levels on the physicochemical and emulsifying properties of a cruciferin protein isolate. *Food Biophysics, 9*, 105–113.

Cheung, L., Wanasundara, J. P. D., & Nickerson, M. T. (2015). Effect of pH and NaCl on the emulsifying properties of a napin protein isolate. *Food Biophysics, 10*, 30–38.

Crouch, M. L., & Sussex, I. M. (1981). Development and storage protein synthesis in *Brassica napus* L. embroyos in vivo and in vitro. *Planta, 153*, 64–74.

Dabrowski, K., & Sosulski, F. W. (1984). Composition of free and hydrolysable phenolic acids in defatted flours of ten oilseeds. *Journal of Agricultural and Food Chemistry, 32*, 128–130.

Dalgalarrondo, M., Robin, J.-M., & Azanza, J.-L. (1986). Subunit composition of the globulin fraction of rapeseed (*Brassic napus*). *Plant Science, 43*, 115–124.

Delisle, J., Amiot, J., Goulet, G., Simard, C., Brisson, G. J., & Jones, J. D. (1984). Nutritive value of protein fractions extracted from soybean, rapeseed and wheat flours in the rat. *Plant Foods for Human Nutrition, 34*, 243–245.

Diosady, L. L., Rubin, L. J., & Tzeng, Y. -M. (1989). *Production of rapeseed protein materials*. US Patent No. 4,889,921.

Diosady, L. L., Xu, L., Chen, B.-K. (2005). *Production of high quality protein isolates from defatted meals of Brasica seeds*. US Patent No. 6,905,713 B2.

Eapen, K. E., Tape, N. W., & Sims, R. P. A. (1968). New process for the production of better-quality rapeseed oil and meal I. Effect of heat treatments on enzyme destruction and color of rapeseed oil. *Journal of American Oil Chemists' Society, 45*, 194–196.

Eapen, K. E., Tape, N. W., & Sima, R. P. A. (1969). New process for the production of better quality rapeseed oil and meal: II. Detoxification and dehulling of rapeseeds – feasibility study. *Journal of American Oil Chemists' Society, 46*, 52–55.

EFSA (2013). Scientific opinion on the safety of "rapeseed protein isolate" as a novel food ingredient. European Food Safety Authority panel on Dietetic Products, Nutrition and Allergies. *EFSA Journal, 11*(10), 3420.

El Nockrashy, A. S., Mukherjee, K. D., & Mangold, H. K. (1977). Rapeseed protein isolates by countercurrent extraction and isoelectric precipitation. *Journal of Agricultural and Food Chemistry, 25*, 193–197.

Fenwick, G. R. (1982). The assessment of a new protein source – Rapeseed. *Proceedings of the Nutrition Society, 41*, 277–288.

Fenwick, G. R., Heaney, R. K., & Mullin, W. J. (1983). Glucosinolates and their breakdown products in food and food plants. *Critical Reviews in Food and Nutrition, 18*, 123–201.

Friedman, M. (1996). Nutritional value of proteins from different food sources: A review. *Journal of Agricultural and Food Chemistry, 44*, 6–29.

Gehrig, P. M., Krzyzaniak, A., Barciszewski, J., & Biemann, K. (1998). Mass spectrometric amino acid sequencing of a mixture of seed storage proteins (napin) from *Brassica napus* products of a multigene family. *Biochemistry, 93*, 3647–3652.

Ghodsvali, A., Khodaparast, M. H., Vosoughi, M., & Diosady, L. L. (2005). Preparation of canola protein materials using membrane technology and evaluation of meals functional properties. *Food Research International, 38*, 223–231.

Grala, W., Buraczewka, L., Wasilewko, J., Verstegen, M. W. A., Tamminga, S., Jansman, A. J. M., ... Korczyński, W. (1998). Flow of endogenous and exogenous nitrogen in different segments of the small intestine in pigd fed diets with soybean concentrate, soybean meal or rapeseed cake. *Journal of Animal Feed Sciences, 7*, 1–20.

Guéguen, J., Bollecker, S., Schwenke, K. D., & Raab, B. (1990). Effect of succinylation on some physicochemical and functional properties of the 12S storage protein from rapeseed (*Brassica napus* L.). *Journal of Agricultural and Food Chemistry, 38*, 61–69.

He, R., Girgih, A. T., Malomo, S. A., Ju, X., & Aluko, R. E. (2013). Antioxidant activities of enzymatic rapeseed protein hydrolysates and the membrane ultrafiltration fractions. *Journal of Functional Foods, 5*, 219–227.

He, R., He, H.-E., Chao, D., Ju, X., & Aluko, R. (2014). Effects of high pressure and heat treatments on physicochemical and gelation properties of rapeseed protein isolate. *Food and Bioprocess Technology, 7*, 1344–1353.

He, R., Malomo, S. A., Alashi, A., Girgih, A. T., Ju, X., & Aluko, R. E. (2013). Purification and hypotensive activity of rapeseed protein-derived renin and angiotensin converting enzyme inhibitory peptides. *Journal of Functional Foods, 5*, 781–789.

Jolivet, P., Boulad, C., Bellamy, A., Larre, C., Barre, M., et al. (2009). Protein compostition of oil bodies from mature *Brassica napus* seeds. *Proteomics, 9*, 3268–3284.

Jones, J. D., & Holme, J. (1979). *Oilseed processing*. US patent No. 4,158,656.

Josefsson, L.-G., Lenman, M., Ericson, M. L., & Rask, L. (1987). Structure of a gene encoding the 1.7S storage proteins, napin from *Brassica napus*. *Journal of Biological Chemistry, 262*, 12196–12201.

Jyothi, T. C., Singh, S. A., & Appu Rao, A. G. (2007). Conformation of napin (*Brassica juncea*) in salts and monohydric alcohols: Contribution of electrostatic and hydrophobic interactions. *Journal of Agricultural and Food Chemistry, 55*, 4229–4236.

Jyothi, T. C., Sinha, S., Singh, S. A., Surolia, A., & Appu Rao, A. G. (2007). Napin from *Brassica juncea*: Thermodynamic and structural analysis of stability. *Biochimica Biophysica Acta, 1774*, 907–919.

Klockeman, D. M., Toledo, R., & Sims, K. A. (1997). Isolation and characterization of defatted canola meal protein. *Journal of Agricultural and Food Chemistry, 45*, 3867–3870.

Kodagoda, L. P., Nakai, S., & Powrie, W. D. (1973). Some functional properties of rapeseed protein isolates and concentrates. *Canadian Institute of Food Science and Technology Journal, 6*, 266–269.

Krause, J. P. (2002). Comparison of the effect of acylation and phosphorylation on surface pressure, surface potential and foaming properties of protein isolates from rapeseed (*Brassica napus*). *Industrial Crops and Products, 15*, 221–228.

Krul, C., Humblot, C., Philippe, C., Vermeulen, M., van Nuenen, M., Havenaar, R., & Rabot, S. (2002). Metabolism of sinigrin (2-propenyl glucosinolate) by the human colonic microflora in a dynamic in vitro large-intestine model. *Carcinogensis, 23*, 1009–1016.

Kvist, S., Carlsson, T., Lawther, J. M., & Basile de Castro, F. (2003). *Process for the fractionation of oilsed press cakes and meals*. WO 03/028473 A1.

Leidt, K.-H., Mörl, L., Pudel, F., Weigel, K., & Zettl, R. (2009). Fluidized bed desolventizer for gentle rapeseed meal processing. *Inform, 20*(11), 731.

Li, F., Huller, M. A. J., Beresford, S. A. A., & Lampe, J. W. (2011). Variation of glucoraphanin metabolism in vivo and ex vivo by human gut bacteria. *British Journal of Nutrition, 106*, 408–416.

Maenz, D. D., Newkirk, R. W., Classen, H. L., & Tyler, R. T. (2004). *Fractionation and processing of oilseeds*. USA Patent No. 6,800,308 B2.

Mahajan, A., & Dua, S. (1994). Comparison of processing treatments on the composition and functional properties of rapeseed preparations (Brassica campestris L. var. Toria). *Die Nahrung, 38*, 578–587.

Mailer, R. J., McFadden, A., Ayton, J., & Redden, B. (2008). Anti-nutritional components, fibre, sinapine and glucosinolate content, in Australian canola (*Brassica napus* L.) meal. *Journal of American Oil Chemists' Society, 85*, 937–944.

Malabat, C., Atterby, H., Chaudhry, Q., Renard, M., & Guéguen, J. (2003). Genetic variability of rapeseed protein composition. In: *Proceedings of 11th international rapeseed congress* (Vol. 4., pp. 205–208). The Royal Veterinary and Agricultural University, Copenhagen, Denmark.

Manamperi, W. A. R., Chang, S. K. C., & Pryor, S. W. (2012). Impact of meal preparation method and extraction procedure on canola protein yield and properties. *Biological Engineering Transactions, 5*, 191–200.

Marczak, E. D., Ohinata, K., Lipkowski, A. W., & Yoshikawa, M. (2006). Arg-Ile-Tyr (RIY) derived from rapeseed protein decreases food intake and gastric emptying after oral administration in mice. *Peptides, 27*, 2065–2068.

Marczak, E. D., Usui, H., Fujita, H., Yang, Y., Yokoo, M., Lipkowski, A. W., & Yoshikawa, M. (2003). New antihypertensive peptides isolated from rapeseed. *Peptides, 24*, 791–798.

Matthäus, B. (1998). Effect of dehulling on the composition on the antinutritive compounds in various cultivars of rapeseed. *Fett/Lipid, 100*, 295–301.

Matthäus, B., Lösing, R., & Fiebig, H.-J. (1995). Determination of phytic acid and it s degradation products in extracts of rapeseed and rapeseed meal. *Journal of High Resolution Chromatography, 18*, 267–268.

Mawson, R., Heaney, R. K., Zdunczyk, Z., & Kozlowska, H. (1995). Rapeseed meal-glucosinolates and their antinutritional effects. Part 6. Taint in end-products. *Die Nahrung, 1*, 21–31.

Mejia, L. A., Korgaonkar, C. K., Schweizer, M., Chengelis, C., Marit, G., Ziemer, E., ... Empie, M. (2009). A 13-week sub-chronic dietary toxicity study of a cruciferin-rich canola protien isolate in rats. *Food Chemical Toxicology, 47*, 2645–2654.

Mejia, L. A., Korgaonkar, C. K., Schweizer, M., Chengelis, C., Novilla, M., Ziemer, E., ... Empie, M. (2009). A 13-week dietary toxicity study in rats of a napin-rich canola protein isolate. *Regulatory Toxicology and Pharmacology, 55*, 394–402.

Mieth, G., Bruckner, J., Kroll, J., & Pohl, J. (1983). Rapeseed: Constituents and protein products. Part 2: Preparation and properties of protein enriched products. *Die Nahrung, 27*, 759–801.

Mills, E. N. C., Madsen, C., Shewry, P. R., & Wichers, H. J. (2003). Food allerges of plant origin-their molecular and evolutionary relationship. *Trends in Food Science and Technology, 14*, 145–156.

Monreal, P., Botey, J., Pena, M., Martin, A., & Eseverri, J. L. (1992). Mustard allergy; Two anaphylactic reactions to ingestion of mustard sauce. *Annals of Allergy, 69*, 317–320.

Monsalve, R. I., Villalba, M., & Rodríguez, R. (2001). Allergy to mustard seeds: The importance of 2S albumins as food allergens. *Internet Symposium on Food Allergens, 3*, 57–69 . <http://www.food-allergens.de>.

Müntz, K. (1998). Deposition of storage proteins. [Review]. *Plant Molecular Biology, 38*, 77–99.

Murray, E. D. (1999). *Oilseed protein extraction*. USA Patent No. 6,005,076.

Murray, E. D. (2005). *Canola protein functionality I*. US Patent No. 2005/0249866 A1.

Murray, E. D., Maurice, T. J., Barker, L. D., & Myers, C. D. (1980). *Process for isolation of proteins using food grade salt solutions at specified pH and ionic strength*. USA Patent No. 4,208,323.

Murray, E. D., Myers, C. D., & Barker, L. D. (1981). *Protein isolate product*. US Patent No. 4,285,862.

Naczk, M., Amarowicz, R., Sullivan, A., & Shahidi, F. (1998). Current research developments on polyphenolics of rapeseed/canola: A review. *Food Chemistry, 62*, 489–502.

Newkirk, R., Classen, H. L., & Edney, M. J. (2003). Effects of prepress solvent extraction on the nutritional value of canola meal for broiler chickens. *Animal Feed Science and Technology, 104*, 111–119.

Newkirk, R. W. (2009). *Canola meal. Feed industries guide* (4th ed.). Winnipeg, Manitoba: Canadian International Grains Institute.

Newkirk, R. W., Maenz, D. D., & Classen, H. L. (2009). *Oilseed processing*. USA Patent No. 7,560,132 B2.

Ochodzki, P., Rakowska, M., Bjergegaard, C., & Sørensen, H. (1995). Studies on enzymatic fractionation, chemical composition and biological effects of dietary fibre in rape seed (*Brassica napus* L.) 1. Chemical composition of seeds and characterization of soluble and insoluble dietary fibre of spring and winter type varieties of double improved oilseed type. *Journal of Animal and Feed Science, 4*, 127–138.

Osborne, T. B., & Mendel, L. B. (1914). Nutritive properties of proteins of the maize kernel. *Journal of Biological Chemistry, 18*, 1–16.

Osborne, T. B. (1897). The amount and properties of the proteids of the maize kernel. *Journal of the American Chemical Society, 19*(7), 525–532.

Pedroche, J., Yust, M. D. M., Lqari, H., Girón-Calle, J., Alaiz, M., Vioque, J., & Millán, F. (2004). *Brassica carinata* protein isolates: Chemical composition, protein characterization and improvement of functional properties by protein hydrolysis. *Food Chemistry, 88*, 337–346.

Pinterits, A., & Arntfield, S. D. (2008). Improvement of canola protein gelation properties through enzymatic modification with transglutaminase. *LWT – Food Science and Technology, 41*, 128–138.

Poikonen, S., Puumalainen, T. J., Kautiainen, H., Palosuo, T., Reunala, T., & Turjanmaa, K. (2008). Stensitization and allergy to turnip tape and oilseed rape in children with atopic dermatitis: A case control study. *Pediatric Allergy and Immunology, 195*, 408–411.

Pudel, F., Tressel, R.-P., & Düring, K. (2015). Production and properties of rapeseed albumin. *Lipid Technology, 27*, 112–114.

Puumalainen, T. J., Poikonen, S., Kotovuori, A., Vaali, K., Kalkkinin, N., Reunala, T., et al. (2006). Napins, 2S albumins are major allergens in oilseed rape and turnip rape. *Journal of Allergy and Clinical Immunology, 117*(2), 426–432.

Puumalainen, T. J., Puustinen, A., Poikonen, S., Turjanmaa, K., Palosuo, T., & Vaali, K. (2015). Proteomic identification of allergenic seed proteins, napin and cruciferin, from cold-pressed rapeseed oils. *Food Chemistry, 175*, 381–385.

Raboy, V. (2003). myo-Inositol-1,2,3,4,5,6-hexakisphosphate. *Phytochemistry, 64*, 1033–1043.

Röbeelen, G. R., Downey, R. K., & Ashri, A. (1989). Brassica species. In G. R. Robeelen, R. K. Downey, & A. Ashri (Eds.), *Oil crops of the world*. New York: McGraw-Hill.

Robin, J. M., Inquello, V., Mimouni, B., & Azanza, J. L. (1991). Relationship between immunological properties and structural model of 11S rapeseed globulin. *Phytochemistry, 30*, 3511–3513.

Rubino, M. I., Arntfield, S. D., Nadon, C. A., & Bernatsky, A. (1996). Phenolic protein interactions in relation to the gelation properties of canola protein. *Food Research International, 29*, 653–659.

Sarwar, G. (1987). Digestibility of protein and bioavailability of amino acids in foods. Effects on protein quality assessment. *World Reviews in Nutrition and Diet, 54*, 26–70.

Schweizer, M., & Green, B. E. (2005). *Oil meal preparation*. USA Patent No. 2005/0031767 A1.

Schwenke, K. D., & Dabrowski, K. (1990). Turbidimetric studies on sinapic acid-rapeseed protein interaction. *Die Nahrung, 34*, 561–567.

Schwenke, K. D., Dahme, A., & Wolter, T. H. (1998). Heat-induced gelation of rapeseed proteins: Implication of electrolytes. In Plant proteins from European crops. In J. Gueguen, & Y. Popineau (Eds.), *Food and Non Food Applications* (pp. 126–130). Berlin: Springer-Verlag.

Schwenke, K. D., Mothes, R., Marzilger, K., Borowska, J., & Koslowska, H. (1987). Rapeseed protein polyanion interactions: Turbidimetric studies in systems with phosphate-containing polyanions, phytic acid and octametaphosphate. *Die Nahrung, 31*, 1001–1013.

Schwenke, K. D., Raab, B., Plietz, P., & Damaschun, G. (1983). The structure of the 12S globulin from rapeseed. *Nahrung, 27*, 165–175.

Schwenke, K. D., Schultz, M., Linow, K.-J., Gast, K., & Zirwer, D. (1980). Hydrodynamic and quasielastic light scattering studies on the 12S globulin from rapeseed. *Journal of Peptide and Protein Research, 16*, 12–18.

Scofield, R., & Crouch, M. J. (1987). Nucleotide sequence of of a member of the napin storage protein family from *Brassica napus*. *Journal of Biological Chemistry, 262*, 12202–12208.

Shewry, P. R., Napler, J. A., & Tatham, A. S. (1995). Seed storage proteins: Structure and biosynthesis. *The Plant Cell, 7*, 945–956.

Simon, A. E., Tenbarge, K. M., Scofield, S. R., Finkelstein, R. R., & Crouch, M. L. (1985). Nucleotide sequence of a cDNA clone of *Brassica napus* 12S storage protein sows homology with legumin from *Pisum sativum*. *Plant Molecular Biology, 5*, 191–201.

Sosulski, F. W., & Bakal, A. (1969). Isolated proteins from rapeseed, flax, and sunflower meals. *Canadian Institute of Food Science and Technology Journal, 2*, 28–32.

Spencer, C. M., Cai, Y., Martin, R., Gaffiney, S. H., Goulding, P. N., Magnolato, D., … Haslam, E. (1988). Polyphenol complexation – some thoughts and observations. *Phytochemistry, 27*, 2397–2409.

Tan, S. H., Mailer, R. J., Blanchard, C. L., & Agboola, S. O. (2011a). Extraction and characterisation of proteins fractions from Australian canola meals. *Food Research International, 44*, 1075–1082.

Tan, S. H., Mailer, R. J., Blanchard, C. L., & Agboola, S. O. (2011b). Canola proteins for human consumption: Extraction, profile, and functional properties. *Journal of Food Science, 76*, R16–R28.

Tan, S. H., Mailer, R. J., Blanchard, C. L., & Agboola, S. O. (2014). Emulsifying properties of proteins extracted form Australian canola meals. *LWT – Food Science and Technology, 57*, 376–382.

Tan, S. H., Mailer, R. J., Blanchard, C. L., Agboola, S. O., & Day, L. (2014). Gelling properties of protein fractions and protein isolate extracted from Australian canola meal. *Food Research International, 62*, 819–828.

Thiyam, U., Stöckmann, H., Zum Felde, T., & Schwarz, K. (2006). Antioxidative effect of the main sinapic acid derivatives from rapeseed and mustard oil by – Products. *European Journal of Lipid Science & Technology, 108*, 239–248.

Thompson, L. U., Allum-Poon, P., & Procope, C. (1976). Isolation of rapeseed protein using sodium hexametaphosphate. *Canadian Institute of Food Science and Technology Journal, 9*, 15–19.

Tzeng, Y.-M., Diosady, L. L., & Rubin, L. J. (1988). Preparation of rapeseed protein isolates using ultrafiltration, precipitation and by diafiltration. *Canadian Institute of Food Science and Technology, 21*, 419–424.

Tzeng, Y. M., Diosady, L. L., & Rubin, L. J. (1990). Production of canola protein materials by alkaline extraction, precipitation, and membrane processing. *Journal of Food Science, 55*, 1147–1151.

Uruapka, F., & Arntfield, S. (2005). Emulsifying caracheritics of commerciall canola protein hydrocolloif system. *Food Research International, 38*, 659–672.

Vioque, J., Sánchez-Vioque, R., Clemente, A., Pedroche, J., Bautista, J., & Millán, F. (1999). Production and characterization of an extensive rapeseed protein hydrolysate. *Journal of the American Oil Chemists' Society, 76*, 819–822.

Vioque, J., Sánchez-Vioque, R., Clemente, A., Pedroche, J., & Millán, F. (2000). Partially hydrolyzed rapeseed protein isolates with improved functional properties. *Journal of the American Oil Chemists' Society, 77*, 447–450.

Visentin, M., Iori, R., Valdicelli, L., & Palmieri, S. (1992). Trypsin inhibitor activity in some rapeseed genotypes. *Phytochemistry, 31*, 3677–3680.

Wallig, M., Belyea, R., & Tumbleson, M. (2002). Effect of pelleting on glucosinolate content of Crambe meal. *Animal Feed Science and Technology, 99*, 205–214.

Wan, L., Ross, A. R. S., Yang, J., Hegedus, D. D., & Kermode, A. R. (2007). Phosphorylation of the 12S globulin cruciferin in wild type and abi1-1 mutant *Arabidopsis thaliana* (thale cress) seeds. *Biochemical Journal, 404*, 247–256.

Wanasundara, J. P. D. (2011). Proteins of Brassicaceae oilseeds and their potential as a plant protein source. *Critical Reviews of Food Science and Nutrition, 51*, 635–677.

Wanasundara, J. P. D., Abeysekara, S. J., McIntosh, T. C., & Falk, K. C. (2012). Solubility differences of major storage proteins of Brassicaceae oilseeds. *Journal of American Oil Chemists' Society, 89*, 869–881.

Wanasundara, J. P. D., & McIntosh, T. C. (2013). *A process of aqueous protein extraction from Brassicaceae oilseeds*. US Patent 8,55,7963.

Wanasundara, J. P. D., & McIntosh, T. C. (2015). Properties of napin from scaled up canola meal fractionation process. In: *Proceedings of 14th international rapeseed congress, Abstract 80, July 05–08, 2015, Saskatoon, Canada*.

Wanasundara, U. N., Amarowicz, R., & Shahidi, F. (1996). Partial characterization of natural antioxidants in canola meal. *Food Research International, 28*, 525–530.

Wang, K., & Arntfield, S. D. (2014). Binding of carbonyl flavours to canola, pea, and wheat proteins using GC/MS approach. *Food Chemistry, 157*, 36–372.

WHO/FAO/UNU (2007). *Protein and amino acid requirement in human nutrition*. Report of a joint WHO/FAO?UNU Expert Consultation 2002. WHO Technical Report 935.

Wijesundera, C., Boiteau, T., Xu, X., Shen, Z., Watkins, P., & Logan, A. (2013). Stabilization of fish oil-in-water emulsions with oleosin extracted from canola meal. *Journal of Food Science, 78*, C1340–C1347.

Wu, J., Aluko, R. E., & Muir, A. D. (2008). Purification of angiotensin I-converting enzyme-inhibitory peptides from the enzymatic hydrolysate of defatted canola meal. *Food Chemistry, 111*, 942–950.

Wu, J., & Muir, A. D. (2008). Comparative structural, emulsifying and biological properties of 2 major canola protiens, cruciferin and napin. *Journal of Food Science, 73*, C210–C216.

Xu, L., & Diosady, L. L. (2000). Interactions between canola proteins and phenolic compounds in aqueous media. *Food Research International, 33*, 725–731.

Yust, M. M., Pedroche, J., Megias, C., Giron-Calle, J., Alaiz, M., Millan, F., & Vioque, J. (2004). Rapeseed protein hydrolysates: A source of HIV proteiase peptide inhibitors. *Food Chemistry, 87*, 387–392.

Zhang, S. B., Wang, Z., & Xu, S. Y. (2008). Antioxidant and antithrombotic activities of rapeseed peptides. *Journal of American Oil Chemists' Society, 85*, 521–527.

Zohary, D., & Hopf, M. (2000). *Domestication of plants in the old world: The origin and spread of cultivated plants in West Asia, Europe and the Nile Valley*. New York: Oxford University Press.

Websites and electronic documents: Accessed during January 1–September 1, 2015

AAFC. *Agriculture and Agri-Food Canada*. (2015). <www.agr.gc.ca/eng/industry-markets-and-trade/statistics-and-market-information/by-product-sector/crops/crops-market-information-canadian-industry/canada-outlook-for-principal-field-crops/canada-outlook-for-principal-field-crops-2015-01-23/?id = 1422296493607>.

ABS. *Australian Bureau of Statistics*. (2015). <www.abs.gov.au/ausstats/abs@.nsf/Lookup/7121.0main + features62012-2013>.

AGCanada.com. (2015). <www.agcanada.com/daily/eu-lifts-wheat-barley-rapeseed-yield-outlook>.

Agricultural Commodities Australia. (2013). <www.abs.gov.au/AUSSTATS/abs@.nsf/Lookup/7121.0Main + Features12013-14>.

Burcon. *Burcon Nutrascience Co.* (2015). <www.burcon.ca>.

CCC. *Canola Council of Canada*. (2015). <www.canolacouncil.org>.

FAO. *Livestock's long shadow – Environmental issues and options*. (2006). <http://www.fao.org/docrep/010/a0701e/a0701e00.HTM>.

FAOSTAT. *Food and Agriculture Organization of the United Nations Statistics Division*. (2015). <http://faostat3.fao.org/home/E>.

FEDIOL. *Protein meals world production 2014*. (2015). <www.fediol.eu/web/world + production + data/1011306087/list1187970075/f1.html>.

GRAS Notice 327. *GRAS notification for crucifeirn-rich and napin-rich protein isolatesderived from canola/rapeseed (Puratein® and Supertein™)*. (2010). <www.fda.gov/Food/FoodIngredientsPackaging/GenerallyRecognizedasSafeGRAS/GRASListings/default.htm>.

LCA Manitoba. (2015). *Life cycle assessment of Canola production in Manitoba. Manitoba Agriculture and Rural Development. (2015)*. <www.gov.mb.ca/agriculture/environment/climate-change/life-cycle-assessment-of-agriculture-in-manitoba.html#canola>.

Ludwig, F., Biemans, H., Jacobs, C., Siupit, I., van Diepen, K., Fawell, J., Capri, E., & Steduto, P. *Water use of oil crops: Current water and future outlooks. Report by the International Life Sciences Institute Europe environment and Health Task Force*. (2011). <www.ilsi.org/Europe/Publications/ILSI-11-009%20WUR%2002.pdf>.

TeuTexx. (2015). <http://teutexx.com/>.

Teutoburger–Oelmuehle. (2015). <www.teutoburger-oelmuehle.com/>.

UK Agriculture. (2015). <www.ukagriculture.com/crops/oil_seed_rape.cfm>.

UniProt. *Universal Protein Resource*. (2015). <www.uniprot.org>.

Chapter 19

Mycoprotein: A Healthy New Protein With a Low Environmental Impact

T. Finnigan, L. Needham and C. Abbott
Quorn Foods, North Yorkshire, United Kingdom

19.1 ORIGINS AND DISCOVERY OF MYCOPROTEIN

According to the FAO (2000), the years 1945–52 saw Europe struggling to restore prewar food production, consumption, and security. Even in the mid-1960s, former levels still had not been reattained in Asia—rightly seen as the highest-risk area, where chronic undernourishment left people extremely vulnerable. Between 23 million and 30 million lives were lost in the Chinese famine of 1960–62. In 1965 and 1966, famine was barely avoided in South Asia. More than 75% of Asians (and probably 90% of undernourishment victims) depended on food production for their income. The late Lord Rank, who as J. Arthur Rank had created the Rank Film Empire, was then chair of the Rank Hovis McDougall (RHM) group of companies and felt that something needed to be done. RHM as a major producer of cereals produced starch as a byproduct. The ideal process therefore would be one that converted abundant carbohydrate into the scarce commodity protein. Food for man was a brave step, but so the search began.

According to Angold, Beech, and Taggart (1989) the search for a suitable microorganism began in a sports field alongside RHM's wheat starch plant in Ashford Kent, United Kingdom. This field was occasionally sprayed with surplus starch and the theory was that this would help to select for those organisms capable of using starch as a substrate. This proved to be correct and a strain of *Penicillium* was isolated with an amino acid profile close to casein. Work progressed on *Penicillium* for 3 years but ultimately it was its inability to grow satisfactorily in continuous culture that resulted in the search for a new organism.

The new search began in 1967 with over 3000 soil samples taken from around the world. Ironically, the organism selected (*Fusarium graminearum* code A3/5) came from a garden in Marlow, Buckinghamshire, within 4 miles of the Lord Rank research center where the project was located. This was later reclassified as *Fusarium venenatum* (PTA 2684) (Yoder & Christianson, 1998) and is a member of the *Ascomycota* branch of the fungi family, mycoprotein can be regarded as the food derived from the mycelium of this *Fusarium*.

Mycoprotein is at the heart of all Quorn foods and given its long history but fairly recent commercial success might be regarded as something of a 50-year overnight success. According to Spector (2015), Quorn represents an excellent present-day example of what our ancestors must have done when first domesticating wild plants for food. Certainly, as we look to a future of increasing food insecurity it seems that we are going to need all of our ingenuity to address the challenges ahead and increased use of existing or newly sourced plant-based proteins must have an important role.

19.2 FOOD SAFETY AND THE REGULATORY FRAMEWORK

Mycoprotein products have been on sale in the United Kingdom since January 1985 and sales in other European countries began in 1991 (Wiebe, 2001; Wiebe, 2004). Mycoprotein now may be sold lawfully in all the countries of the European Union (EC 1997), and also has approvals in Switzerland, Norway, Taiwan, Canada, South Africa, Australia, and New Zealand. In the United States, Marlow Foods submitted a Generally Recognized as Safe (GRAS) Self-affirmation Petition to the Food and Drug Administration (FDA) in 2001. This was accepted by the FDA and Quorn products entered the United States market in 2002.

TABLE 19.1 Typical Composition of Mycoprotein

Nutrient	Typical Composition of Mycoprotein per 100 g	
	Dry Mycoprotein	Mycoprotein Ingredient (Wet Weight)
Moisture (g)	0	75
Protein (g)	45	11.25
Fat (g)	13	3.25
Fiber (g)	25	6.25
Carbohydrate (g)	10	3
Energy (kcal)	340	85
Ash (g)	3.4	0.85

The chemical analysis of mycoprotein demonstrates that it contains a wide spectrum of nutrients. Typically, the dry matter in 100 g mycoprotein contains 45 g protein, 25 g fiber, 13 g fat, 10 g available carbohydrate, and a range of vitamins and minerals. When used as a food ingredient with a solids content of about 25%, 100 g of mycoprotein typically contains about 11 g protein, 6 g fiber, 3 g fat, 3 g carbohydrate, and 85 kcal of energy, as summarized in Table 19.1.

An extensive database, consisting of thorough analytical data on identity and composition, manufacturing process, analysis for possible impurities, animal studies, digestibility, and nutritional evaluation and human studies, has been used to support the safety assessment. Animal toxicology studies have demonstrated that there are no health concerns from acute or chronic exposure and that mycoprotein supports normal growth and development in animal species. Assurance of safety was established from the analysis of all these data and subsequent clinical studies with human subjects that verified availability of nutrients and assessed tolerance.

The evaluation of all available analytical, animal, and human safety data, as well as market information on typical levels and frequency of consumption of mycoprotein, leads to the conclusion that the use of mycoprotein will not produce any acute or chronic adverse effects in individuals consuming these food products under the intended conditions of use.

Human volunteer studies have shown that mycoprotein contains high-quality protein with a biological value similar to milk protein. It has a protein digestibility corrected amino acid score (PDCAAS) close to 1.0. Its fiber content has no adverse effect on mineral absorption. Extensive experience in use has shown mycoprotein to be a very well-tolerated food. A small proportion of the population may exhibit intolerance towards mycoprotein, but levels of intolerance are orders of magnitude lower than to foods such as soya and egg. At least some of these individuals are sensitive to other fungal foods and recent expert opinion suggests that there could be a small subgroup where rapid fermentation of fiber in the large intestine may be involved (Hunter, 2014).

Clinical studies also have demonstrated that mycoprotein has a range of potential physiological benefits. It is unusual in that it is rich in both protein and fiber and that it is low in carbohydrate with a fat content that is largely unsaturated. Mycoprotein has been shown to lower total and low-density lipoprotein (LDL) cholesterol, induce satiety, and can reduce the glycemic response when present with carbohydrate-rich foods.

19.3 CULTIVATION AND PROCESSING OF MYCOPROTEIN

19.3.1 Fungal Fermentation Technology

To manufacture mycoprotein, the filamentous organism, *F. venenatum*, PTA-2684, is grown axenically in a continuous fermentation. The fermentation medium comprises food-grade carbohydrate together with other ingredients that are of food-grade quality and purity which are appropriate for the growth of the mycelium. The liquid and gaseous feeds are sterilized prior to addition to the fermenter. The inoculum is prepared starting from stock cultures which are available in lyophilized form from the American Type Culture Collection, Washington, DC, as PTA-2684 (Fig. 19.1).

An inoculum of pure culture is introduced after initial filling of the sterilized fermentation vessel. After a period of batch growth of the organism, a continuous feed of nutrients and simultaneous removal of fermenter broth is established. In the continuous fermentation process, constant environmental conditions are maintained by continuous automatic control.

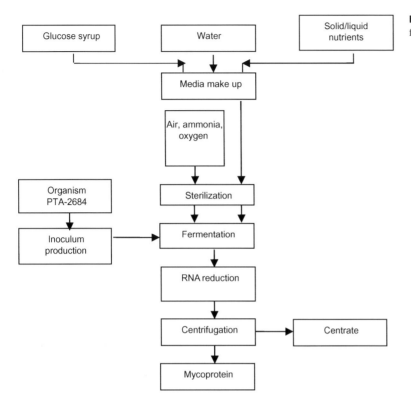

FIGURE 19.1 Schematic of the fermentation process for the production of mycoprotein.

TABLE 19.2 Average Amino Acid Composition Typical for the Centrate (g/100 g Dry Weight)					
Aspartic acid	1.6	Threonine	0.8	Methionine	0.3
Serine	0.8	Alanine	1.9	Lysine	1.2
Glutamic acid	4.7	Proline	0.8	Isoleucine	0.6
Glycine	1.3	Cystine	0.3	Leucine	1.0
Histidine	0.5	Tyrosine	0.4	Phenylalanine	0.6
Argenine	1.4	Valine	0.8		

The plant is designed and the process operated so as to avoid contamination. Temperature and pH are controlled, and the flow of nutrients is adjusted to maintain an excess in the supernatant. Flows of other medium components are set to maintain the specified supernatant conditions. The process is aerobic, so the supply of air and any supplementary oxygen is adjusted in response to measured dissolved oxygen levels. Biomass concentration is controlled by adjustment of total flow of medium into the fermenter and is inferred from the carbon dioxide evolution rate and checked by on-line analysis; the fluid level in the fermenter is maintained by control of exit flow. The collected fermenter broth is then heat-shocked to induce the natural nuclease enzymes in the mycelium (Ward, 1996). The action of these enzymes reduces the RNA content of the mycelium from approximately 10% to below 2%, by dry weight. The broth is then centrifuged to produce a mycelium paste of approximately 75% water. At this point the paste is termed mycoprotein and it is then quickly chilled ready for use in the manufacture of food products. This process renders the source organism nonviable. However, the effect of the RNA reduction step is to render the cell membrane leaky, resulting in losses of up to 30% of the biomass into the centrate (liquid discharged from the centrifuge). The composition of centrate is shown in Tables 19.2 and 19.3. Centrate typically will have a total solids level of ca 1.3 g/100 mL and is thus a fairly dilute waste containing interesting biomolecules but with an expensive extraction/dewatering process to get at them. Nevertheless, the content of 5′ nucleotides and amino acids produces an exciting natural flavoring with proven umami impact (Dermiki et al., 2013; Rodger et al., 1998).

TABLE 19.3 Average Typical Values for Chemical Composition of Centrate

	Concentration (g/L)	Dry Weight (%)
Carbohydrate (total)[a]	4.8	37
Nucleic acid (5′ GMP)	1.6	12 (2–3%)
Protein (amino N × 6.25)	2.2	17
Inorganic salts	3.6	28
Others	0.8	6
Total	13	

[a]Mannitol c.1.5 g/L.

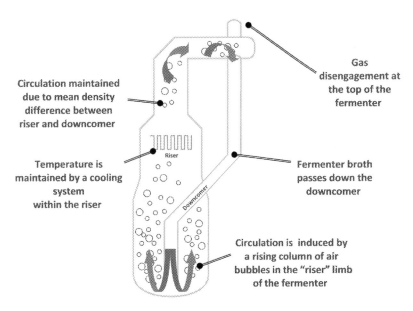

FIGURE 19.2 Schematic representation of air lift fermentation.

19.3.1.1 Air Lift Fermentation

Fusarium venenatum for mycoprotein production is grown under strictly defined conditions, with temperature, pH, nutrient concentration, dissolved oxygen, and growth rate all maintained constant (Trinci, 1991). In early development RHM had used stirred tank fermentation for scale-up. However, because of their filamentous morphology, cultures of fungi are more viscous than bacterial cultures (Righelato, 1979) and are more difficult to mix. This was eventually solved by the formation of a joint venture with ICI in 1984 and the development of the current air lift fermentation technology. Fig. 19.2 shows that air lift fermentation possesses an elegant simplicity that relies on the introduction of air at the base of the fermenter column creating millions of microbubbles that then rise up the full height of the fermenter column at which point the gas disengages, causing a density difference and the liquid to fall and the process to begin once again. Current fermenter volumes are c.155 m^3 at a height of c.50 m.

According to Trinci (1992), in a continuous-flow culture, growth of the fungus can be restricted by the supply of any nutrient but is usually limited by the concentration of the carbon and energy source (eg, glucose) with all other nutrients present in excess. However, continuous-flow cultures avoid the fluctuating conditions inherent in batch cultures (Pirt, 1975) and enable perpetual exponential growth of the organism to be maintained at a specific growth rate approaching its maximum rate of growth for the prevailing conditions. In practice, mycoprotein fermentations are run for about 6 weeks, which yields a productivity some fivefold greater than what could be achieved by a series of separate batch fermentations (Sadler, 1988). In this way and starting with just a few milligrams of pure culture it is possible to grow from this to produce over 1500 tonnes of mycoprotein before the fermenter run is terminated. Current practice in mycoprotein production is to terminate the fermentation when more highly branched variants begin to supplant the sparsely branched culture (Simpson, 1996).

(A)
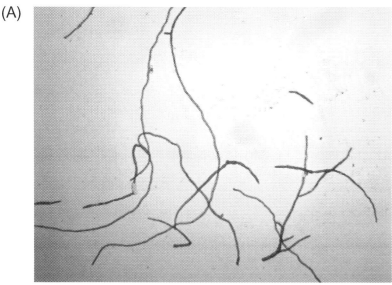

(B)
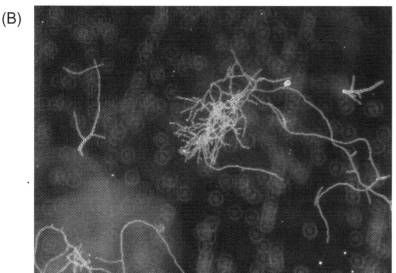

FIGURE 19.3 Filamentous and branched nature of mycoprotein: (A) filamentous variant; (B) branched colonial variant.

It is common for relatively sparsely branched strains of microfungi to be supplanted by shorter, more highly branched variants during long-term continuous culture. Many of these variants have a transient existence at low levels, normally <1% of population on colony-forming unit basis (Trinci, Robson, Wiebe, Cunliffe, & Naylor, 1990). The filamentous nature of mycoprotein and the highly branched nature of the colonial variant are depicted in Fig. 19.3A and B.

19.3.2 Mycoprotein and the Creation of Meat-Like Texture

Fig. 19.4 depicts the production process for the creation of Quorn mince and pieces from mycoprotein.

From receipt of mycoprotein the production process is batch continuous. In the production of Quorn mince, mycoprotein is mixed with a little egg albumen, some roasted barley malt extract, and water. The process for Quorn pieces is similar at this point except no malt is added but a natural flavoring is mixed in to give a savory character. Mixing is carried out at low shear on batch sizes approaching two tonnes. The apparent simplicity of this process masks the challenge of dispersing a powder of complex hydration characteristics such as egg albumen into a viscoelastic material such as mycoprotein. In addition, a little calcium is added to the mix. This has been shown to change the rheology of the mix presumably by interhyphal crosslinking, which improves the meat-like texture of the finished product.

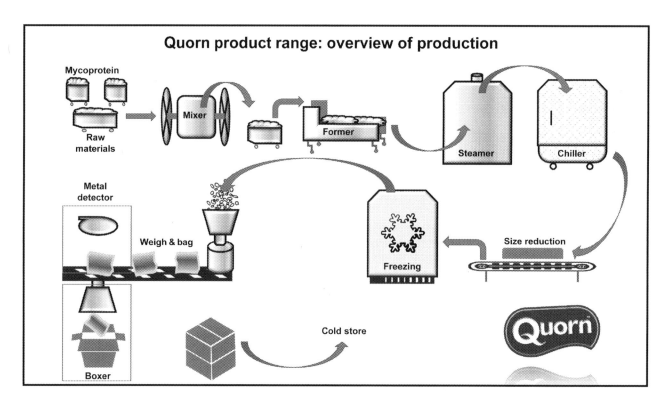

FIGURE 19.4 Schematic representation of the process for converting mycoprotein into Quorn mince or pieces.

After mixing, the mass is discharged into equipment common to the food industry used to produce shaped blocks by forming under pressure. It is at this point that the flow characteristics of the mix begin to introduce laminations which can be considered as textural precursors for the final meat-like textural attributes achieved in the final product.

The formed blocks are then raised to 85–90°C by live steam. This denatures the native proteins and the blocks are then chilled and frozen to approximately −18°C. Freezing is carried out over c.30 min. Freezing is a critical process in the creation of the desirable meaty texture. The controlled growth of ice crystals effectively pushes the filamentous hyphae together to create fibrous bundles with a resultant texture that can be described as meat-like. In addition, this finished product texture is remarkably stable both to end-use environment, for example, pH and processing (Knight, Roberts, & Shelton, 2001) allowing relatively unconstrained food product development.

Fig. 19.5 compares the microscopic structure of textured soya, chicken, and Quorn. The larger more cable-like fibers typical of texture vegetable protein promote a rubbery texture on chewing which is not desirable. In this way it can be seen that poultry and Quorn, with their tightly packed laminations, promote a less rubbery and more fibrous eating quality in a way that textured vegetable protein cannot.

19.3.2.1 Hypotheses on Texture Creation

Fig. 19.3 has already shown us the filamentous structure of mycoprotein. Indeed, the filamentous nature of mycoprotein is exploited in the creation of meat-like textures by the creation of a fiber–gel composite through controlled heat denaturation of native proteins, such as egg albumen, when mixed with mycoprotein fibers, followed by freeze texturization where the controlled growth of ice crystals creates fibrous bundles that emulate the texture of whole muscle meat, as depicted in Fig. 19.5. Fig. 19.3 also shows the morphology of the so-called colonial variant which appears after about 30 days of continuous fermentation and whose more globular format is less able to reproduce meat-like texture.

As mentioned, this ability to create fibrous bundles from the filamentous hyphae differentiates mycoprotein from other meat-free proteins in its ability to introduce fibrosity—a highly desirable sensory characteristic within the overall challenge to emulate the eating quality of meat. The simplistic material science definition of fibrosity in food is "compression-fracture" happening repeatedly as the food is chewed and on this basis it can be imagined that creating fibrous bundles with mycoprotein helps to fulfill this requirement.

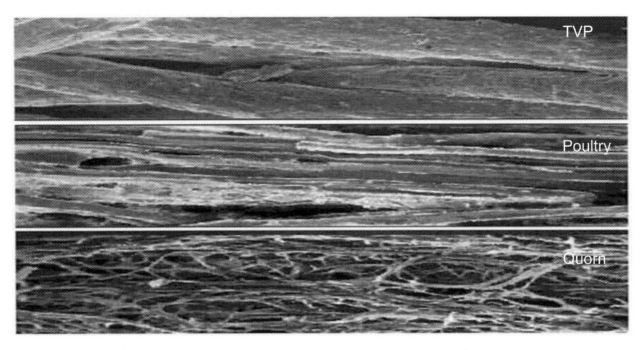

FIGURE 19.5 Microscopic view comparison of Quorn with textured vegetable protein and poultry muscle tissue.

The strength of the mycoprotein and egg system can be visualized as being dependent on the properties of both the entangled fibers and the gelled protein—a fiber gel composite. If we assume (and only for the sake of argument) that the rigidity of the hyphae and strength of the gel are constant then what other factors impact on overall system strength. There are some interesting hypotheses to consider here.

19.3.2.2 Hyphal Morphology

Hyphal aspect ratio and degree of branching will intuitively affect the degree of entanglement—if the aspect ratio were 1 for example, as with a sphere, it would be somewhat difficult to create an entangled mass.

We have also observed that below c.400 microns in length there is a tendency to increase the bitty sensory characteristic which is undesirable in finished product eating quality and leads to descriptors such as "cakey" and "short." Indeed, the correlations of overall hyphal morphology (length and branch frequency) with eating quality are a subject of continuous and ongoing research but could be argued to be somewhat academic given that producing a single "ideal" hyphal geometry during fermentation is not yet possible.

19.3.2.3 Interaction Between Hyphae

Apart from the physical nature of hyphal entanglement there will also be a degree of interaction between the "surface chemistry" of the hyphae and also the amount of interaction with the gelled interstitial albumen. In addition, if we were to imagine pulling an individual hyphae out from the biomass then the resistance to pulling the hyphae out is determined both by the entanglement and the adhesive forces of the albumen gel (its gel strength). This has recently been demonstrated by Finnigan, Akintoye, and Mousavi (2015) in the use of calcium to impact hyphal rheology presumably by interhyphal bridging and the creation of improved meat-like texture.

Thus, the nature and scope of the entanglement and the adhesive forces created by the albumen must be correlated with eating quality but remains the topic for further research.

19.3.2.4 Orientation and Dispersion of the Hyphae

If the hyphae could be aligned totally then the response of the system to any applied force would depend on whether the hyphae were parallel or perpendicular to the applied force. If randomly entangled then no such effect would occur. Thus, dispersion is important since if the hyphae are dispersed as clumps then it will be the behavior of 'the clump' that will be most important and given that clumps tend to have an aspect ratio of 1, then we risk a preponderance of nonentangled clumps. In addition, water trapped within the clumps becomes unavailable for solute dissolution, for example flavor and albumen.

19.3.2.5 Hyphal Pressure

The amount of hyphal pressure (turgor) that remains within the hyphae post RNA reduction must impact on eating quality either through a correlation with features such as entanglement, system strength, surface properties, or by the degree of "expressible water" that the cells possess and impact on degree of solute dissolution. Hyphal turgor will be influenced most significantly by the nature of the RNA reduction process where the temperature is elevated in order to allow the endogenous nuclease to degrade RNA to levels below c.2% (dry weight). The time–temperature combinations involved can impact overall yield dramatically, presumably by altering the cell membrane structure and characteristics which can result in losses of intercellular material of up to 30%.

19.3.2.6 Phase Volume

The packing fraction of a system of rigid rods will be 0.5. However, the flexible hyphae might be argued to achieve 0.6 (ie, 60 g hyphae occupy 100 mL). But how important is this, and what is in the "space" not occupied by the hyphae? Suboptimal distribution of the albumen binder, for example, within this matrix will lead to binder-starved regions and product weakness. Thus, hyphal properties will impact on the packing density that can be achieved.

19.3.3 Process Variables That Impact Quality

Whilst the physical properties of the hyphae including surface charge can be argued to impact finished product quality, the interactions with process are also a key determinant of the successful development of meat-like textures.

19.3.3.1 Mixing

The challenge for mixing technology is that mycoprotein is essentially a viscoelastic paste into which we are adding powdered ingredients of variable hydration characteristics and expecting effective dispersion at a production mixer scale of 2 tonnes, such that uniform dispersion must be achieved at the functional consumer unit of c.10–15 g. Rheological properties of mycoprotein will, of course, be highly correlated with the previously described RNA reduction process as well as the level of solids achieved in the final harvested biomass.

19.3.3.2 Fiber Alignment

It is known that fiber alignment occurs during induced extensional flow of mycoprotein (Miri, 2004; Miri, Barigou, Fryer, & Cox, 2005). Within the manufacturing process this begins during the forming process precook and the process must be optimized to develop the correct flow patterns that are effectively precursors to the final meat-like texture.

19.3.3.3 Thermal Gel Creation

Heat setting is a key unit process. Any mixing effects and fiber alignments are "fixed" at this point, converting a soft and dough-like texture to a rubbery precursor to meat-like eating quality.

We know that hyphae respond differently to heat setting by steaming than to heat setting by microwaving for example. In the latter, the hyphae tend to be plumper and protein dispersion is more uniform at the surface and formation of a gel is heavily influenced by environmental conditions such as mixedness, ionic strength, and rate of heating and cooling.

We know that air inclusion within the mix can cause air pockets to form on heating, promoting areas of softer texture. This can be a particular problem if CO_2 has been used to cool and has not been adequately removed by vacuum. Recent work is also pointing to the significance of the gel properties post freezing in the creation of meat-like texture.

19.3.3.4 Freezing and Frozen Storage

Of all the unit processes employed in the production of Quorn none is more impactful than freezing and frozen storage (Evans, 1996). In fact, for optimal texture we require relatively slow freezing (compared with conventional food freezing processes), as the development of ice crystals appears to compress the mycoprotein fibers into bundles that convey meat-like texture in the mouth (Rodger & Angold, 1991). We also know that "Ostwald ripening" of these crystals appears to improve "meatiness" over time in storage but that lengthy storage can result in product defects, typically a change in the distribution of expressible water giving rise to high initial juiciness but then a dry and woody chew.

19.3.4 Creation of Granular Comminute Texture

Mycoprotein can also behave as a continuous phase into which previously textured mycoprotein (or other textured proteins) can be dispersed. Finnigan and Stephens (1996) have demonstrated this ability in the creation of so-called comminuted textures such as burgers and sausage where the whole muscle-like texture is not appropriate. This has allowed the commercial application of mycoprotein in creating a range of textures beyond the characteristic whole-muscle texture of Quorn fillets or pieces through to the more granular comminuted textures of Quorn burgers and sausages. More recently, exciting developments in the creation of textured vegetable proteins from new sources and processes has further improved the quality of the products achieved in synergy with mycoprotein, highlighting the importance of technical collaboration in this space.

19.3.5 Fat Mimetics

When a dispersion of mycoprotein in water at c.20% w/v is subjected to very high-pressure homogenization (in excess of 20,000 psi) we observe significant conformational change to the hyphae. The effect of this pressure is to change the aspect ratio of the hyphae and to create particles that when mixed into certain food systems have the ability to behave as fat mimetics. Finnigan and Blanchard (2009) demonstrated this effect in the creation of frozen ice creams at c.4% total fat but with a creamy mouthfeel suggestive of a more indulgent high-fat system.

19.4 NUTRITIONAL CHARACTERISTICS OF MYCOPROTEIN

19.4.1 Nutritional Properties

The chemical analysis of mycoprotein demonstrates that it contains a wide spectrum of nutrients. The general nutrition properties of mycoprotein have been the subject of various publications (Edelman, Fewell, & Solomons, 1983; Edwards, 1993; Sadler, 1990, 1991; Wheelock, 1993).

Overall, mycoprotein is a source of good-quality protein which is combined with low-energy and high-fiber content. Its fat consists of largely unsaturated fatty acids, predominantly ω-6 and ω-3, linoleic and linolenic acids, respectively. The fiber is a mixture of chitin and β-glucans that performs physiologically as dietary fiber and does not have any adverse effect on mineral status.

19.4.1.1 Protein

The intended use of mycoprotein in products that form the center of a meal requires that mycoprotein provide high-quality protein. Analyses of the amino acid composition, represented in Table 19.4, demonstrate that mycoprotein contains all of the essential amino acids.

Bioassays in chicks have shown that methionine and lysine are highly available. The sulfur amino acids, methionine and cysteine, are the first limiting ones, and lysine is particularly important for growth. Rat bioassays have demonstrated that the protein efficiency ratio (PER) and net protein utilization (NPU) are both in excess of 85% of the values for casein (Jonker, 1995). Slope ratio assays in rats gave similar or better results in comparison with casein.

A human volunteer study at the Massachusetts Institute of Technology (MIT) confirmed that the results of the animal assays could be extrapolated to man (Udall, Lo, Young, & Scrimshaw, 1984). The results are summarized in Table 19.5. In comparison to skimmed milk protein, mycoprotein had the same biological value (BV), whilst the NPU was calculated to be slightly lower as a result of the somewhat lower digestibility (D) and the content of nonprotein nitrogen.

Subsequently, a study in ileostomy subjects at the Dunn Clinical Nutrition Centre, Cambridge, United Kingdom, was completed in 1989 (Cummings, 1990). The study included measurements of nitrogen digestibility which were higher (89.8%) than the earlier human data in Table 19.5, generated at MIT.

A PDCAAS of 0.91 had been calculated using the protein digestibility data from MIT (Miller & Dwyer, 2001). As ileal digestibility is recognized to be a better measure than whole-gut digestibility, the PDCAAS was recalculated using the most recent data from the Dunn study. A conservative digestibility value of 86% was used for the calculation because analytical data suggested that around 10% nonprotein nitrogen (from glucosamine) may have been digested, though this is uncertain. The resulting figure was 0.996 (Edwards & Cummings, 2010).

TABLE 19.4 Typical Amino Acid Analysis of Mycoprotein

Amino Acid	g/100 g Protein	Amino Acid	g/100 g Protein
Lysine	8.3	Histidine	3.5
Methionine	2.1	Arginine	7.3
Cystine	0.8	Tyrosine	4.0
Threonine	5.5	Aspartic acid	10.3
Tryptophan	1.6	Serine	5.1
Valine	6.2	Glutamic acid	12.5
Leucine	8.6	Proline	4.5
Isoleucine	5.2	Glycine	4.5
Phenylalanine	4.9	Alanine	6.0

TABLE 19.5 Typical Protein Quality of Mycoprotein

Test Material	Protein Quality of Mycoprotein				
	In Rat		In Human		
	PER	NPU	Digestibility	Biological Value	NPU (Calculated)
Mycoprotein	2.4	61	78	84	65
Mycoprotein + methionine	3.4	82	79	92	73
Casein	2.5	70	–	–	–
Skimmed milk	–	–	95	85	80

NPU, net protein utilization; *PER*, protein efficiency ratio.

19.4.1.2 Fat

The fat in mycoprotein is very low in saturates and high in mono- and polyunsaturated fatty acids. As mycoprotein is low in available carbohydrate, approximately one-third of its energy content is contributed by fat, typically containing 13 g/100 g on a dry basis and 3.25 g/100 g as consumed (25% solids). Typically, 40% of the fat in mycoprotein consists of polyunsaturates, 11% monounsaturates, and 11% saturates. Each 100 g of dry mycoprotein provides 4.3 g of the ω-6 fatty acid linoleic acid (c.18:2) together with a relatively high concentration (6.9 g) of ω-3, linolenic acid (c.18:3). Data concerning the fatty acid composition of mycoprotein are summarized in Table 19.6.

Of the total lipid content, 65% is in the form of triglycerides and diglycerides and 30% as phospholipids. The remaining 5% consists of sterols and unsaponifiables.

19.4.1.3 Fiber

The cell wall components contribute a dietary fiber content of about 25 g/100 g of mycoprotein dry matter, which is over 6 g/100 g on a 25% solids basis. This gives mycoprotein the unusual combination of being a source of protein which is not only low in fat, but also rich in fiber. The amount and composition of the fiber were confirmed in research undertaken at the Dunn Clinical Nutrition Centre, Cambridge, United Kingdom. It is largely insoluble fiber, consisting of approximately one-third chitin (poly-N-acetyl glucosamine) and two-thirds β-glucans. A study in ileostomy patients demonstrated that the fiber remained largely undigested in the small intestine, and in vitro microbiological investigations indicated that it would be fermented in the large intestine. Thus, both analytically and physiologically the cell wall components have been confirmed to possess characteristics consistent with their classification as dietary fiber (Table 19.7).

TABLE 19.6 Typical Fatty Acid Composition of Mycoprotein

Fatty Acid Composition of Pycoprotein		
Fatty Acid		g/100 g
Palmitic	16:0	1.3
Stearic	18:0	0.2
Oleic	18:1	1.4
Linoleic	18:2	4.3
Linolenic	18:3	0.9

TABLE 19.7 Typical Nonstarch Polysaccharide Content of Mycoprotein

Analysis of Mycoprotein Nonstarch Polysaccharides		
Component	Soluble (g/100 g Dry Matter)	Insoluble (g/100 g Dry Matter)
N-acetyl galactosamine	0.25	0.09
N-acetyl glucosamine	0.43	9.31
Arabinose	0.16	0.06
Mannose	0.63	2.67
Galactose	0.37	0.77
Glucose	0.58	8.22
Uronic acid	0.43	2.00
Subtotals	3.22	23.12
Total fiber	26.34	

TABLE 19.8 Typical Mineral Content of Mycoprotein

Mineral	mg/kg	Mineral	mg/kg
Calcium	1700	Iron	30
Phosphorus	1050	Zinc	400
Potassium	4000	Copper	20
Sodium	200	Manganese	250
Magnesium	1850		

19.4.1.4 Minerals

Mycoprotein contains a range of minerals, as summarized in Table 19.8.

As background consumption of the fiber in mycoprotein is limited because intakes of similar sources such as mushroom fiber and arthropod chitin are generally low, the question of possible effects on mineral absorption has been investigated. No adverse effect on mineral balance was found with regard to calcium, phosphorus, magnesium, iron, copper, and zinc.

TABLE 19.9 Apparent Absorption of Minerals Following a Digestibility Study in Ileostomy Patients

Mineral Absorption	Diet		
	Mycoprotein	PSF	Bread
Calcium (%)	31.5	28.3	29.5
Phosphorus (%)	80.3	74.4	73.5
Magnesium (%)	48.4	42.8	42.1
Iron (%)	46.7	40.5	49.8
Zinc (%)	19.3	23.8	24.4

PSF, polysaccharide-free diet.

TABLE 19.10 Typical Vitamin Content of Mycoprotein

Vitamin	mg/kg
Thiamin	0.4
Riboflavin	9
Niacin	14
Pyridoxine	5
Pantothenic acid	10
Folic acid	0.4
Biotin	0.6

The fiber research at the Dunn Clinical Nutrition Centre included an examination of mineral absorption during the digestibility study involving ileostomy patients. There was no significant effect on the apparent absorption of calcium, magnesium, phosphorus, iron, and zinc in comparison with a polysaccharide-free diet (PSF) and wholemeal bread (see Table 19.9).

19.4.1.5 Vitamins

Mycoprotein contains a range of water-soluble, B vitamins as shown in Table 19.10.

19.4.2 Nutrition Research

The nutrition research into mycoprotein has been reviewed by Denny, Aisbitt, and Lunn (2008).

19.4.2.1 Effects on Total Cholesterol, LDL Cholesterol, and High-Density Lipoprotein Cholesterol

Clinical studies performed with mycoprotein have demonstrated that it has the ability to lower total and LDL blood cholesterol.

The first demonstration that mycoprotein has the ability to lower blood cholesterol was in the tolerance study by Udall et al. (1984), where the only significant change in blood analysis was a lowering of blood cholesterol during the mycoprotein phase of the study. Two studies by Turnbull, Leeds, and Edwards (1990, 1992), at King's College, University of London, demonstrated that mycoprotein lowers total and LDL cholesterol in subjects with slightly raised cholesterol levels under both clinically controlled and free-living conditions. In the first study, 17 subjects were provided with clinically prepared meals in which mycoprotein was incorporated at 190 g/day for 3 weeks

(Turnbull et al., 1990). Total cholesterol and LDL blood cholesterol were significantly reduced, and high-density lipoprotein (HDL) cholesterol increased. Furthermore, the apolipoproteins A1 and B decreased in subjects receiving the mycoprotein compared to baseline. In the second study, 21 subjects were provided 27 g dry weight of mycoprotein (approximated to 130 g of regular moisture mycoprotein) per day in biscuit form as part of their normal diets for 8 weeks (Turnbull et al., 1992). Blood was collected at baseline, 4, and 8 weeks. Total cholesterol and LDL cholesterol decreased over the 8-week study, though no statistically significant differences were observed in HDL cholesterol and apolipoproteins. Studies in Japanese subjects confirmed these effects, even though the subjects generally had lower starting cholesterol levels (Homma et al., 1995; Ishikawa et al., 1995; Nakamura et al., 1994).

19.4.2.2 Effects on Satiety

Studies by Burley, Paul, and Blundell (1993) and Turnbull, Walton, and Leeds (1993) demonstrated that when subjects received a nutritionally comparable lunch based on either chicken or mycoprotein, those receiving mycoprotein felt less hungry during the afternoon and when offered an ad libitum evening meal consumed less than those who had previously eaten chicken. A further study by Burley (unpublished) showed that the effect was still evident after repeated administration of mycoprotein.

In a more recent study at the Pennington Research Center, Baton Rouge, United States, the effects of a preload of mycoprotein, tofu, or chicken prior to a test meal were measured (Williamson et al., 2006). In addition, the effect on subsequent intake at a later, ad libitum meal was also measured. Compared to chicken, mycoprotein reduced food intake of the test meal and there was no compensation for this at the later, ad libitum meal. In other words, subjects receiving mycoprotein consumed less at their next meal and did not eat any more at the following meal. Tofu had a similar effect. Recent work at Imperial (Bottin, 2014) has again demonstrated proof of principle that diets rich in mycoprotein can exert a positive effect on appetite regulation. An interesting working hypothesis is now being explored looking at the production of short-chain fatty acids from gut digestion of fiber in mycoprotein and their link with appetite regulation.

19.4.2.3 Effects on the Glycemic Response

Mycoprotein also has the ability to reduce the glycemic response, that is, the rate of change in blood glucose, following its inclusion in a standard test meal (Turnbull & Ward, 1995). In this study, 19 subjects were asked to fast overnight and on the next day they received a single serving of a control milkshake containing soya flour and dried skim milk, or an experimental milkshake containing 20 mg of mycoprotein. Blood samples were taken at fasting and in 30-min intervals up to 120 min postprandial. The postprandial serum glucose response was statistically lower in subjects receiving the mycoprotein milkshake compared to controls, and the serum insulin response also exhibited a similar trend, with statistical significance achieved at 30 and 60 min postprandial. The areas under the curve for serum glucose and insulin were significantly lower in subjects receiving mycoprotein. The authors concluded that mycoprotein would be a beneficial supplement to diets of healthy and diabetic individuals.

19.5 MYCOPROTEIN AND ENVIRONMENTAL IMPACT

The world is going to need many solutions to the complex issues of providing sustainable solutions to global food security. Opinion leaders are now talking with increasing clarity about the so-called trilemma (Tilman & Clark, 2014) where separating our dietary choices from their impact on both human health and the health of the planet is no longer tenable. Mycoprotein offers an important example of a healthy new protein with a low environmental impact and as such one of the many solutions we will need to address this issue of our generation.

By 2050 world population is set to increase to above 9 billion, which is over 30% higher than today (FAO, 2009). In order to feed this larger, wealthier, and more urban population, food production will need to rise by 70% (FAO, 2009). This means an increase in cereal cultivation of over 1 billion tonnes and an increase in meat production of over 200 million tonnes (FAO, 2009). Much of the increased demand for meat is forecast to come from the Asian markets, with China already consuming more meat than either the United States or the European Union even though its per capita consumption is currently only half that found in these markets.

In 2013, the UK government's report on food security reinforced the need for a change in behavior such that meat is promoted as an occasional treat rather than an everyday staple (House of Commons, 2013). Meanwhile, as demand begins to outstrip supply, so meat prices will continue to rise, placing excessive strain on the supply chain and leaving us vulnerable to issues such as the "horsemeat scandal." In fact, there is now worldwide recognition that this increase in demand for meat simply cannot be met. Many reports are now highlighting that continued focus on intensification of existing agriculture to provide a solution risks both catastrophic impacts for our health and for the environment (Lymbery & Oakeshott, 2014) as well as increasing the potential for conflict over vital resources such as land and water.

Our understanding of climate change continues to grow. Recent reports from the IPCC suggest a significant deepening of concern with predictions that "nobody will be untouched by the impacts of climate change" (IPCC, 2014). In addition, science is now telling us that agriculture and food production have a surprisingly important role within this and represent around 25–32% of global anthropogenic greenhouse gas (GHG) emissions (Steinfeld, et al., 2006), with livestock alone emitting 11–18% of global emissions (de Vries & de Boer, 2010). Whilst reductions in emissions are possible these impacts could also increase as demand for meat grows, damaging the very ecosystems needed to produce crops for animal feed. In fact, the production of meat from plant proteins is inherently inefficient with huge amounts of grain and crops being used to feed livestock when it could be fed directly to humans. Currently, more than 90% of global soya production is used as animal feed, with analysts estimating that nearly 40% of cereals are also used in this way, representing a highly inefficient use of this food and the land required to grow it (D'Silva & Webster, 2010). Reports also show that over 15,000 liters of water (Dibb & Fitzpatrick 2014) are required to produce one kilo of beef and that if meat consumption continues to rise as predicted then the amount of water required to grow animal feed will need to double by the middle of this century. With over 2.5 billion people already living in areas of water stress (McKinney, Schoch, & Yonavjak, 2013) and with global warming predicted to further reduce its availability, conflicts over water are expected to become more acute.

Our appetite for more and cheaper meat is also driving a whole industry of chemicals used extensively as fertilizers and pesticides, with concerns that this is altering much of the balance of nature and biodiversity. In addition, whilst some nations are working to restrict and control the use of antibiotics as growth promoters in the production of meat, their widespread use has caused many now to talk of a new era of antibiotic-resistant bacteria and the return of pandemic disease in humans (Lymbery & Oakeshott, 2014).

19.5.1 Environmental Impact

Agriculture and food production contribute up to 29% of all global greenhouse gases, with around half of this generated by the production of livestock (Bailey, Froggatt, & Wellesley, 2014).

Hypothetically, products made from mycoprotein should inherently have a lower environmental impact than meat and in order to investigate this hypothesis, initial life cycle analysis (LCA) research carried out in conjunction with De Montfort University in 2010 revealed that Quorn mince may have half the embedded carbon when compared with beef (Allen et al., 2009; Finnigan et al., 2010).

The acknowledged health benefits of mycoprotein combined with lower levels of embedded carbon compared with meat therefore suggested a valuable role for Quorn with consumers who may wish to reduce meat consumption. Further analysis began in 2011 as part of a Knowledge Transfer Partnership involving Sheffield Hallam University and Innovate UK, with a view to improving the quality of the LCA data of this initial scoping study by completing product carbon footprints for mycoprotein and best-selling Quorn retail products.

Continuing research begins to establish the wider environmental impacts of Quorn products; assessing not only the embedded GHG emissions associated with the products but also the water and land use footprints associated with Quorn Foods' supply chain—all with a continued commitment to independent certification and validation.

19.5.1.1 Product Carbon Footprint

Quorn Foods are the first global meat-alternative company to achieve third-party certification of its product carbon footprint figures. This enabled the business through analysis of the entire product lifecycle of individual products to communicate confidently the GHG emissions of mycoprotein and the finished products Quorn Mince and Quorn Chicken-style Pieces. Further benefits relate to the analysis of supply-chain carbon "hotspots" and associated evaluation of alternative product formulations.

Fundamentally though, achieving this level of data assurance allows for confident and consistent communication of product lifecycle emissions as well as a standardized approach to product comparison and reporting. Understanding where the carbon footprint of Quorn products may fit within the wider sustainable diets debate and specifically when compared to animal-based protein production systems is of real value.

As part of the communications strategy for this research, the Carbon Reduction Label is used both on-pack and as part of corporate communications to highlight the rigor and comparability of the product carbon footprinting undertaken.

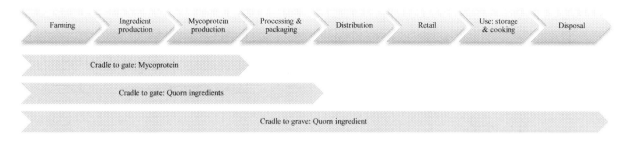

FIGURE 19.6 Boundaries for product carbon footprint analysis.

TABLE 19.11 Carbon Emission Reduction 2012–15 (Carbon Trust, 2015)

Product	Country	Reduction
Mycoprotein	United Kingdom	15%
Quorn Mince (frozen)	United Kingdom	10%
Quorn Pieces (frozen)	United Kingdom	11%

19.5.1.1.1 Methodology

The footprinting exercise completed in 2012 consisted of a "footprint–preassess–certify–communicate" process. The scope of analysis covered both cradle-to-grave and cradle-to-gate investigations for mycoprotein and key Quorn retail products (see Fig. 19.6). Research analysis was carried out internally, therefore allowing not only for supply chain analysis to be carried out with complete transparency but also for capacity building within the business; allowing for continued and more varied environmental analyses to continue as knowledge develops.

Independent certification provided by the Carbon Trust complies with the requirements of internationally recognized standards (BSI 2008): PAS 2050: 2011; the Product Carbon Footprint Protocol parts 1 & 2; and the certification requirements of the Carbon Trust's Footprint Expert Guide (v4.1). Third-party certification allowed for the research to benefit from a consistent verification method applied to the models, as well as an impartial and independent evaluation. It verified the footprint models and data as certified to the standards mentioned and also ensured quality assurance of the traceability, assumptions, and activity data assessed.

The underlying quality and validity of the data compiled to complete this analysis were fundamental and were assessed using the data quality assessment of the Carbon Trust's product carbon footprinting software package (Footprint Expert). This framework sets out requirements stipulating, for example, that certification requires Grade A-quality data to be used to support at least 70% of emissions, Grade B to support a maximum of 25%, and C a maximum of 5. Data quality attributes considered are either of an intrinsic or an application nature. Based on Section 7.2 of PAS 2050, intrinsic qualities consider, for example: complete, consistent, reproducible and precise data, whilst application quality queries the age, geographical area, and technology applied.

Initially certified in 2012 by the Carbon Trust, the recertification process and a number of new product certifications were completed in 2015. The recertification process established that a number of energy and resource efficiency activities carried out throughout both the direct operations of Quorn Foods and also its supply chain, resulted in a reduction of up to 15% of the certified product carbon footprints (Table 19.11).

19.5.1.1.2 Results and Key Comparisons

The importance of independent certification cannot be underestimated when the wider aim is to share product carbon footprint results. In the case of the data shown in Table 19.12, such results may then be discussed in relation to the sustainable diets debate and responsibly contribute to consideration around the GHG emissions impacts of the dietary choices we make.

TABLE 19.12 Certified Carbon Emissions per kg (Carbon Trust, 2015)

Product	Cradle-to-Gate kgCO$_2$e Rounded	Cradle-to-Grave kgCO$_2$e Rounded
Mycoprotein[a]	1.6	
Quorn Mince (frozen)[b]	2.4	3.6
Quorn Mince (chilled)[a]	4.5	5.5
Quorn Pieces (frozen)[b]	2.2	3.8
Quorn Pieces (chilled)[a]	4.5	5.5

[a]United Kingdom only.
[b]United Kingdom, Nordic, South Africa, Australia, and New Zealand markets.

Livestock is estimated to contribute to more than 14% of GHG emissions (Bailey et al., 2014)—a greater share than transport. Therefore it is apparent that an understanding of the environmental impacts of alternative proteins be part of the overall commentary on sustainable diets.

For comparisons to be made in a consistent and measured way, a third-party report was commissioned in 2014 to identify credible carbon, water, and land use footprinting information for, firstly, beef and chicken, and contrast this with data for the Quorn equivalent products; Quorn mince and pieces. The analysis used consistent boundaries (cradle to processing gate) and also took account of the variation in farming systems that can lead to significant differences in environmental efficiency, especially when considering beef production. Indeed the approach to comparisons commits itself to a truly conservative approach, that is, figures for the better performing farms or systems are the ones used for comparison.

Beef The product carbon footprint of Quorn mince can be considered to be at least 10 times lower than that of beef. The analysis report used a methodology developed by the Carbon Trust and based upon the dairy guidelines (Dairy UK, Dairy Co., & The Carbon Trust, 2010) and is fully compatible with IDF guidelines (IDF, 2010) and FAO beef studies (Gerber et al., 2013; Opio, 2013). It has been used over 100,000 times on nearly 40,000 farms in the United Kingdom and Ireland (EBLEX, 2012). The boundary for analysis includes all feed production, manure storage/spreading, and enteric methane of four generic beef production systems in the United Kingdom, though the two of particular interest concern "intensive mixed" and "extensive grazing."

Chicken The product carbon footprint of Quorn pieces can be considered to be at least four times lower than that of chicken. Data from FAO analysis (MacLeod et al., 2013) as well as PAS 2050-certified industry data for both United Kingdom and Irish systems, applied via methodology that takes account of the additional waste burden (eg, bones) that would derive a comparable edible meat yield footprint for comparison to Quorn—as opposed to published data referring only to carcass weight.

Therefore, it is clear that Quorn products may well have a significant role to play in addressing the challenges of our food system and its associated GHG impacts.

19.5.1.2 Water Footprint

Water is a scarce resource and will come under increasing pressure as the global population increases. It is estimated that 92% of all fresh water used by humankind relates to agriculture and food production. The changes in global economic structure have seen a parallel increase in the demand for meat and this is set to continue to grow, and through water footprinting it has been shown that meat production uses significantly more water than food of plant origin per nutritional unit (Gerbens-Leenes, Mekonnen, & Hoekstra, 2013).

Water footprinting follows a cradle-to-gate approach, from raw materials, including the origin and growing of feed for animal-sourced products, up to the processing and packing of the finished product. Water footprinting divides water use into three categories:

- Blue water—this is surface and ground water, found in rivers and lakes;
- Green water—this is the water held by the land in soil and is the proportion associated with crop growth;
- Gray water—defined as the volume of freshwater required to dilute pollutants created throughout a production supply chain to maintain water quality standards.

TABLE 19.13 Water Footprint per Unit of Weight and per Unit of Nutritional Value

Food Source	Green Water (L/kg)	Blue Water (L/kg)	Gray Water (L/kg)	Total (L/kg)	Energy (L/kcal)	Protein (L/g)
Mycoprotein	540	35	202	777	0.9	6
Quorn Mince	1500	60	400	1960	1.9	14
Quorn Pieces	1300	60	350	1710	1.9	12
Frozen soya beans[a]	2037	70	37	2145	1.4	19
Tofu[a]	2397	83	44	2523	3.5[d]	31
Cereals[a]	1232	228	184	1644	0.5	21
Pulses[a]	3180	141	734	4055	1.2	19
Vegetables[a]	194	43	85	322	1.34	26
Milk[a]	863	86	72	1021	1.82	31
Eggs[a]	2592	244	429	3265	2.29	29
Global beef[a]	14414	550	451	15415	10	112
UK beef average[b]	20700	100	3700	24500	16	178
UK beef mixed[c]	15500	250	4000	19750	13	143
UK beef grazed[c]	16500	300	5000	21800	14	158
Chicken[a]	3545	313	467	4325	3	34

[a]Hoekstra (2013).
[b]Chatterton, Hess, and Williams (2011).
[c]Carbon Trust Comparison Report (2014).
[d]Mccance and Widdowson (2002).

To evaluate and understand the water impact of mycoprotein and Quorn product footprinting, research has been conducted throughout the supply chain. This research gives transparency on the use of water, allowing on-going plans for the reduction of water per unit, and enabling benchmarking and comparisons with other food products. The results of this research are detailed in Table 19.13.

The results confirm that Quorn can play an important role providing protein and energy more efficiently than meat, utilizing limited water resources. Whilst the level of water used in the production of meat will vary by location, animal, and method of production, currently available data suggest that the water footprint of beef could be 10 times greater than Quorn mince, and chicken up to three times greater than Quorn pieces. What is notable is that of the plant and animal products reviewed, Quorn requires the lowest quantity of water per gram of protein produced.

19.5.1.3 Land Use

With over 70% of agricultural land currently used for livestock production, the growing demand for meat means that more efficient solutions are needed as land becomes scarcer. There are many published studies, the results of which vary significantly between approaches, however, in all studies protein produced from plants seems to be much more land-efficient per unit than from livestock.

Quorn Foods have investigated the land required to make their leading ingredient products, again following a cradle-to-gate approach from agriculture to finished product. For the basis of comparison, a Carbon Trust report (Carbon Trust, 2014) assessed the land use requirements for a range of beef and chicken production systems.

For beef, this analysis and the main modeling criteria thereof take account of a wide variety of factors—chiefly varying herd management and feeding regimens but also incorporating nutrition type (grass-based or with a proportion of supplementary feed), impact of seasonality on this, variable kill out ratios and finished weights, relative digestibility

TABLE 19.14 Comparative Land Use per kg of Product

Source	Land (ha/kg)
Mycoprotein	0.00017
Quorn Mince (frozen)	0.0004
Quorn Pieces (frozen)	0.0003
Beef—mixed feeding	0.0035
Beef—grazed	0.0049
Chicken	0.0007

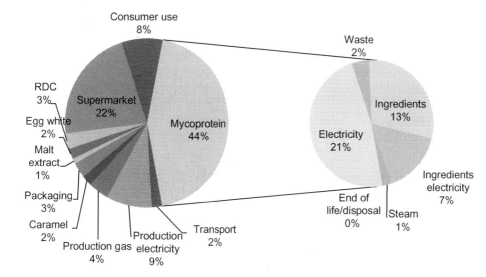

FIGURE 19.7 Breakdown of CO_2e emissions by various aspects of Quorn mince production.

of the diets, and, of course, the productivity of the animal is key to understanding this metric. Sources such as EBLEX (2011) and DEFRA (2014) were used for data relating to, for example, dry matter requirements. The results suggest that land used for the production of Quorn mince is up to 10 times lower than for beef (see Table 19.14).

To establish the average land requirements for chicken farming systems, Williams, Audsley, and Sandars (2006) and Carbon Trust industry data formed the basis of the analysis. Factors including feed ingredients for both broiler and layer systems, yield and typical United Kingdom feed amounts to produce a kilogram of meat were used to thereby estimate ha/kg of chicken meat. The results suggest that land used for the production of Quorn pieces is at least two times lower than for chicken.

Studies have shown that between 12 and 24 kg of feed are required to produce 1 kg of edible beef (Ramirez, Patel, & Blok, 2006). Poultry has a higher conversion efficiency but typically requires 2–4 kg (Pimental & Pimental, 2003) and in both cases more protein is fed to the animal than is actually produced. The production of mycoprotein simply takes the carbohydrate from the grain and converts it to protein—without the need for animals. In fact, because the original grain protein remains available, the Quorn process actually increases the overall protein balance.

19.5.2 How Low Can We Go?

Work continues in driving down the environmental impacts of the organization further, whilst investment in projects that contribute to increasingly efficient supply chain systems for mycoprotein and finished Quorn products will thereby result in improvements to comparison metrics such as GHG emissions, water and land use, not to mention more efficient use of resources, reduction in waste, and redistribution of food waste.

Analysis to date is vital in understanding where we can improve. Fig. 19.7 reveals the breakdown of emissions of Quorn Mince from cradle to grave. Almost half of the emissions associated with the full lifecycle of this product are attributable to mycoprotein. Of this segment, it is clear that wheat farming and electricity usage are most significant. Indeed, this full "farming to consumer" scope of analysis reveals that around 60% of total product emissions are created by electricity use—thereby both a key risk and also an opportunity for the business.

In 2013, Quorn Foods established the organizational footprint of the business and its Scope 1 and 2 emissions at a corporate level. This work modeled the future position of the company based on growth targets, recognized that the carbon intensity of the business had fallen (2010−12), and evaluated options for emissions mitigation. This allowed for a realistic target to be set of 14% reduction in carbon emissions per tonne of production by 2016 based on a 2012 baseline; a target that was surpassed with achievement of a 14% reduction already by December 2014.

In addition, the organizational water footprint for the Quorn Foods business and factories has been established and evaluated. Quorn Foods have demonstrated a steady reduction in annual water use achieved through factory and supply chain projects, with water usage now over 20% below that measured in 2011 per tonne of product. The scope for further and ongoing reduction is under constant review.

19.5.2.1 Cradle to Cradle Approach

This lifecycle approach to the analysis of Quorn products is beneficial, not only to understand and therefore reduce use of resources and environmental impacts but, more generally, to offer a complete and multifaceted view of the economic, social, and environmental dimensions of the organization and its value chain. By adopting this approach and applying it to the program of research projects ongoing, one can seek to answer the question of—just how much more sustainable could Quorn Foods aspire to become?

Process optimization and yield improvement plans are core to the current business approach. This yields fascinating projects, particularly at our Billingham fermentation site and with the production of mycoprotein; whereby strategies to improve harvesting techniques, reduce operational downtime, explore alternative raw materials and introduce new technologies are continuing to challenge current methods of production and strive for improvements.

An example of this is the culmination of many years' research into the alternative gelling agents appropriate for Quorn products where the use of egg albumen was to be reduced or avoided, the latter to access vegan consumers. After extensive research and development, a number of alternative plant-based proteins were found to be appropriate in achieving a suitable texture capability in combination. These proteins also offer a more sustainable option; particularly as they avoid the use of animal-based farming systems and the inherant inefficiencies. A range of vegan products have now been launched in UK retailers and are building good distribution. More launches are planned within international markets, which will widen the appeal and accessibility of the Quorn product range to consumers.

A research project investigating a range of hybrid meat products (part meat−part plant-based protein such as Quorn) is also in progress and will offer interesting case studies in terms of related benefits to the consumer's diet on a nutritional, physiological, and environmental basis.

We are aiming to establish value from materials previously defined as waste. For example, our fermentation technology is being scrutinized in order to establish the ways in which elements of the liquid waste stream could be utilized in other industries for significant value. Whether this relates to flavor components, nucleotides, or protein elements, this could certainly be fascinating with regards to the potential impact on the current economic and environmental structure of the business.

This makes for a very exciting vision of the future for Quorn Foods—who aim to challenge established boundaries at all stages of the supply chain and also actively collaborate and share information.

REFERENCES

Allen, B., Ozawa-Meida, L., Lemon, M., & Paton, I. (2009). *Phase 1 Report: Scoping study to investigate the Quorn production process and identify comparisons with the production of beef and chicken products.* Institute of Energy and Sustainable Development. De Montfort University. Personal Communication.

Angold, R., Beech, G., & Taggart, J. (1989). *Mycoprotein: A case study, and mycoprotein: The process. Food Biotechnology* (pp. 87−122). Cambridge: Cambridge University Press.

Bailey, R., Froggatt, A., & Wellesley, L. (2014). *Livestock − climate change's forgotten sector.* Global Public Opinion on Meat and Dairy Consumption.

Bottin, J. (2014). *Nutritional and surgical influences on appetite regulation and body composition in overweight and obese humans.* Ph.D. thesis. Imperial College London.

BSI (2008). *Guide to PAS 2050. How to assess the carbon footprint of goods and services.* London: BSI.

Burley, V. J., Paul, A. W., & Blundell, J. E. (1993). Influence of a high-fibre food (myco-protein) on appetite: Effects on satiation (within meals) and satiety (following meals). *European Journal of Clinical Nutrition, 47*(6), 409–418.

Carbon Trust (The) (2014). *Quorn, beef and chicken footprints*. Internal Company Report.

Carbon Trust (The) (2015). Report to Marlow Foods on product carbon footprint certification.

Chatterton, J. C., Hess, T. M., & Williams, A. G. (2011). *The water footprint of English beef and lamb production*. UK: Cranfield University.

Cummings, J. H. (1990). *Final report of the studies of the digestion of mycoprotein in the human stomach and small intestine*. Dunn Clinical Nutrition Centre (unpublished).

Dairy UK, Dairy Co., & The Carbon Trust (2010). *Guidelines for the carbon footprinting of dairy products in the UK*.

DEFRA (2014). *Statistics about the structure of the agriculture industry*.

Denny, A., Aisbitt, B., & Lunn, J. (2008). Mycoprotein and health. *British Nutrition Bulletin, 33*, 298–310.

Dermiki, M., Mounayar, R., Suwankanit, C., Scott, J., Kennedy, O., Mottram, D., ... Methven, L. (2013). Maximising umami taste in meat using natural ingredients: effects on chemistry, sensory perception, and hedonic liking in young and old consumers. *J Sci Fd Agric, 93*, 3312–3321.

De Vries, M., & De Boer, I. J. M. (2010). Comparing environmental impacts for livestock products: A review of life cycle assessments. *Livestock Science, 128*(1), 1–11.

Dibb, S., & Fitzpatrick, I. (2014). *Let's talk about meat: Changing dietary behaviour for the 21st century*. Eating Better, UK.

D'Silva, J., & Webster, J. (2010). Introduction. In J. D'Silva, & J. Webster (Eds.), *The meat crisis: Developing more sustainable production and consumption* (p. 2). London: Earthscan.

EBLEX (2011). *Making grass silage for better returns*. UK: Agriculture & Horticulture Development Board.

EBLEX (2012). *Down to Earth. The beef & sheep roadmap phase three*. UK: Agriculture & Horticulture Development Board.

EC (1997). Regulation No 258/97 of the European Parliament and of the Council of 27 January concerning novel foods and novel food ingredients. *Official Journal L, 43*(14/02), 0001–0006.

Edwards, D. G. (1993). The nutritional evaluation of mycoprotein. *International Journal of Food Sciences and Nutrition, 44*(Suppl. 1), S37–S43, UK.

Edwards, D. G., & Cummings, J. H. (2010). The protein quality of mycoprotein. *Proceedings of the Nutrition Society, 69*(OCE4), E331.

Edelman, J., Fewell, A., & Solomons, G. L. (1983). *Mycoprotein—A new food. Nutrition abstracts and reviews in clinical nutrition* (Vol. 53, pp. 471–480).

Evans, J. (1996). *The control and effects of ice crystal growth in a mycelial system. Ph.D. thesis*. University of Nottingham.

Finnigan, T. J. A., Akintoye, M., & Mousavi, R. (2015). GB Patent GB2516491B.

Finnigan, T. J. A., & Blanchard, R. (2009). *Edible fungi*. US Patent 7,635,492B2.

Finnigan, T. J. A., Lemon, M., Allen, B., & Paton, I. (2010). Mycoprotein LCA and Food 2030. *Aspects of Applied Biology, 102*, 81–90.

Finnigan, T. J. A., & Stephens, J. (1996). *Texturized foodstuffs from gelled edible fungus and hydrocolloid mixtures*. WO Patent 96/21362.

Food and Agricultural Organisation (2009). *How to feed the world in 2050*. Rome: Food and Agriculture Organization of the United Nations (FAO).

Gerbens-Leenes, P. W., Mekonnen, M. M., & Hoekstra, A. Y. (2013). The water footprint of poultry, pork and beef: A comparative study in different countries and production systems. *Water Resources and Industry, 1*, 25–36.

Gerber, P. J., Steinfeld, H., Henderson, B., Mottet, A., Opio, C., Dijkman, J., ... Tempio, G. (2013). *Tackling climate change through livestock – A global assessment of emissions and mitigation opportunities*. Rome: Food and Agriculture Organization of the United Nations (FAO).

Hoekstra, A. Y. (2013). *The water footprint of modern consumer society* (1st ed.). Oxford, UK: Routledge.

Homma, Y., Nakamura, H., Kumagai, Y., Ryuzo, A., Saito, Y., Ishikawa, T., ... Inadera, H. (1995). Effects of eight week ingestion of mycoprotein on plasma levels of lipids and apo (lipo) proteins. *Progress in Medicine, 15*(3), 183–195.

House of Commons (2013). *Global food security: First report of session 2013–14* (Vol. 1London: House of Commons.

Hunter, J. (2014). *Investigation of symptoms reported after eating mycoprotein. Interim report of 2 year study*. Marlow Foods Document.

International Dairy Federation (2010). *A common carbon footprint approach for dairy. The IDF guide to standard lifecycle assessment methodology for the dairy sector*. Bulletin of the International Dairy Federation 445/2010.

IPCC (2014). Summary for policymakers. In C. B. Field, V. R. Barros, D. J. Dokken, K. J. Mach, M. D. Mastrandrea, T. E. Bilir, M. Chatterjee, K. L. Ebi, Y. O. Estrada, R. C. Genova, B. Girma, E. S. Kissel, A. N. Levy, S. MacCracken, P. R. Mastrandrea, & L. L. White (Eds.), *Climate Change 2014: Impacts, Adaptation, and Vulnerability. Part A: Global and Sectoral Aspects. Contribution of Working Group II to the Fifth Assessment Report of the Intergovernmental Panel on Climate Change* (pp. 1–32). Cambridge, United Kingdom and NewYork, NY, USA: Cambridge University Press.

Ishikawa, T., Ohsuzu, F., Yoshida, H., Yamashita, T., Miyajima, E., Nakamura, H., ... Kaji, D. (1995). The effect of mycoprotein intake (12 and 24 g per day) over 4 weeks on serum cholesterol levels. *Progress in Medicine, 15*, 61–74.

Jonker, D. (1995). *Determination of the net protein utilisation, digestibility, and biological value of three samples of freeze dried mycoprotein in rats. (Report V95, 134)*. The Hague, The Netherlands: TNO Nutrition and Food Research Institute.

Knight, N., Roberts, G., & Shelton, D. (2001). The thermal stability of Quorn pieces. *International Journal of Food Science & Technology, 36*(1), 47–52.

Lymbery, P., & Oakeshott, I. (2014). *Farmageddon: The true cost of cheap meat*. London, UK: Bloomsbury Publishing.

MacLeod, M., Gerber, P., Mottet, A., Tempio, G., Falcucci, A., Opio, C., ... Steinfeld, H. (2013). *Greenhouse gas emissions from pig and chicken supply chains – A global life cycle assessment*. Rome: Food and Agriculture Organization of the United Nations (FAO).

Marlow Foods (2001). *GRAS notification for mycoprotein*. (Submitted as: U.S. FDA, 2002 – GRN 091). Submitted by: North Yorkshire, UK: Marlow Foods Ltd.

McCance and Widdowson's The Composition of Foods Integrated Dataset (2002). Food Standards Agency, UK.

McKinney, M. L., Schoch, R. M., & Yonavjak, L. (2013). *Environmental science: Systems and solutions* (5th ed.). Burlington, MA: Jones & Bartlett Learning.

Miller, S. A., & Dwyer, J. T. (2001). Evaluating the safety and nutritional value of mycoprotein. *Food Technology, 55*(7), 42–47.

Miri, T. (2004). *Rheology and microstructure of mycoprotein filamentous paste. Ph.D. thesis*. University of Birmingham.

Miri, T., Barigou, M., Fryer, P. J., & Cox, P. W. (2005). Flow induced fibre alignment in mycoprotein paste. *Food Research International, 38*, 1151–1160.

Nakamura, H., Ishikawa, T., Akanuma, M., Nishiwaki, M., Yamashita, T., Tomiyasu, K., ... Miyajima, E. (1994). Effect of myco-proteins intake on serum lipids of healthy subjects. *Progress in Medicine, 14*(7), 1972–1976.

Opio, C. G. (2013). *Greenhouse gas emissions from ruminant supply chains – A global life cycle*. Rome: Food and Agriculture Organization of the United Nations (FAO).

Pimentel, D., & Pimentel, M. (2003). Sustainability of meat-based and plant-based diets and the environment. *The American Journal of Clinical Nutrition, 78*(3), 660S–663S.

Pirt, S. J. (1975). *Principles of microbe and cell cultivation*. Oxford, UK: Blackwell Scientific Publications.

Ramirez, C. A., Patel, M., & Blok, K. (2006). How much energy to process one pound of meat? A comparison of energy use and specific energy consumption in the meat industry of four European countries. *Energy, 31*(12), 2047–2063.

Righelato, R. C. (1979). The kinetics of mycelial growth. In J. H. Burnett, & A. P. J. Trinci (Eds.), *Fungal Walls and Hyphal Growth* (pp. 385–401). Cambridge, UK: Cambridge University Press.

Rodger, G. W., & Angold, R. E. (1991). *The effect of freezing on some properties of Quorn mycoprotein. Food Freezing* (pp. 87–95). London: Springer.

Rodger, G. W., Cordell, G. B., & Mottram, D. S. (1998). *Flavouring materials*. WO Patent 99/030579.

Sadler, M. (1988). Quorn. *Nutrition and Food Science, 112*, 9–11.

Sadler, M. (1990). Myco-protein—A new food. *Nutrition Bulletin, 15*(3), 180–190.

Sadler, M. (1991). Mycoprotein in the British diet. *General Practitioners Yearbook*, , 515–518.

Simpson, D. R. (1996). *Characterisation of morphological mutants arising during production of Quorn mycoprotein. Ph.D thesis*. University of Manchester.

Spector, T. (2015). *The diet myth*. Weidenfeld and Nicolson.

Steinfeld, H., Gerber, P., Wassenaar, T., Castel, V., Rosales, M., & Haan, C. D. (2006). *Livestock's long shadow: Environmental issues and options*. Food and Agriculture Organization of the United Nations (FAO).

Tilman, D., & Clark, M. (2014). Global diets link environmental sustainability and human health. *Nature, 515*(7528), 518–522.

Trinci, A. P. J. (1991). Quorn mycoprotein. *Mycologist, 5*(3), 106–109.

Trinci, A. P. J. (1992). Mycoprotein: A twenty-year overnight success story. *Mycological Research, 96*(1), 1–13.

Trinci, A. P. J., Robson, G. D., Wiebe, M. G., Cunliffe, B., & Naylor, T. W. (1990). *Growth and morphology of* Fusarium graminearum *and other fungi in batch and continuous culture*. Special Publications of the Society for General Microbiology.

Turnbull, W. H., Leeds, A. R., & Edwards, G. D. (1990). Effect of mycoprotein on blood lipids. *American Journal of Clinical Nutrition., 52*, 646–650.

Turnbull, W. H., Leeds, A. R., & Edwards, D. G. (1992). Mycoprotein reduces blood lipids in free-living subjects. *The American Journal of Clinical Nutrition, 55*(2), 415–419.

Turnbull, W. H., Walton, J., & Leeds, A. R. (1993). Acute effects of mycoprotein on subsequent energy intake and appetite variables. *The American Journal of Clinical Nutrition, 58*(4), 507–512.

Turnbull, W. H., & Ward, T. (1995). Mycoprotein reduces glycemia and insulinemia when taken with an oral-glucose-tolerance test. *The American Journal of Clinical Nutrition, 61*(1), 135–140.

Udall, J. N., Lo, C. W., Young, V. R., & Scrimshaw, N. S. (1984). The tolerance and nutritional value of two microfungal foods in human subjects. *The American journal of clinical nutrition, 40*(2), 285–292.

Ward, P. (1996). *A process for the reduction of nucleic acid content of a fungus imperfectus*. WO Patent 95/23843.

Wheelock, V. (1993). Quorn: Case study of a healthy food ingredient. *British Food Journal, 95*(5), 40–44.

Wiebe, M. G. (2001). Mycoprotein from *Fusarium venenatum*: A well-established product for human consumption. *Applied Microbiology and Biotechnology, 58*, 421–427.

Wiebe, M. G. (2004). Quorn mycoprotein – Overview of a successful fungal product. *Mycologist, 18*(1), 17–20.

Williams, A., Audsley, E., & Sandars, D. (2006). *Determining the environmental burdens and resource use in the production of agricultural and horticultural commodities*. Defra Project Report IS0205.

Williamson, D. A., Geiselman, P. J., Lovejoy, J., Greenway, F., Volaufova, J., Martin, C. K., ... Ortego, L. (2006). Effects of consuming mycoprotein, tofu, or chicken upon subsequent eating behavior, hunger, and satiety. *Appetite, 46*, 41–48.

Yoder, W. T., & Christianson, L. M. (1998). Species-specific primers resolve members of Fusarium section Fusarium: Taxonomic status of the edible "Quorn" fungus reevaluated. *Fungal Genetics and Biology, 23*(1), 68–80.

Chapter 20

Heterotrophic Microalgae: A Scalable and Sustainable Protein Source

B. Klamczynska and W.D. Mooney
TerraVia Holdings Inc., South San Francisco, CA, United States

20.1 INTRODUCTION

Single-cell algae, also known as microalgae, have been in existence for over a billion years and have been a vital part of the food chain. In fact, microalgae are the world's original oil producers and the ancestors from which all plants have descended (Fig. 20.1). They have the same oil-producing machinery as all plants, giving them the ability to produce any kind of plant oil. They also have the capability of producing other nutrients found in higher-order plants such as protein, fiber, starch, vitamins, and antioxidants. In total, there are more than 15,000 novel compounds that originate from algae biomass (Cardozo et al., 2007).

There is evidence that microalgae were consumed as early as 2000 years ago. More recently, in the early 20th century, interest and exploration of algae as a source of human nutrition rose, in part due to the versatility and flexibility of microalgae. This interest especially grew after World War II as the human population was growing rapidly and shortages in resources were of increasing concern. Historically, *Chlorella* has been the microalgae of choice due to its prolific growth and adaptability to different conditions.

Early work in the 1950s by the Carnegie Institute and Stanford University in the United States (Burlew, 1953), as well as work in Germany, Israel, Japan, and Italy, showed promise for the cultivation of *Chlorella* in open ponds, utilizing photosynthesis. However, there were significant obstacles to making this technology economically viable at larger scale. During that time, advances in traditional agriculture, like increased yields, made this platform less interesting.

Currently, *Spirulina* and *Chlorella* are the predominant whole-cell microalgae that are used for consumption. They are often consumed in the form of tablets, capsules, and liquids (Becker, 2004; Pulz & Gross, 2004; Spolaore, Joannis-Cassan, Duran, & Isambert, 2006). Although microalgae in general, and *Chlorella* in particular, have been part of human nutrition for a long time, utilization of microalgae as a protein source in mainstream foods was hampered by strong green flavor and lack of consistent, high-quality supply. This chapter will discuss recent developments in algae protein designed to overcome those obstacles.

20.2 *CHLORELLA* CLASSIFICATION

Algae constitute a group of ~40,000 species. Algae can be unicellular (microalgae) or multicellular (macroalgae), commonly referred to as seaweed. Most microalgae are capable of photosynthesis, but many are mixotrophic or heterotrophic. The *Chlorella* genus is a microalga and belongs to the group of green algae, the Chlorophyta.

Chlorella is a common inhabitant of fresh waters and soils. The cells are spherical and 2–10 µm in diameter. The cell typically contains a nucleus, one or more chloroplasts, and other structures suspended in a cytoplasm. The chlorophyll and carotenoid pigments are localized in the chloroplasts, or plastids. The cell is usually surrounded by a cell wall. The mode of reproduction is asexual, via the production of autospores which are identical to the parent cell.

Thus, the term "growth" applied to microalgae refers to the increase of a population, rather than increase in mass of individual cells.

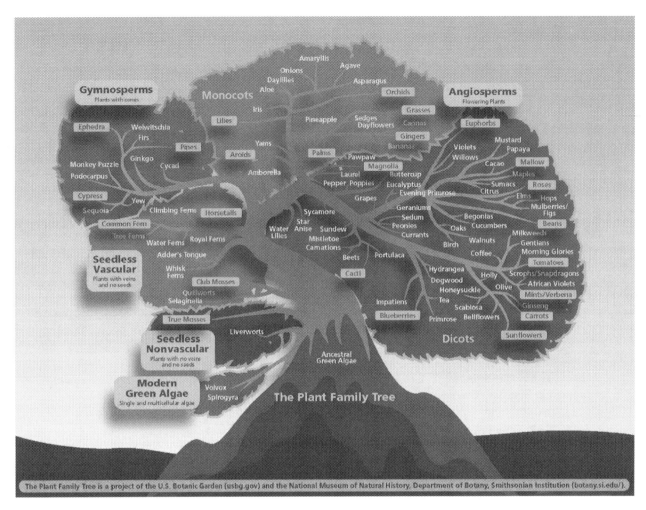

FIGURE 20.1 Phylogenic tree.

20.3 PRODUCTION

The traditional and common method of cultivating microalgae is in open ponds that mimic the natural environments of microalgae. Those systems take advantage of sunlight and would appear to have relatively low initial costs. Water consumption, land use, and energy costs to operate open pond systems must be considered to understand the full monetary and environmental costs of open pond systems. For example, water consumption can be quite significant.

In order for the microalgae to grow, they need consistent environmental conditions and nutrient supply, which are challenging to maintain in an open pond system. Additional significant challenges include contamination, dependence on weather conditions, maintaining a consistent concentration of carbon dioxide, and limited light penetration beyond the surface. Closed systems, by contrast, avoid most of the shortfalls of an open pond by providing full control of the growth conditions. Microalgae can be grown in closed systems either photoautotrophically, mixotrophically, or heterotrophically.

Photo bioreactors utilize sunlight for energy, and coupled with a controlled environment, can give consistent, high-purity product. However, the system requires extensive surface area due to the low penetration rates of the light in the culture medium (Borowitzka, 1999).

Heterotrophic cultivation takes place in a closed fermentation process and relies on renewable plant sugars as a source of energy for the microalgae that grow in the absence of light. Heterotrophic cultivation has been in use for some time. One of the best-developed applications is in the production of long-chain polyunsaturated fatty acids. A distinct advantage of heterotrophic cultivation is that the growth conditions can be precisely controlled, allowing for rapid growth and consistent product quality. Microalgae grown heterotrophically are capable of utilizing a wide variety of sugar sources ranging from sugar beets, corn, and sugar cane, to cellulosic sugars.

Certain microalgae are able to change their metabolism to adapt to changes in the type and amount of nutrients, as well as the conditions during growth. Thus, the chemical composition in microalgae can vary within the same species due to environmental factors such as seasonality, nutrients, temperature, photoperiod, salinity, carbon source and intensity, and color of light, among others.

This adaptability of microalgae can be used to vary the outcomes of the growth cycle. For example, microalgae with protein content above 60% or microalgae with 80% oil content can be produced in a matter of days depending on the type of microalgae used and conditions during cultivation. The microalgae can be left whole, or further processed to extract specific compounds. For the use as whole cells, there is very minimal processing required—just washing and drying of the cells.

20.4 SUSTAINABILITY PROFILE

20.4.1 Case Study: TerraVia Inc.

The sustainability profiles for these different production systems can vary widely. For the purpose of this chapter, we will review one case study for heterotrophic microalgae in a closed fermentation process. One of the leading producers of microalgae products using this system is the California-based company, TerraVia Holdings Inc. (TerraVia). TerraVia is a producer of a wide variety of algae-based products, including algae oil and whole algae products, such as whole algae protein.

Currently, TerraVia has two production facilities. Their largest manufacturing operations take place in Orindiúva, Brazil at the Solazyme Bunge Renewable Oils joint venture facility. They also produce oils and whole-algae products at a facility Peoria, Illinois.

To manufacture these products, TerraVia first selects the best microalgae for the application. Different strains are used depending on the desired product such as whole algae protein, or the production of lauric oil, which is an alternative to unsustainably harvested palm oil. The microalgae are fed renewable plant sugars in stainless steel fermentation tanks where they then grow. For whole algae protein, the whole cells are then dried and milled. This process is further illustrated in Fig. 20.2.

TerraVia's process is flexible and can use a variety of sugar feedstocks. Currently, TerraVia is focused on using Brazilian sugarcane and dextrose derived from US corn. Brazilian sugarcane is sourced through the Solazyme Bunge Renewable Oils joint venture. The Solazyme Bunge Renewable Oils facility is colocated with the Bunge Moema sugar mill in São Paulo State. The manufacturing facility in Peoria, Illinois, uses readily available dextrose (sugar). TerraVia's goal is to use sugar derived from cellulosic feedstocks to produce its products.

This manufacturing process allows TerraVia to produce a wide range of products from a variety of sugar feedstocks at a single location in a matter of days. This process means that whole algae protein production can have a lower environmental impact than other sources of protein—from beef and whey, to other vegan sources. In addition, the flexibility and versatility of this process can be revolutionary in providing new solutions needed to address climate change and nutrition security.

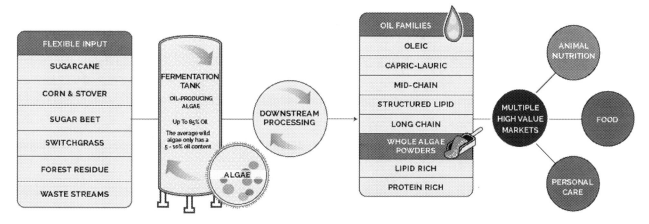

FIGURE 20.2 TerraVia production process.

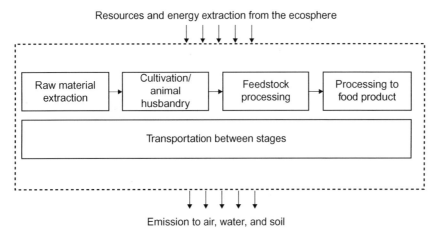

FIGURE 20.3 Cradle-to-gate lifecycle assessment scope. *Source: thinkstep (2015) Cradle-to-Gate Assessment of Whole Algal Protein Products. Preliminary analysis pending critical review (14044, Section 6.3).*

TABLE 20.1 System Boundaries of Cradle-to-Gate Lifecycle Assessment

Included	Excluded
✓ Cultivation of crops	✗ Human labor
✓ Animal husbandry	✗ Manufacturing facilities overhead
✓ Processing of sugarcane to sugar	✗ Packaging
✓ Processing of sugar to whole algae protein	✗ Construction of capital equipment
✓ Processing of crops to proteins	✗ Maintenance and operations of support equipment (eg, forklifts)
✓ Ancillary raw materials	✗ Transportation of employees
✓ Upstream energy production	✗ Use and end-of-life
✓ Intermediate transport	✗ Transport of product from facility gate to point-of-use
✓ Treatment of coproducts by economic allocation	

Source: thinkstep (2015) Cradle-to-Gate Assessment of Whole Algal Protein Products. Preliminary analysis pending critical review (14044, Section 6.3).

20.4.2 A Low Environmental Impact

When considering the environmental impact of a product, there are often three primary indicators: greenhouse gas (GHG) emissions, water consumption, and land use efficiency. Independent lifecycle assessments (LCAs) are an important tool for assessing the impact in these categories. TerraVia approached thinkstep (formerly PE International) to conduct a comprehensive cradle-to-gate study of AlgaVia whole algae protein, considered for production at the Solazyme Bunge Oils facility utilizing sugarcane as a feedstock. The preliminary results for this LCA are described below. As a cradle-to-gate study, the LCA considered the impact of the production process, from sourcing raw materials, cultivation and/or animal husbandry, and processing, as illustrated in Fig. 20.3 and Table 20.1.

The study also includes a comparative analysis for common sources of protein, including beef, whey, rice, soy, and pea protein. The study compared each LCA on a per kilogram of protein produced basis, and not per kilogram of product. The typical protein content for each source is listed in Table 20.2.

Overall, the study found that whole algae protein has a lower carbon and water footprint than beef and whey, and lower or on par with the vegan sources considered. A separate analysis looking at land use efficiency (ie, the amount of protein produced per hectare of feedstock) found that whole algae protein produced more protein per hectare than all other sources compared.

TABLE 20.2 Protein Content of Comparative Protein Products

Product	Percent Protein by Mass (%)
AlgaVia whole algae protein	65
Whey protein	90
Rice protein isolate	77
Pea protein isolate	80
Soy protein isolate	90
Beef	25

Source: thinkstep (2015) Cradle-to-Gate Assessment of Whole Algal Protein Products. Preliminary analysis pending critical review (14044, Section 6.3).

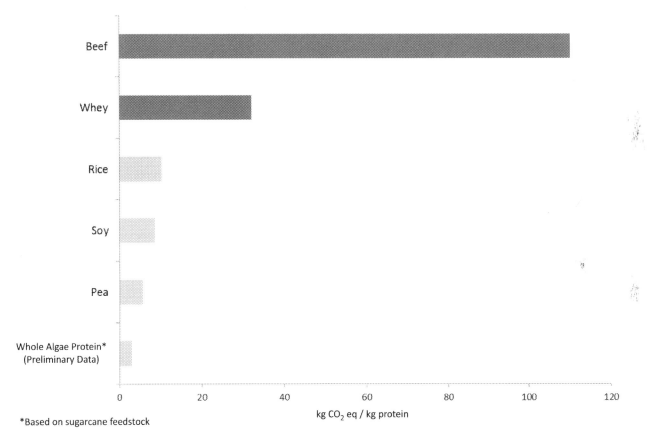

FIGURE 20.4 Estimated Carbon footprint of whole algae protein produced in Brazil versus other protein sources. *From thinkstep (2015) Cradle-to-Gate Assessment of Whole Algal Protein Products. Preliminary analysis pending critical review (14044, Section 6.3).*

20.4.2.1 GHG Emissions

The GHG emissions associated with producing whole algae protein at the Solazyme Bunge Oils facility is lower than beef and whey, and likely lower or on par with the vegan sources considered in the analysis (Fig. 20.4). In fact, producing 1 kg of beef protein results in over 3500% more GHG emissions than a kg of whole algae protein. While emissions from whey protein production were much lower than beef, they were still nearly 1000% higher than the emissions from the production of whole algae protein.

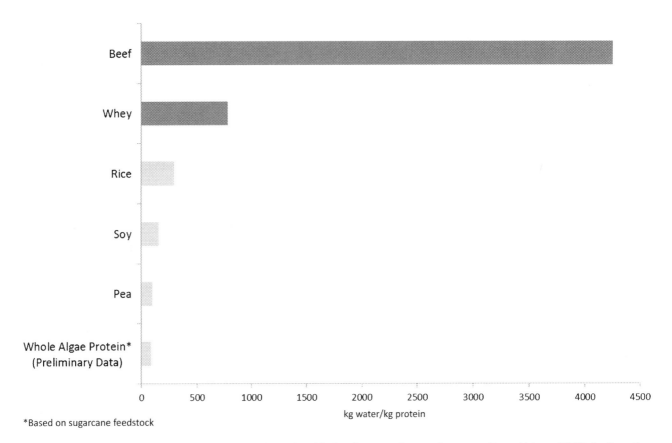

FIGURE 20.5 Water consumption of whole algae protein produced in Brazil versus other protein sources. *From thinkstep (2015) Cradle-to-Gate Assessment of Whole Algal Protein Products. Preliminary analysis pending critical review (14044, Section 6.3).*

The higher GHG emissions for whey and beef are primarily driven by emissions from cultivation and animal husbandry. The cultivation emissions come from the production of corn and soy required to feed the livestock, while animal waste causes most of the animal husbandry emissions. Thinkstep's analysis was based on the use of sugarcane. Sugarcane cultivation in Brazil has a relatively low carbon footprint and contributes to the low GHG emissions for production of whole algae protein. Further, the waste sugarcane material (bagasse) provides all the energy to power both the Bunge sugarcane mill and the Solazyme Bunge Oil facility, driving GHG emissions to low levels. For plant-based proteins, the energy required for protein processing was the largest contributor to the GHG emissions in the LCA.

20.4.2.2 Water Consumption

Water consumption is a net measure of water use—the water lost from a watershed as a result of evaporation, evapotranspiration, product integration, water transfers to different watersheds, or release of water to sea. Water consumption is an appropriate indicator of the water impacts from activities such as protein production because it accounts for the water which is actually made unavailable for future use within the watershed.

Whole algae protein produced at the Solazyme Bunge Oil facility consumes less water than beef and whey, and likely less or on par with the vegan sources considered (see Fig. 20.5). Again, beef and whey's impact is much higher than the other sources of protein. Water consumption required for beef production is over 4800% higher than for production of whole algae protein. Water consumption for whey production is 810% higher. Pea protein had the second lowest water consumption, which was about 17% higher than whole algae protein.

The low water consumption for whole algae protein production is due to the fact that the sugarcane supply is rainfed and uses a contained fermentation process. Furthermore, much of the treated wastewater coming from the fermentation facility is returned back to the sugarcane fields as "fertigation." The treated wastewater contains valuable nutrients for next season's sugarcane crop, such as potassium, and returning treated wastewater to the fields replenishes water and nutrients back into the cane fields.

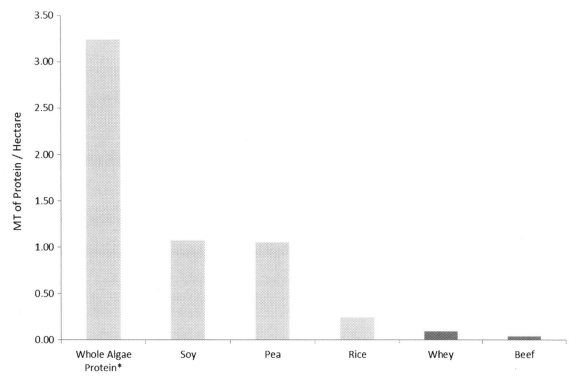

FIGURE 20.6 Protein yield per hectare. *Calculated from FAO and USDA Statistical Databases; Redefining Agricultural Yields: from tonnes to people nourished per hectare, Cassidy et al. (2013); Proteins From Land Plants—Potential resources for human nutrition and food security, Li Day (2013).*

20.4.2.3 Land Efficiency

Land efficiency, or yield, is another important measure and will become increasingly so as global population continues to rise. In order to adequately feed, clothe, and shelter nine billion people, producers will need to do more with fewer resources.

The Solazyme Bunge production process has the ability to produce more protein per hectare of land than the other sources of protein. This is primarily due to the high yield of the sugarcane feedstock, as well as the high protein content of the microalgae (Fig. 20.6).

20.4.3 Climate Change Adaptation and Resilience

TerraVia's production process may also provide a solution to the challenges of climate change. Fundamentally, TerraVia's process takes what the world has in abundance (plant sugars) to produce what it needs every day (oil and protein). As technology for producing cost-effective cellulosic sugars develops, TerraVia's processes can utilize nonfood sources of sugar (eg, municipal green waste), and turn them into nutritious foods, such as whole algae protein. This operational flexibility provides the ability to respond to changes in demand and needs in real time. By simply switching out microalgae strains, high oleic oil can be produced at the beginning of the week and a high-protein product can be produced at the end of the week.

This also fundamentally decouples geography and seasonality from oil and protein production. Not only can multiple oils and protein be produced from any renewable sugar feedstock source, they can be produced anywhere at any time, allowing for production closer to consumers and away from threatened ecosystems.

20.5 NUTRITIONAL VALUE AND SAFETY

20.5.1 Nutritional Value

Spirulina and *Chlorella* are probably the best-known examples of microalgae currently used in human nutrition. They are mostly grown in open pond systems, and typically have 50–60% protein content. The vivid color coming from high

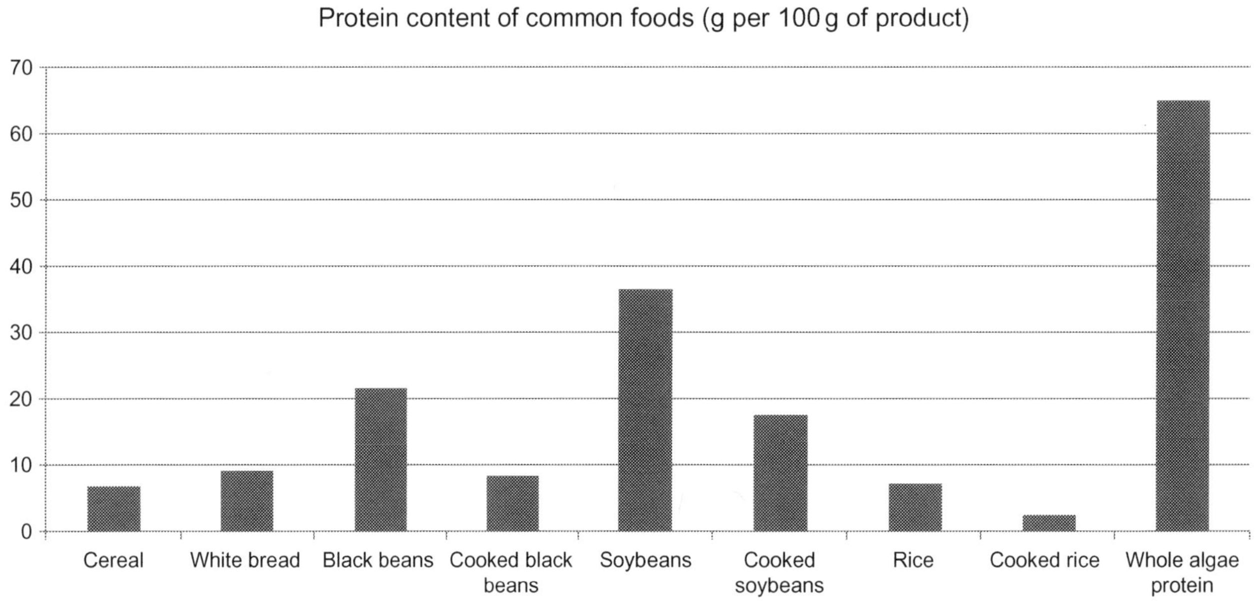

FIGURE 20.7 Protein content of common foods. *From USDA National Nutrient Database http://ndb.nal.usda.gov.*

chlorophyll content coupled with the strong flavor prevents their use in mainstream foods, limiting microalgae mostly to the supplement aisle. Their nutritional value, utilization, and growing have been reviewed in detail previously (Chronakis & Madsen, 2011; Conde, Balboa, Parada, & Falqué, 2013).

Microalgae growth through an enclosed heterotrophic process limits the development of chlorophyll since it is no longer needed for the metabolic processes. By ensuring a steady nitrogen supply, the protein content can be further increased.

The whole algae protein from TerraVia, Inc. contains around 65% protein by dry cell weight. Because the product is a whole-cell product, all of the cellular components are still present. In addition, fiber (15%), micronutrients such as lutein and zeaxanthin, and lipid high in polyunsaturated fatty acids (10%) are present in the cells. The intact cell walls protect the proteins and other nutrients, but are thin enough to allow for easy digestion. In an in vitro study using the Tiny-TIM model, protein digestibility was found to be 88%. There was no significant difference in protein digestibility between intact and disrupted cells (unpublished study).

As seen in Fig. 20.7, the protein content of whole algae protein is very high in comparison to common food staples. On a 100 g dry basis, whole algae protein has almost double the protein content of soybeans and 10 times the protein of rice. Coupled with ease of use, this gives whole algae protein the potential as an excellent whole-food protein source, but also ideal for supplementing diets lacking in proteins.

Whole algae protein contains all the essential amino acids. The amino acid breakdown of whole algae protein as compared to rice, beans, and soy is shown in Fig. 20.8. The glutamic acid and arginine levels are double or triple compared to other proteins. These two amino acids have been shown to have health benefits, such as muscle recovery and heart health.

Although whole algae protein contains all essential amino acids, the PDCASS is around 0.5 due to the very high levels of nonessential amino acids. This is consistent with other whole-food protein sources (nonisolated protein), like pulses, rice, wheat, or corn (Boye, Wijesinha-Bettoni, & Burlingame, 2012). In plant proteins, the PDCASS can usually be improved by isolating the protein and modifying the amino acid composition to match the recommended levels. But this requires significant further processing and the isolated, processed protein is not a whole food.

An important fact to consider is that it is very rare for humans to rely on only one protein source, as most diets contain protein from variety of different foods. Thus, the PDCASS should not be the only consideration, but rather the breadth of other nutrients supplied along with the protein, as well as the whole formulation and overall diet. As discussed further below, whole algae protein provides fiber, healthy lipids, and other micronutrients as well as functional properties and manufacturing efficiencies.

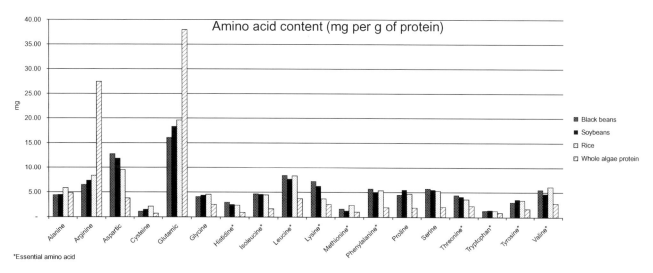

FIGURE 20.8 Amino acid composition of whole algae protein.

20.5.2 Safety

Chlorella has been in the human food supply for centuries, and it is recognized as safe. *Chlorella vulgaris* and *Chlorella pyrenoidosa* are considered not novel in the EU (Regulation (EC) No 258/97). Recently, *Chlorella protothecoides* was recognized as Generally Regarded as Safe and a "no questions" letter was received from the Food and Drug Administration (FDA) in the United States (FDA, 2014).

The whole-cell *C. protothecoides* was evaluated for dietary safety in a 13-week feeding trial in rodents, as well as evaluated for food allergy potential. No adverse effects related to the whole algae protein were reported (Szabo, Matulka, & Chan, 2013). In another study, an enzymatic protein hydrolysate from *C. vulgaris* was tested in the nutritional recovery of malnourished mice. The study showed no negative effects from *C. vulgaris* (Morris et al., 2011).

20.6 PROPERTIES AND APPLICATIONS OF WHOLE ALGAE PROTEIN

Most commercially available proteins on the market are either concentrates (>65% protein) or isolates (>90% protein). They are obtained by processing and fractionating the respective food sources. The protein content of the unprocessed, raw foods is fairly low. Thus, it is only economical to produce the protein when it is a coproduct from processing the other product streams. For example, soy protein isolates are produced because soya is processed into dozens of other industrial and food products.

In contrast, TerraVia's *C. protothecoides* contains 65% protein without the need to further process the material or isolate the protein. This has significant implications for its properties and functionality. While isolated proteins can have several functional characteristics, like water absorption, gelling, foaming, and emulsification, whole algae protein is unique in that the algae cells are still intact, and the protein is protected inside by the cell walls. This renders the protein nonfunctional. Another important property of isolated protein is its isoelectric point, which is the pH at which the protein exhibits the lowest solubility. This property has significant implications when fortifying products at low pH—usually stabilizers need to be employed to prevent the protein from precipitating. Again, the advantage of using the whole algae protein lies in the fact that the protein is protected inside the cell and not affected by changes in pH.

Unlike traditional *Chlorella* strains used in tablets and supplements, heterotrophically grown whole algae protein can be used to fortify virtually any food products. It is due not only to the neutral color and flavor, but also because of the whole-cell nature of whole algae protein which exhibits low water absorption and minimal interactions with other ingredients. In food matrices where competition for water plays a role, like bars or crackers, the whole-cell protein does not influence rheology and reduces the tendency for hardening over time. For example, in a cracker application, whole algae protein was used at 20% of the formulation, partially replacing wheat flour. This resulted in doubling the protein content of the cracker. There was no significant impact on dough rheology and sheetability of the dough. Gummies and caramels are additional examples of low water activity applications where the protected nature of protein and minimal water absorption allow for successful application.

The multicomponent nature of whole cell gives food formulators the benefit of achieving several nutritional benefits at once. As an example, a chocolate-flavored beverage was fortified with whole algae protein to contain 11 g of protein per serving. This amount of whole algae protein also provided 4 g of fiber and 3 g of lipid, eliminating the need to add additional ingredients to the formulation.

Most low-pH protein-fortified beverages require use of gums and stabilizers to protect the protein from precipitation. A low-pH beverage formula fortified with whole algae protein does not require any gums or stabilizers since the protein is protected inside the cell walls. Even though the whole algae protein component can settle overtime, the beverage retains smooth mouthfeel without the grittiness normally associated with low-pH protein systems.

The small particle size and excellent dispersability make the whole algae protein a good component for powdered blends where it provides a very smooth mouthfeel to the finished food. Further, the particle size of whole algae protein is so small that it has been used to fortify chocolate and compound coatings.

A high glutamic acid level gives the whole algae protein a distinctive umami flavor, and plays a very important role in flavor perception and delivery. For example, it can be used to enhance savory flavors without adding monosodium glutamate. Also, chocolate and tropical flavors can benefit from some umami notes, however, it should be noted that other flavors might not be as compatible.

20.7 CONSUMER ACCEPTANCE

With a wide variety of uses in food, an impressive nutritional profile and low environmental footprint, microalgae ingredients such as whole algae protein have many advantages in the market. Of course, one key area for any new product is consumer acceptance. Microalgae ingredients already fit into some rising consumer trends that food producers are seeing today, such as a desire for cleaner labels, more sustainable and plant-based diets, eating lower on the food chain, where possible, and cutting back on saturated fats.

Most consumers (about 58% in one internal study) admit that they do not know much about algae as an ingredient. Nevertheless, consumers have a positive association for algae, as being natural, environmentally friendly, and healthy (Figs. 20.9 and 20.10).

On learning about algae and its ability to provide essential nutrients such as healthy oils, fiber, and protein, a majority of survey participants became much more positive about algae. In fact, more than half of the consumers (58%) surveyed were more likely to buy food products that contained algae. This is especially true for younger consumers, who tend to be more socially and environmentally conscious. An increase in millennials' share of the market, coupled with greater understanding of microalgae, can help ingredients such as whole algae protein gain wider acceptance in a variety of food products (Figs. 20.11 and 20.12).

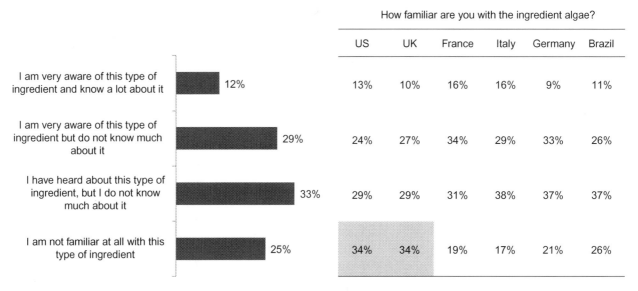

FIGURE 20.9 Initial consumer awareness of algae as an ingredient.

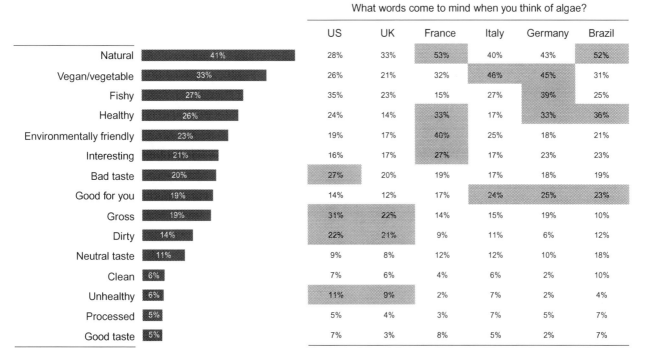

FIGURE 20.10 Initial consumer reaction to algae as an ingredient.

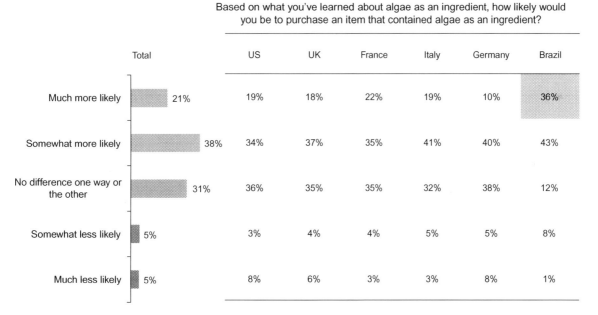

FIGURE 20.11 Consumer acceptance after learning more.

20.8 FUTURE DEVELOPMENTS

While there are many advantages of whole-cell algae protein, there might be a need in the market for other protein products derived from *Chlorella*. From a nutritional perspective, protein isolates can be useful for fortification as well as unlocking interesting functional properties.

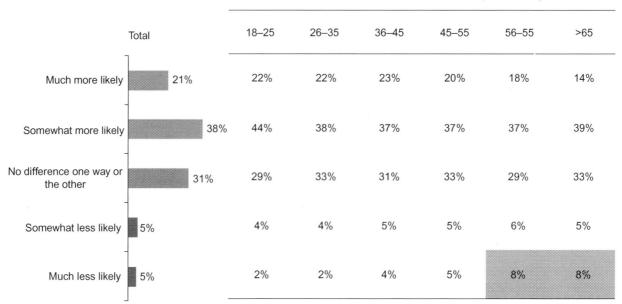

FIGURE 20.12 Consumer acceptance by age group.

There has been very limited research on protein in microalgae as related to food functionality to date. Some recent studies explored isolation and fractionating protein from *Chlorella* and *Spirulina*. Protein isolated from *C. vulgaris* was found to have emulsifying properties and protein stability comparable to sodium caseinate (Ursu et al., 2014). The extraction of protein was achieved by disrupting the cell walls and solubilization at neutral or alkaline pH. The recovery was achieved by subsequent precipitation at acidic pH and ultrafiltration. In another study, protein extracted from *C. pyrenoidosa* was hydrolyzed using commercially available enzymes: Alcalase, papain, trypsin, showing the potential of algae protein to be further modified to suit nutritional or functional needs (Wang & Zhang, 2012). There are also reports of unique proteins in algae with potential health benefits. A lutein−protein complex extracted from *Chlorella* has shown antioxidant activity and inhibition of lipid peroxidation in vitro (Cai, Huang, & Wang, 2015).

Additional research is needed into the functionality, nutrition profile, and other benefits of the protein and micronutrients in microalgae. This will help unlock the potential range of applications for microalgae-based protein.

20.9 CONCLUSION

With a global population growing and demanding more protein, heterotrophic microalgae is a scalable and sustainable source of protein. The closed-system growth process allows for consistent and clean production, and avoids issues with color and strong flavor often associated with microalgae grown via photosynthesis. Due to the flexibility in the types of renewable plant sugars that can be fed to the microalgae, future production may not be constrained by geography. And finally, recent data indicate that microalgae grown on sugarcane feedstock can produce a highly sustainable source of protein. Whole algae protein has had success in the marketplace and is being sold commercially today as an ingredient in a variety of products. Additional research into the functionality of the protein and other micronutrients in microalgae will help to expand the range of applications for microalgae-based protein.

REFERENCES

Becker, W. (2004). Microalgae in human and animal nutrition. In A. Richmond (Ed.), *Handbook of microalgae culture* (pp. 312−351). Oxford: Blackwell.

Borowitzka, M. A. (1999). Commercial production of microalgae: Ponds, tanks, tubes and fermenters. *Journal of Biotechnology*, 70, 313−321.

Boye, J., Wijesinha-Bettoni, R., & Burlingame, B. (2012). Protein quality evaluation twenty years after the introduction of the protein digestibility corrected amino acid score method. *British Journal of Nutrition*, 108, S183−S211.

Burlew, J. S. (Ed.), (1953). *Algae culture from laboratory to pilot plant.* Washington, DC: Carnegie Institute, Publication Number 600.

Cai, X., Huang, Q., & Wang, S. (2015). Isolation of a novel lutein-protein complex from *Chlorella vulgaris* and its functional properties. *Food & Function, 6*(6), 1893–1899.

Cardozo, K. H., Guaratini, T., Barros, M. P., Falcão, V. R., Tonon, A. P., Lopes, N. P., ... Pinto, E. (2007). Metabolites from algae with economical impact. *Comparative Biochemistry and Physiology C Toxicology and Pharmacology, 146*(1–2), 60–78.

Chronakis, I. S., & Madsen, M. (2011). Algae proteins. In G. O. Phillips, & P. A. Williams (Eds.), *Handbook of food proteins* (pp. 353–394), Woodhead Publishing Series in Food Sciences, Technology and Nutrition.

Conde, E., Balboa, E. M., Parada, M., & Falque, E. (2013). Algal proteins, peptides and amino acids. In H. Dominguez (Ed.), *Functional ingredients from algae for foods and nutraceuticals* (Edition: 1st, pp. 135–180). Woodhead Publishing Series in Food Science, Technology and Nutrition, No. 256.

European Parliament Regulation (EC) No 258/97 of the European Parliament and of the Council of 27 January 1997 concerning novel foods and novel food ingredients Official Journal L 043, 14/02/1997, pp. 0001–0006.

FDA. (2014). Agency Response Letter GRAS Notice No. GRN 000519 2014.

Morris, H. J., Carrillo, O. V., Alonso, M. E., Bermúdez, R. C., Almarales, Á., Llauradó, G., ... Fontaine, R. (2011). Oral administration of an enzymatic protein hydrolysate from the green microalga *Chlorella vulgaris* enhances the nutritional recovery of malnourished mice. *Journal of Medicinal Food, 14*(12), 1583–1589.

Pulz, O., & Gross, W. (2004). Valuable products from biotechnology of microalgae. *Applied Microbiology and Biotechnology, 65*, 635–648.

Spolaore, P., Joannis-Cassan, C., Duran, E., & Isambert, A. (2006). Commercial applications of microalgae. *Journal of Bioscience and Bioengineering, 101*, 87–96.

Szabo, N. J., Matulka, R. A., & Chan, T. (2013). Safety evaluation of Whole Algalin Protein (WAP) from *Chlorella protothecoides*. *Food and Chemical Toxicology, 59*, 34–45.

Ursu, A. V., Marcati, A., Sayd, T., Sante-Lhoutellier, V., Djelveh, G., & Michaud, P. (2014). Extraction, fractionation and functional properties of proteins from the microalgae *Chlorella vulgaris*. *Bioresource Technology, 157*, 134–139.

Wang, X., & Zhang, X. (2012). Optimal extraction and hydrolysis of *Chlorella pyrenoidosa* proteins. *Bioresource Technology, 126*, 307–313.

Chapter 21

Edible Insects: A Neglected and Promising Food Source

A. Van Huis[1] and F.V. Dunkel[2]
[1]*Wageningen University, Wageningen, The Netherlands,* [2]*Montana State University, Bozeman, MT, United States*

21.1 INTRODUCTION

Interest in the practice of eating insects in the Western world is very recent. This is remarkable considering that insects are common food in the tropics. In the Western world there is the erroneous perception that eating insects is practiced by people in extreme poverty who eat insects out of necessity. This attitude of considering it "a poor person's diet" and a primitive behavior created an "embarrassment factor" that has made insect-eating people in tropical countries not mention it to Westerners. This is also one of the reasons that international and donor agencies have not given much attention to the use of insects as human food. Robert Pemberton reminded us in 1999 that "East Asian cultures have a more balanced perspective regarding insects than in the West. Entomophobia is uncommon in Asia, as is the idea among many Western people that most insects are related to filth or are dangerous" (Pemberton, 1999). In East Asia, it seems clearly understood that some insect species are pests, some make important medicinal preparations, others are interesting companion animals, some are subjects of sport, and others are fine food.

Until very recently in the Western world it has not been considered as a serious alternative to our chicken, pork, or beef. In 1885, Vincent M. Holt published a small pamphlet entitled "Why not eat insects?" (Holt, 1995). Bodenheimer (1951) in his book "Insects as Human Food: A Chapter of the Ecology of Man," lists an impressive number of examples of eating insects being practiced all over the world. Gene DeFoliart founded the Food Insects Newsletter in 1988 and continued as editor until 1995 (DeFoliart, Dunkel, & Gracer, 2009) and wrote an online bibliography (DeFoliart, 2012). Thanks to DeFoliart, an awareness in the Western world was created as he outlined the benefits of insects as human food and animal feed (DeFoliart, 1989). In 2005, a book on mini-livestock was published (Paoletti, 2005), and in 2008 the Food and Agricultural Organization (FAO) of the United Nations organized an edible insect workshop in Thailand with a strong bias towards Asia (Durst, Johnson, Leslie, & Shono, 2010). In May 2013, the FAO published as the result of a world consultancy, a book "Edible Insects: Future Prospects for Food and Feed Security," which was downloaded 2.3 million times within 24 h. The figure now stands at more than 7 million downloads and the book has been translated into Chinese, French, Italian, and Korean (Van Huis et al., 2013). This book has been cited numerous times in scientific and popular articles. In May 2014, a conference "Insects to feed the world" was held in the Netherlands and attracted 450 participants from 45 countries (Van Huis & Vantomme, 2014). In the last few years the interest in edible insects in the Western world has been increasing exponentially. This is not just the interest of the scientific community or the public media, but also of private companies who are launching businesses to produce and market insect products either for human consumption or for animal feed. Government authorities are now faced with how to deal with insects as food or feed with legislative frameworks that were not designed or updated to accommodate this rapid growth in acceptance.

We will give some examples of the practice of eating insects from different parts of the world and answer the following questions. Are there environmental benefits of producing this mini-livestock (insects) compared to conventional livestock? If we want to promote the consumption of edible insects can we continue harvesting from nature or should insects be farmed? How does the nutritional value of insects compare to conventional meat? Are there food risks when consuming insects? Is it possible to convince Western consumers to incorporate insects into their diet and what is necessary to make this possible? What kind of insect products can be brought to the market? Is the legislative framework in place to make this all possible? What are the prospects of edible insects to become a new agricultural and food sector?

21.2 ETHNO-ENTOMOLOGY

Considerable information on the eating of insects worldwide is available in the publications of Bodenheimer (1951) and DeFoliart (2012). Jongema (2015) produced a list of edible insect species around the world. He listed 2039 different species belonging to the following insect groups: beetle larvae (31%), caterpillars (18%), wasps, bees and ants (15%), crickets, grasshoppers and locusts (14%), true bugs (11%), termites (3%), dragonflies, flies and others (9%). Other arthropod groups such as spiders are also eaten. A world map has also been produced on the occurrence of edible insects based on refereed literature data. However, caution has to be taken as the number of species often reflects research intensity rather than actual figures. For example, Ramos Elorduy in Mexico produced an impressive number of articles on the topic (Ramos-Elorduy, 1993; Ramos-Elorduy & Morales, 1989) and Malaisse in the Democratic Republic of Congo listed quite some numbers of edible insects species, in particular caterpillars (Malaisse, 1997).

Insect species are often seasonally available. For example, from social insects such as termites and ants often the reproductives (winged ones) are eaten, which appear with the first rains after the dry season. Others, such as caterpillars depend on host plants. Many aquatic species are available throughout the year, for example, the giant waterbug, *Lethocerus indicus* (Hemiptera: Belostomatidae) in Southeast Asia.

There are numerous techniques to collect insects. As an example, for grasshoppers, this ranges from manual collection by women early in the morning when the cold-blooded animals are still rather sessile, up to commercially light-trapping the edible grasshopper *Ruspolia nitidula* in East Africa (Agea, Biryomumaisho, Buyinza, & Nabanoga, 2008). There are numerous techniques to trap winged termites, but most often they are caught by using a light above a pan or other water receptacle.

Some cases of insect eating are very specific. Aboriginal people living in central and southern Australia eat the contents of the apple-sized galls (abnormal outgrowths of plant tissue caused by an insect laying an egg in it) of *Cystococcus pomiformis* (Hemiptera: Eriococcidae) commonly called bush coconuts or bloodwood apples (Gullan & Cranson, 2005); the latter name because the galls occur on the bloodwood eucalypts (*Corymba* species). Each mature gall contains a single adult female up to 4 cm long. Aboriginals relish the watery female insects and her nutty-flavored larvae, then scrape out and consume the white coconut-like flesh of the inner gall.

Honey is a product of bees, however honey is sometimes collected by ants. Aboriginals in Australia and local people in Mexico collect honey from honeypot ants (in the first country *Melophorus* sp. and *Camponotus* sp., and in the latter *Myrmcocystus* sp.). These ants, called honeypot ants, serve as honey reservoirs, which in their abdomens store the honey that other workers collect from, for example, aphids, in their huge extended crops.

Caterpillars are eaten all over the world and in particular in Africa, However, Australia is one of the few countries in the world where the adults (butterflies) were eaten, namely, the Bogong moth (*Agrotis infusa*) (Flood, 1980). The moths spend the dry season in rocky crevices in the Bogong high plains. They are smoked out of the crevices and collected on kangaroo skins. They are eaten after the scales, wings, and legs are roasted off.

Edible insect resources can be threatened because of overexploitation and habitat degradation (Ramos-Elorduy, 2006; Yen, 2015). Habitat degradation can happen because of pesticide use. In Japan, the grasshopper *Oxya* spp. occurring in rice fields, is a main insect consumed today, but in the final quarter of the 20th century its abundance declined; both sellers and consumers attribute this trend to the use of pesticides (Payne, 2015). Populations of the popular Korean snack, rice field grasshoppers, or "mettugi," plummeted due to pesticide use, and returned to normal when Koreans began to require organic rice (Pemberton, 2002). A similar story was recorded in Thailand where the Bombay locust (*Patanga succincta*) was a widespread and destructive pest of maize. After a program to promote its use as food it is now a popular food and not considered a pest anymore (Hanboonsong, 2010). To the contrary, 170 tons are now imported annually from Cambodia (Ratanachan (2009) cited in Hanboonsong, Jamjanya, and Durst (2013)). Forestry resources are sometimes compromised when collectors cut down trees in national parks to facilitate harvesting of edible insects. This happens with the mopane caterpillar *Imbrasia belina* (Lepidoptera: Saturniidae) in southern Africa. In such cases, sustainable harvesting practices need to be developed (Gondo, Frost, Kozanayi, Stack, & Mushongahand, 2010). Because an increased demand for edible insects will put pressure on the wild-harvested populations (92% of the species), Yen (2015) proposed to investigate the effects on food webs, and also the effect of mass trapping techniques (such as light traps) on nontarget species, including possible ecosystem effects.

Most edible insects in the tropics are collected from nature. There are examples of enhancing the harvestability of insects species and examples have been given by Van Itterbeeck and Van Huis (2012). For example, eggs of aquatic Hemiptera in Mexico are semicultivated by water management and by providing egg-laying sites. Palm trees may be cut deliberately, to trigger palm weevils (*Rhynchophorus* spp.; Col.: Curculionidae) to oviposit on the trunk. In the Central African Republic, collection of arboreal, foliage-consuming caterpillars is facilitated by manipulating host tree distribution and abundance, shifting cultivation, fire regimens, host tree preservation, and manually introducing caterpillars to a designated area. Costa Neto (2015) mentions from Latin America the semidomestication of scale insects (*Dactylopius* spp.), ants (*Atta* spp.), and wasps (*Polybia* spp.). In northern Thailand, collectors leave some larvae of the bamboo caterpillar (*Omphisa fuscidentalis*) to mature from bamboo culms into adults in order to assure a next generation (Hanboonsong et al., 2013).

Because of the seasonality of many edible insect species, the only way to keep them available longer is to use conservation practices (like the drying of mopane caterpillars and migratory locusts in North Africa), converting them into insect meal, or tinning them. The best way, however, would be to rear them as mini-livestock and, as such, they would not threaten the natural resource.

21.3 ENVIRONMENT

It is generally recognized that for multiple environmental reasons, alternative protein sources are needed. One reason is the jeopardizing of the natural, wild habitats. Another reason is the unsustainable use of land (and its related water and air resources) currently in agricultural production. At this time, livestock production causes land degradation, greenhouse gas (GHG) emissions (namely, CO_2, CH_4, and NO_2 are responsible for 9, 35–40%, and 65% of global emissions, respectively), 64% of global NH_4 emissions, water depletion and pollution, and biodiversity loss (Steinfeld et al., 2006). Other concerns of livestock production are animal welfare as exemplified in the book *Farmageddon* (Lymbery, 2014) and zoonotic infections transmissible from animals to humans (Tomley & Shirley, 2009). For the environmental concerns, a number of mitigation measures have been proposed, such as improving efficiency in crop and animal production; reducing enteric CH_4 emissions, reducing emissions from manure management, sequestering of soil carbon, and changing human consumption of animal-source food (De Boer et al., 2011; Gerber et al., 2013). Eating insects instead of the common production animals is an option if producing edible insects would be environmentally advantageous. The problem is that the variety of insect species that can be eaten is much larger than that for conventional livestock and it is difficult to generalize.

The number of quantitative studies published on GHG emissions produced by farmed food and feed insects is limited. Oonincx et al. (2010) showed that the amount of greenhouse gases emitted per kg of mass gain of three edible insect species, the yellow mealworm (*Tenebrio molitor*), the house cricket (*Acheta domesticus*), and the migratory locust (*Locusta migratoria*) was lower than that for pigs and much lower for than that for cattle. The production of NH_3 by these insects was also lower than for conventional livestock species. However, a better and widely accepted method to assess GHG emissions, land use, and fossil energy use between animal protein sources is a lifecycle assessment. It takes into account not only direct GHG emissions through respiration, but also GHG emissions related to feed production and transportation, as well as emissions due to the heating of the climate-controlled rearing facility. When the production of 1 kg of edible protein of two mealworm species was compared to that of milk, chicken, pork, or beef, GHG emissions were lower, similar amounts of energy, and much less land were required (Oonincx & De Boer, 2012). The feed for the insects had a large impact on these figures: 56% of GHG emissions, 44% of energy use, and 99% of land use. Considering the latter, mealworms require only 18 m^2 to produce 1 kg of protein, which is considerably less than for milk, chicken, pork, and beef (2.5, 2.6, 3.0, and 11.0 times less, respectively).

Insects are efficient converters of feed into body weight, probably because they are cold-blooded and do not need feed to maintain body temperature. Van Huis (2013) calculated that for producing 1 kg of edible product, crickets needed 2.1 kg of feed, which is 2.1 times more efficient than chicken, 4.3 times more than pigs, and 11.9 times more than cattle. The food conversion efficiency has also been calculated for different mealworm species and it was around 3 on high-protein products (Van Broekhoven, 2015), compared to 4.0 for poultry, 9.1 for pigs, and 25.0 for beef, when only the edible portion is taken into account (100% for mealworms; 55% for poultry and pigs, and 40% for cattle) (Smil, 2002).

A large advantage of edible insects in comparison to conventional livestock is that a number of species can successfully be grown on organic side-streams, converting low-value organic byproducts into high-value proteins. This conversion is particularly important considering that one-third of all our agricultural produce and food is wasted; globally 1.3 billion tons each year annually (FAO, 2011) costing US$750 billion (Economist, 2014). Ramos-Elordy, Gonzalez, Hernandez, and Pino (2002) demonstrated this usefulness of edible insects in waste management by using waste fruits and vegetables for mealworms. However, when diets composed of products from beer brewing, bread/cookie baking, potato processing, and bioethanol production which are low in protein and high in starch, insect development time and mortality increases, and weight gain decreases compared to diets high in yeast-derived proteins (Van Broekhoven, Oonincx, Van Huis, & Van Loon, 2015).

There has been no study that evaluated the water requirements of edible insect species compared to traditional sources of protein (beef, pork, chicken). Very likely water consumption by insects will be considerably less than for common livestock species. Agriculture consumes about 70% of fresh water worldwide. For the production of 1 kg of livestock product, water requirements are the following: 4300 L for chicken, 6000 L for pigs, 10,400 L for sheep, and 15,400 L for cattle (Mekonnen & Hoekstra, 2010). For cattle, pastures make up 72%, crop ingredients 23%, fodder crops 4%, while for cattle drinking water less than 1% is used. For insects (except migratory locust) pastures and fodder crops are not used, so the water requirements would be much less. And again, insects can be raised on organic byproducts.

21.4 FARMING INSECTS

In order to get a predictable and continuous harvest of edible insects, they need to be farmed. Apart from the semi-domestication practices as described above, attempts have been made to farm insects.

It has been estimated that the mopane woodlands produce 9500 million mopane worms with a market value of US $84 million (Styles, 1994). However, the abundance of the mopane caterpillar is erratic and therefore the possibility of domestic farming has been investigated. Although it was demonstrated that it is possible to establish and maintain a captive population over 3 years, the costs are high and virus infections were a major problem (Ghazoul, 2006). Other problems like parasitoids can be tackled by using protective sleeves over the branches, as has been done with the silkworm *Anaphe panda* (Mbahin, Raina, Kioko, & Mueke, 2010).

Rearing of crickets such as the domestic house cricket (*Acheta domesticus*) and the common cricket or field cricket (*Gryllus bimaculatus*) is advanced in Thailand and 20,000 farms produced 7500 tons/year (Hanboonsong et al., 2013). Also, in the Lao People's Democratic Republic, these cricket species have been reared (Hanboonsong & Durst, 2014). Most farmers feed their crickets high-protein commercial chicken feed, which accounts for as much as half of total production costs (Durst & Hanboonsong, 2015). Large agribusiness firms in Thailand now produce specialized cricket feed. Some farmers reduce costs by feeding their maturing crickets local fruits and vegetables; fresh pumpkin or squash gives them a more attractive golden color and taste when they are mature (Durst & Hanboonsong, 2015).

Farmers in southern Thailand also produce the palm weevil, *Rhynchophorus ferrugineus*. They rear the insect in sections of palm of about 0.5 m in length. Adult weevils are released in drilled holes into the stem, which then reproduce, and the harvest is about 2 kg of larvae per stem and per cycle. Some farmers are now rearing palm weevils using plastic containers, filled with ground palm stems and mixed with pig feed (Durst & Hanboonsong, 2015).

Insects are an integral and widely accepted component of the diets of many cultures in Southeast Asia. Silk moth pupae, an important "byproduct" of the silk industry, has documented consumption in China at least as early as the first millennium (Durst & Hanboonsong, 2015). In Thailand the eating of silkworm pupae has now entered into commercial markets, and local production is unable to satisfy the demand, requiring the importation of large volumes from China (Durst & Hanboonsong, 2015). In Thailand, economic and population growth has been accompanied by a rising demand for insects for human consumption.

When it comes to the Western world then, there are a number of insect-rearing companies that produce many insect species as pet food for captive reptiles, fish, and birds, or as bait for fishing. In the West, there are also companies that produce beneficial insects and market those to control arthropod pests of agricultural crops. However, feedstock companies that produce for aquaculture and the livestock industry need to be assured of large and continuous quantities of standard quality. The cost of insect products needs to be competitive with current protein sources.

Some insect-rearing companies in the Netherlands now have specialized to produce insects for human food. This specialization means that they have set up special production lines, in which protocols are followed as if producing normal food, which means respecting hygiene and making sure each batch of the product is uniquely identified and a tracking system is carefully implemented. As the volume is still limited, prices are still high. For example, the cost price per kg of protein from mealworms at a farm in the Netherlands was US$35 compared to US$2.2 for grains (Meuwissen, 2011). The high price is mainly because of the high costs of labor and only automation can reduce the price. The insect species offered for human consumption in the Netherlands are the migratory locust (*Locusta migratoria*), the house cricket (*Acheta domesticus*), the yellow mealworm (*Tenebrio molitor*), and the lesser mealworm (*Alphitobius diaperinus*). In the United States, the most popular retail products currently are energy bars and cricket power or cricket meal. These sell for $3 to $3.50 for a 54–60-g bar, which is similar to the high-end noninsect energy bars. Roasted cricket powder retails at $35 for 9 kg which is, of course, four times more expensive than wheat flour, but comparable to the various flour ingredients needed for a gluten-free baked item (cake or cookies). Cricket products, as are all pure insect products, gluten-free.

Infections by several kinds of microorganisms may occur when producing insects for food and feed and these are: viruses, bacteria, microsporidia, fungi, and nematodes (carrying pathogenic bacteria). We know quite a lot about entomopathogens as control agents of agricultural insect pests, but very little about pathogens that occur while mass-rearing insects. One well-known pathogen is the *Acheta domestica* densovirus, endemic in Europe for 35 years (Liu et al., 2011). Since 2009, epizootics have also been reported from American commercial rearing and, for that reason, Weissman, Gray, Pham, and Tijssen (2012) suggested replacing the house cricket for commercial production with the resistant species *Gryllodes sigillatus*. Other crickets like the Jamaican cricket, *Gryllus assimilis*, and the European field cricket, *Gryllus bimaculatus*, were also found to be resistant (Szelei et al., 2011). Eilenberg, Vlak, Nielsen-LeRoux, Cappellozza, and Jensen (2015) mention an example of virus diseases that are infective to crabs and also to *A. domesticus*, indicating that invertebrate viruses sometimes can cross the species barrier. Concerning food safety, Eilenberg et al. (2015) indicate that insect pathogens are generally specific for invertebrates and do not harm vertebrates. They also gave recommendations to prevent and control insect diseases: be observant and diagnose any problem, keep production facilities clean, separate production stock into different facilities, maintain wide genetic variability in populations (quarantine new breeding stock insects for some time), and maintain several different lines for reproduction in a population as a reservoir of genetic variability (Eilenberg et al., 2015).

Sikorowski and Lawrence (1994) stressed applying good practices in insect rearing. Change in diet, exposure to elevated temperature, humidity, or toxins may cause microorganisms to multiply in the tissues of weakened hosts and cause a severe or fatal disease. Microbial degradation of the diet may also reduce the number of insects per unit of diet and the quality of insects produced. On the other hand, inclusion of antimicrobials often used in insect mass rearing diets, such as sorbic acid, are often growth inhibitors for the insects themselves (Dunkel & Read, 1991).

It is expected that large-scale mass rearing (tons/day) will first be developed for insects as feed. The focus is on the domestic house fly (*Musca domestica*) and the black soldier fly (*Hermetia illuscens*). Huge numbers will be required for fish, chicken, and pig feed. With larger volumes, economies of scale will be achieved, and it is believed that a number of companies are already able to produce these protein feed ingredients for prices similar or lower than fishmeal in the United States, Malaysia, and South Africa. In exploring the microbial safety of this source of feed, it was actually found that the black soldier fly reduces *Escherichia coli* in dairy manure (Liu et al., 2008). One US feed company, Enviroflight, driven by a passion for retaining the wild fisheries of the oceans, has as its mission to develop sustainable animal and plant nutrients using regionally available, low-value materials. EnviroFlight uses the coproduct from breweries, ethanol production, and preconsumer food waste as a feedstock for black soldier fly larvae (*Hermetia illuscens*), a food and feed insect (NexusMedia, 2014).

21.5 NUTRITION

The main problem with generalizing nutritional advantages is there are many species (over 2000) of edible insects and much variation in their nutrient content between species and within species with different diets. There are many publications dealing with nutritional values of edible insect species. Several of those publications have reviewed the literature for human consumption (Bukkens, 2005; Nowak, Persijn, Rittenschober, & Charrondiere, 2014; Rumpold & Schlüter, 2013; Xiaoming, Ying, Hong, & Zhiyong, 2010) or insectivores in general (Finke & Oonincx, 2014). Nutritional value depends on many factors such as such as gender, stage of development, diet, environmental factors such as temperature, day length, humidity, light intensity, and spectral composition (Finke & Oonincx, 2014). Processing methods can also affect the nutritional composition (Ekpo, 2011; Kinyuru, Kenji, Njoroge, & Ayieko, 2010; Madibela, Mokwena, Nsoso, & Thema, 2009).

21.5.1 Protein Content and Amino Acids

Protein content is commonly determined by multiplying the amount of nitrogen by 6.25, known as the crude protein content. This method may lead to a slight overestimation of true protein content because of the presence of other nitrogen-containing compounds, for example, chitin. The average protein content of insect orders varied between 35% for Isoptera (termites) and 61% for Orthoptera (crickets, grasshoppers, locusts). Among the latter group were species with protein contents up to 77% (Rumpold & Schlüter, 2013). The same study indicates that almost all insect orders generally meet the requirements recommended by the WHO/FAO/ONU for amino acids, and high values have been obtained for phenylalanine and tyrosine and some insects are rich in tryptophan, lysine, and threonine (WHO, 2007).

21.5.2 Fats and Fatty Acids

The average fat content per insect order ranged from 13% for Orthoptera (grasshoppers, crickets, locusts), 33% for Coleoptera (beetles, grubs) and true bugs (Hemiptera), termites (Isoptera), Blattodea (cockroaches), and, in some cases, caterpillars (Lepidoptera) are also rich in fat (between 28% and 33%) (Rumpold & Schlüter, 2013). Terrestrial edible insects seem to be a better source of long-chain polyunsaturated fatty acids, in particular the ω-6 fatty acids than aquatic ones (Fontaneto et al., 2013). The first are also easier to collect. Mealworm fat content and fatty acid profile depend on the diet consumed (Van Broekhoven et al., 2015). Mealworm larvae and crickets are high in palmitic acid, oleic acid, and linoleic acid (Finke, 2002; Tzompa-Sosa, Yi, Van Valenberg, Van Boekel, & Lakemond, 2014; Van Broekhoven et al., 2015). polyunsaturated fatty acids (PUFAs) are important for human health (Kouba & Mourot, 2011), particularly to avert depression (Sarri et al., 2008) and increase cognitive function (Stonehouse et al., 2010). High amounts of linoleic and/or linolenic acids are essential and cannot be synthesized by humans. Beef and pork contain very little PUFA and consist mainly of monounsaturated fatty acids (MUFAs) (Rumpold & Schlüter, 2013). Wang, Fu, Yan, and Zhao (2014) investigated the effect of *T. molitor* PUFA on obesity and found the PUFA to reduce body weight and cholesterol in a study using obese mice. The ratio between ω-6 and ω-3 PUFAs (n6/n3 ratio) is also of importance for human health, with an optimal ratio being 5:1 or lower (Kouba & Mourot, 2011) and the FAO recommendation being 10:1 (FAO, 2010). Mealworm n6/n3 ratio exceeded 18:1 (Van Broekhoven et al., 2015) and crickets 16:1. (Tzompa-Sosa et al., 2014). Because the fatty acid profile can be altered by diet, this requires further study.

21.5.3 Chitin

Chitin is the second most abundant polysaccharide in nature, and is commonly found in lower organisms such as fungi, crustaceans, and insects, but not in mammals. It has always been assumed that the fiber in insects is mainly chitin, but amino acids account for 9–33% of the weight of acid detergent fiber (ADF) content (Finke, 2007). This means that using ADF to estimate insect chitin results in an overestimation of insect chitin content. House crickets and the larvae of the yellow mealworm chitin content was between 1.6% and 2.0% (Finke, 2007). In comparison the adult yellow mealworm contained 7.4% chitin. Paoletti, Norberto, Damini, and Musumeci (2007) demonstrated that chitin digestion by humans is possible. They found chitinases in several human tissues and their role has been associated with defense against parasite infections and to some allergic conditions. Chitin and chitin derivatives have nonspecific antiviral and antitumor activities and it was shown to have an effect on innate and adaptive immune responses including the ability to recruit and activate innate immune cells (Lee, Silva, Lee, Hartl, & Elias, 2008).

21.5.4 Minerals

Among people in developing countries, deficiencies of important minerals such as iron and zinc are widespread. These deficiencies are caused by the low bioavailability in staple foods such as cereals and legumes due to the considerable amount of phytic acid and other antinutrients and the lack of animal foods with higher content and bioavailability. Anemia affects one-quarter of the world's population and is concentrated in preschool-aged children and women (McLean, Cogswell, Egli, Wojdyla, & De Benoist, 2009). Of the world's population 17.3% is at risk to inadequate intakes of zinc (Gibson, 2015), which is responsible for at least 450,000 deaths in Africa (58%), Asia (40%) and Latin America (2%) (Fischer Walker, Ezzati, & Black, 2008). In Kenya, it was shown that crickets and termites have a high iron and zinc content (Christensen et al., 2006). It is, however, unknown to what extent the minerals are bioavailable. In the Democratic Republic of Congo, a cereal made with caterpillars was used as a supplement to complement feedings in infants between 6 and 18 months of age. Compared with the usual diet, the supplemental feeding did not reduce the prevalence of stunting at 18 months, suggesting that factors other than dietary deficiencies also contribute to stunting. However, the infants in the supplement cereal group had higher Hb concentration and fewer were anemic (Bauserman et al., 2015).

21.5.5 Vitamins

Edible insects can be rich in vitamins but species have to be specifically selected for the exact desired vitamins (Rumpold & Schlüter, 2013). One generalization is that insects are a good source of B vitamins (Finke & Oonincx, 2014). Furthermore, it has been suggested that the content of vitamins in edible insects can be controlled via feed.

21.6 CONSUMER ATTITUDES

As people in Western cultures may not be familiar with insects as food, food neophobia can be expected. Besides, in the Western world insects are often viewed as dirty, disgusting, and dangerous (Looy, Dunkel, & Wood, 2014), and often viewed as pests and transmitters of diseases. This may be a misconception since only 5000 species of the one million species described can be considered harmful to either plants, animals, or humans (Van Lenteren, 2006). The Western attitude towards eating insects is a cultural bias that has been considered a hindrance towards acceptance of insects as normal food and, as such, a possible contribution to food insecurity (DeFoliart, 1999; Looy & Wood, 2015; Yen, 2009). Insect cuisine, for Westerners, has even been considered a threat to their psychological and cultural identity (Looy et al., 2014). Westerners have coined the anthropological term "entomophagy" as an alien habit by primitive people. However, if we consider insects as normal food, we should not use this term anymore.

Concerning unfamiliar foods, Fischer and Frewer (2009) found that perceptions of benefit are best predicted by familiarity or personal experience with the food, while risk information plays a more important role in perceptions of risk. They indicated that risk–benefit communication should be proactive rather than reactive as attitudes are less amenable to information interventions once they have been established. People interested in insects in Belgium (50% of respondents visiting an insectarium) showed a willingness to eat insects (Caparros Megido et al., 2014). Based on the survey, the authors recommended for popularization of insect products: stress the proximity of insects and crustaceans; introduce experimental tasting; and consider organoleptic qualities (taste, smell, and texture). Hartmann, Shi, Giusto, and Siegrist (2015) compared consumers' willingness to eat different insect-based, processed (eg, cookies based on cricket flour) and unprocessed (eg, crickets) food in China and Germany. While the Chinese rated all insect-based food more favorably than Germans, the latter reported higher willingness to eat the processed insect-based foods compared to the unprocessed foods. Insects as a normal but not mentioned part of familiar food, for example, figs and fig bars, do not seem to matter. Once a food enters into a "desired food" category, even, its true origins or contents make no difference in acceptability. The introduction of insects as a food source in Western societies seems more likely to succeed if insects are incorporated into familiar food items, which will reduce neophobic reactions and negative attitudes towards insect-based foods.

In the most recent Western culture cookbook, *The Insect Cookbook*, Kofi Annan the former Secretary General of the United Nations was interviewed about insect eating and his opinion was that it is a matter of educating the public (Van Huis, Van Gurp, & Dicke, 2014). This seemed to be confirmed in a study on the acceptance of insect eating by Dutch and Australian participants (Lensvelt & Steenbekkers, 2014). Providing information and giving consumers an opportunity to try eating insects increased consumer acceptance. Although making insects unrecognizable seems to make it less "scary," consumers are also interested in trying the whole insect.

Tan et al. (2015) compared consumer acceptance of insects by Dutch and Thai participants. While many Dutch participants were motivated by sustainable food consumption, the Thai participants considered insects more in terms of their taste and familiarity. Thai participants were strongly repulsed by mealworms, due to the association with larvae that they often see in decaying matter—an association that was absent amongst the Dutch participants who were more familiar with mealworms as food and less familiar with the observation of larvae in decaying matter than the Thai participants.

Dunkel et al. (unpublished data) conducted a longitudinal study of undergraduate US students' acceptance of edible insects. Each year for 23 years, students were given a similar set of informational sessions and similar insect-containing cuisine to sample (Dunkel, 1996). In 1991 student acceptance was 46% and nutritional information was significantly more important to their acceptance than environmental issues. By 1993 student acceptance was 77% and nutritional and environmental aspects were equally important in their acceptance. There has been little change in student acceptance in the last few years (2013–14) when acceptance rose to 88%. For Euro-Americans to overcome their aversion to eating insects, students suggested that dispelling their stereotype was more important than nutritional or environmental information. After an information and sampling session in 2014, Montana secondary school family consumer science teachers and sous chef instructors had an acceptance rate of only 45%, reminiscent of university students over two decades ago. In 2015, the Montana State University campus community, consisting of professors, staff, and students who did not have an informational session prior to their sampling experience had an 85% consumer acceptance rate.

Even when stressing the environmental, nutritional, and food safety aspects, and even if insect-based food products have an excellent taste, Western culture consumers may not be convinced. In the Western world, insects have rarely been considered food. However, there are some unusual edible insects in Western cultures such as the Sardinian cheese with insect larvae, "casu marzu" (also called "casu modde," "casu cundídu," "casu fràzigu" in Sardinian, or in Italian "formaggio marcio" (rotten cheese)) is a traditional Sardinian sheep milk cheese, notable for containing live insect larvae (maggots). Although found mostly in the island of Sardinia, the cheese is also found in the nearby Corsica, where it goes by the name of "casgiu merzu." Derived from Pecorino, "casu marzu" goes beyond typical fermentation to a stage most would consider decomposition, brought about by the digestive action of the larvae of the cheese fly *Piophila casei*. Cultural acceptance has to do with emotions and with psychology.

However, with globalization it is possible that currently hesitant consumers may adapt to edible insects, as has been shown in the cases of sushi and lobster. In the 1980s and 1990s, Euro-Americans shifted sushi from aversion to a restaurant preference and gourmet-meal-at-home choice. In North America, the American lobster did not achieve popularity until the mid-19th century, when New Yorkers and Bostonians developed a taste for it. Prior to this time, American lobster was deemed worthy only of being used as fertilizer or fish bait. By the mid-20th century lobster was viewed as a staple in restaurants and groceries (Johnson, 2007). Now, even US consumers who are vegetarian are modifying their diet to include insects once they learn of the nutritional and environmental benefits, and, particularly, the deliciousness that insects can have.

21.7 FOOD SAFETY

Food safety deals with both insects directly used for human consumption and meat products of livestock given insects as feed. The long history of human consumption of insects in the tropics suggests, with little evidence to the contrary, that insects harvested for human consumption do not cause any significant health problems (DeFoliart, 1992).

Several authors have reviewed the potential hazards of a range of contaminants, like heavy metals, mycotoxins, pesticide residues, and pathogens (Belluco et al., 2013; Van der Spiegel, Noordam, & Van der Fels-Klerx, 2013). The hazards may be caused by the insect itself or because of production methods, preservation, and processing conditions.

Similar to other animal-derived products, insects are rich in nutrients and moisture. Insect gut microflora provide a medium for growth of unwanted microorganisms in certain conditions. This makes insects susceptible to microbiological hazards if adequate heat treatment or storage conditions are not applied. Therefore, edible insects need to be processed and stored with care as one would any dry food product. Klunder, Wolkers-Rooijackers, Korpela, and Nout (2012), focusing on mealworms (*Tenebrio molitor*) and crickets (*Acheta domesticus* and *Brachytrupes* sp.), analyzed the insects as fresh, boiled, roasted, and stored (both refrigerated and in the ambient environment). They showed that a short heating step was sufficient to eliminate Enterobacteriaceae such as *E. coli* and *Salmonella*. However, some spore-forming bacteria will remain a potential risk in cooked insects probably introduced through soil contact (eg, the mopane caterpillar is dried on the soil) and cannot be fully eliminated by boiling. Lactic fermentation of composite flour/water mixtures containing 10% or 20% powdered roasted mealworm larvae resulted in successful acidification and was demonstrated effective in safeguarding shelf-life and safety by the control of enterobacteria and bacterial spores.

For insects used as animal feed, one study provided data on larvae fed a range of waste substrates in the United Kingdom, China, Mali, and Ghana. The following chemical contaminants were considered: veterinary medicines, pesticides, heavy metals, dioxins and polychlorinated biphenyls, polyaromatic hydrocarbons, and mycotoxins (Charlton et al., 2015). Chemical contaminants were below recommended maximum concentrations suggested by bodies such as the European Commission, the World Health Organization and Codex. Only the toxic heavy metal cadmium was found in three of the housefly (*Musca domestica*) samples analyzed above the lowest European Union (EU) limit in animal feed (500 µg/kg).

Recently it was shown that insects and crustaceans, long considered widely separated branches of the arthropod family tree, actually belong together (Pennisi, 2015). That also means that cross-reactivity between insects and crustaceans may be likely. For example, the allergen arginine kinase was found to cross-react between the cricket *Gryllus bimaculatus* and the freshwater shrimp *Macrobrachium* spp. (Srinroch, Srisomsap, Chokchaichamnankit, Punyarit, & Phiriyangkul, 2015). Safety of yellow mealworms (*Tenebrio molitor* L.) for human consumption was tested and the major cross-reactive proteins were identified as not only arginine kinase, but also tropomyosin, both well-known allergens in noninsect arthropods. In vitro cross-reactivity studies showed that there is a realistic possibility that house dust mites and crustacean allergic patients may react to food containing yellow mealworm proteins (Verhoeckx et al., 2014). Broekman et al. (2015) also found in in vivo and in vitro tests that shrimp allergic patients are at risk for developing allergic reactions when consuming food containing mealworm proteins.

The global demand for meat from 2005/07 to 2050 will increase by 76% (Alexandratos & Bruinsma, 2012). However, this increased demand in this time period will be mainly from developing countries (113%) and less from developed countries (27%). The question then is whether changing Western attitudes towards increased insect consumption will have an impact. According to DeFoliart (1999) it is because acculturation toward Western lifestyles tends to cause a reduction in the use of insects. Deroy, Reade, and Spence (2015) believe that even the occasional consumption of insects by Westerners, if it comes with a positive re-evaluation of their status as a nutritious food source would mean a big change—one that potentially reached far beyond these occasional consumers. They believe that a sensory-driven strategy stands a much greater chance of people deciding to eat insects on a regular basis. Taste is the actual motivator. The turn—or better said return—to entomophagy in this sense, needs to be driven by a psychologically realistic motivation and gastronomic interest.

21.8 PROCESSING AND MARKETING

The mopane caterpillar is a food item that is marketed in large quantities in southern Africa, and therefore the adding value process is described below (Kozanayi & Frost, 2002). Collection of the mopane caterpillar is done in the mopane forests. There they are processed (which includes having their gut contents emptied) and dried. Batches of processed and dried caterpillars are then transported to the consumer markets either by the collectors themselves or through intermediate traders, who then sell on wholesale markets. Wholesalers may repackage their stock into smaller, sealed and labeled packs for sale in formal outlets (shops and supermarkets) or sell the bulk directly to retailers in open markets. Retailers, whether trading with consumers through the formal or the informal market sector, can also obtain stocks direct from intermediate traders. Small traders in bars, restaurants, or open-air markets may further added value by cooking caterpillars or adding spices before selling them to consumers.

In Kenya, termites and lake flies were processed into readily acceptable consumer products by baking, boiling, and steam cooking under pressure (Ayieko, Oriamo, & Nyambuga, 2010). The processed products included crackers, muffins, sausages, and meat loaf. These processed products were readily accepted, making commercialization easier. Also in Kenya, 5% of the wheat flour was replaced with ground termites and the buns produced using this fortified flour had similar aroma and taste as the control and were well accepted by consumers (Kinyuru, Kenji, & Njoroge, 2009).

In the Netherlands, freeze-dried insects have been on the market for a number of years (migratory locust, the yellow mealworm, and the lesser mealworm). They are produced by three rearing companies in the Netherlands who normally produce insects as pet food and as feed for animals in zoos. However, they have set up special production lines to rear insects for human consumption and they have self-imposed regulations (eg, hygienic measures and a batch ID and tracing system), which are also used for other animal food commodities. These freeze-dried insects can be bought in specialized shops and through the Internet. In 2015, one supermarket chain in the Netherlands with more than 500 outlets started in 2015 by selling hamburgers, nuggets, and schnitzels which contain 16% ground lesser mealworms. The commercialization is done by a Belgium company while the insects are produced by one of the above-mentioned rearing companies in the Netherlands. To facilitate marketing, an insect cookbook was produced, first in Dutch and later in English (Van Huis et al., 2014). The cookbook not only contains recipes but also information about eating insects in different parts of the world and interviews with persons such as chef Rene Redzepi, owner of the Noma restaurant (Copenhagen, Denmark), which was ranked in 2010, 2011, 2012, and 2014, as the best restaurant in the world by Restaurant Magazine.

Since 2010, the number of launchings of companies with new food insect products or kits to produce food insects in a small scale has steadily risen. United States and Canadian start-up companies are mainly basing their products on *Acheta domesticus*, roasted and ground into a fine powder or a coarse meal. A similar trend of lauchings has occurred in Europe during the past 5 years, but focused on other insect species.

The main commercial food insects in the United States are the house cricket, *Acheta domesticus*, the wax moth, *Galleria melonella*, and the yellow mealworm, *Tenebrio molitor*, the giant mealworm (*Zophobas atratus*), and the lesser mealworm (*Alphitobius diaperinus*). All are sold live, shipped from several food suppliers in various locations directly to the consumer. Crickets are supplied at any stage from "pinheads" to adults. The other two commercial food insects are only sold as larvae. In the United States, there seems to be a commercial preference for crickets and cricket products. Since 2012, the company Chapul, has produced in its own factory, cricket bars made from cricket flour and markets those in different flavors, also internationally. The founder of Chapul, Patrick Crowley, is professionally a hydrologist who is passionate about retaining the wild waterways of the western United States and also realized that macro-livestock and the production of their feed is threatening water availability. He sought to make a statement about water and the future and this led to the creation of a new source of protein, the cricket-based Chapul bar. There are also other companies that produce cricket bars in different flavors such as Exo since 2013. Six Foods produces "Chirps," a chip made from cricket flour, and has sold those commercially since May 2015. In Austin, Texas, the Aspire Food Group focuses on commercial-scale farming of organic crickets exclusively for human consumption. This is currently a rapidly expanding market throughout the United States.

Others wishing to make an environmental statement including universities and private companies (Little Herds LLC, Austin, TX), are trying to ameliorate the "disgust factor" among the general public. Montana State University Catering Service, Bozeman, Montana, has created a new cuisine based on cricket flour. MSU catering service now uses cricket flour to fill orders for brownies, cookies, and smoothies that are gluten-free and high in complete protein as well as calcium, zinc, and iron.

Most of the 27 restaurants serving insects in the United States in 2014 were in California and New York. Don Bugito in San Francisco, CA, has imported some of the culinary ideas from Mexico, one of the best culinary regions in the Americas for edible insects. The Portland OR restaurant, Sushi Mazi, has combined two new-to-Western-culture-palates, sushi and grasshoppers. The grasshoppers are steamed, though, not raw.

Well-known cookbooks from the Americas are: *Entertaining with Insects* by Ronald Taylor and Barbara Carter (Taylor & Carter, 1996); *Eat a Bug Cookbook* by David George Gordon (Gordon, 1998); and *Creepy, Crawly Cuisine* by Julieta Ramos-Elorduy (Ramos-Elorduy, 1998). Other books have had culinary sections and recipes as well. *Edible* by Daniella Martin (Martin, 2014), and Chronicle of a Changing Culture: *The Food Insects Newsletter* (DeFoliart et al., 2009).

21.9 LEGISLATION

In the Western world, edible insects have only recently been considered as food for human consumption and as feed for livestock. Consumption guidelines and regulations have not yet been incorporated into policy documents and have been largely omitted from regulatory frameworks. A first overview on legislative issues was provided in an FAO discussion paper (Halloran & Münke, 2014). International recommendations specific to the use of insects in food and feed are yet to be developed. No standards in the Codex Alimentarius (the international reference standard for food and feed established by the FAO and the WHO) specifically refer to the use of insects in animal feed or food.

The state of the art of European legislation was discussed by Van der Spiegel et al. (2013) and Belluco et al. (2013). Even in nations where there is a tradition of consuming a variety of insect species, they do not appear explicitly in dietary guidelines (Halloran, Vantomme, Hanboonsong, & Ekesi, 2015). A recent paper reviews various actions taken or underway in Thailand, Canada, Kenya, and Switzerland concerning regulations and legislation governing the use of insects as food and feed (Halloran et al., 2015).

People who want to advance insects as food and feed find legislative issues the biggest hurdle in advancing edible insects in the agricultural and food sector. For example, questions like "How can the prohibition of eating insects be justified since hundreds of millions of people have consumed insects for millennia" or "How can a free-roaming chicken be allowed to pick and eat uncertified insects from the soil and when we propose to serve them certified insects, it is not allowed." The simple fact is that in the Western world, when the food and feed legislation was made, nobody thought about insects as either food or feed. And to adapt the legislation takes time. Also, when in the legislation the word "animal" was used, few people considered that insects are also animals. One clear example of a deficient legislation in the EU is the following (Byrne, 2015; Koeleman, 2014): Insect protein was given the green light for use in aquaculture in the EU in June 2013. However, the condition is that animals are killed in an official registered slaughterhouse (Annex IV to Regulation (EC) No 999/2001). As insects are animals, they also fall under this regulation. This then prevents the use of insects in fish farming. However, it also affects the permission to kill insects for human consumption.

In EU food product applications, the most important question for food producers is whether or not the product is considered a novel food. If so, the producer has to provide a Novel Food Dossier, among others, proving the product is safe for the consumer. Halloran et al. (2015) concluded "Addressing insects as a novel food focuses primarily on food safety and consumer protection. While these issues are highly relevant, they can also undermine the importance of nature conservation, traditional food systems, and economic development" and "The development of future legislation must take into consideration the multi-dimensional nature of insects as food and feed."

US legislation affecting edible insects has developed differently than that of the EU. Insects or products from insects used for food must have as their water source, clean, pure, uncontaminated, drinking water. Their food sources must be fresh and clean. This is always interesting to explain to students or entrepreneurs in the edible insect area, since no such restrictions apply to the close cousins of insects, the Crustacea, such as lobster, crab, and shrimp. Certainly the detritus and decaying flesh normally consumed by free-ranging lobster would not pass FDA standards. Throughout New England these enormous Crustacea were an easy supply of protein, but they were not valued. "Their plenty makes them little esteemed and seldom eaten," wrote William Wood in *New England's Prospect*, 1634. In the 1600s, 1700s, and 1800s, abundance bred contempt, so the colonists often only used lobster to fend off hunger and as cheap food for indentured servants, prisoners, and slaves. Servants specified in employment agreements that they would not eat lobster more than twice per week (Johnson, 2007). Lobsters were fed to pigs and used as fertilizer and fish bait. In the 1900s, lobsters became a prized food for humans. Now lobsters are moving off the menu until more humane killing procedures can be developed for them (Johnston, 2004).

US legislation affecting insects used as feed is complex. Although insects are a preferred part of the diet of free-ranging chickens and fish, and certainly an occasional part of the diet of other ruminant and nonruminant human food animals, insects' presence in commercial food formulations is carefully controlled by the US Food and Drug Administration (FDA). This commonly known piece of nonhuman animal behavior was not considered in developing US feed regulations. The Federal Food, Drug, and Cosmetic Act (FFDCA) requires that any substance added to or expected to become a component of animal food, either directly or indirectly, must be used in accordance with a food additive regulation unless it is generally recognized as safe (GRAS) for that intended use. Typical feed ingredients such as forages, grains, and most minerals and vitamins are GRAS as sources of nutrients. Insects are typically a natural food and source of nutrients for chickens, fish, and other nonruminants. It seems that insects of specific species should be considered GRAS by the definition of the US FDA. The legal definition for a food additive is found in Section 201 (s) of the FFDCA. Feed regulations for human food may not contain insects if the feed is sold in interstate commerce. Feed produced on-farm with insects can be fed to animals used for human food if the insects are produced on the same farm where the human food animals are being raised. Yet, no regulation has been issued for figs in interstate and international commerce, all of which, by definition, contain edible insects, fig wasps, and their parasitoid wasps. These are small, microscopic insects, but without pollination by the fig wasp, a fig cannot develop. After pollination, all the male fig wasps and the previous generation of fig wasps, and their parasitoid wasps are trapped inside the fig. There are 900 species of fig wasps, and each is responsible for pollinating one or two species of fig plant. Without these tiny insects, there would be no figs. Some vegetarians and vegans refuse to eat figs and fig products based on the possibility of insect content. Actually, insects contaminate most agricultural products upon harvest and on the way to market. From canned corn to curry paste, from premium coffee to peanut butter, most foods contain insects. For example, when tomato ketchup qualifies for the highest USDA grade standard possible, it is required to contain no more than 30 fruit fly eggs per every 100 grams (3.5 ounces) (Meyer, 2003). For some people, no amount of explaining is sufficient.

Legislation clearly does not affect all food insects. Certainly it is time for insects to take their place beside fish, chickens, pigs, lobster, shrimp, and cattle as a normal source of protein in use in the world at this time.

21.10 THE WAY FORWARD

One of the major hurdles currently is the legislative framework. The International Platform of Insects for Food and Feed (IPIFF) was established on the April 13, 2015. It is made up of insect-producing companies from the Netherlands, France, Germany, and South Africa. Their main concern is the removal of the legislative roadblocks in the EU, and this involves the EU Commission's Directorate General for Health and Consumers (DG Sanco) and the Scientific Committee of the EU's food safety authority (EFSA). "The insect producing business is an industry-in-waiting and that is ready to explode once the application areas become wide open," according to a spokesman of IPIFF (Byrne, 2015).

A major problem of starting a new sector such as the one of edible insects is the trust and cooperation between entrepreneurs, which is one of the main challenges for the success of a start-up dealing with a radical innovation (Pascucci, Dentoni, & Mitsopoulos, 2015). Production processes can be difficult to patent, although it occurs (Aldana et al., 2015), making cooperation sometimes difficult. Economies of scale will make the insect products less expensive and automation will probably happen first in the sector of insect as feed, as huge volumes are required.

Consumers in the Western world may have psychological difficulties in accepting insects as food even when environmental benefits, high nutritional value, excellent organoleptic qualities, and low price are mentioned. However, increasing exposure to this new food item will likely trigger a change, and providing information about the sustainability of the product, giving people a tasting experience, incorporating ground insects into familiar products (eg, burgers), and making insect products delicious are key. However, at a global scale, it is more important that in emerging economies the value of edible insects is realized as most demand for more meat will be from those countries. It is also urgent that the Western world overcome these barriers so that nutritionally at-risk countries trying to adopt Western culture ways do not lose their insect-eating practices due to an "embarrassment factor."

The key to success is the golden triangle, the collaboration of government, industry, and academia. It is an innovative challenge. The cooperation between biological disciplines (multidisciplinarity) is required to create insect products, while the cooperation of socioeconomic disciplines (interdisciplinarity) and the public at large (transdisciplinarity) are required for marketing and public acceptance. Edible insects have an exceptionally high potential to contribute to a more sustainable and socially more equitable global food security.

REFERENCES

Agea, J. G., Biryomumaisho, D., Buyinza, M., & Nabanoga, G. N. (2008). Commercialization of *Ruspolia nitidula* (Nsenene grasshoppers) in Central Uganda. *African Journal of Food Agriculture and Development, 8*, 319–332.

Aldana, J., Quan, E., Vickerson, A., Marchant, B., Kaulfuss, O., & Radley, R. (2015). *Contained systems to provide reproductive habitat for Hermetia illucens*. United States Patent Application 20150122182. http://www.freepatentsonline.com/y2015/0122182.html.

Alexandratos, N., & Bruinsma, J. (2012). *World agriculture towards 2030/2050: The 2012 Revision*. Global Perspective Studies Team. ESA Working Paper No. 12–03. Rome: Agricultural Development Economics Division of the Food and Agriculture Organization of the United Nations.

Ayieko, M. A., Oriamo, V., & Nyambuga, I. A. (2010). Processed products of termites and lake flies: Improving entomophagy for food security within the Lake Victoria region. *African Journal of Food, Agriculture, Nutrition and Development, 10*, 2085–2098.

Bauserman, M., Lokangaka, A., Gado, J., Close, K., Wallace, D., Kodondi, K.-K., ... Bose, C. (2015). A cluster-randomized trial determining the efficacy of caterpillar cereal as a locally available and sustainable complementary food to prevent stunting and anaemia. *Public Health Nutrition, 18*, 1785–1792.

Belluco, S., Losasso, C., Maggioletti, M., Alonzi, C. C., Paoletti, M. G., & Ricci, A. (2013). Edible insects in a food safety and nutritional perspective: A critical review. *Comprehensive Reviews in Food Science and Food Safety, 12*, 296–313.

Bodenheimer, F. S. (1951). *Insects as human food: A chapter of the ecology of man*. The Hague: Dr. W. Junk Publishers.

Broekman, H., Knulst, A., Den Hartog-Jager, S., Gaspari, M., de Jong, G., Houben, G., & Verhoeckx, K. (2015). Shrimp allergic patients are at risk when eating mealworm proteins. *Clinical and Translational Allergy, 5*(Suppl. 3), 77.

Bukkens, S. G. F. (2005). Insects in the human diet: Nutritional aspects. In M. G. Paoletti (Ed.), *Ecological implications of minilivestock: Role of rodents, frogs, snails, and insects for sustainable development* (pp. 545–577). Enfield: Science Publishers, Inc, Chapter 28.

Byrne, J. (2015). *Insect feed producers align to remove EU regulatory roadblocks*. Feed Navigator. <http://www.feednavigator.com/Regulation/Insect-feed-producers-align-to-remove-EU-regulatory-roadblocks>.

Caparros Megido, R., Sablon, L., Geuens, M., Brostaux, Y., Alabi, T., Blecker, C., ... Francis, F. (2014). Edible insects acceptance by Belgian consumers: Promising attitude for entomophagy development. *Journal of Sensory Studies, 29*, 14–20.

Charlton, A. J., Dickinson, M., Wakefield, M. E., Fitches, E., Kenis, M., Han, R., ... Smith, R. (2015). Exploring the chemical safety of fly larvae as a source of protein for animal feed. *Journal of Insects as Food and Feed, 1*, 7–16.

Christensen, D. L., Orech, F. O., Mungai, M. N., Larsen, T., Friis, H., & Aagaard-Hansen, J. (2006). Entomophagy among the Luos of Kenya: A potential mineral source? *International Journal of Food Sciences and Nutrition, 57*, 198–203.

Costa-Neto, E. M. (2015). Anthropo-entomophagy in Latin America: An overview of the importance of edible insects to local communities. *Journal of Insects as Food and Feed, 1*, 17–23.

De Boer, I. J. M., Cederberg, C., Eady, S., Gollnow, S., Kristensen, T., Macleod, M., ... Zonderland-Thomassen, M. A. (2011). Greenhouse gas mitigation in animal production: Towards an integrated life cycle sustainability assessment. *Current Opinion in Environmental Sustainability, 3*, 423–431.

DeFoliart, G. R. (1989). The human use of insects as food and as animal feed. *Bulletin of the Entomological Society of America, 35*, 22–35.

DeFoliart, G. R. (1999). Insects as food: Why the western attitude is important. *Annual Review of Entomology, 44*, 21–50.

DeFoliart, G. (1992). Insect as human food: Gene DeFoliart discusses some nutritional and economic aspects. *Crop Protection, 11*, 395–399.

DeFoliart, G. (2012). *The human use of insects as a food resource: A bibliographic account in progress*. http://www.food-insects.com/.

DeFoliart, G., Dunkel, F. V., & Gracer, D. (2009). *The food insects newsletter: Chronicle of a changing culture*. Salt Lake City: Aardvark Global Publishing.

Deroy, O., Reade, B., & Spence, C. (2015). The insectivore's dilemma, and how to take the West out of it. *Food Quality and Preference, 44*, 44–55.

Dunkel, F. V., & Read, N. R. (1991). Review of the effect of sorbic acid on insect survival in rearing diets with reference to other antimicrobials. *American Entomologist, 37*, 172–178.

Dunkel, F. (1996). Incorporating food insects into undergraduate entomology courses. *The Food Insects Newsletter, 9*, 1–4.

Durst, P. B., & Hanboonsong, Y. (2015). Small-scale production of edible insects for enhanced food security and rural livelihoods: Experience from Thailand and Lao People's Democratic Republic. *Journal of Insects as Food and Feed, 1*, 25–31.

Forest insects as food: Humans bite back In P. B. Durst, D. V. Johnson, R. N. Leslie, & K. Shono (Eds.), *Proceedings of a workshop on Asia-Pacific resources and their potential for development, 19–21 February 2008, Chiang Mai, Thailand* Bangkok: Regional Office for Asia and the Pacific of the Food and Agriculture Organization of the United Nations.

Economist (2014). *Food loss and its intersection with food security. Global food security index 2014*. London: Special Report of the Intelligence Unit of the Economist.

Eilenberg, J., Vlak, J. M., Nielsen-LeRoux, C., Cappellozza, S., & Jensen, A. B. (2015). Diseases in insects produced for food and feed. *Journal of Insects as Food and Feed, 1*, 87–102.

Ekpo, K. E. (2011). Effect of processing on the protein quality of four popular insects consumed in Southern Nigeria. *Archives of Applied Science Research, 3*, 307–326.

FAO (2010). *Fats and fatty acids in human nutrition: Report of an expert consultation, 10–14 November 2008, Geneva. Food and nutrition paper no. 91*. Rome: Food and Agriculture Organization of the United Nations.

FAO (2011). *Global food losses and food waste – Extent, causes and prevention*. Rome: Food and Agriculture Organization of the United Nations.

Finke, M. D. (2002). Complete nutrient composition of commercially raised invertebrates used as food for insectivores. *Zoo Biology, 21*, 269–285.

Finke, M. D. (2007). Estimate of chitin in raw whole insects. *Zoo Biology, 26*, 105–115.

Finke, M. D., & Oonincx, D. (2014). Insects as food for insectivores. In J. Juan Morales-Ramos, G. Rojas, & D. I. Shapiro-Ilan (Eds.), *Mass production of beneficial organisms* (pp. 583–616). San Diego: Academic Press, Chapter 17.

Fischer, A. R. H., & Frewer, L. J. (2009). Consumer familiarity with foods and the perception of risks and benefits. *Food Quality and Preference, 20*, 576–585.

Fischer Walker, C. L., Ezzati, M., & Black, R. E. (2008). Global and regional child mortality and burden of disease attributable to zinc deficiency. *European Journal of Clinical Nutrition, 63*, 591–597.

Flood, J. (1980). Of moths and men. In J. Flood (Ed.), *The moth hunters: Aboriginal prehistory of the Australian Alps*. Canberra: Australian Institute of Aboriginals Studies, Chapter 6.

Fontaneto, D., Tommaseo-Ponzetta, M., Galli, C., Risé, P., Glew, R. H., & Paoletti, M. G. (2013). Differences in fatty acid composition between aquatic and terrestrial insects used as food in human nutrition. *Ecology of Food and Nutrition, 50*, 351–367.

Gerber, P. J., Steinfeld, H., Henderson, B., Mottet, A., Opio, C., Dijkman, J., ... Tempio, G. (2013). *Tackling climate change through livestock – A global assessment of emissions and mitigation opportunities*. Rome: Food and Agriculture Organization of the United Nations.

Ghazoul, J. (2006). *Mopani woodlands and the mopane worm: Enhancing rural livelihoods and resource sustainability. Final technical report*. London: DFID.

Gibson, R. S. (2015). *Dietary-induced zinc deficiency in low income countries: Challenges and solutions. The Avanelle Kirksey Lecture at Purdue University,* . Nutrition Today (50, pp. 49–55).

Gondo, T., Frost, P., Kozanayi, W., Stack, J., & Mushongahand, M. (2010). Linking knowledge and practice: Assessing options for sustainable use of mopane worms (*Imbasia belina*) in southern Zimbabwe. *Journal of Sustainable Development in Africa, 12*, 281–305.

Gordon, D. G. (1998). *The eat-a-bug cookbook: 33 ways to cook grasshoppers, ants, water bugs, spiders, centipedes, and their kin*. Berkeley: Ten Speed Press.

Gullan, P. J., & Cranson, P. S. (2005). Insects as food. In P. J. Cranston, & P. S. Cranson (Eds.), *The insects: An outline of entomology* (3rd ed., pp. 10–13). Victoria: Blackwell Publishing Ltd.

Halloran, A., & Münke, C. (2014). *Discussion paper: Regulatory frameworks influencing insects as food and feed*. Rome: Food and Agriculture Organization of the United Nations.

Halloran, A., Vantomme, P., Hanboonsong, Y., & Ekesi, S. (2015). Regulating edible insects: The challenge of addressing food security, nature conservation, and the erosion of traditional food culture. *Food Security, 7*, 739–746.

Hanboonsong, Y. (2010). Edible insects and associated food habits in Thailand. In P. B. Durst, D. V. Johnson, R. L. Leslie, & K. E. Shono (Eds.), *Forest insects as food: Humans bite back* (pp. 173–182). Bangkok: Regional Office for Asia and the Pacific of the Food and Agriculture Organization of the United Nations.

Hanboonsong, Y., & Durst, P. B. (2014). *Edible insects in Lao PDR: Building on tradition to enhance food security. RAP publication 2014/12*. Bangkok: Regional Office for Asia and the Pacific of the Food and Agriculture Organization of the United Nations.

Hanboonsong, Y., Jamjanya, T., & Durst, P. B. (2013). *Six-legged livestock: Edible insect farming, collection and marketing in Thailand*. Bangkok: Regional Office for Asia and the Pacific of the Food and Agriculture Organization of the United Nations.

Hartmann, C., Shi, J., Giusto, A., & Siegrist, M. (2015). The psychology of eating insects: A cross-cultural comparison between Germany and China. *Food Quality and Preference, 44*, 148–156.

Holt, V. M. (1995). *Why not eat insects?* Oxford, Thornton's. Text reset from the original 1885 edition by Meeuws, D. H., Oxford (July/August 1993).

Johnston, B. (2004). *Italian animal rights law puts lobster off the menu*. London: The Daily Telegraph, March 6, 2004.

Johnson, P. (2007). Lobster. In *Fish Forever: The Definitive Guide to Understanding, Selecting, and Preparing Healthy, Delicious, and Environmentally Sustainable Seafood*, (pp. 163–175). John Wiley & Sons, ISBN 978-0-7645-8779-5.

Jongema, Y. (2015). List of edible insect species of the world. Laboratory of Entomology. Wageningen: Wageningen University. <http://www.wageningenur.nl/en/Expertise-Services/Chair-groups/Plant-Sciences/Laboratory-of-Entomology/Edible-insects/Worldwide-species-list.htm/>.

Kinyuru, J. N., Kenji, G. M., & Njoroge, M. S. (2009). Process development, nutrition and sensory qualities of wheat buns enriched with edible termites (*Macrotermes subhylanus*) from Lake Victoria region, Kenya. *African Journal of Food and Agriculture Nutrition and Development, 9*, 1739–1750.

Kinyuru, J. N., Kenji, G. M., Njoroge, S. M., & Ayieko, M. (2010). Effect of processing methods on the in vitro protein digestibility and vitamin content of edible winged termite (*Macrotermes subhylanus*) and grasshopper (*Ruspolia differens*). *Food and Bioprocess Technology, 3*, 778–782.

Klunder, H. C., Wolkers-Rooijackers, J., Korpela, J. M., & Nout, M. J. R. (2012). Microbiological aspects of processing and storage of edible insects. *Food Control, 26*, 628–631.

Koeleman, E. (2014). Insects crawling their way into feed regulation. *AllAboutFeed, 22*, 18–21.

Kouba, M., & Mourot, J. (2011). A review of nutritional effects on fat composition of animal products with special emphasis on n-3 polyunsaturated fatty acids. *Biochimie, 93*, 13–17.

Kozanayi, W., & Frost, P. (2002). *Marketing of mopane worm in Southern Zimbabwe. Mopane worm market survey: Southern Zimbabwe*. Harare: Institute of Environmental Studies.

Lee, C. G., Silva, C. A. D., Lee, J.-Y., Hartl, D., & Elias, J. A. (2008). Chitin regulation of immune responses: An old molecule with new roles. *Current Opinion in Immunology, 20*, 684–689.

Lensvelt, E. J. S., & Steenbekkers, L. P. A. (2014). Exploring consumer acceptance of entomophagy: A survey and experiment in Australia and the Netherlands. *Ecology of Food and Nutrition, 53*, 543–561.

Liu, Q., Tomberlin, J. K., Brady, J. A., Sanford, M. R., & Yu, Z. (2008). Black Soldier Fly (Diptera: Stratiomyidae) larvae reduce *Escherichia coli* in dairy manure. *Environ. Entomol, 37*, 1525–1530.

Liu, K., Li, Y., Jousset, F.-X., Zadori, Z., Szelei, J., Yu, Q., ... Tijssen, P. (2011). The *Acheta domesticus* Densovirus, Isolated from the European house cricket, has evolved an expression strategy unique among parvoviruses. *Journal of Virology, 85*, 10069−10078.

Looy, H., Dunkel, F. V., & Wood, J. R. (2014). How then shall we eat? Insect-eating attitudes and sustainable foodways. *Agriculture and Human Values, 31*, 131−141.

Looy, H., & Wood, J. R. (2015). Imagination, hospitality, and affection: The unique legacy of food insects? *Animal Frontiers, 5*, 8−13.

Lymbery, P. (2014). *Farmageddon: The true cost of cheap meat*. London: Bloomsbury Publishing.

Madibela, O. R., Mokwena, K. K., Nsoso, S. J., & Thema, T. F. (2009). Chemical composition of mopane worm sampled at three different sites in Botswana and subjected to different processing. *Tropical Animal Health and Production, 41*, 935−942.

Malaisse (1997). *Se Nourir en Foret Claire Africaine: Approche Ecologique et Nutritionnelle*. Les Presses Agronomiques de Gembloux.

Martin, D. (2014). *Edible. An adventure into the world of eating insects and the last great hope to save the planet*. New York: New Harvest.

Mbahin, N., Raina, S. K., Kioko, E. N., & Mueke, J. M. (2010). Use of sleeve nets to improve survival of the Boisduval silkworm, *Anaphe panda*, in the Kakamega Forest of western Kenya. *Journal of Insect Science, 10*, 6. Available from http://dx.doi.org/10.1673/031.010.0601.

McLean, E., Cogswell, M., Egli, I., Wojdyla, D., & de Benoist, B. (2009). Worldwide prevalence of anaemia, WHO Vitamin and Mineral Nutrition Information System, 1993−2005. *Public Health Nutrition, 12*, 444−454.

Mekonnen, M. M., & Hoekstra, A. Y. (2010). *The green, blue and grey water footprint of farm animals and animal products. Value of Water Research Report Series No. 48*. Delft: UNESCO-IHE.

Meuwissen, P. (2011). *Insecten als nieuwe eiwitbron - Een scenarioverkenning van de marktkansen (insects as a new protein source - an exploration of market opportunities)*. s-Hertogenbosch: ZLTO projecten.

Meyer, J. (2003). *Insects in food*. Department of Entomology, North Carolina State University. http://www.cals.ncsu.edu/course/ent425/text18/food.html%20accessed%205%20October%202005, http://www.cals.ncsu.edu/course/ent425/text18/food.html. Accessed 5 October 2005.

Nexus Media (2014). Soldier flies: The new food for farm fish. October 24, 2014. http://www.scientificamerican.com/video/soldier-flies-the-new-food-for-farm-fish/.

Nowak, V., Persijn, D., Rittenschober, D., & Charrondiere, U. R. (2014). Review of food composition data for edible insects. *Food Chemistry, 193*, 39−46.

Oonincx, D., & De Boer, I. (2012). Environmental impact of the production of mealworms as a protein source for humans − A life cycle assessment. *PLoS One, 7*, e51145.

Oonincx, D. G. A. B., Van Itterbeeck, J., Heetkamp, M. J. W., Van den Brand, H., Van Loon, J. J. A., & Van Huis, A. (2010). An exploration on greenhouse gas and ammonia production by insect species suitable for animal or human consumption. *PLoS One, 5*, e14445.

Paoletti, M. G. (2005). *Ecological implications of minilivestock: Potential of insects, rodents, frogs and snails*. Enfield: Science Publisher, Inc..

Paoletti, M. G., Norberto, L., Damini, R., & Musumeci, S. (2007). Human gastric juice contains chitinase that can degrade chitin. *Annals of Nutrition and Metabolism, 51*, 244−251.

Pascucci, S., Dentoni, D., & Mitsopoulos, D. (2015). The perfect storm of business venturing? The case of entomology-based venture creation. *Agricultural and Food Economics, 3*, 1−11.

Payne, C. L. R. (2015). Wild harvesting declines as pesticides and imports rise: The collection and consumption of insects in contemporary rural Japan. *Journal of Insects as Food and Feed, 1*, 57−65.

Pemberton, R. W. (1999). Insects and other arthropods used as drugs in Korean traditional medicine. *Journal of Ethnopharmacology, 65*, 207−216.

Pemberton, R. W. (2002). Wild-gathered foods as countercurrents to dietary globalisation in South Korea. In K. Cwiertka, & B. Boudewijn Walraven (Eds.), *Asian food: The global and the local* (pp. 76−94). Abingdon: Routledge.

Pennisi, E. (2015). All in the (bigger) family revised arthropod tree marries crustacean and insect fields. *Science of The Total Environment, 347*, 220−221.

Ramos-Elorduy, J. (1993). Insects in the diet of tropical Forest People in Mexico. In C. M. Hladik, A. Hladik, O. F. Linares, H. Pagezy, A. Semple, & M. Hadley (Eds.), *Food and nutrition in the tropical forest. Biocultural interactions and applications to development* (pp. 205−212). Paris: UNESCO.

Ramos-Elorduy, J. (1998). *Creepy crawly cuisine: The gourmet guide to edible insects*. Rochester, Vermont: Park Street Press.

Ramos-Elorduy, J. (2006). Threatened edible insects in Hidalgo, Mexico and some measures to preserve them. *Journal of Ethnobbiology and Ethnomedicine, 2*, 51. Available from http://dx.doi.org/10.1186/1746-4269-2-51.

Ramos-Elorduy, J., Gonzalez, E. A., Hernandez, A. R., & Pino, J. M. (2002). Use of *Tenebrio molitor* (Coleoptera: Tenebrionidae) to recycle organic wastes and as feed for broiler chickens. *Journal of Economic Entomology, 95*, 214−220.

Ramos-Elorduy, J., & Morales, J. M. P. (1989). *Los Insectos Comestibles en el México Antiguo (estudio etnoentomológico)*. Mexico: A.G.T. Editor.

Rumpold, B. A., & Schlüter, O. K. (2013). Nutritional composition and safety aspects of edible insects. *Molecular Nutrition & Food Research, 57*, 802−823.

Sarri, K. O., Linardakis, M., Tzanakis, N., & Kafatos, A. G. (2008). Adipose DHA inversely associated with depression as measured by the Beck Depression Inventory. *Prostaglandins Leukotrienes and Essent Fatty Acids, 78*, 117−122.

Sikorowski, P. P., & Lawrence, A. M. (1994). Microbial contamination and insect rearing. *American Entomologist, 40*, 240−253.

Smil, V. (2002). Worldwide transformation of diets, burdens of meat production and opportunities for novel food proteins. *Enzyme and Microbial Technology, 30*, 305−311.

Srinroch, C., Srisomsap, C., Chokchaichamnankit, D., Punyarit, P., & Phiriyangkul, P. (2015). Identification of novel allergen in edible insect, *Gryllus bimaculatus* and its cross-reactivity with *Macrobrachium* spp. allergens. *Food Chemistry, 184*, 160−166.

Steinfeld, H., Gerber, P., Wassenaar, T., Castel, V., Rosales, M., & De Haan, C. (Eds.), (2006). *Livestock's long shadow. Environmental Issues and Options*. Rome: Food and Agriculture Organization of the United Nations.

Stonehouse, W., Conlon, C. A., Podd, J., Hill, S. R., Minihane, A. M., Crystal, H., & Kennedy, D. (2010). DHA supplementation improved both memory and reaction time in healthy young adults: a randomized controlled trial. *The American Journal of Clinical Nutrition, 97*, 1134–1143.

Styles, C. V. (1994). The big value in mopane worms. *Farmer's Weekly, 22 July*, 20–22.

Szelei, J., Woodring, J., Goettel, M. S., Duke, G., Jousset, F. X., Liu, K. Y., ... Tijssen, P. (2011). Susceptibility of North-American and European crickets to *Acheta domesticus* densovirus (AdDNV) and associated epizootics. *Journal of Invertebrate Pathology, 106*, 394–399.

Tan, H. S. G., Fischer, A. R. H., Tinchan, P., Stieger, M., Steenbekkers, L. P. A., & Van Trijp, H. C. M. (2015). Insects as food: Exploring cultural exposure and individual experience as determinants of acceptance. *Food Quality and Preference, 42*, 78–89.

Taylor, R. L., & Carter, B. J. (1996). *Entertaining with insects*. Yorba Linda: Salutek Publishing Company.

Tomley, F. M., & Shirley, M. W. (2009). Livestock infectious diseases and zoonoses. *Philosophical Transactions of the Royal Society B: Biological Sciences, 364*, 2637–2642.

Tzompa-Sosa, D. A., Yi, L., Van Valenberg, H. J. F., Van Boekel, M. A. J. S., & Lakemond, C. M. M. (2014). Insect lipid profile: Aqueous versus organic solvent-based extraction methods. *Food Research International, 62*, 1087–1094.

Van Broekhoven, S., Oonincx, D. G. A. B., Van Huis, A., & Van Loon, J. J. A. (2015). Growth performance and feed conversion efficiency of three edible mealworm species (Coleoptera: Tenebrionidae) on diets composed of organic by-products. *Journal of Insect Physiology, 73*, 1–10.

Van der Spiegel, M., Noordam, M. Y., & Van der Fels-Klerx, H. J. (2013). Safety of novel protein sources (insects, microalgae, seaweed, duckweed, and rapeseed) and legislative aspects for their application in food and feed production. *Comprehensive Reviews in Food Science and Food Safety, 12*, 662–678.

Van Huis, A. (2013). Potential of insects as food and feed in assuring food security. *Annual Review of Entomology, 58*, 563–583.

Van Huis, A., Van Gurp, H., & Dicke, M. (2014). *The insect cookbook*. New York: Columbia University Press.

Van Huis, A., Van Itterbeeck, J., Klunder, H., Mertens, E., Halloran, A., Muir, G., & Vantomme, P. (2013). Edible insects: Future prospects for food and feed security. *FAO forestry paper 171*. Rome: Food and Agriculture Organization of the United Nations.

Van Huis, A., & Vantomme, P. (2014). Conference report: Insects to feed the world. *Food Chain, 4*, 184–192.

Van Itterbeeck, J., & Van Huis, A. (2012). Environmental manipulation for edible insect procurement: A historical perspective. *Journal of Ethnobiology and Ethnomedicine, 8*, 1–19.

Van Lenteren, J. C. (2006). Ecosystem services to biological control of pests: Why are they ignored? *Proceedings of the Netherlands Entomological Society Meeting, 17*, 103–111.

Verhoeckx, K. C. M., Van Broekhoven, S., Den Hartog-Jager, C. F., Gaspari, M., De Jong, G. A. H., Wichers, H. J., ... Knulst, A. C. (2014). House dust mite (Der p 10) and crustacean allergic patients may react to food containing yellow mealworm proteins. *Food and Chemical Toxicology, 65*, 364–373.

Wang, L., Fu, Y., Yan, S., & Zhao, Y. (2014). Reducing fat of *Tenebrio molitor* polyunsaturated fatty acid. *Journal of Northeast Forestry University Year, 2014*, 132–135.

Weissman, D. B., Gray, D. A., Pham, H. T., & Tijssen, P. (2012). Billions and billions sold: Pet-feeder crickets (Orthoptera: Gryllidae), commercial cricket farms, an epizootic densovirus, and government regulations make for a potential disaster. *Zootaxa, 3504*, 67–88.

WHO (2007). Protein and amino acid requirements in human nutrition. Report of a joint FAO/WHO/UNU expert consultation. WHO Technical Report Series 935. World Health Organization, Food and Agriculture Organization of the United Nations, United Nations University. ISBN 92-4-120935-6.

Xiaoming, C., Ying, F., Hong, Z., & Zhiyong, C. (2010). Review of the nutritive value of edible insects. In P. B. Durst, D. V. Johnson, R. L. Leslie, & K. E. Shono (Eds.), *Forest insects as food: Humans bite back*. Bangkok: Regional Office for Asia and the Pacific of the Food and Agriculture Organization of the United Nations.

Yen, A. L. (2009). Edible insects: Traditional knowledge or western phobia? *Entomological Research, 39*(5), 289–298.

Yen, A. L. (2015). Insects as food and feed in the Asia Pacific region: Current perspectives and future directions. *Journal of Insects as Food and Feed, 1*, 33–55.

Part III

Consumers and Sustainability

Chapter 22

Meat Reduction and Plant-Based Food: Replacement of Meat: Nutritional, Health, and Social Aspects

M. Neacsu, D. McBey and A.M. Johnstone
University of Aberdeen, Aberdeen, United Kingdom

22.1 TRANSITION TOWARDS PLANT-BASED PROTEIN SUPPLEMENTATIONS

The main source of protein in the Western world diet is of animal origin, followed by dairy, and scarcely from plant sources. In the United Kingdom, according to the National Diet and Nutrition Survey, for adults aged 19–64 years, the main protein intake was from animal sources, especially meat and processed meat, as follows: from chicken and turkey 20.3%, followed by beef and veal 15.5%, other types of meat and processed meat 17%, fish (oily and white) 9.3%, and eggs 6.7%. The only plant-based protein source mentioned in the survey was baked beans at 7.0% (Henderson, Gregory, Irving, & Swan, 2003). Sans and Combris have recently published a review which encompassed worldwide meat consumption pattern over the last 50 years, observing that this rose from 23.1 kg per person per year in 1961 to 42.20 kg/person/year in 2011. The same trend was observed for proteins from dairy foods (Sans & Combris, 2015). These changes happened mostly by replacing plant-based foods from the diet; so much so that in recent times plants are not even regarded as sources of protein.

Developed countries have thus achieved, on average, levels of animal-based protein consumption that exceed standard nutritional needs. This has also translated, in some cases, into overconsumption of calories. This overconsumption of animal-based protein was mainly in the form of meat and has surged worldwide, driven by economic development and urbanization (Sans & Combris, 2015). If we look at the Food and Agriculture Organization of the United Nations (FAO) and Biodiversity International definition of sustainable diet, as: "those diets with low environmental impacts which contribute to food and nutrition security and to healthy life for present and future generations" (FAO, 2010 and Biodiversity International), it is easily recognizable that this trend of animal-based protein consumption is unsustainable considering the plethora of publications and reports dealing with diet and protein supply in the context of the sustainability and food security (Aiking, 2011; Aiking, 2014; Beverland, 2014; Kneafsey, Dowler, Lambie-Mumford, Inman, & Collier, 2013; Macdiarmid, 2013; Macdiarmid et al., 2012; Sabaté & Soret, 2014; Sage, 2013; SCAR Report, 2011; Tomlinson, 2013). Other various publications deal with the environmental effects of meat and dairy production and with associated moral and religious grounds (Carlsson-Kanyama, 1998; de Bakker & Dagevos, 2012; Garnett, 2009; González, Frostell, & Carlsson-Kanyama, 2011; Goodland, 1997; McMichael, Powles, & Butler, 2007; Orlich et al., 2013; Pluhar, 2010; Steinfeld et al., 2006). Consequently, the international scientific community is making urgent calls for a transition towards plant-based diets (Vinnari & Vinnari, 2014) and a reduction in animal-based protein sources (Macdiarmid et al., 2011).

Besides the environmental and ethical considerations mentioned above, a transition towards plant-based diets is also supported by public health considerations (Vinnari & Vinnari, 2014). The World Health Organization (WHO) actively promotes an increase in consumption of fruits and vegetables, legumes, whole grains, and nuts among other dietary recommendations for nutrient intakes in order to prevent chronic diseases (WHO, 2015). The FAO-WHO Group of Experts also established dietary recommendations which indicated that proteins must not exceed 15% of total calories, carbohydrates constituting no more than 60% of total calories (3% as fiber) and no more than 25% of total calories derived from lipids and that 75% of total calories should be obtained from plant foods and 25% derived from animal foods (Nishida, Uauy, Kumanyika, & Shetty, 2004). In the first part of this chapter, the nutritional and especially the health aspects of plant-based protein consumption is reviewed.

22.2 PLANT PROTEIN SOURCES: NUTRITIONAL ADEQUACY ASPECTS

There are many nutritious plant and alternative protein sources with varying degrees of worldwide availability. Legumes and pulses are among the most conventional, nutritious, and accessible protein sources. Therefore, the following sections in this chapter are dedicated primarily to legumes and pulses. Legumes are plants belonging to the family *Leguminosae* and are commonly subdivided into pulses, which, in addition to protein, store high levels of carbohydrate (>60%) and low amounts of lipid (<6%) in their dry seeds; and leguminous oilseeds, which boast higher lipid, but lower carbohydrate contents than pulses (Michaels, 2004). The most consumed staple foods worldwide, such as beans, soybeans, lentils, peas, and chickpeas, are all legumes. Proteins in legume seeds represent from about 20% of dry weight in pea and beans up to 38–40% in soybean and lupin (Derbyshire, Wright, & Boulter, 1976; Guéguen & Cerletti, 1994). This high protein content of legumes contrasts with the lower protein content of cereals, which is about 7–13%, and is more similar to that of meats (18–25%) (FAOSTAT Database, 2015; Table 22.1).

From a nutritional point of view, all legume-derived proteins are relatively low in sulfur-containing amino acids, methionine, cysteine, and tryptophan, but the amounts of other essential amino acids, such as lysine, are much greater than in cereal grains (Table 22.1; Ampe et al., 1986; Rockland & Radke, 1981). Pulses contain higher concentrations of lysine (around 1500–3000 mg/100 g) relative to cereals (around 700 mg/100 g), and similar to the content of lysine from meat and fish (Table 22.1). Cereals however contain higher concentrations of cysteine in comparison to that found in pulses. Regarding lysine and sulfur-containing amino acid contents, legume and cereal proteins complement each other, so diets containing both types of food ingredients are nutritionally balanced. For that reason, it can be concluded that in order to achieve a diet balanced in amino acids, complementation and diversification of plant-based proteins would be a feasible and sustainable solution. Therefore, understanding amino acid balance is key to recognizing the protein contribution pulses can make to complement cereal protein. Together, they can replace part of the animal protein in human diet.

Amino acid balance in a particular protein source can be scored against that of a reference protein, typically hen's egg (regarded as well-balanced in relation to adult human metabolic needs) or milk (Michaels, 2004). Plant-based proteins cannot replicate this balance on their own, because each type of plant protein displays a characteristic set of limiting amino acids.

Nine amino acids are classified as dietary essentials in human nutrition (histidine, isoleucine, leucine, lysine, methionine, phenylalanine, threonine, tryptophan, and valine) (Tome, 2012). However, the amino acid composition of foods only represents the potential quality of a protein food and not its quality in practice. A critical factor is the bioavailability of the amino acids within the human body after ingestion, which offers the required supply of amino acids in human diet. A lack of bioavailability could represent a serious problem for the full exploitation of these alternative sources of protein. Several factors have been identified which could affect the bioavailability of amino acids from plant-based proteins, impair their digestion, and increase endogenous nitrogen excretion. These factors are related to their low content of sulfur-containing amino acids, the compact proteolysis-resistant structure of the native seed proteins, the structure and conformation of the proteins, the presence of nonprotein compounds (dietary fiber, tannins, phytates) and/or antiphysiological proteins (protease inhibitors, lectins), suggesting that plant proteins could have a lower overall nutritional quality than animal proteins (Aw & Swanson, 1985; Bressani, Elias, & Braham, 1982; Carbonaro, Marletta, & Carnovale, 1992; Chang & Satterlee, 1981; Deshpande & Nielsen, 1987; Evans & Bauer, 1978; Jansman, Hill, Huisman, & van der Poel (1988); Liener, 1976; Sarwar & Peace, 1986).

Heat treatment, that is, cooking, can inactivate antinutritional components from plant protein sources (protease inhibitors, lectins), and at the same time could affect the structural properties of the protein (legume protein oligomerization factors lead to the disruption of the multimeric structure, followed by the denaturation of the monomers, initiating further rearrangement and/or aggregation) and therefore limit its digestion (Jansman et al., 1988; Kinsella, Damodaran, & German, 1985). Although legume proteins become generally less soluble after cooking (Carbonaro, Marletta, & Carnovale, 1993, 1997), cooking could have a differential effect on protein digestibility: heating glycoprotein II from *Phaseolus vulgaris* L. has been found to have no effect on either the extent or the rate of proteolysis (Sgarbieri, Clarke, & Pusztai, 1982); the protein digestibility of common bean was increased (Carbonaro et al., 1997) upon cooking and that of lentil was unchanged, and that of fava bean was significantly decreased. However, recent work has shown that microwave cooking could be recommended for legume preparation, resulting in increased in vitro protein digestibility and improved nutritional quality due to better retention rates of both B vitamins and minerals and a reduction in the level of antinutritional factors.

TABLE 22.1 Protein Content and Amino Acid Composition of Selected Cereal, Legume, and Animal Foods

Food	Protein (g/100 g)	Amino Acids Content (mg/100 g Product)																		
		Ile	Leu	Lys	Met	Cys	Phe	Tyr	Thr	Trp	Val	Arg	His	Ala	Asx	Glux	Gly	Pro	Ser
Barley (*Hordeum vulgare*) whole seed, hulls removed	11	421	784	406	196	267	603	365	389	180*	592	555	248	464	666	2771	453	1282	476
Buckwheat (*Fagopyrum sagittatum*) hulled, groats, dark flour	12.2	415	720	464	183	293	464	293	439	152*	817	1195	255	573	1084	2114	780	525	610
Maiz (*Zea mays*) grain or whole meal	9.5	350	1190	254	182	147	464	363	342	67	461	398	258	716	596	1800	351	850	473
Oats (*Avena sativa*) meal	13	526	1012	517	234	372	698	459	462	176*	711	876	292	633	1075	2919	656	723	656
Quinoa (*Chenopodium quinoa*)	12	432	720	672	240	-	492	336	420	127*	540	841	288	564	876	1428	624	372	444
Rice (*Oryza* spp.) brown or husked	7.5	300	648	299	183	84	406	275	307	98*	433	650	197	474	808	1622	393	369	427
Rye (*Secale cereale*) whole meal	11	414	728	401	172	225	522	227	395	87*	561	541	261	503	845	2856	512	1108	510
Wheat (*Triticum* spp.) whole grain	12.2	426	871	374	196	332	589	391	382	142*	577	602	299	472	644	3900	512	1298	600
Bean (*Phaseolus vulgaris*)	22.1	927	1685	1593	234	188	1154	559	878	223*	1016	1257	627	927	2648	3271	839	789	1228
Broad bean (*Vicia faba*)	23.4	936	1659	1513	172	187	1011	749	786	202*	1030	2082	554	976	2628	3527	966	932	1048
Chickpea (*Cicer arietinum*)	20.1	891	1505	1376	209	238	1151	589	756	174*	913	1891	531	872	2332	3187	807	849	1023
Cowpea (*Vigna* spp.)	23.4	895	1647	1599	273	255	1209	610	842	254	1060	1498	764	962	2580	3845	876	914	1003
Lentil (*Lens culinaris*)	24.2	1045	1847	1739	194	221	1266	789	960	231*	1211	2101	662	1041	2798	4013	1022	1033	1273
Lima bean (*Phaseolus lunatus*)	19.7	977	1604	1466	246	199	1195	637	823	199	1015	1169	621	917	2421	2578	826	924	1289
Lupine (*Lupinus* spp.)	31.2	1369	2241	1652	235	434	1153	1103	1138	314	1258	2965	814	1103	3420	6849	1293	1283	1582
Pea (*Pisum sativum*)	22.5	961	1530	1692	205	252	1033	616	914	202*	1058	2142	514	918	2466	3632	911	878	976
Soybean (*Glycine max*) seed	38	1889	3232	2653	525	552	2055	1303	1603	532	1995	3006	1051	1769	4861	7774	1736	2281	2128
Beef and veal (*Bos taurus*) edible flesh	17.7	852	1435	1573	478	226	778	637	812	198*	886	1118	603	1033	1590	2703	860	668	713
Chicken (*Gallus gallus*) edible flesh	20	1069*	1472*	1590*	502*	262*	800*	669*	794*	205*	1018*	1114*	525*	682*	1834*	3002*	1059*	829*	781*

(*Continued*)

TABLE 22.1 (Continued)

Food	Protein (g/100 g)	Amino Acids Content (mg/100 g Product)																
		Ile	Leu	Lys	Met	Cys	Phe	Tyr	Thr	Trp	Val	Arg	His	Ala	Asx	Glux	Gly	Pro	Ser
Pork (*Suidae*) edible flesh	11.9	608*	897*	961*	321*	133*	496*	426*	583*	162*	616*	756*	391*	654*	1060*	1718*	676*	542*	496*
Hen egg, whole	12.4	778	1091	863	416	301	709	515	634	184*	847	754	301	733	1190	1576	410	515	946
Fish, fresh, all types	18.8	900	1445	1713	539	220	737	689	861	211*	1150	1066	665	1126	1947	2655	906	692	816
Clupeiformes salmonoidei (including trout, salmon, whitefish, smelt)	18	815	1259	1604	469	181	671	547	786	199*	959	1017	547	1123	1547	2382	1045	683	700
Gadiformes (including cod, hake, haddock, ling, torsk)	17	797	1450	1703	574	199	860	666	879	-	889	1121	500	1134	1817	2687	794	666	849
Perciformes scombroidei (including tuna, mackerel, swordfish, skipjack, albacore)	27	1197	1836	2328	657	294	916	968	1067	320*	1784	1374	1348	1344	2497	3577	985	834	968
Cow, pasteurized	3.5	219	430	248	86	-	239	218	153	50*	255	88	118	140	233	633	79	283	188

All values are based on data from FAOSTAT Database, http://www.fao.org/ag/; where (*) are amino acid values evaluated with microbiological method determination; the rest of food items amino acids' content was determined by column chromatographic methods.

22.3 PLANT-BASED PROTEIN SOURCES: HEALTH AND WELLBEING ASPECTS

22.3.1 Systemic and Gut Health Impacts

There is an increased awareness of the association between good health and regular consumption of plant foods. Numerous epidemiological studies have demonstrated the beneficial effects in the prevention of cancer, coronary heart disease (CHD), and/or many other chronic diseases (Anderson & Major, 2002; Bazzano et al., 2001; Bellisle & Slama, 2002; Champ, 2002; Dillard & German, 2000; Rizkalla, Bazzano, Tees, & Nguyen, 2008; Rochfort & Panozzo, 2007).

Human studies of epidemiology and intervention have also indicated an inverse correlation between legume consumption and the risk of CHD (Bazzano et al., 2001), type II diabetes mellitus, obesity (Rizkalla et al., 2002), and a significant decrease in low-density lipoprotein (LDL) cholesterol and triglycerides and increase in high-density lipoprotein (HDL) cholesterol (Anderson & Major, 2002; Bazzano et al., 2008; Neacsu, Fyfe, Horgan, & Johnstone, 2014). Further associations have been made between the frequency of legume consumption and CHD and cardiovascular disease (CVD); legume consumption four or more times per week compared with less than once a week has been associated with 22% and 11% lower risk of CHD and CVD, respectively (Flight & Clifton, 2006). Anderson and Major (2002), produced a meta-analysis of clinical trials looking at the emerging evidence that indicates that regular intake of pulses, as part of a heart-healthy diet, significantly decreases risk for CVD. They found that the intake of pulses decreases serum cholesterol or LDL cholesterol by 7% and serum triacylglycerols by more than 10%, however pulses do not significantly affect serum HDL cholesterol values.

The hypocholesterolemic effects of legumes appear to be related to their soluble dietary fiber, vegetable protein, oligosaccharides, isoflavones, phospholipids and fatty acids, and saponins (Anderson & Major, 2002). Research data have confirmed that soy protein can lower LDL cholesterol to a small but significant degree (5–6%); isoflavones may play a small role in cholesterol-lowering and in lowering heart disease rates (Flight & Clifton, 2006). It is also considered that the bile acid binding and increased excretion of bile acids may play a prominent role in the hypocholesterolemic effects of pulses. Another finding of the meta-analysis conducted by Anderson and Major was that intake of pulses, with their low glycemic index (GI) and mineral content, has favorable effects on blood pressure, glycemic regulation, and weight management (Anderson & Major, 2002).

Pulses contain 14–32% fiber, of which 55–88% is insoluble and the remainder is soluble (Tosh & Yada, 2010). Soluble viscous fiber in particular contributes to satiety by slowing the transit of digested foodstuffs in the upper gastrointestinal tract, resulting in a more gradual absorption of dietary constituents, including glucose. These actions can prevent rapid spikes and falls in blood glucose levels.

The ability of food to moderate blood glucose is known and is directly related to fiber content. It was more than 25 years ago when legumes were identified as low GI foods (Jenkins et al., 1981, 1983; Thorne, Thompson, & Jenkins, 1983); leguminous vegetables having the lowest score on the scale made by Bornet et al. in 1997, where plant-based foods were classified based on their GI index. Pulses have a low GI, which provides for slow release of energy and a delayed response to hunger, both of which are critical for weight loss and maintenance diets (Foster-Powell, Holt, & Brand-Miller, 2002). Low-GI diets have been shown to reduce fasting and postprandial insulin, glucose, triacylglycerol, and nonesterified fatty acid concentrations, and to increase HDL cholesterol and decrease total cholesterol, while improving in vivo and in vitro insulin-mediated glucose uptake (Brand et al., 1991; Behall & Howe, 1995; Frost, Keogh, Smith, Akisanya & Leeds, 1996; Järvi et al., 1999; Jenkins et al., 1985, 1987; Wolever, Jenkins, Vuksan, Jenkins, & Buckley, et al., 1992; Wolever, Jenkins, Vuskan, Jenkins, Wong, et al., 1992). Low-GI diets are therefore associated with a wide range of health benefits with respect to established metabolic risk factors.

Metabolic syndrome is a cluster of metabolic and cardiovascular risk factors associated with altered postprandial metabolism (Rizkalla et al., 2002). Metabolic syndrome is associated with the subsequent development of type II diabetes and CVD. Epidemiological studies have documented that nutritional factors may affect the prevalence of the metabolic syndrome. The beneficial effects of low-GI foods on postprandial metabolism might be useful not only for the treatment, but also for the prevention of this condition. The metabolic syndrome is an identifiable and potentially modifiable risk state for both type II diabetes and cardiovascular disease and could be prevented by adopting a healthy dietary pattern that satisfies all the strategies for reducing CHD risk.

Plant foods are also a rich source of carbohydrates like starch, fiber, and oligosaccharides. Starch can be classified, according to its digestibility, as soluble, insoluble, or resistant. Englyst, Kingman, and Cummings (1992) referred to resistant starch as the proportion of starch that is not hydrolyzed or digested as it passes through the gastrointestinal tract. Resistant starch has a physiological function similar to that of dietary fiber and can be considered a probiotic acting as a substrate for microbiological fermentation that produces short-chain fatty acids, methane, and carbon dioxide and in doing so confers benefits to human colonic health. Besides the resistant starch, the nonstarch polysaccharide and oligosaccharide fractions of pulses also provide substrates for the bowel microflora, and are extensively fermented within that organ (Goodlad & Mathers, 1990; Key & Mathers, 1995).

Oligosaccharides are nondigestible fibers with prebiotic effects—the ability to stimulate the growth and/or activate "good microflora," also known as bifidobacteria. Fermentation of oligosaccharides by certain bifidobacteria produces short-chain fatty acids too, which can be oxidized and used for energy in preference to glucose. Short-chain fatty acids resulting from metabolic products of anaerobic bacterial fermentation consist mainly of butyrate, propionate, and acetate (Andoh, Tsujikawa, & Fujiyama, 2003), and are the preferred respiratory fuel of the colonocytes lining the colon. These cells serve to increase blood flow, lower luminal pH, and help prevent abnormal colonic cell populations (Topping & Clifton, 2001).

Regarding systemic health, many studies have not shown an independent effect of fiber alone on CHD events and/or deaths (Flight & Clifton, 2006). Therefore, there are emerging results which support that health benefits derived from different food components other than just fiber; wholegrains are nutritionally more important because they deliver a whole package of nutrients and phytochemicals that may work synergistically to promote health.

Legumes, pulses, and cereals, in addition to being an important source of macronutrients and minerals, also contain a rich variety of bioactive phytochemicals, including phytosterols and natural antioxidants (Amarowicz & Pegg, 2008; Rochfort & Panozzo, 2007), that are increasingly being recognized for their potential benefits for human health. However, plant-based foods are also associated with a series of compounds, known as antinutrients, such as protease inhibitors, α-galactosides, vicine, convicine, tannins, saponins, alkaloids, and phytates (Muzquiz, 2000). These compounds interfere with the assimilation of some nutrients and in some cases these can be toxic or cause undesirable physiological effects, for example, flatulence (Muzquiz et al., 2012). There is a balance between deleterious and beneficial effects of these plant components depending on their chemical structure, concentration, bioavailability, time of exposure, and their interaction with other dietary components. Consequently, they are classed as antinutrients or not displaying negative and/or positive effects on health (Champ, 2002; Campos-Vega, Loarca-Pina, & Oomah, 2010).

Saponins have been reported in many edible legumes, like lupins (Woldemichael, Montenegro, & Timmermann, 2003), lentils (Morcos, Gabriel, & El-Hafez, 1976; Ruiz et al., 1996), chickpeas (El-Adawy, 2002), and beans and peas (Shi et al., 2004). Recent evidence suggests that legume saponins may possess anticancer activity (Shi et al., 2004), be beneficial for hyperlipidemia (Shi et al., 2004), and reduce the risk of heart disease in humans (Geil & Anderson, 1994). Investigations on colon cancer cells suggest that the biological activity of saponins is attributed to its aglycones, that is, the lipophilic saponin cores, released by the colonic microflora after hydrolysis (Gurfinkel & Rao, 2003).

Plant-based foods in general and pulse grains in particular are a dietary source of phytates, also known as myoinositol phosphates, having the capacity to form complex compounds with inorganic cations (Sendberg, 2002), with proteins (thus decreasing protein solubility), and also appear to bind with starch through phosphate linkages (Lajolo, Genovese, Pryme & Dale, 2004). However, some myoinositol phosphates, including phytic acid (IP6), have been suggested to have beneficial health effects, such as amelioration of heart disease by controlling hypercholesterolemia and atherosclerosis, and to reduce the risk of colon cancer (Champ, 2002). IP6 has been suggested to be responsible for the epidemiological link between high-fiber diets (rich in IP6) and low incidence of some cancers (Campos-Vega et al., 2010). Recent studies (Letcher, Schell, & Irvine, 2008; Wilson, Bulley, Pisani, Irvine, & Saiardi, 2015) on phytate bioavailability and metabolism showed that no myoinositol phosphate isomers are present at systemic level, that is, in plasma after consumption of diets rich in plant-based foods. This suggests that probably the phytate bioactivity is attributed to the myoinositol moiety. However, further studies are necessary to support this theory. More relevant research summarizing systemic and gut health benefits of plant-based foods are presented in Table 22.2.

22.3.2 Satiety and Weight Management

Observational studies have examined the potential associations between pea, bean, and pulse consumption and weight status, and consistently show that individuals with lower body mass index (BMI) consume more pulses. Using data from National Health and Nutrition Examination Survey (NHANES) 1999–2002, individuals who regularly consumed beans weighed less, had a 23% reduced risk of increased waist size and a 22% reduced risk of being obese. In addition, they consumed significantly higher intakes of dietary fiber, potassium, magnesium, iron, and copper. Such results require further experimental confirmation to determine whether pulses have independent effects on body weight (Papanikolaou & Fulgoni, 2008).

TABLE 22.2 Summary of Relevant Research Briefing Systemic and Gut Health Benefits and Satiety Aspects Involving Plant-Based Foods

Plant Source/Component	Role or Bioactivity	References
Plant-based diets (in general)	• Prevention of coronary heart disease (CHD) and hyperlipidemia	Rao and Al-Weshahy (2008)
Plant dietary fiber (nonstarch polysaccharide, oligosaccharide, and resistant starch)	• Reduce the risk of colorectal cancer	Cassidy, Bingham, and Cummings (1994) and Topping and Clifton (2001)
Plant foods (rich in phytates, myoinositol phosphates)	• Reduce the risk of colorectal cancer	Champ (2002)
Plant foods (phytic acid IP6)	• Amelioration of heart disease	Champ (2002)
Plant foods (as base of a low-GI diet)	• Reduce fasting and postprandial insulin, glucose, triacylglycerol, and nonesterified fatty acid concentrations • Increase high-density lipoprotein (HDL) cholesterol • Decrease total cholesterol • Improving in vivo and in vitro insulin-mediated glucose uptake	Behall and Howe (1995), Brand et al. (1991), Frost et al. (1996), Järvi et al. (1999), Jenkins et al. (1985, 1987, 1988), Wolever, Jenkins, Vuksan, Jenkins, & Buckley, et al. (1992), and Wolever, Jenkins, Vuskan, Jenkins, Wong, et al. (1992)
Pseudo cereals (buckwheat rich foods)	• Modulate gastrointestinal satiety hormones	Stringer, Taylor, Appah, Blewett, and Zahradka (2013)
Wholegrain cereals	• Reduce the risk of cardiovascular disease (CVD)	Anderson (2002, 2003)
Cereal grain, legumes (general)	• Weight management	Williams, Grafenauer, and O'Shea (2008)
Legumes consumption (in general)	• Reduce the risk of CHD	Bazzano et al. (2001) and Flight and Clifton (2006)
	• Reduce the risk of type II diabetes mellitus	
	• Reduce the risk of obesity	Rizkalla et al. (2002)
	• Decrease in low-density lipoprotein (LDL) cholesterol and increase in HDL cholesterol	Anderson and Major (2002), Bazzano et al. (2008), and Neacsu et al. (2014)
	• Decrease in LDL cholesterol and triglycerides	Anderson and Major (2002)
Wholegrain legumes	• Decrease insulin and sugar glucose	
Legumes (as saponin rich diets)	• Anticancer activity	Gurfinkel and Rao (2003)
Legume diet (rich in saponins)	• Anticancer activity	Ellington, Berhow and Singletary (2006), Shi et al. (2004), Xiao, Huang, Zhu, Ren & Zhang (2007), and Zhu, Xiong, Yu, and Wu (2005)
	• Beneficial for hyperlipidemia	Shi et al. (2004)
Legume (soy as isoflavone-rich sources)	• Decrease in LDL cholesterol	
Legume (soy tofu)	• Decrease in LDL cholesterol and triglycerides	

(Continued)

TABLE 22.2 (Continued)

Plant Source/Component	Role or Bioactivity	References
Pulses	• Decrease in LDL cholesterol and triglycerides, no effect on HDL cholesterol	Anderson and Major (2002)
	• Favorable effects on blood pressure, glycemic regulation, and weight management	
Pulses	• Potential for breast and colon cancer prevention	Mathers (2002)
Pulses (whole)	• Weight loss	Abete, Parra, and Martinez (2009), Hermsdorff, Zulet, Abete, and Martínez (2011), McCrory, Hamaker, Lovejoy, and Eichelsdoerfer (2010), and Sichieri, Condo, Saura, and Albino (1993)
Pea, beans, and pulses consumption (in general)	• Satiety—hunger, weight loss	McCrory et al. (2010) and Papanikolaou and Fulgoni (2008)
Pulses (low GI foods)	• Prevention of CHD, blood glycemic control, cholesterol control	Rizkalla et al. (2002)
Pulses (dietary fiber)	• Hunger, weight maintenance	Saris (2003)
Pulse phytochemicals (phytosterols, isoflavones, saponins)	• Improve the cholesterol and triglyceride levels, relieve the symptoms of menopause	Rochfort and Panozzo (2007)
Pulses isolates/extracts	• Weight loss	Celleno, Tolaini, D'Amore, Perricone, and Preuss (2007), Koike, Koizumi, Tang, Takahara and Saitou (2005), Opala, Rzymski, Pischel, Wilczak, and Wozniak (2006), Thom (2000), Udani, Hardy and Madsen (2004)
Pea protein, pulses	• Satiety—hunger	Diepvens, Häberer and Westerterp-Plantenga (2008) and Sufian, Hira, Asano, and Hara (2007)
Plant protein and peptides	• Potential for CVD prevention (impact regulatory pathway associated with cardiovascular homeostasis)	Cam and Gonzales de Mejia (2012)

Some components in pulses may contribute to weight control by inhibiting intestinal absorption of carbohydrates and other energy-yielding nutrients like protein (McCrory et al., 2010). An increase in the release of cholecystokinin (CCK), a gut hormone secreted in response to fat and protein which helps to slow gastric emptying and increase satiety, has been reported following bean consumption. Satiety may be enhanced through upregulation of CCK brain receptors as peptides present in beans show very potent in vitro CCK stimulating activity. Therefore, pulses may influence satiety through modulation of intestinal hormones and stimulation of satiety receptors in the brain (Sufian et al., 2007). Consumption of a beverage containing a pea protein hydrolysate increased satiety by reducing hunger, the desire to eat and thirst scores in overweight men and women (Diepvens et al., 2008). Following the pea supplement, baseline hunger returned after 117–151 min in comparison to 100–128 min with the consumption of a whey protein beverage. After 240 min of consuming the beverages, less hunger was reported from pea protein consumers compared to whey protein consumers (Diepvens et al., 2008).

Short-term studies (mostly single-meal studies) indicate reduced hunger and increased satiety 2–4 h after pulse consumption including canned beans, lentils, bean puree, and bread made with chickpea flour, when meals were controlled for energy, but not when controlled for available carbohydrate (McCrory et al., 2010). This suggests that at least part of the effect of pulses on satiety may be mediated by available carbohydrate amount or composition.

The gastric and intestinal bulking effects of insoluble fiber in pulses also result in greater satiety and thus reduced energy consumption (Saris, 2003). Short-chain fatty acids obtained after fiber fermentation by gut may also suppress hepatic glucose production. A more stable glucose metabolism can result, which may lead to greater satiety and subsequent reductions in energy intake. The production of the short-chain fatty acid propionate may also stimulate satiety (McCrory et al., 2010). There do not seem to be differential effects of pea protein on hunger and satiety compared to other meat and dairy proteins when fed at similar amounts as preloads (Lang, Bellisle, & Oppert, 1998). Similar conclusions were found when comparing equivalent amounts of protein consumption derived from soy- and meat-based foods (Neacsu et al., 2014).

Several human intervention studies (Abete et al., 2009; Hermsdorff et al., 2011; Karlström et al., 1987; McCrory et al., 2010; Sichieri et al., 1993) tested the effectiveness of whole pulses for weight loss during intentional caloric restriction. Most of these studies reported significant effects on body weight from pulse treatments versus nonpulse control diets. These studies ranged from 6–8 weeks long and pulse treatments varied, including eating rice and beans twice a day to incorporating mixed pulses, approximately 3–5 cups/week. Weight losses were in the range of 3.6–8.2 kg.

There are a number of human clinical studies (Celleno et al., 2007; Koike et al., 2005; Opala et al., 2006; Thom, 2000; Udani et al., 2004; Udani & Singh, 2007) which have examined the effects of dietary supplementation with pulse "extracts" on body weight. Intervention length ranged from 4 to 12 weeks. All trials resulted in greater weight loss in the treatment group with mean weight loss being 0.4 ± 0.2 kg/week compared with 0.2 ± 0.2 kg/week in the placebo groups. There are authors suggesting that these findings could be also attributed to α-amylase inhibitors found in pulses, specifically dry beans (up to 2–4 g/kg), which reduce starch digestibility and thus energy availability. Isolated α-amylase inhibitor was found to lower postprandial glycemic responses (Lajolo & Genovese, 2002), but could be inactivated during cooking (Lajolo & Genovese, 2002). These arguments justify the use of pulse extracts prepared with processing methods aimed to retain the amylase inhibitor activity (McCrory et al., 2010). More relevant research on satiety and weight management involving plant-based foods is presented in Table 22.2.

22.4 MEAT REPLACEMENT: SOCIAL ASPECTS

It seems clear that, from both an environmental and public health perspective, it would be beneficial to reduce the quantity of meat and increase the volume of plant foods eaten by the average Westerner. This leads us to the question of how likely those in the West are to adopt such dietary change. To attempt to answer this question, we now turn to look at three factors which may impact the likelihood of any large-scale dietary change: (1) the complex nature of food choice; (2) the difficulties encountered when trying to convince a nation to change its behavior; and (3) the special status that is afforded to meat.

22.4.1 The Complexity of Food Choice

Food choice is an extremely complex phenomenon (Sobal & Bisogni, 2009). It is influenced by both physiological and psychosocial impulses (Sobal, Bisogni, & Jastran, 2014), is both a conscious and an unconscious process, is affected by both internal and external (ie, social) forces, and has been approached from a myriad of theoretical positions and disciplines—psychologists, behavioral economists, social scientists, public health researchers, and neuroscientists are all represented in the quest to better understand why we choose to eat what we do. With over 200 food choices made by a person each day (Wansink & Sobal, 2007), the task of unpicking and evaluating the motivations that drive these choices seems daunting.

There have been attempts to develop frameworks through which food choice can be better understood. Steptoe, Pollard, and Wardle (1995) developed a food choice questionnaire that identified nine factors that affected food choice: health, mood, convenience, sensory appeal, natural content, price, weight control, familiarity, and ethical concern. Of these, sensory appeal, health, convenience, and price were found to be the most salient factors for the majority of food consumption decisions, although the authors stress the multidimensional character of food choice. A combination of some or all of these factors may play a role. Furthermore, each of these factors was more or less important dependent on demographic characteristics such as sex, age, and income. Furst, Connors, Bisogni, Sobal, and Falk (1996) argued that life course, influences, and personal systems were the main determinants of food choice. Life course influences were deemed to form the bedrock of food choice, and are those which result from the personal experience of living in a particular cultural and social era—for example living with rationing during a war may lead one to become less particular with the foods that they eat. Influences refers to the interconnected "ideals, personal factors, resources, social framework and food context" (Furst et al., 1996, p. 252) that lead individuals to make food choices. Finally, personal systems are comprised of value negotiations, which are considerations towards taste, cost, convenience, ethics, etc., and strategies, which are the habits and routines which are formed and employed in food purchasing, preparation, and consumption.

Even considering these two examples of efforts to understand food choice only, it is clear that although there is some overlap in the different components that the authors deem relevant in food choice behaviors, there is also a great deal of difference. This serves to highlight how difficult it is to make sense of why we choose to eat what we do. When specifically considering food choice concerning meat- and plant-based alternatives, we can see that factors such as the taste and enjoyment derived from eating meat, the perceived "naturalness" of humans consuming meat, and lack of knowledge and time to prepare alternatives are all important. These intricacies are relevant when we consider how to go about changing eating patterns on a societal level.

22.4.2 Changing the Diet of a Nation

Perhaps because of the complexity of food choice, previous efforts to change dietary patterns appear to have been largely unsuccessful. There are a range of measures that can be adopted when trying to change public behavior, and these have been ranked in the ladder of intervention which has been developed by the Nuffield Council on Bioethics. The top of the ladder involves measures in which the government curbs individual freedoms, so that each intervention that is to be made involves weighting any potential benefits with this curbing of freedoms. In short, there is a debate about what (if any) role the state should play in ensuring that individuals lead healthy lives (Box 22.1).

With regards to public eating patterns, most attempts to bring about change have involved measures that fall near the bottom of the intervention ladder. The most common methods applied to bring about dietary change have been public information and education campaigns (Mazzochi, Traill, & Shogren, 2009), and while these appear to increase public awareness of the campaign messages, actual behavioral change seems to be limited at best (Brambila-Macias et al., 2011; Capacci et al., 2012). However, Gordon, McDermott, Stead, and Angus (2006) argue that social marketing campaigns, whereby the techniques and tools used by marketers are adopted to promote socially beneficial behavioral change, can be a successful method in changing the eating habits of a populace, and a sustained social marketing campaign in Australia seemed to lead to an increase in fruit and vegetable consumption (Pollard et al., 2008). Any such campaigns may highlight the environmental benefits of reducing meat consumption, as consumers seem unaware, or skeptical of, the positive environmental impact of reducing meat consumption, and those who consumed most meat were also least likely to believe that reducing consumption would have a positive effect on the environment (Tobler, Visschers, & Siegrist, 2011).

Box 22.1 Ladder of Intervention

- *Eliminate choice*. Regulate in such a way as to entirely eliminate choice, for example through compulsory isolation of patients with infectious diseases.
- *Restrict choice*. Regulate in such a way as to restrict the options available to people with the aim of protecting them, for example removing unhealthy ingredients from foods, or unhealthy foods from shops or restaurants.
- *Guide choice through disincentives*. Fiscal and other disincentives can be put in place to influence people not to pursue certain activities, for example through taxes on cigarettes, or by discouraging the use of cars in inner cities through charging schemes or limitations of parking spaces.
- *Guide choices through incentives*. Regulations can be offered that guide choices by fiscal and other incentives, for example offering tax-breaks for the purchase of bicycles that are used as a means of traveling to work.
- *Guide choices through changing the default policy*. For example, in a restaurant, instead of providing chips as a standard side dish (with healthier options available), menus could be changed to provide a more healthy option as standard (with chips as an option available).
- *Enable choice*. Enable individuals to change their behaviors, for example by offering participation in an NHS "stop smoking" programme, building cycle lanes, or providing free fruit in schools.
- *Provide information*. Inform and educate the public, for example as part of campaigns to encourage people to walk more or eat five portions of fruit and vegetables per day.
- *Do nothing or simply monitor the current situation*.

From Nuffield Council on Bioethics. (2007). *Public health: Ethical issues*. London: Nuffield Council on Bioethics. Available from: <http://nuffieldbioethics.org/wp-content/uploads/2014/07/Public-health-ethical-issues.pdf> Accessed 27.10.15.

More "invasive" techniques, such as fiscal interventions (eg, taxes on high-fat or high-sugar foods), although less prevalent appear to potentially offer more effective ways to change food behaviors (Brambila-Macias et al., 2011; Capacci et al., 2012). However, a recent recommendation by Public Health England that a tax on sugar could help to cut childhood obesity was seemingly dismissed by the UK government, who instead signaled their intention to look at other measures such as regulating the advertising of sugary products (Campbell & Mason, 2015). This could be due to conservative reluctance to raise taxes and reduce state interference, and these issues coupled with governmental commitments to the broad livestock industry mean that any such tax on meat is problematic (Nordgren, 2012). Further complications are also foreseeable, as in Finland where it has been announced that a similar tax on sugar is to be scrapped as it breaks European Union competition rules (Finland: Tax on Sweets and Ice Cream Scrapped, 2015). Furthermore, an important caveat with such measures is that they must be rigorously designed to help mitigate the effect of such taxes on lower-income households (Bødker, Pisinger, Toft, & Jørgensen, 2015; Madden, 2015).

Other methods to change dietary patterns should also be considered. Better nutritional labeling may lead to improved food choices (Capacci et al., 2012), although more research needs to be undertaken to better understand how consumers use and understand nutritional labels in their everyday lives (Grunert & Wills, 2007). One source of advertising that may be employed to convince people to eat less, but better quality, meat may be the use of on-pack certification labels (eg, fairtrade, little red tractor). Studies have found that consumers want clear labeling that includes country of origin, certification, GM and pesticide status, and system of production, amongst other things (Bernués, Olaizola, & Corcoran, 2003; Bernabéu & Tendero, 2005; Ehmke, Lusk, & Tyner, 2008). However, the public seems to be largely unaware of the meaning of many of these labels and it is argued that work needs to be done in order to make them more useful and informative to the public.

Changing food consumption behaviors seems an onerous task. Coupled with this, the eating of meat seems to hold a special status in many societies, and as such it may be particularly difficult to convince people to eat less.

22.4.3 Decreasing Meat Consumption

With regards to decreasing meat consumption, and increasing plant-based alternatives, previous research points to a general reluctance to make such a change. Although it has been suggested that industrialized nations may be reducing their meat intake (Fresco, 2009), overall global meat consumption is expected to rise as more countries modernize and mimic Western dietary patterns (FAO, 2006; Henchion, McCarthy, Resconi, & Troy, 2014). As the GDP of a country increases, so does the demand for meat (Schroeder, Barkley, & Schroeder, 1996). Therefore if and when more nations modernize we can expect global demand for meat to increase significantly. One explanation for this may be the symbolic value of meat as a marker of prosperity (Heinz & Lee, 1998). However, this is not the only symbolic value that we associate with meat, with advertising used as a means to create and spread these symbolic meanings. These symbols have the effect of separating us from a more accurate picture of the meat we consume (ie, factory farming techniques, slaughterhouses, etc.) (Heinz & Lee, 1998). Meat is depicted as a vital part of a healthy diet (Heinz & Lee, 1998), and eating meat is portrayed as part of human nature, and the reason that humans are the dominant species on the planet (Peace, 2008). Meat advertisements also frequently employ the symbolism of meat as a masculine activity, in contrast to the feminization of men through ideas such as metrosexuality (Rogers, 2008; Buerkle, 2009).

There is a dearth of research looking at the factors affecting meat consumption. In a review of previous studies, Latvala et al. (2012) found that men eat more meat than women, meat consumption decreases with age, and people with high incomes eat more meat than those on low incomes. Taste, healthiness, price, and the safety of meat were all found to be important factors in meat consumption, with animal welfare becoming more so and environmental questions generally not asked. Clearly, more research is required to discover meat consumption patterns.

There are potential opportunities to be explored for reducing meat consumption. It would be wrong to assume a meat eater/vegetarian dichotomy, with consumers instead sitting somewhere on a meat-eating to meat-avoiding continuum. Up to 40% of the UK population were found to be "meat reducers," with the primary reason for a reduction in meat consumption being concerns regarding health (Baker, Thompson, & Palmer-Barnes, 2002). Flexitarians are individuals who have reduced their meat consumption but do not identify as vegetarians (Dagevos & Voordouw, 2013). Better understanding of the motivations and circumstances of such individuals may open up pathways for more widespread meat reduction and adoption of more plant-based diets. The generally negative perception of current meat alternatives can also be used as a stimulus to develop new plant-based protein products (de Boer & Aiking, 2011). Making such products with greater similarity to meat may also tempt those who currently consume most meat (Hoek et al., 2011).

This section has sought to briefly introduce some of the key problems that need to be addressed if people are to be convinced to reduce their meat intake and concurrently increase the amount of plant-foods that they eat.

22.5 OVERALL CONCLUDING REMARKS

Diets with less animal proteins and more sustainable plant-based foods can possibly supply sufficient balanced macronutrient content in the human diet, provided that a varied choice of plant foods is consumed. The main current sources of plant proteins are pulses and whole-grain cereals. A reduction in the consumption of animal protein-rich foods is an efficient and possibly unavoidable way to reduce the negative impact of human behavior on the environment and ultimately to improve human health in a sustainable manner.

Although food choice research points out a multitude of different directions, one clear message that runs throughout all studies is that food choice is complex. However, it is vital to understand this complexity if effective and lasting public dietary change strategies are to be created. It may be that people are simply unwilling to alter their habits, and if this is the case, and if there is sufficient political appetite for such change, then more forceful measures such as taxation may have to be considered. The evidence seems to suggest that when it comes to eating meat, any attempts to convince people to limit their intake may be fraught with difficulties.

However, to address and achieve all these aspects, broad interdisciplinary research efforts and actions are necessary, involving nutritionists, social scientists, the international development community, and economists to ultimately be driven by the main stakeholders.

REFERENCES

Abete, I., Parra, D., & Martinez, J. A. (2009). Legume, fish, or high-protein-based hypocaloric diets: Effects on weight loss and mitochondrial oxidation in obese men. *Journal of Medicinal Med Food, 12*, 100–108.

Aiking, H. (2011). Future protein supply. *Trends in Food Science and Technology, 22*(2), 112–120.

Aiking, H. (2014). Protein production: Planet, profit, plus people? *American Journal of Clinical Nutrition, 100*(Suppl.), 483S–489S.

Amarowicz, R., & Pegg, R. B. (2008). Legumes as a source of natural antioxidants. *European Journal of Lipid Science and Technology, 110*, 865–878.

Ampe, C., Van Damme, J., de Castro, A., Sampaio, M. J., Van Montagu, M., & Vanderkerckhove, J. (1986). The amino acid sequence of the 2S sulfur-rich proteins from seeds of Brazil nut (Bertholletia excelsa H.B.K.). *European Journal of Biochemistry, 159*, 597–604.

Anderson, J. W. (2002). Whole-grains intake and risk for coronary heart disease. In L. Marquart, J. L. Slavin, & R. G. Fulcher (Eds.), *Whole-grain foods in health and disease* (pp. 187–200). St Paul, Minnesota, USA: American Association of Cereal Chemists.

Anderson, J. W. (2003). Whole grains protect against atherosclerotic cardiovascular disease. *Proceedings of the Nutrition Society, 62*, 135–142.

Anderson, J. W., & Major, A. W. (2002). Pulses and lipaemia, short-and long-term effect: Potential in the prevention of cardiovascular disease. *British Journal of Nutrition, 88*(S3), 263–271.

Andoh, A., Tsujikawa, T., & Fujiyama, Y. (2003). Role of dietary fiber and short-chain fatty acids in the colon. *Current Pharmaceutical Design, 9*, 347–358.

Aw, T. L., & Swanson, B. G. (1985). Influence of tannin on *Phaseolus vulgaris* protein digestibility and quality. *Journal of Food Science, 50*(1), 67–71.

Baker, S., Thompson, K. E., & Palmer-Barnes, D. (2002). Crisis in the meat industry: A values-based approach to communications strategy. *Journal of Marketing Communications, 8*(1), 19–30.

Bazzano, L. A., He, J., Ogden, L. G., Loria, C., Vupputuri, S., Myers, L., & Whelton, P. K. (2001). Legume consumption and risk of coronary heart disease in US men and women: NHANES I epidemiologic follow-up study. *Archives of Internal Medicine, 161*(21), 2573–2578.

Bazzano, L. A., Tees, M. T., & Nguyen, C. H. (2008). Effect of non-soy legume consumption on cholesterol levels: A meta-analysis of randomized controlled trials. *Circulation, 118*, S1122.

Behall, K., & Howe, J. (1995). Effect of long-term consumption of amylose vs amylopectin starch on metabolic variables in human subjects. *American Journal of Clinical Nutrition, 61*, 334–340.

Bernabéu, R., & Tendero, A. (2005). Preference structure for lamb meat consumers. A Spanish case study. *Meat Science, 71*(3), 464–470.

Bernués, A., Olaizola, A., & Corcoran, K. (2003). Labelling information demanded by European consumers and relationships with purchasing motives, quality and safety of meat. *Meat Science, 65*(3), 1095–1106.

Beverland, M. B. (2014). Sustainable eating: Mainstreaming plant-based diets in developed economies. *Journal of Macromarketing, 34*(3), 369–382.

Bødker, M., Pisinger, C., Toft, U., & Jørgensen, T. (2015). The Danish fat tax—Effects on consumption patterns and risk of ischaemic heart disease. *Preventive Medicine, 77*, 200–203.

Bornet, F. R., Billaux, M. S., & Messing, B. (1997). Glycaemic index concept and metabolic diseases. *International Journal of Biology Macromolecules, 21*, 207–219.

Brambila-Macias, J., Shankar, B., Capacci, S., Mazzocchi, M., Perez-Cueto, F. J., Verbeke, W., & Traill, W. B. (2011). Policy interventions to promote healthy eating: A review of what works, what does not, and what is promising. *Food and Nutrition Bulletin, 32*(4), 365–375.

Brand, J. C., Colagiuri, S., Crossman, S., Allen, A., Roberts, D. C., & Truswell, A. S. (1991). Low-glycemic index foods improve long term glycemic control in NIDDM. *Diabetes Care*, *14*, 95−101.

Bressani, R., Elias, L. G., & Braham, J. E. (1982). Reduction of digestibility of legume proteins by tannins. *Journal of Plant Foods*, *4*, 43−55.

Buerkle, C. W. (2009). Metrosexuality can stuff it: Beef consumption as (heteromasculine) fortification. *Text and Performance Quarterly*, *29*(1), 77−93.

Cam, A., & de Mejia, E. G. (2012). Role of dietary proteins and peptides in cardiovascular disease. *Molecular nutrition and food research*, *56*(1), 53−66.

Campbell, D., & Mason, R. *David Cameron faces pressure to back sugar tax.* (2015). Retrieved from www.theguardian.com/society/2015/oct/22/david-cameron-faces-pressure-to-back-sugar-tax Accessed 28.10.15.

Campos-Vega, R., Loarca-Pina, G. F., & Oomah, B. D. (2010). Minor components of pulses and their potential impact on human health. *Food Research International*, *43*, 461−482.

Capacci, S., Mazzocchi, M., Shankar, B., Macias, J. B., Verbeke, W., Pérez-Cueto, F. J., … Traill, W. B. (2012). Policies to promote healthy eating in Europe: A structured review of policies and their effectiveness. *Nutrition Reviews*, *70*(3), 188−200.

Carbonaro, M., Cappelloni, M., Nicoli, S., Lucarini, M., & Carnovale, E. (1997). Solubility-digestibility relationship of legume proteins. *Journal of Agricultural and Food Chemistry*, *45*, 3387−3394.

Carbonaro, M., Marletta, L., & Carnovale, E. (1992). Factors affecting cystine reactivity in proteolytic digests of *Phaseolus vulgaris*. *Journal of Agricultural and Food Chemistry*, *40*, 169−174.

Carbonaro, M., Marletta, L., & Carnovale, E. (1993). Protein solubility of raw and cooked bean (*Phaseolus vulgaris*): Role of the basic residues. *Journal of Agricultural and Food Chemistry*, *41*, 1169−1175.

Carlsson-Kanyama, A. (1998). Climate change and dietary choices—How can emissions of greenhouse gases from food consumption be reduced? *Food Policy*, *23*, 277−293.

Cassidy, A., Bingham, S. A., & Cummings, J. H. (1994). Starch intake and colorectal cancer risk: An international comparison. *British Journal of Cancer*, *69*, 937−942.

Celleno, L., Tolaini, M. V., D'Amore, A., Perricone, N. V., & Preuss, H. G. (2007). A dietary supplement containing standardized *Phaseolus vulgaris* extract influences body composition of overweight men and women. *International Journal of Medical Sciences*, *4*, 45−52.

Champ, M. M. (2002). Non-nutrient bioactive substances of pulses. *The British Journal of Nutrition*, *88*, 307−319.

Chang, K. C., & Satterlee, L. D. (1981). Isolation and characterization of the major protein from Great Northern Beans (*Phaseolus vulgaris* L.). *Journal of Food Science*, *46*, 1368−1373.

Dagevos, H., & Voordouw, J. (2013). Sustainability and meat consumption: Is reduction realistic. *Sustainability: Science, Practice, and Policy*, *9*(2), 60−69.

De Bakker, E., & Dagevos, H. (2012). Reducing meat consumption in today's consumer society: Questioning the citizen-consumer gap. *Journal of Agricultural and Environmental Ethics*, *25*, 877−894.

De Boer, J., & Aiking, H. (2011). On the merits of plant-based proteins for global food security: Marrying macro and micro perspectives. *Ecological Economics*, *70*, 1259−1265.

Derbyshire, E., Wright, D. J., & Boulter, D. (1976). Legumin and vicilin, storage proteins of legume seeds. *Phytochemistry*, *15*(1), 3−24.

Deshpande, S. S., & Nielsen, S. S. (1987). In vitro enzymatic hydrolysis of phaseolin, the major storage protein of *Phaseolus vulgaris* L. *Journal of Food Science*, *52*(5), 1326−1329.

Diepvens, K., Häberer, D., & Westerterp-Plantenga, M. (2008). Different proteins and biopeptides differently affect satiety and anorexigenic/orexigenic hormones in healthy humans. *International Journal of Obesity*, *32*(3), 510−518.

Dillard, C. J., & German, J. B. (2000). Phytochemicals: Nutraceuticals and human health. *Journal of the Science of Food and Agriculture*, *80*(12), 1744−1756.

Ehmke, M. D., Lusk, J. L., & Tyner, W. (2008). Measuring the relative importance of preferences for country of origin in China, France, Niger, and the United States. *Agricultural Economics*, *38*(3), 277−285.

El-Adawy, T. A. (2002). Nutritional composition and antinutritional factors of chickpeas (*Cicer arietinum* L.) undergoing different cooking methods and germination. *Plant Foods for Human Nutrition*, *57*, 83−97.

Ellington, A. A., Berhow, M. A., & Singletary, K. W. (2006). Inhibition of Akt signalling and enhanced ERK1/2 activity are involved in induction of macroautophagy by triterpenoid B-group soyasaponins in colon cancer cells. *Carcinogenesis*, *27*, 289−306.

Englyst, H. N., Kingman, S. M., & Cummings, J. H. (1992). Classification and measurement of nutritionally important starch fractions. *European Journal of Clinical Nutrition*, *46*(Suppl. 2), S33−50.

European Commission − Standing Committee on Agricultural Research (SCAR) (2011). Sustainable food consumption and production in a resource-constrained world. In: *The 3rd SCAR foresight exercise*.

Evans, R. J., & Bauer, D. H. (1978). Studies of the poor utilization of the rat of methionine and cystine in heated dry bean seed (*Phaseolus vulgaris*). *Journal of Agricultural and Food Chemistry*, *26*, 779−784.

FAO (2006). *World agriculture: Towards 2030/2050*. (71Rome: Interim Report, Food and Agriculture Organization of the United Nations (FAO).

FAO. (2010). http://www.fao.org/ag/humannutrition/23781-0e8d8dc364ee46865d5841c48976e9980.pdf.

FAOSTAT Database. (2015). http://www.fao.org/docrep/005/AC854T/AC854T03.htm#noteA, http://www.fao.org/ag/ Accessed 06.10.15.

Finland: Tax on Sweets and Ice Cream Scrapped (2015). In www.bbc.co.uk. Retrieved from http://www.bbc.co.uk/news/blogs-news-from-elsewhere-34389928 Accessed 28.10.15.

Flight, I., & Clifton, P. (2006). Cereal grains and legumes in the prevention of coronary heart disease and stroke: A review of the literature. *European Journal of Clinical Nutrition*, 60, 1145–1159.

Foster-Powell, K., Holt, S. H., & Brand-Miller, J. C. (2002). International table of glycemic index and glycemic load values: 2002. *The American Journal of Clinical Nutrition*, 76(1), 5–56.

Fresco, L. O. (2009). Challenges for food system adaptation today and tomorrow. *Environmental Science and Policy*, 12(4), 378–385.

Frost, G., Keogh, B., Smith, D., Akisanya, K., & Leeds, A. (1996). The effect of low-glycemic carbohydrate on insulin and glucose response in vivo and in vitro in patients with coronary heart disease. *Metabolism: Clinical and Experimental*, 45, 669–672.

Furst, T., Connors, M., Bisogni, C. A., Sobal, J., & Falk, L. W. (1996). Food choice: A conceptual model of the process. *Appetite*, 26(3), 247–266.

Garnett, T. (2009). Livestock-related greenhouse gas emissions: Impacts and options for policy makers. *Environmental Science and Policy*, 12, 491–503.

Geil, P. B., & Anderson, J. W. (1994). Nutrition and health implications of dry beans: A review. *Journal of the American College of Nutrition*, 13, 549–558.

González, A., Frostell, B., & Carlsson-Kanyama, A. (2011). Protein efficiency per unit energy and per unit greenhouse gas emissions: Potential contribution of diet choices to climate change mitigation. *Food Policy*, 36, 562–570.

Goodlad, J. S., & Mathers, J. C. (1990). Large bowel fermentation in rats given diets containing raw peas (*Pisum sativum*). *British Journal of Nutrition*, 64, 569–587.

Goodland, R. (1997). Environmental sustainability in agriculture: Diet matters. *Ecological Economics*, 23, 189–200.

Gordon, R., McDermott, L., Stead, M., & Angus, K. (2006). The effectiveness of social marketing interventions for health improvement: What's the evidence? *Public Health*, 120(12), 1133–1139.

Grunert, K. G., & Wills, J. M. (2007). A review of European research on consumer response to nutrition information on food labels. *Journal of Public Health*, 15(5), 385–399.

Guéguen, J., & Cerletti, P. (1994). Proteins of some legume seeds, soybean, pea, fababean and lupin. In B. J. F. Hudson (Ed.), *New and developing sources of food proteins*. New York: Chapman and Hall.

Gurfinkel, D. M., & Rao, A. V. (2003). Soyasaponins: The relationship between chemical structure and colon anticarcinogenic activity. *Nutrition and Cancer*, 47, 24–33.

Heinz, B., & Lee, R. (1998). Getting down to the meat: The symbolic construction of meat consumption. *Communication Studies*, 49(1), 86–99.

Henchion, M., McCarthy, M., Resconi, V. C., & Troy, D. (2014). Meat consumption: Trends and quality matters. *Meat Science*, 98(3), 561–568.

Henderson, L., Gregory, J., Irving, K., & Swan, G. (2003). *The National Diet & Nutrition Survey: Adults aged 19 to 64 years* (Vols. 1–4). Norwich: HMSO.

Hermsdorff, H. H. M., Zulet, M. Á., Abete, I., & Martínez, J. A. (2011). A legume-based hypocaloric diet reduces proinflammatory status and improves metabolic features in overweight/obese subjects. *European Journal of Nutrition*, 50(1), 61–69.

Hoek, A. C., Luning, P. A., Weijzen, P., Engels, W., Kok, F. J., & de Graaf, C. (2011). Replacement of meat by meat substitutes. A survey on person- and product-related factors in consumer acceptance. *Appetite*, 56(3), 662–673.

Jansman, A. J. M., Hill, G. D., Huisman, J., & van der Poel, A. F. B. (Eds.), (1988). *Recent advances of research in antinutritional factors in legume seeds* The Netherlands: Wageningen Pers.

Järvi, A. E., Karlström, B. E., Granfeldt, Y. E., Björck, I. E., Asp, N. G., & Vessby, B. O. (1999). Improved glycemic control and lipid profile and normalized fibrinolytic activity on a low-glycemic index diet in type 2 diabetic patients. *Diabetes Care*, 22(1), 10–18.

Jenkins, D. J., Wolever, T., Kalmusky, J., Giudici, S., Giordano, C., Patten, R., ... Csima, A. (1987). Low glycemic index diet in hyperlipidemia: Use of traditional starch foods. *American Journal of Clinical Nutrition*, 46, 66–71.

Jenkins, D. J., Wolever, T. M., Jenkins, A. L., Thorne, M. J., Lee, R., Kalmusky, J., ... Wong, G. S. (1983). The glycemic index of food tested in diabetic patients. A new basis for carbohydrate exchange favouring the use of legumes. *Diabetologia*, 24, 257–264.

Jenkins, D. J., Wolever, T. M., Kalmusky, J., Giudici, S., Giordano, C., Wong, G. S., ... Buckley, G. (1985). Low glycemic index carbohydrate foods in the management of hyperlipidemia. *The American Journal of Clinical Nutrition*, 42(4), 604–617.

Jenkins, D. J., Wolever, T. M., Taylor, R. H., Barker, H. M., Fielden, H., & Jenkins, A. L. (1981). Effect of guar crispbread with cereal products and leguminous seeds on blood glucose concentrations of diabetics. *British Medical Journal*, 281, 1248–1250.

Karlström, B., Vessby, B., Asp, N. G., Boberg, M., Lithell, H., & Berne, C. (1987). Effects of leguminous seeds in a mixed diet in non-insulin-dependent diabetic patients. *Diabetes Research (Edinburgh, Scotland)*, 5(4), 199–205.

Key, F. B., & Mathers, J. C. (1995). Digestive adaptations of rats given white bread and cooked haricot beans (*Phaseolus vulgaris*): Large-bowel fermentation and digestion of complex carbohydrates. *British Journal of Nutrition*, 74, 393–406.

Kinsella, J. E., Damodaran, S., & German, B. (1985). Physicochemical and functional properties of oilseed proteins with emphasis on soy proteinsIn A. M. Altschul, & H. L. Wilcke (Eds.), *New Proteins Foods* (Vol. 5, pp. 107–179). New York: Academic Press.

Kneafsey, M., Dowler, E., Lambie-Mumford, H., Inman, A., & Collier, R. (2013). Consumers and food security: Uncertain or empowered? *Journal of Rural Studies*, 29, 101–112.

Koike, T., Koizumi, Y., Tang, L., Takahara, K., & Saitou, Y. (2005). The anti-obesity effect and the safety of taking "Phaseolamin™ 1600 diet". *Journal of New Remedies and Clinics, 54*, 1−16.

Lajolo, F. M., & Genovese, M. I. (2002). Nutritional significance of lectins and enzyme inhibitors from legumes. *Journal of Agricultural and Food Chemistry, 50*, 6592−6598.

Lajolo, F. M., Genovese, M. I., Pryme, I. F., & Dale, M. (2004). Beneficial (antiproliferative) effects of different substances. In M. Muzquiz, G. D. Hill, M. M. Pedrosa, & C. Burbano (Eds.), *Proceedings of the fourth international workshop on antinutritional factors in legume seeds and oilseeds* (pp. 123−135). Wageningen: EAAP Publication No. 110.

Lang, V., Bellisle, F., & Oppert, J. M. (1998). Satiating effect of proteins in healthy subjects: A comparison of egg albumin, casein, gelatin, soy protein, pea protein, and wheat gluten. *American Journal of Clinical Nutrition, 67*(6), 1197−1204.

Letcher, A., Schell, M., & Irvine, R. (2008). Do mammals make all their own inositol hexakisphosphate? *Biochemical Journal, 416*, 263−270.

Liener, I. E. (1976). Legume toxins in relation to protein digestibility: A review. *Journal of Food Science, 41*(5), 1076−1081.

Muzquiz, M., Varela, A., Burbano, C., Cuadrado, C., Guillamo, E., Muzquiz, M., ... Pedrosa, M. M. (2012). Bioactive compounds in legumes: Pronutritive and antinutritive actions. Implications for nutrition and health. *Phytochemistry Reviews, 11*(2−3), 227−244.

Macdiarmid, J., Kyle, J., Horgan, G., Loe, J., Fyfe, C., Johnstone, A., & McNeill, G. (2011). *Livewell: A balance of healthy and sustainable food choices. WWF report.* Scotland: WWF.

Macdiarmid, J. I. (2013). Is a healthy diet an environmentally sustainable diet? *Proceedings of the Nutrition Society, 72*(01), 13−20.

Macdiarmid, J. I., Kyle, J., Horgan, G. W., Loe, J., Fyfe, C., Johnstone, A., & McNeill, G. (2012). Sustainable diets for the future: Can we contribute to reducing greenhouse gas emissions by eating a healthy diet? *The American Journal of Clinical Nutrition, 96*(3), 632−639.

Madden, D. (2015). The poverty effects of a 'fat-tax' in Ireland. *Health Economics, 24*(1), 104−121.

Mathers, J. C. (2002). Pulses and carcinogenesis: Potential for the prevention of colon, breast and other cancers. *British Journal of Nutrition, 88*(S3), 273−279.

Mazzochi, M., Traill, W. B., & Shogren, J. F. (2009). *Fat economics: Nutrition, health and economic policy.* Oxford: Oxford University Press.

McCrory, M. A., Hamaker, B. R., Lovejoy, J. C., & Eichelsdoerfer, P. E. (2010). Pulse consumption, satiety, and weight management. *Advances in Nutrition: An International Review Journal, 1*(1), 17−30.

McMichael, J., Powles, C., & Butler, R. (2007). Food, livestock production, energy, climate change, and health. *Lancet, 370*, 1253−1263.

Michaels, T. E. (2004). *Pulses, overview. Encyclopedia of grain science* (pp. 494−501). USA: Elsevier Ltd.

Morcos, S. R., Gabriel, G. N., & El-Hafez, M. A. (1976). Nutritive studies on some raw and prepared leguminous seeds commonly used in the Arab Republic of Syria. *Zeitschrift fuer Ernaehrungswissenschaft, 15*, 378−386.

Muzquiz,, M. (2000). Factores antinutricionales en fuentes proteicas. In J. Vioque,, A. Clemente,, J. Bautista,, & F. Millan, (Eds.), *Jornada internacional sobre proteínas alimentaras.* Spain: Universidad de Sevilla.

Neacsu, M., Fyfe, C., Horgan, G., & Johnstone, A. M. (2014). Appetite control and biomarkers of satiety with vegetarian (soy) and meat-based high-protein diets for weight loss in obese men: A randomized crossover trial. *The American Journal of Clinical Nutrition, 100*(2), 548−558.

Nishida, C., Uauy, R., Kumanyika, S., & Shetty, P. (2004). The joint WHO/FAO expert consultation on diet, nutrition and the prevention of chronic diseases: Process, product and policy implications. *Public Health Nutrition, 7*(1a), 245−250.

Nordgren, A. (2012). A climate tax on meat? In T. Potthast, & S. Meisch (Eds.), *Climate Change and Sustainable Development, Ethical Perspectives on Land Use and Food Production* (pp. 109−114). Wageningen: Wageningen Academic Publishers.

Nuffield Council on Bioethics (2007). *Public health: Ethical issues.* London: Nuffield Council on Bioethics. Available from: <http://nuffieldbioethics.org/wp-content/uploads/2014/07/Public-health-ethical-issues.pdf> Accessed 27.10.15.

Opala, T., Rzymski, P., Pischel, I., Wilczak, M., & Wozniak, J. (2006). Efficacy of 12 weeks supplementation of a botanical extract-based weight loss formula on body weight, body composition and blood chemistry in healthy, overweight subjects − A randomised double-blind placebo-controlled clinical trial. *European Journal of Medical Research, 11*, 343−350.

Orlich, M. J., Singh, P. N., Sabate, J., Jaceldo-Siegl, K., Fan, J., Knutsen, S., ... Fraser, G. E. (2013). Vegetarian dietary patterns and mortality in adventist health study. *JAMA Internal Medicine, 173*(13), 1230−1238.

Papanikolaou, Y., & Fulgoni, V. L., III (2008). Bean consumption is associated with greater nutrient intake, reduced systolic blood pressure, lower body weight, and a smaller waist circumference in adults: Results from the National Health and Nutrition Examination Survey 1999−2002. *Journal of the American College of Nutrition, 27*(5), 569−576.

Peace, A. (2008). Meat in the genes. *Anthropology Today, 24*(3), 5−10.

Pluhar, E. B. (2010). Meat and morality: Alternatives to factory farming. *Journal of Agricultural and Environmental Ethics, 23*, 455−468.

Pollard, C. M., Miller, M. R., Daly, A. M., Crouchley, K. E., O'Donoghue, K. J., Lang, A. J., & Binns, C. W. (2008). Increasing fruit and vegetable consumption: Success of the Western Australian Go for 2and5® campaign. *Public Health Nutrition, 11*(03), 314−320.

Rao, V., & Al-Weshahy, A. (2008). Plant-based diets and control of lipids and coronary heart disease risk. *Current Atherosclerosis Reports, 10*(6), 478−485.

Rizkalla, S. W., Bellisle, F., & Slama, G. (2002). Health benefits of low glycaemic index foods, such as pulses, in diabetic patients and healthy individuals. *British Journal of Nutrition, 88*, S255−S262.

Rochfort, S., & Panozzo, J. (2007). Phytochemicals for health, the role of pulses. *Journal of Agricultural and Food Chemistry, 55*, 7981−7994.

Rockland, L. B., & Radke, T. M. (1981). Legume protein quality. *Food Technology, 28*, 79−82.

Rogers, R. A. (2008). Beasts, burgers, and hummers: Meat and the crisis of masculinity in contemporary television advertisements. *Environmental Communication, 2*(3), 281−301.

Ruiz, R. G., Price, K. R., Arthur, A. E., Rose, M. E., Rhodes, M. J. C., & Fenwick, R. G. (1996). Effect of soaking and cooking on the saponin content and composition of chickpeas (*Cicer arietinum*) and lentils (*Lens culinaris*). *Journal of Agricultural and Food Chemistry, 44*, 1526–1530.

Sabaté, J., & Soret, S. (2014). Sustainability of plant-based diets: Back to the future. *The American Journal of Clinical Nutrition, 100*(Suppl. 1), 476S–482S.

Sage, C. (2013). The interconnected challenges for food security from a food regimes perspective: Energy, climate and malconsumption. *Journal of Rural Studies, 29*, 71–80.

Sans, P., & Combris, P. (2015). World meat consumption patterns: An overview of the last fifty years (1961–2011). *Meat Science, 109*(2015), 106–111.

Saris, W. H. (2003). Glycemic carbohydrate and body weight regulation. *Nutrition Reviews, 61*, S10–S16.

Sarwar, G., & Peace, R. W. (1986). Comparisons between true digestibility of total nitrogen and limiting amino acids in vegetable proteins fed to rats. *The Journal of Nutrition, 116*(7), 1172–1184.

Schroeder, T. C., Barkley, A. P., & Schroeder, K. C. (1996). Income growth and international meat consumption. *Journal of International Food and Agribusiness Marketing, 7*(3), 15–30.

Sendberg, A. S. (2002). Bioavailability of minerals in legumes. *British Journal of Nutrition, 88*, S281–S285.

Sgarbieri, V., Clarke, E. M. V., & Pusztai, A. (1982). Proteolytic breakdown of kidney bean (*P. vulgaris*) storage proteins: Nutritional implications. *Journal of the Science of Food and Agriculture, 33*, 881–891.

Shi, J., Arunasalam, K., Yeung, D., Kakuda, Y., Mittal, G., & Jiang, Y. (2004). Saponins from edible legumes: Chemistry, processing, and health benefits. *Journal of Medicinal Food, 7*, 67–78.

Sichieri, R., Condo, A. N., Saura, S. K. I., & Albino, C. C. (1993). Reducao de peso com dieta de baixo teor de gordura baseada em arroz e feijao. *Arquivos Brasileiros de Endocrinologia and Metabologia, 37*, 135–138.

Sobal, J., & Bisogni, C. A. (2009). Constructing food choice decisions. *Annals of Behavioral Medicine, 38*(1), 37–46.

Sobal, J., Bisogni, C. A., & Jastran, M. (2014). Food choice is multifaceted, contextual, dynamic, multilevel, integrated, and diverse. *Mind, Brain, and Education, 8*(1), 6–12.

Steinfeld, H., Gerber, P., Wassenaar, T., Castel, V., Rosales, M., & de Haan, C. (2006). *Livestock's long shadow—Environmental issues and options.* Rome: Food and Agriculture Organization of the United Nations.

Steptoe, A., Pollard, T. M., & Wardle, J. (1995). Development of a measure of the motives underlying the selection of food: The food choice questionnaire. *Appetite, 25*(3), 267–284.

Stringer, D. M., Taylor, C. G., Appah, P., Blewett, H., & Zahradka, P. (2013). Consumption of buckwheat modulates the post-prandial response of selected gastrointestinal satiety hormones in individuals with type 2 diabetes mellitus. *Metabolism: Clinical and Experimental, 62*(7), 1021–1031.

Sufian, M. K., Hira, T., Asano, K., & Hara, H. (2007). Peptides derived from dolicholin, a phaseolin-like protein in country beans (*Dolichos lablab*), potently stimulate cholecystokinin secretion from enteroendocrine STC-1 cells. *Journal of Agricultural and Food Chemistry, 55*, 8980–8986.

Thom, E. (2000). A randomized, double-blind, placebo-controlled trial of a new weight-reducing agent of natural origin. *Journal of International Medical Research, 28*, 229–233.

Thorne, M. J., Thompson, L. U., & Jenkins, D. J. A. (1983). Factors affecting starch digestibility and the glycemic response with special reference to legumes. *American Journal of Clinical Nutrition, 38*, 481–488.

Tobler, C., Visschers, V. H., & Siegrist, M. (2011). Eating green. Consumers' willingness to adopt ecological food consumption behaviors. *Appetite, 57*(3), 674–682.

Tome, D. (2012). Criteria and markers for protein quality assessment – A review. *British Journal of Nutrition, 108*(S2), S222–S229.

Tomlinson, I. (2013). Doubling food production to feed the 9 billion: A critical perspective on a key discourse of food security in the UK. *Journal of Rural Studies, 29*, 81–90.

Topping, D. L., & Clifton, P. M. (2001). Short-chain fatty acids and human colonic function: Roles of resistant starch and nonstarch polysaccharides. *Physiologival Review, 81*, 1031–1064.

Tosh, S. M., & Yada, S. (2010). Dietary fibres in pulse seeds and fractions: Characterization, functional attributes, and applications. *Food Research International, 43*(2), 450–460.

Udani, J., & Singh, B. B. (2007). Blocking carbohydrate absorption and weight loss: A clinical trial using a proprietary fractionated white bean extract. *Alternative Therapies in Health and Medicine, 13*, 32–37.

Udani, J., Hardy, M., & Madsen, D. C. (2004). Blocking carbohydrate absorption and weight loss: A clinical trial using phase 2 brand proprietary fractionated white bean extract. *Alternative Medicine Review, 9*, 63–69.

Vinnari, M., & Vinnari, E. (2014). A framework for sustainability transition: The case of plant-based diets. *Journal of Agricultural and Environmental Ethics, 27*(3), 369–396.

Wansink, B., & Sobal, J. (2007). Mindless eating the 200 daily food decisions we overlook. *Environment and Behavior, 39*(1), 106–123.

Williams, P. G., Grafenauer, S. J., & O'Shea, J. E. (2008). Cereal grains, legumes, and weight management: A comprehensive review of the scientific evidence. *Nutrition Reviews, 66*(4), 171–182.

Wilson, M. S., Bulley, S. J., Pisani, F., Irvine, R. F., & Saiardi, A. (2015). A novel method for the purification of inositol phosphates from biological samples reveals that no phytate is present in human plasma or urine. *Open Biology, 5*(3), 150014.

Woldemichael, G. M., Montenegro, G., & Timmermann, B. N. (2003). Triterpenoidal lupin saponins from the Chilean legume *Lupinus oreophilus* Phil. *Phytochemistry, 63*, 853–857.

Wolever, T., Jenkins, D., Vuksan, V., Jenkins, A., Buckley, G., Wong, G., & Josse, R. (1992a). Beneficial effect of low glycemic index diet in type 2 diabetes. *Diabetic Medicine, 9*, 451–458.

Wolever, T., Jenkins, D., Vuskan, V., Jenkins, A., Wong, G., & Josse, R. (1992b). Beneficial effect of low-glycemic index diet in overweight NIDDM subjects. *Diabetes Care, 15*, 562–564.

World Health Organisation (2015). *Obesity and overweight*. http://www.who.int/mediacentre/factsheets/fs311/en/.

Xiao, J. X., Huang, G. Q., Zhu, C. P., Ren, D. D., & Zhang, S. H. (2007). Morphological study on apoptosis HeLa cells induced by soyasaponins. *Toxicology in Vitro, 21*, 820–826.

Zhu, J., Xiong, L., Yu, B., & Wu, J. (2005). Apoptosis induced by a new member of saponin family is mediated through caspase-8-dependent cleavage of Bcl-2. *Molecular Pharmacology, 68*, 1831–1838.

Chapter 23

Flavors, Taste Preferences, and the Consumer: Taste Modulation and Influencing Change in Dietary Patterns for a Sustainable Earth

S.R. Nadathur[1] and M. Carolan[2]

[1]*Givaudan Flavors, Cincinnati, OH, United States,* [2]*Colorado State University, Ft. Collins, CO, United States*

23.1 CONSUMERS: DIETARY AND PURCHASE HABITS

Our diets differ based on several factors such as culture, upbringing, our environment, and health. A meat-based diet is more prevalent in the developed economies, while a plant-based diet is more common in parts of Asia (http://www.healthy.net/Health/Article/Cultural_Diets/1700). With an increase in affluence and multinational companies, fast foods and high-caloric choices are trending up in other parts of the globe including the two most populous countries, India and China. Due to fast-paced lives, processed foods find a common place in the pantry for many people and in the United States, about 70% of the diet is composed of processed foods (Marketplace, 2013). Common dietary patterns today are generally omnivore and vegetarian, with vegan diets increasing in popularity. In addition to our dietary patterns, promotions of food fads arise as people seek a simple path to treating certain health issues. Although each type of dietary habit has its benefits and disadvantages, practitioners of such trends swear by their effectiveness. These trends have included the low-carbohydrate diet, high-fat diet, and the current propensity towards high-protein diets. Dietary protein is the source for nitrogen, a vital component for our body and intracellular functions. Amino acids, which are broken down from plant- or animal-derived protein, form proteins for various tissues, fluids, enzymes, hormones, and numerous cellular activities. In addition to protein, people should consume a balanced diet including sources of fat and carbohydrates for proper nutrition. "In general, mankind, since the improvement in cookery, eats twice as much as nature requires" (Benjamin Franklin). In the developed economies, it is common to eat three meals during the day, though a huge swath of the global populace gets by on one meal or even go hungry. In fact, there is an overabundance of food portions and calories in the United States, while one in seven goes without food around the globe (World Food Programme, 2015). "The spirit cannot endure the body when overfed, but, if underfed, the body cannot endure the spirit" (St. Frances de Sales). Developed economies average 3300 calories per day, while in developing economies consumption is lower by at least 1000 calories. Western-style diets are rich in calories and high in animal protein, fats, and sugars. These foods increase the likelihood of an increase in body mass and obesity. This increase in body weight can affect our health and normal metabolic functioning leading to systemic or chronic conditions.

"Let food be thy medicine, thy medicine shall be thy food" (Hippocrates). Irrespective of the type of diet, or choices we make, flavors and taste, are key attributes to relish food. Various participants in a study (Glanz, Basil, Maibach, Goldberg, & Snyder, 1998), reported taste as their main influence on food choices, followed by cost. Products with consumer appeal had sweet, salty, and fatty tastes (Drewnowski & Almiron-Roig, 2010), while consumers disliked bitter-tasting products (Drewnoski & Gomez-Carneros, 2000). With an increased awareness on the effect of food habits on health issues, consumers are demanding healthier options. Manufacturers have responded by developing alternate products to satisfy consumer demands. These include low-fat, low-sugar, low-sodium, allergen-free, and high-protein products. In the current trend towards high proteins, plant proteins such as soy and pea are common ingredients in many related food products. However, consumers expect that these products taste like their regular counterparts. In the case of plant protein-based products, off-tastes are a common issue, while in reduced sugar products, bulking agents such as starch or dextrin change the product matrix, and alter the predominance of taste attributes. Therefore, healthier products often have off-tastes or lack the sensorial experience (aroma, taste, and mouthfeel) found in a regular-calorie product (Clark, 1998).

Cost and product labels were also critical factors when consumers choose between similar products. With limited space on store shelves, competition between branded products and private labels, consumers have been leaning towards the less expensive private labeled versions. Increased food quality and recessionary periods have encouraged this switch. Low-income consumers tend to buy products which are unhealthy and calorie-rich (http://www.institutefornaturalhealing.com/2011/04/the-economics-of-obesity-why-are-poor-people-fat/). Sale prices however help increase healthier food items including vegetables and fruits. Price reductions on carrots and fresh fruits increased their sales at least twofold (French, 2003). The study also found that the greater the price reduction, the higher the increase in sales of low-fat snacks. Other factors influencing consumer choice include the fear of trying new foods and the throwing away of such purchased foods. Hence, there is a tendency for many consumers to opt for the foods with which they are familiar (http://www.sciencedaily.com/releases/2012/12/121211130442.htm).

Food manufacturers thus rely on unique flavors and ingredients to help their products resonate with targeted consumer groups. Each country or region has its preferred flavors that people are accustomed to eating. Flavors provide the aroma and taste to create the first sensorial experience for the customer and ease the reluctance toward new product introduction. In addition, flavors help reduce the complexities of adding the appropriate fruit or vegetable to enable a stable product matrix. Flavors can also deliver the impact that a ripe fruit provides at a fraction of the cost, while reducing the natural variability of crops. In the case of high-protein products, reducing off-tastes such as beany notes in soy or earthy taste of pea isolates via taste modulation would be important.

23.2 FLAVOR AND TASTE

Anthelme Brillat-Savarin, a renowned 18th century French lawyer and epicure noted that "... and tastes are in fact but a single composite sense, whose laboratory is the mouth and its chimney, the nose...." Aroma, along with the visual image is one of the initial drivers of liking and disliking for new foods. Olfaction is the sense of smell and has two pathways, orthonasal and retronasal. Orthonasal olfaction is the detection of aroma components directly via the nasal passage, such as the aroma of fresh-cut grass or the fatty smell of French fries. This detection of aroma is an important function and aids in the identification of both beneficial and harmful components. Retronasal olfaction is the detection of aroma, which emanates during the eating process. When food is ingested, molecules are released, which are then detected by the olfactory cells. The aroma molecules travel up the nasopharynx passage, and consequently, this detection is possible only when we breathe air out of the nose. Together, ortho- and retronasal olfaction provide the sensorial experience for the enjoyment of food.

23.2.1 Physiology of Taste

In addition to the aroma, multiple factors affect our taste and enjoyment of food (Rozin, 1990). Taste molecules are detected by chemoreceptors on the tongue. Thus, tasting is a sensation and the brain receives electrical signals from the taste buds or papillae. Each taste bud is a combination of several receptor cells and basal cells. There are about 2000–8000 taste buds on the tongue and another 2000 supporting cells on the roof, sides of the mouth, and under the tongue. Replacement of taste buds occurs every 2 weeks, with the total number of taste buds steadily declining with age. A number of factors contribute to this reduction, such as age, our eating habits, smoking, and health conditions (NIH Medline Plus (https://www.nlm.nih.gov/medlineplus/ency/article/004013.htm)). Supertasters have many more papillae than the normal populace and are reported to have an enhanced ability to discern certain basic tastes. However, this ability may not cover all taste sensations.

There are four basic taste sensations, salt, sweet, sour, and bitter. In addition, detection of glutamates has led to umami (savory) being the fifth basic taste. Recently, a fat receptor was identified and may become the sixth basic taste. In addition, kokumi was also in consideration as another taste sensation. Though there are a few different interpretations, kokumi enhances taste sensations, acting via the calcium receptor (Maruyama, Yasuda, Kuroda, & Eto, 2012). Although it was thought that the tongue was split into zones of taste perception, recent research has shown that detection of sensations occurs throughout the tongue and that parts of the tongue are more responsive to certain tastes.

Sweet (T1R2, T1R3) and bitter (T2R) tastes are perceived via G-protein-coupled receptors and thus create a sensory response. G-protein couplings create a cascade of events, which involve GTPase. Salty and sour tastes are thought to be perceived by ion channels, whereby proton (H^+) and sodium ions (Na^+) pass through specific channels. G-protein coupling is also involved for the T1R3 receptor-mediated umami taste. There is increasing research on a fat-detecting receptor, which detects long-chain fatty acids via a G-protein GPR120 (Gallindo et al., 2012). Gene CD36 is involved in the liking of fats based on a study on rats (Degrace-Passily & Besnard, 2012). Astringency, the sensation of pungent (or spicy) and cooling compounds are trigeminal perceptions. Ion-specific TRP channels were found to play a role in detecting these sensations (Viana, 2011). TRPM8 was identified for detecting cooling, TRPV1 for capsacin, and TRPA1 for nonpungent compounds.

Many consumers dislike bitter and astringent tastes. In addition, these taste attributes are associated with many recently developed plant protein-based products. As this book is devoted to the topic of sustainable proteins, we will limit discussion to these two taste attributes.

23.2.1.1 Bitter Taste

Consumers typically dislike bitter tastes. Bitter-sensitive taste buds are located in the back of the tongue and thought to be a defense mechanism. Bitter tastes come from a variety of compounds, many of which are medicinal. Examples include quinine, caffeine, and acetaminophen. In addition, certain peptides in plant proteins, or minerals added to protein beverages are often bitter. Bitter peptides have hydrophobic amino acid side chains. The bitter taste in soybeans is likely due to genistein, an isoflavone glucoside (Chang, Huan, & Ho, 1990). Though isoflavones have antioxidant properties, they also contribute an undesirable taste to soy products. Other beans, such as kidney and navy, also contain bitter glucosides, while saponins in quinoa can add bitterness as well.

23.2.1.2 Astringency

This sensation is a drying of the mouth involving the interaction of salivary proteins and phenolic components. Sometimes astringency and bitterness may seem related to each other since the presence of bitter compounds may lead to an astringent perception. Astringency is a tactile response, and can occur via phenolic compounds such as tannic acids present in tea or plant proteins such as pea. These phenolic compounds bind to a class of salivary proteins called proline-rich proteins (PRP) to form a complex. This creates a drying sensation in the mouth, due to a reduction in the flow of saliva. Protein-based products are also fortified with minerals, which can also have a metallic and/or astringent taste. A more prevalent taste in protein-rich foods is the chalkiness, or mineral taste. Chalkiness may occur due to peptides, an aggregate of small/fine particles, or mineral fortification, especially calcium. Aggregates of small particles often form in dairy protein-based products, due to high processing temperature. Thus ultra-high temperature (UHT) processed milk has a high degree of chalkiness and similar scenarios are possible with plant protein-based products when processed at high temperatures.

23.3 WHY WE EAT WHAT WE EAT: TASTE PREFERENCES AND INFLUENCES

"Tell me what you eat, and I will tell you who you are" (Brillat-Savarin). Our taste preferences develop from prenatal times and evolve with age. Factors such as genetics, cultural upbringing, and the environment further play a role. These factors are depicted in Fig. 23.1.

Flavors from foods consumed by the mother during pregnancy influence the preferences of the child later in adulthood. In babies, the intake of sweet liquids led to a satisfied expression, while bitter and sour liquids were rejected with a negative expression. Infants fed either soy hydrolysate formulation or milk hydrolysate formulation preferred the formula they were accustomed to consuming. They did not like the other formula, which was unfamiliar to them (Menella & Beauchamp, 2005). As children grow older, foods such as pizza and ice cream were favored over vegetables and fruits (Cooke & Wardle, 2005). In addition, aversion exists to taste unfamiliar foods, as it is comforting to consume familiar foods. Much of these influences can be traced to genetic factors, as well as family environment (Wardle & Cooke, 2008). Pirastu et al. (2012) studied 400 participants in five countries to identify genetic involvement in taste preferences. Many genes were involved in the liking or disliking of foods and these variants were responsible for whether people like sheep cheese versus coffee. The authors concluded that understanding these influences will help identify methods to provide nutrients to those who dislike certain foods. There are also structural expectations to meals that shape taste preferences. For instance in the West, meat holds a privileged place in how meals are presented and organized (Douglas & Nicod, 1974). When a meal can only be considered a "meal" when meat is present, a significant barrier is present for those looking to introduce into meal structures alternative protein sources.

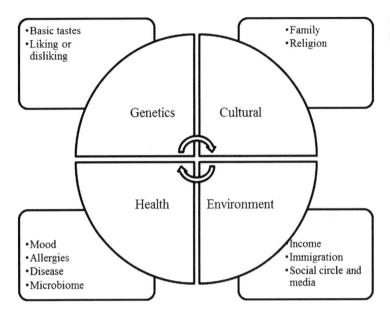

FIGURE 23.1 Depiction of influences on consumer taste preferences and food choices.

23.3.1 Genetics and Food Choices

Taste preferences start from prenatal times, and many of those taste preferences stay with people through adulthood. Studies have shown that there is a difference in the ability to detect bitter-tasting compounds, phenylthiocarbamide (PTC) and 6-propylthiouracil (PROP). PTC or PROP tastes either clean or bitter based on an individual's genetic markers (Sun-wei & Reed, 2001). Certain populations are unable to taste these compounds including people from West Africa. The rate increases to the single digits for Chinese, while 40% of people from India are unable to taste PTC (Garcia-Bailo, Toguri, Eny, & El-Sohemy, 2007). Variation in the bitter taste of PROP appears linked to phenotypic differences in a taste gene TAS2R38 (Mennella, Pepino, & Reed, 2005). In addition, the differences in this gene account for the liking of sweet-flavored products among children. Those able to detect PROP were also likely supertasters. Coffee was another food item linked to the bitter receptor (Pirastu et al., 2014).

Avoiding bitter foods is also akin to avoiding toxic substances. In fact, several plants have off-tastes built in for their survival. This ability to distinguish bitter-tasting foods is likely to affect food habits and the consequential influences on health (Beckett et al., 2014). Women who could readily detect PROP disliked cruciferous vegetables, grapefruit, and soy products (Drewnoski, 2001). Although bitter substances are rejected as harmful, they may contain beneficial compounds such as anticarcinogens present in cruciferous vegetables. The differences in this ability to reject bitter products may relate to genetic variants of the individual's genes and these variances may prompt manufacturers to develop targeted food products (El-Sohemy et al., 2007).

The taste of coriander or cilantro seemed soapy to people from East Asia, Europe, and parts of Africa. However, South Asians loved coriander and included it as an important herb in daily cooking (Mauer & El-Sohemy, 2012). The origins of the different responses to coriander were traced to the olfactory response gene OR6A2, which carried a varied sensitivity to aldehydes. A team of scientists also found an association for cilantro taste to several genes including a bitter taste receptor. The dislike for cilantro was related to the aroma, more than taste (Wysocki, 2010).

Understanding some of these genetic influences on taste may help in the development of foods specific for some people. In fact, personalization of foods is one area that will continue to grow and evolve. However, personalization requires gathering information about target customers. This could well raise privacy issues (Gorman, 2006). Genetics and cultural preferences for food are typically related and one influences the other. Next, we will discuss how culture and the environment affect our food preferences.

23.3.2 Our Upbringing and Cultural Influence on Food Choices

"The French cook; we open tins" (John Galsworthy, English novelist). Culture and dietary habits go in tandem. Countries and regions within the country consume a wide-ranging menu. Typically, recipes are handed down through generations and each family has its own unique twist to basic recipes. Immigration has introduced regional cuisines to other parts of the globe, and these cuisines have been adapted to local tastes. Religious and cultural influences can become intertwined and these habits are likely to shape our diets. Vegetarian diets have strong links to religious beliefs and subsects of these philosophies further restrict the eating of certain foods. The West has since adopted such diets due to the beneficial impact on health. Conversely, the advent of globalism has introduced fast foods from the West into many parts of the globe. These foods have negatively affected other countries, which have traditionally consumed healthier foods.

Studies showed that children from various countries have different food preferences. A majority of kids (70%) from Germany liked biscuits with a lot of fat versus only 35% of kids from Cyprus. In addition, children from Germany liked plain apple juice whereas kids from neighboring countries like Italy and France enjoyed apple juice with added sugar and flavors (Lanfer et al., 2013). Cultural trends were found to be different in European countries. In particular, France ate cheese with more microorganisms (live cheese) compared to Denmark and Sweden who favored more pasteurized cheese. Rare meat was consumed in France, whereas Sweden and Denmark liked it well-cooked (Bouchet, 1998).

Diets of immigrants often changed when they moved to another country. Many immigrants adapted to the local culture and foods, which frequently carried negative associations. Chinese moving to a Western country had a higher likelihood of cardiovascular diseases once fast food became a major part of their diet (Rosenmöller, Gasevic, Seidell, & Lear, 2011). Hispanic immigrants altered their diets to move away from traditional menus to high-fat and high-sugar diets with long-term health implications (McArthur, Anguiano, & Nocetti, 2001). Similar results were found for South Asians moving to Europe (Holmboe-Ottensen & Wandel, 2012). With the advent of Western diets to all parts of the globe, high-fat, high-sugar diets are displacing traditional local diets that were high in grains, legumes, and vegetables. The growing affluence in countries like China and India has resulted in the adoption of food convenience, leading to obesity and chronic diseases (http://www.hsph.harvard.edu/obesity-prevention-source/obesity-trends/obesity-rates-worldwide/).

As more attention is paid to sustainable protein sources, it can be expected that interest in entomophagy (edible insects) will grow. Yet, when new insect-based foods are developed and consumer tested, they overwhelmingly induce feelings of disgust. These feelings can be so strong that prospective eaters often refuse to even try the new foods (Bednářová, Borkovcová, Mlček, Rop, & Zeman, 2013; Looy & Wood, 2006). Studies involving students in the United States document that whereas a majority is willing to touch insects with their hands, a majority refuse touching them with their lips (Rozin, Haidt, McCauley, Dunlop, & Ashmore, 1999). In comparisons of different protein alternatives, it was shown that visible insects—insect-based food that still looked like insects—were the least preferred (Schösler, De Boer, & Boersema, 2012). Some studies explore the degree to which this aversion is due to a lack of familiarity with these novel protein sources. To that end, one study held multiple "educational bug banquets" for junior high, high school, and university students in Canada. The results, according to the study's authors, "suggest that educational bug banquets have complex and subtle effects on attitudes that may depend on age, but they may help prepare people to respond more positively to future encounters with these species" (Looy & Wood, 2006). Other research suggests the importance of "flavor familiarity" when introducing new foods—like insects—into one's diet. A recent study examining consumer acceptance of edible insects (specifically mealworms and crickets) finds increased acceptance when those foods are prepared using spices and other flavoring agents that draw upon an eater's existing culinary background (Caparros Megido et al., 2014).

There is also evidence that expectations not only shape preferences but can also alter how consumers experience flavors. We generally expect, for example, food presented as "unhealthy" to taste better; effects that persist even after the foods are consumed (Raghunathan, Naylor, & Hoyer, 2006). These expectations, in other words, appear to make food taste better. Consumers repeatedly rated the taste of Coca-Cola higher when they knew what they were drinking (Woolfolk, Castellan, & Brooks, 1983). The same was true with McDonald's French fries, chicken nuggets, hamburgers, milk, and apple juice: children consistently preferred the taste of those presented in McDonald's packaging over those served in a plain-white wrapping (Mirsky, 2007).

Building on a point mentioned above, there are a number of interesting historical cases pointing to the role of familiarity in taste. In other words, the acquiring of taste preferences takes time. Through repeated exposures individuals are given the time to work through aversions, stereotypes, and tactile sensations associated with particular foods. This was observed, for instance, during World War I. As soldiers became repeatedly exposed to canned foods on a daily basis most went from disliking the food to actually desiring it, as evidenced by the growth of canned food purchases in households once the soldiers returned to civilian life after the war (Bruegel, 2002).

A similar story has been described with soy. In the first year that soy proteins were allowed into school meal programs, US schools served 23 million pounds of vegetable protein, the vast majority of which came from the soybean (Johnson, Myers, & Burden, 1992; see also McCloud, 1974). By the mid-1990s, soy protein constituted approximately 30% by weight of meat products served through the National School Lunch Program, which translates into over

50 million pounds of soy protein per year (Ensminger, 1993). In addition to changes to the chemical properties of soy to alter their bitterness, these school programs, which exposed generations to soy proteins beginning at a very young age, have been described as playing a major role in helping Americans overcome their initial aversion to soy-based foods (DuBois, 2008).

23.3.3 Affording a Healthy Diet

Financial conditions affect our food purchases. The poor tend to buy caloric-dense food items such as fast foods in many parts of the globe, in part due to the reality than many live in urban food deserts (http://www.foodsafetynews.com/2010/05/few-healthy-food-choices-in-urban-food-deserts/#.Vlz1VfmrSM8). Places that food deserts occur have significant disadvantages due to location, the type of population, and lack of transportation in that region. Food deserts tend to have correlation to poverty and lower education and these factors affect peopleese fac choices (Dutko, Ver Ploeg, & Farrigan, 2012). Such foods were likely to be highly processed and loaded with unhealthy fats and carbohydrates. In addition, there was a lack of fresh vegetables, produce, and healthier food choices. There is also a correlation between financial poverty and time poverty (Warren, 2003). The working poor especially lack the resources, including the resource of time, to learn about new foods and the new preparation and cooking techniques they often require.

Families who earned slightly more than a median income and considered middle class consumed more fast food than those families who earned around $30,000 (Leigh, 2011). The study also found that visits to fast food restaurants decreased as income increased beyond $60,000, although the use of promotions, toys, and other giveaways enticed customers. A study with over 100,000 children in several European countries found that consumption of fruit was higher in wealthier homes, while soft drinks led the way in homes with lesser incomes. These factors increased obesity in kids and adolescents (Vereecken, Inchley, Subramanian, Hublet, & Maes, 2005).

There is an inverse correlation with respect to the consumption of healthy food and the occurrence of chronic health conditions (Drewnowski & Darmon, 2005). The overconsumption of fast food diets may increase obesity and thus cause the development of diabetes and cardiovascular disease. Consumption of healthier foods is critical for reducing the incidence of chronic health issues. Combinations of grains and legumes provide a complete amino acid profile along with various nutrients and minerals. The availability of such foods must involve simple items and easily prepared recipes which are part of many cultures. Any attempt to incentivize the consumption of alternative protein sources thus must include components tied to their access, as it is impossible to learn about and become familiar with certain foods if you do not have contact with them. In addition, the poor often have less access to education and awareness of healthy eating habits may be limited. Thus, the tendency to buy familiar foods is prevalent. Worries about the wasting of time and money may prevent the inclination to purchase novel foods. Policies must be sensitive to these socioeconomic barriers when seeking to encourage the consumption of alternative protein sources. Merely telling people to eat differently, in other words, in a strict nutrition literacy sense, is rarely enough to alter behaviors (Carolan, 2011).

23.3.4 Ice Cream, Broccoli, or Nuts?

Our food consumption patterns directly influence our health. Proteins are critical for a variety of bodily functions. A balanced diet containing proteins, carbohydrates, and fat is vital for our wellbeing. Many diets such as those in India or China include various grains, vegetables, herbs, and spices for their medicinal value. Good eating habits, even in times of stress, aid in boosting our immune systems. Unhealthy eating habits, such as high intake of fat and sugar, lead to chronic and systemic health conditions. Studies found that the harmful effects to the immune system continue for a period even after a change to healthier diets (Van Kempen, Jaminon, van Berkel, & van Eck, 2014). Labels help us understand the nutrition components in the foods we select. Those trying to eat healthily when faced with a medical condition chose products based on their nutrition labels. Such recognition improved food choices and enabled better eating habits and lifestyles in African-Americans (Satia, Galanko, & Neuhouser, 2005).

Our mood also influences the choice of food we consume. Stress, sadness, or a depressive feeling can cause overeating of higher-fat and sugary foods. These foods are termed comfort foods, as they are rich and indulgent. Consequently, this results in a craving when faced with stressful situations (Harvard Health Publication, 2012). These higher-fat and sweet foods counter the release of stress hormones and calm brain activity (Gibson, 2006). Consumption of healthy foods rich in proteins and good fats such as pulses, nuts, and whole grains aided a positive mood (Dallman, 2010). A likely reason may be the release of tryptophan, which forms serotonin for a calmer mood.

Health conditions may also change people's dietary patterns. Diseases such as diabetes and cardiovascular conditions have led people to healthier habits, as the consequences of not changing their diet would be detrimental.

In such situations, health concerns override the taste aspects and, in fact, bitter food consumption increased in quantity due to their perceived benefits.

Food allergies occur primarily due to the body's inability to digest proteins. Proteins documented to elicit an allergenic response are present in nuts, seeds, fish, shellfish, eggs, beans, and grains (Food Allergy Research and Resource Program (http://farrp.unl.edu/for-consumers)). Depending on each individual's situation, restricted diets require implementation to reduce immune responses, some of which can be fatal. In many cases, allergenic responses are not to just one class, but can go across several categories. Gluten-free, soy-free, and nut-free products are especially important to cater to the diets of those with known allergies to these foods.

23.4 SUSTAINABLE PROTEIN SOURCES IN FOODS AND THEIR CHALLENGES

Plant and animal sources provide proteins and these include grains, pulses, nuts, dairy, and meat. However, animals need to consume plant protein to make meat or milk. There is a growing awareness of the negative health aspects of eating red meat. More importantly, the environmental aspects of meat production contribute to climate change while we face an immense challenge to feed a rapidly growing population. The challenges facing the growing global population have been discussed in the introductory chapter. Varieties of proteins are available from plants and alternate sources such as mycoproteins, algae, and insects. Food products containing these proteins are gaining momentum from consumer awareness in both health and the environment. These protein sources, such as pea, lentil, and even insects are standard menu items in many Asian and Latin-American cultures. Traditional African-American foods included a variety of grains, beans, and leafy greens, which formed a complete diet. Now these plant proteins are becoming part of Western-style snack, beverage, and meal stock-keeping units (SKUs). Product developers still face some challenges to create foods with great appeal, though this is true for all types of goods. Mere inclusion of plant protein sources may not help the sale of these products, as consumers may reach for their familiar food or beverage. In developing a protein beverage, research showed that consumers could differentiate between several types of protein levels and many types of protein. It was important that the protein beverage had to taste great for widespread acceptance (Oltman, Lopetcharat, Bastian, & Drake, 2015). Flavor and taste were key attributes for product success, despite health claims. Hence, developers need to understand the changing taste preferences and cultural factors in order to launch a successful product.

23.4.1 Off-Tastes Associated With Plant Proteins

Most plant-based proteins have certain off-tastes, though milk proteins also develop off-flavors such as cardboard, astringent, and chalky. For example, soybean has a beany aftertaste, while pea proteins have an earthy aroma. In addition, protein isolates or concentrates may taste bitter or astringent depending on the peptide breakdown or the presence of other compounds. Introduction of plant proteins has been via familiar products such as beverages and snack bars. In these products, off-tastes are more "visible" and require modulation. Cultures where plant protein sources are prevalent understand the presence of these "off-tastes." In fact, these off-tastes, such as the beany note of soy, are inherent and accepted as such. Cooking methods minimize these "off-tastes" by the inclusion of spice blends or Maillard browning notes formed during sautéing. For example, batters made of various dried pea and lentil flours have an earthy aroma, but the cooked crepe is no longer earthy, and has a pleasant browned taste.

Flavor off-tastes occur via the breakdown of fat and protein. Unsaturated fats in soybeans are broken down to form aldehydes, ketones, and alcohols. Lipoxygenase converts polyunsaturated fatty acids (linoleic acid) to hydroperoxide intermediates, which break down to form hexanal, trans-2 hexenal, cis-3 hexenol, pentanol, hexanol, 2-pentyl furan, and ethyl vinyl ketone. These compounds contributed to the off-tastes associated with soy protein (Rackis, Sessa, & Honig, 1979). Rice protein provides a pleasant nutty taste. However, oxidation of residual rice bran oil can cause unpleasant aldehydes and ketones similar to those formed in soybeans. In addition, oxidation products of the conjugated fatty acids added bitterness (Baur, Grosch, Wieser, & Jugel, 1977). Genistein and daidzein formed in soymilk by the oxidation of isoflavones and these compounds were bitter and astringent. Flaxseed contains high amounts of linoleic and linolenic acids and is prone to oxidation. Hence, it is advisable that full-fat or partially deoiled flaxseed meal, along with rice proteins be refrigerated and used within a short time to reduce off-tastes in finished products. An earthy note in navy bean is developed from the formation of geosmin (Buttery, Guadagni, & Ling, 1976). Quinoa contains a saponin coating, which tastes bitter. Washing quinoa aids in the removal of this component to provide a cleaner-tasting product.

Sorghum and millets have little off-tastes and are used widely to make a variety of both savory and sweet products. Hemp protein has a nutty taste and is suitable for many baked goods and beverages. Mycoprotein is a mild-tasting product and may have slight off-tastes. This enables the addition of a variety of flavors to make mycoprotein suitable for a variety of applications. Insect proteins and flours may have more of the unappealing factor than any major off-tastes. Though insects are consumed as snacks or toppings in Mexico and other countries, the consumption in the United States will require the protein be masked to ensure a clean-tasting product. Algal protein (from *Chlorella*), has high glutamic and aspartic acids content and is perceived as savory and umami. Hence, algal proteins may find ready use in sauces, dips, and salty foods. However, use of this protein from algal sources broadly in nonsavory applications will require masking of the umami taste. The presence of off-flavors in plant and alternate protein sources is no different from those found in dairy protein-based products. Consumers do not desire to eat products which are astringent or bitter. Overcoming these off-tastes is key to making better-tasting consumer products, especially if we need to encourage more consumption of plant protein products.

23.4.2 Role of Flavors in Modulating Off-Notes in Protein-Based Products

Flavors aid in the acceptance or dislike of foods. Flavors help to mask or suppress the undesirable off-tastes and increase the palatability of an otherwise unappealing product. Masking or taste modulation uses flavors that contain several ingredients, which aid the perception of a desirable product. These ingredients may be aroma molecules or natural extracts, or other proprietary components derived from taste receptor studies. A masking flavor can function in many ways. It can bind to the protein while modulating the taste, enhance desirable notes, suppress off-tastes, and counter bitterness and astringency. Addition of a masking flavor provides a neutral-tasting base product making characterizing flavors such as strawberry or chocolate profiles more visible.

In addition to protein, food products contain other components and additives. These include fats, sugars or sweeteners, salts, acids, vitamins, and minerals. Off-tastes can arise from a combination of these components and it is important to modulate them including basic tastes for a product with broad customer appeal. Hence, flavors may require inclusion of additional components to combat off-tastes present in the finished product. As bitter and astringency are some of the primary off-tastes in protein-based products requiring modulation, the discussion is limited to these two attributes.

23.4.2.1 Bitter Taste Modulation

A potential strategy for bitter taste modulations would be using compounds to interfere with the ability of the bitter substance to bind within the T2R receptor. A novel small molecule can reduce bitterness by preventing activation of T2R receptors caused by artificial sweeteners, saccharin, and acesulfame K (Slack et al., 2010). Maillard reaction products of catechin were found to modulate the bitterness of caffeine (Zhang, Xia, & Peterson, 2014). The causative molecules were spiroglycosides, and one of the six molecules had the most ability to reduce bitterness. Cocoa powder was found to contain these spiro compounds. Probenecid, a molecule used to treat gout, binds nearby the T2R receptors and affects the ability of bitter molecules to interact with the T2R receptor (Greene et al., 2011). This interaction likely affects the cascade of steps that occur once the G-protein is coupled. Addition of cyclodextrin to products can help dissolve flavonoids and reduce bitter taste (Szejtki & Szente, 2005). Cyclodextrins form complexes with bitter compounds from a variety of sources to eliminate bitter taste. Suppression of bitterness by various salts was studied (Keast, Breslin, & Beauchamp, 2001). Bitterness suppression varied with the cation, and on the source of bitterness. In addition, sodium salt increased sweetness by suppressing bitterness. Thus, salt in low amounts can alter the flavor perceptions of a food matrix.

23.4.2.2 Astringency Modulation

Astringency correlates negatively to liking of plant-based food products (Lesschaeve & Noble, 2005). Salivary proteins are bound to astringent compounds, reducing the flow of saliva. A process that restores this flow can have a modulating effect on astringency. Sugar or sweet substances positively affect the reduction of astringency. Acidic pH reduced the flow of saliva and increased astringency of whey protein beverages (Ye et al., 2011). Thus, modulation of acidic taste may aid in the acceptance of whey protein-based products. In the case of chalkiness, adding an emulsifier can disperse large aggregates and blend in the small aggregates resulting in reduced chalkiness. Inclusion of fats also helps to minimize chalkiness in protein drinks, as the coating of fat on the tongue prevents the formulation of the fine powders to collect and cause the sensation. Hence, flavors, along with masking components are essential for formulating an acceptable product.

23.4.3 Binding of Flavors by Proteins

Proteins also bind flavors and change the flavor profile with time. Globular proteins such as whey proteins bind flavor molecules by hydrophobic bonding. When these globular proteins denature, the peptide chain unfolds leading to increased binding of a variety of molecules. Most of the binding is reversible and occurs via hydrogen bonding. However, irreversible binding of straight-chain aldehydes occurred, which caused loss of flavor impact (Lubbers, Landy, & Voilley, 1998). Relative to molecular size, longer-chain compounds had a greater affinity for binding. Thus, the binding of some of the flavor molecules will affect the perceived flavor profile resulting in an unbalanced flavor. Consequently, it may be desirable to prevent flavor binding to prevent loss of flavor components and maintain flavor profile during shelf-life.

Similar flavor-binding results were found with plant proteins such as soy or legumes. Studies done with hexyl acetate showed differential binding with soy protein. Acid denaturation of the protein resulted in very little binding of the ester, while heat denaturation retained the ability to bind hexyl acetate (Semonova, Antipova, Misharina, & Golovnya, 2002). Deamidation is the conversion of amino groups on the protein to carboxylic groups, which can alter or improve the functionality of proteins. In addition, the reduction in amide groups can decrease flavor loss, especially vanillin that is an important component of vanilla flavor. Deamidation of soy protein isolate by protein glutamidase led to less flavor binding of vanillin and maltol (Suppavorasatit & Calwallader, 2012). This reduction in flavor loss would help the product retain the named flavor profile (eg, strawberry) over a longer time. Developing neutral-tasting plant protein concentrates and isolates can create new research for purification as well as to modify the proteins. This would be especially useful for beverages, baked products, and snack items.

23.5 INTRODUCTION OF NEW FOODS AND CHANGING CONSUMER HABITS

Current products on the market utilize plant protein concentrates and isolates to replace dairy protein or eggs in traditional or familiar products of Western societies. New-generation meat alternates or substitutes are in development to rival the taste and texture of meat. Clearly, these products will aid in the switch of dietary habits from an animal protein-based diet. Any reduction in meat consumption will also lessen the resources required to produce animal feed including land, water, and energy.

To achieve a major dent in environmental and socioeconomic aspects would entail changes in dietary patterns towards plant-based diets. This presents a transformational opportunity for the current global citizens, especially in Western societies. With a major increase in population causing ever more exploitation of natural resources, it is vital that we reduce meat consumption towards a plant-based diet. Cultures around the globe have been consuming a variety of grains, legumes, seeds, nuts, and vegetables, all of which provide adequate protein, and other vital nutrients and minerals. This consumption occurred for centuries and even had a health connotation. Purifying proteins would also strip away these valuable nutrients while adding cost.

Understanding prevailing cultural influences and learning to overcome neophobic tendencies would create a significant moment in our lifetime to encourage people from around the globe to consume the variety the earth has to offer. Social media can aid in this movement via promotion of recipes and trends, while encouraging the switch to an environmentally friendly diet. People would not only enjoy great foods, but also improve their health and reduce the ill effects of a high-caloric Western diet. This switch would greatly affect land use and rather than growing crops for animal feed, farmers can cultivate them for direct human consumption. Further, fertilizer, water, and fossil energy use will lessen with a consequential reduction in greenhouse gas emission.

Changing food habits is a difficult process and many factors play a role including social, cultural, and neophobic tendencies. Those with a need such as a medical condition, may accept these difficult food choices more readily than if the situation was hypothetical. Typically, beneficial foods are likely to be bitter or have some off-taste associated with them. Though our instincts tell us to avoid bitter foods, they help reduce blood sugar and contain several phytonutrients that boost our ability to fight off diseases (Weill, 2014). In addition, bitter components increase bile secretion, which increases the availability of fat-soluble vitamins.

However, plant-based foods have some disadvantages, which are not unique. Bitterness, off-tastes in purified plant protein, and flatus require explanation for Western diets to change (Kay, 1998). We have discussed options to reduce bitterness in plant protein isolates or concentrates. Protein purification and taste modulation methods are certainly the best options for utilizing these proteins in beverages, bars, and cultured products. However, societies from around the globe have consumed these grains, legumes, and seeds for centuries utilizing a variety of herbs and spices to make tasteful dishes. Introducing and encouraging those foods made from other cultures could be a major initiative, which can wean away the Western societies from a meat-based diet. Although large cities in the United States and Europe are more accepting of these foods, understanding the cultural influences and using demographic changes to create a completely new menu for the next generation would be a prudent choice.

Relative to beans and legumes, which are often associated with flatus, dairy products cause more flatus due to the breakdown of lactose. Though this is natural, most people relate a vegetarian diet to flatus and shy away from consuming them. An option may be to add baking soda to the water during cooking of the beans or to sprout them. Germination or sprouting resulted in the reduction of oligosaccharide level, which is the source of flatulence-causing gas (Jood, Mehta, Singh, & Bhat, 1985). Yet, diets rich in beans, legumes, greens, and grains support health in multiple ways. These sources provide proteins, vitamins, and minerals, which aid the normal functioning of several organs and reduce the incidence of cancer, diabetes, and kidney failure.

The benefits of eating healthy and supporting the environment can be accomplished at the same time. People can be given incentives, lectured, or be part of the discussion to change. Knowing that food is nutritionally beneficial did not influence people to consume them (Wansink & Chan, 2001). During World War II, a study tried to determine the best methods to encourage the inclusion of organ meats in soldier's diets. The discussion-decision method to include organ meat was more influential than a lecture method (Lewin, 1951). Thus, varieties of options need consideration in order to influence people in Western societies to include more plant-based foods. It is also important that those eating more plant-based diets resist the switch to a Western-style diet. Such switches will exacerbate climate change issues and affect their health as well and thereby requiring lots more resource allocation.

Global warming, climate change, reducing meat consumption, are all akin to "someone else's problems." However, shifting eating habits is not an easy task to accomplish. Encouraging people in Western societies to participate via discussion rather than a professorial method is crucial (Wansink, 2002). In addition, recognizing the link between food and cultural habits is very important. Chef Jamie Oliver from the United Kingdom attempted to create a healthier lunch menu for schools in the United States in 2014. He found that changing habits of kids to eat healthy foods requires overcoming resistance. With time, he understood the cultural dimension in that region of the United States, and used incentives to develop better eating among the kids (Von Post, 2011). Changing habits involves providing the background facts so the consumer can make the proper choice, such as the harmful effects of climate change. Behavioral changes are difficult and it will require providing more information on the need to change habits. People do not need to give up meat altogether, but make a decision to reduce consumption to a few times a week rather than daily. There are many other related decisions that can help make the earth a better place, and impact climate change. If many people join in, these reductions can add up to making a meaningful impact. We mean that quite literally: the enrollment of *many people*. The literature is clear on the effectiveness of when families and communities begin making dietary changes together (eg, Ashida, Wilkinson, & Koehly, 2012). It is a virtuous cycle. People are more likely to adopt new behaviors (and indeed even tastes) when others within their social network do so (Carolan, 2011). That is why, for instance, targeting school-aged kids in schools is so appealing (Mcisaac, Read, Veugelers, & Kirk, 2013). If it were to become "normal" to eat alternative proteins you can bet school-aged children would start eating them at greater rates. Moreover, that ought to be the goal: to reach a point were sustainable protein consumption is the normal thing to do.

23.6 CONCLUSIONS

Consumers are influenced by the aroma and taste of various foods, while several factors affect their purchase choices including income, education, and costs. Consumers also eat certain foods and these choices relate to their upbringing, genetics, and culture. It is imperative that people, especially in Western societies, reduce meat consumption and move towards a plant-based diet for their protein needs. This change requires broad understanding of taste preferences, modulating tastes, and cultural influences to enable switching diets for the greater good.

DISCLAIMER

The views and opinions expressed in this chapter are those of the authors and do not reflect the official policy or position of the affiliated organizations.

REFERENCES

Ashida, S., Wilkinson, A. V., & Koehly, L. M. (2012). Social influence and motivation to change health behaviors among Mexican-origin adults: Implications for diet and physical activity. *American Journal of Health Promotion*, 26(3), 176–179.

Baur, C., Grosch, W., Wieser, H., & Jugel, H. (1977). Enzymatic oxidation of linoleic acid: Formation of bitter tasting fatty acids. *Zeitschrift für Lebensmittel-Untersuchung und – Forschung*, 164, 171–176.

Beckett, E. L., Martin, C., Yates, Z., Veysey, M., Duesing, K., & Lucock, M. (2014). Bitter taste genetics – The relationship to tasting, liking, consumption and health. *Food Function*, 5(12). Available from http://dx.doi.org/10.1039/C4FO00539B.

Bednářová, M., Borkovcová, M., Mlček, J., Rop, O., & Zeman, L. (2013). Edible insects-species suitable for entomophagy under condition of Czech Republic. *Acta Universitatis Agriculturae et Silviculturae Mendelianae Brunensis, 61*(3), 587–593.

Bouchet, D. (1998). Differences in food culture – Traditions and trends. exemplified with the cultural differences between France-Denmark-Sweden. In C. Heggun (Ed.), *Quality and risk management. Proceedings of the 25th international dairy congress (21–24 September 1998, Aarhus, Denmark)* (pp. 210–216). Aarhus: The Danish National Committee of the IDF, 1999.

Bruegel, M. (2002). How the French learned to eat canned food, 1809–1930. In W. Belasco, & P. Scranton (Eds.), *Food nations: Selling taste in consumer societies* (pp. 113–130). New York: Routledge.

Buttery, R. G., Guadagni, D., & Ling, L. (1976). Geosmin, a musty off-flavor of dry beans. *Journal of Agriculture and Food Chemistry, 24*(2), 419–420.

Caparros Megido, R., Sablon, L., Geuens, M., Brostaux, Y., Alabi, T., Blecker, C., ... Francis, F. (2014). Edible insects acceptance by Belgian consumers: Promising attitude for entomophagy development. *Journal of Sensory Studies, 29*(1), 14–20.

Carolan, M. (2011). *Embodied food politics*. Burlington, VT: Ashgate.

Chang, S. S., Huan, A. S., & Ho, C. T. (1990). Isolation and identification of bitter compounds in defatted soybean flour. In R. L. Rouseff (Ed.), *Bitterness in foods and beverages: Developments in food science 25* (pp. 267–274). Amsterdam: Elsevier.

Clark, J. E. (1998). Taste and flavour: Their importance in food choice and acceptance. *Proceedings of the Nutrition Society, 57*, 639–643.

Cooke, L. J., & Wardle, J. (2005). Age and gender differences in children's food habits. *British Journal of Nutrition., 93*, 741–846.

Dallman, M. F. (2010). Stress-induced obesity and the emotional nervous system. *Trends in Endocrinology and Metabolism, 21*(3), 159–165.

Degrace-Passilly, P., & Besnard, P. (2012). CD36 and taste of fat. *Current Opinion in Clinical Nutrition and Metabolic Care., 15*(2), 107–111.

Douglas, M., & Nicod, M. (1974). Taking the biscuit: The structure of British meals. *New Society, 30*(637), 744–747.

Drewnoski, A. (2001). The science and complexity of bitter taste. *Nutrition Review, 59*(6), 163–169.

Drewnowski, A., & Almiron-Roig, E. (2010). Human perceptions and preferences for fat-rich foods. In J. P. Montmayeur, & J. le Coutre (Eds.), *Fat detection: Taste, texture, and post ingestive effects*. Boca Raton, FL: CRC Press. Chapter 11. Available from: <http://www.ncbi.nlm.nih.gov/books/NBK53528/>.

Drewnowski, A., & Darmon, N. (2005). The economics of obesity: Dietary energy density and energy cost. *American Journal of Clinical Nurition, 82* (Suppl.), 265S–273S.

Drewnoski, A., & Gomez-Carneros, C. (2000). Bitter taste, phytonutrients, and the consumer: A review. *American Journal of Clinical Nutrition., 72*, 1424–1435.

DuBois, C. (2008). Social context and diet: Changing soy production and consumption in the United States. In C. DuBois, C.-B. Tan, & S. Mintz (Eds.), *The world of soy* (pp. 208–233). Urbana and Chicago, IL: University of Illinois.

Dutko, P., Ver Ploeg, M., & Farrigan, T. (2012). *Characteristics and influential factors of food deserts*. Washington, DC: United States Department of Agriculture Economic Research Service, Economic Research Report No. 140.

El-Sohemy, A., Stewart, L., Khataan, N., Fontaine-Bisson, B., Kwong, P., Ozsungur, S., & Cornelis, M. C. (2007). Nutrigenomics of taste – Impact on food preferences and food production. *Forum Nutrition, 60*, 176–182.

Ensminger, A. (1993). *Foods and nutrition encyclopedia*. Boca Raton, FL: CRC Press.

French, S. A. (2003). Pricing effects on food choices. *Journal of Nutrition, 133*(3), 841S–843S.

Gallindo, M. M., Voigt, N., Stein, J., van Lengerich, J., Raguse, J.-D., Hofmann, T., ... Behrens, M. (2012). G-protein-coupled receptors in human fat taste perception. *Chemical Senses., 37*(2), 123–139.

Garcia-Bailo, B., Toguri, C., Eny, K. M., & El-Sohemy, A. (2007). Genetic variation in taste and its influence on food selection. *Journal of Integrative Biology, 13*(1), 69–80.

Gibson, E. L. (2006). Emotional influences on food choice: Sensory, physiological and psychological pathways. *Physiology and Behavior, 89*, 53–61.

Glanz, K., Basil, M., Maibach, E., Goldberg, J., & Snyder, D. (1998). Why Americans eat what they eat: Taste, nutrition, cost, convenience, and weight control concerns as influences on food consumption. *Journal of the American Dietetic Association., 98*(10), 1118–1126.

Gorman, U. (2006). Ethical issues raised by personalized nutrition based on genetic information. *Genes Nutrition, 3*(1), 14–22.

Greene, T. A., Alarcon, S., Thomas, A., Berdougo, E., Doranz, B. J., Breslin, P. A. S., & Rucker, J. B. (2011). Probenecid inhibits the human bitter taste receptor TAS2R16 and suppresses bitter perception of salicin. *PLoS One, 6*(5), e20123 . (http://doi.org/10.1371/journal.pone.0020123)

Harvard Health Publication. *Why stress causes people to overeat*. (2012). <http://www.health.harvard.edu/newsletter_article/why-stress-causes-people-to-overeat>.

Holmboe-Ottensen, G., & Wandel, M. (2012). Changes in dietary habits after migration and consequences for health: A focus on South Asians in Europe. *Food and Nutrition Research, 56*, 18891. Available from http://dx.doi.org/10.3402/fnr.v56i0.18891.

Johnson, L. A., Myers, D. J., & Burden, D. J. (1992). Soy protein's history, prospects in food, feed. *International News on Fats, Oils, and Related Materials, 3*(4), 429–444.

Jood, S., Mehta, G., Singh, R., & Bhat, C. (1985). Effect of processing on flatus-producing factors in legumes. *Journal of Agriculture and Food Chemistry, 33*(2), 268–271.

Kay, T. (1998). The preparation of soy-bean foods for use in rural communities of the developing world. *Journal of Tropical Pediatrics, 44*, 251–252.

Keast, R., Breslin, P., & Beauchamp, G. (2001). Suppression of bitterness using sodium salts. *Chimia: International Journal for Chemistry, 55*(5), 441–447.

Lanfer, A., Bammann, K., Knof, K., Buchecker, K., Russo, P., Veidebaum, T., ... Ahrens, W. (2013). Predictors and correlates of taste preferences in European children: The IDEFICS study. *Food Quality and Preference, 27*(2), 128–136. ISSN 0950-3293, http://dx.doi.org/10.1016/j.foodqual.2012.09.006

Leigh, J. P. (2011). *UC Davis study shows that fast-food dining is most popular for those with middle incomes, rather than those with lowest incomes*. <http://www.ucdmc.ucdavis.edu/publish/news/newsroom/5673>.

Lesschaeve, I., & Noble, A. C. (2005). Polyphenols: Factors influencing their sensory properties and their effects on food and beverage preferences. *American Journal of Clinical Nutrition, 81*(Suppl.), 330S−335S.

Lewin, K. (1951). *Field theory in social science: Selected theoretical papers*. New York: Harper & Row.

Looy, H., & Wood, J. R. (2006). Attitudes toward invertebrates: Are educational "Bug Banquets" effective? *The Journal of Environmental Education, 37*(2), 37−48.

Lubbers, S., Landy, P., & Voilley, A. (1998). Retention and release of aroma compounds in foods containing proteins. *Food Technology, 52*, 68−74, 208−214

Marketplace (2013). <http://www.marketplace.org/topics/life/big-book/processed-foods-make-70-percent-us-diet>.

Maruyama, Y., Yasuda, R., Kuroda, M., & Eto, Y. (2012). Kokumi substances, enhancers of basic tastes, induce responses in calcium-sensing receptor expressing taste cells. *PLoS One, 7*, 1−8. Available from http://dx.doi.org/10.1371/journal.pone.0034489.

Mauer, L., & El-Sohemy, A. (2012). *Flavor*. <http://www.nature.com/news/soapy-taste-of-coriander-linked-to-genetic-variants-1.11398>.

McArthur, L. H., Anguiano, R. P. V., & Nocetti, D. (2001). Maintenance and change in the diet of Hispanic immigrants in Eastern North Carolina. *Familiy and Consumer Sciences Research Journal, 29*(4), 309−335.

McCloud, J. T. (1974). Soy protein in school feeding programs. *Journal of the American Chemists' Society, 51*(1), 141A−142A.

Mcisaac, J. L. D., Read, K., Veugelers, P. J., & Kirk, S. F. L. (2013). Culture matters: A case of school health promotion in Canada. *Health Promotion International, 31*. Available from http://dx.doi.org/10.1093/heapro/dat055.

Menella, J. A., & Beauchamp, G. A. (2005). Understanding the origin of flavor preferences. *Chemical Senses, 30*(Suppl. 1), 242−243.

Mennella, J. A., Pepino, M. Y., & Reed, D. R. (2005). Genetic and environmental determinants of bitter perception and sweet preferences. *Pediatrics, 115*(2), 216−222.

Mirsky, S. (2007). Carrots, sticks and robot picks. *Scientific American, 297*(4), 48.

Oltman, A. E., Lopetcharat, K., Bastian, E., & Drake, M. A. (2015). Identifying key attributes for protein beverages. *Journal of Food Science, 80*, S1383−S1390. Available from http://dx.doi.org/10.1111/1750-3841.12877.

Pirastu, N., Kooyman, M., Traglia, M., Robino, A., Willems, S. M., Pistis, G., ... Gasparini, P. (2014). Association analysis of bitter receptor genes in five isolated populations identifies a significant correlation between *TAS2R43* variants and coffee liking. *PLoS One, 9*(3), e92065. Available from http://dx.doi.org/10.1371/journal.pone.0092065.

Pirastu, N., Robino, A., Lanzara, C., Athanasakis, E., Esposito, L., Tepper, B. J., & Gasparini, P. (2012). Genetics of food preferences: A first view from silk road populations. *Journal of Food Science, 77*(12), S413−S418.

Rackis, J. J., Sessa, D. J., & Honig, D. H. (1979). Flavor problems of vegetable proteins. *Journal of American Oil Chemists Society, 56*, 262−271.

Raghunathan, R., Naylor, R. W., & Hoyer, W. D. (2006). The unhealthy tasty intuition and its effects on taste inferences, enjoyment, and choice of food products. *Journal of Marketing, 70*(4), 170−184.

Rosenmöller, D. L., Gasevic, D., Seidell, J., & Lear, S. A. (2011). Determinants of changes in dietary patterns among Chinese immigrants: A cross-sectional analysis. *International Journal of Behavioral Nutrition and Physical Activity, 8*, 42. Available from http://dx.doi.org/10.1186/1479-5868-8-42.

Rozin, P. (1990). Development in the food domain. *Developmental Psychology, 26*(4), 555−562.

Rozin, P., Haidt, J., McCauley, C., Dunlop, L., & Ashmore, M. (1999). Individual differences in disgust sensitivity: Comparisons and evaluations of paper-and-pencil versus behavioral measures. *Journal of Research in Personality, 33*(3), 330−351.

Satia, J. A., Galanko, J. A., & Neuhouser, M. L. (2005). Food nutrition label use is associated with demographic, behavioral and psychosocial factors and dietary intake among African Americans in North Carolina. *Journal of American Dietetic Association, 105*(3), 392−402.

Schösler, H., De Boer, J., & Boersema, J. J. (2012). Can we cut out the meat of the dish? Constructing consumer-oriented pathways towards meat substitution. *Appetite, 58*(1), 39−47.

Semonova, M. G., Antipova, A. S., Misharina, T. A., & Golovnya, R. V. (2002). Binding of aroma compounds with legumin. I. Binding of hexyl acetate with 11S globulin depending on the protein molecular state in aqueous medium. *Food Hydrocolloids, 16*(6), 557−564.

Slack, J. P., Brockhoff, A., Batram, C., Menzel, S., Sonnabend, C., Born, S., ... Meyerhof, W. (2010). Modulation of bitter taste perception by a small molecule hTAS2R antagonist. *Current Biology, 20*(12), 1104−1109. Available from http://dx.doi.org/10.1016/j.cub.2010.04.043.

Sun-wei, G., & Reed, D. (2001). The genetics of phenylthiocarbamide perception. *Annals of Human Biology, 28*(2), 111−142.

Suppavorasatit, I., & Calwallader, K. (2012). Effect of enzymatic deamidation of soy protein by protein-glutaminase on the flavor-binding properties of the protein under aqueous conditions. *Journal of Agriculture and Food Chemistry, 60*(32), 7817−7823.

Szejtki, J., & Szente, L. (2005). Elimination of bitter, disgusting tastes of drugs and foods by cyclodextrins. *European Journal of Pharmaceutics and Biopharmaceutics, 61*(3), 115−125.

Van Kempen, E., Jaminon, A., van Berkel, T. J. C., & van Eck, M. (2014). Diet-induced (epigenetic) changes in bone marrow augment atherosclerosis. *Journal of Leukocyte Biology, 96*(50), 833−841.

Vereecken, A. C., Inchley, J., Subramanian, S. V., Hublet, A., & Maes, L. (2005). The relative influence of individual and contextual socio-economic status on consumption of fruit and soft drinks among adolescents in Europe. *European Journal of Public Health, 15*(3), 224−232.

Viana, F. (2011). Chemosensory properties of the trigeminal system. *American Chemical Society Neuroscience, 2*, 38−50.

Von Post, R. (2011). Eat your peas: A recipe for culture change. *Strategy & Business, 2011*(63). <http://www.strategy-business.com/article/11205?gko=ac42d>

Wansink, B. (2002). Changing eating habits on the home front: Lost lessons from World War II Research. *Journal of Public Policy and Marketing*, *21*(1), 90–99.

Wansink, B., & Chan, N. (2001). Relation of soy consumption to nutritional knowledge. *Journal of Medical Food*, *4*, 145–150.

Wardle, J., & Cooke, L. J. (2008). Genetic and environmental determinants of children's food preferences. *British Journal of Nutrition*, *99*(Suppl. 1), S15–S21.

Warren, T. (2003). Classand gender-based working time? Time poverty and the division of domestic labour. *Sociology*, *37*(4), 733–752.

Weill, A. (2014). *Why bitter is better*. <http://www.huffingtonpost.com/andrew-weil-md/bitter-foods_b_5206909.html>.

Woolfolk, M. E., Castellan, W., & Brooks, C. I. (1983). Pepsi versus Coke: Labels, not tastes, prevail. *Psychological Reports*, *52*(1), 185–186.

World Food Programme (2015). <http://www.wfp.org/videos/7-billionth-child-1-7-chance-being-hungry>.

Wysocki, C. J. (2010). Vile weed or essential ingredient? *CEN Newsletters*, *88*(6), 72.

Ye, A., Streicher, C., & Singh, H. (2011). Interactions between whey proteins and salivary proteins as related to astringency of whey protein beverages at low pH. *Journal of Dairy Science*, *98*(12), 5842–5850.

Zhang, L., Xia, Y., & Peterson, D. G. (2014). Identification of bitter modulating maillard-catechin reaction products. *Journal of Agriculture and Food Chemistry*, *62*, 10092–10100.

Chapter 24

Food Security and Policy

M. Carolan
Colorado State University, Ft. Collins, CO, United States

24.1 INTRODUCTION

According to the United Nations, global agricultural production will need to be *at least* 60% higher in 2050 than 2007 levels (FAO, 2012). This is a smaller increase than the agriculture sector has achieved over the past half century. But before we let out a collective sigh of relief it is questionable whether these increases can be achieved, let alone achieved sustainably (see Fig. 24.1).

A 2013 study examined yields of four key staple crops—maize, rice, wheat, and soybeans (Ray, Mueller, West, & Foley, 2013). The findings are not encouraging, as it notes that yields are increasing by only about 0.9–1.6% a year. That would lead to an overall yield increase of somewhere between 38% and 67% by 2050. This means there may be enough food to eat in 2050 if (1) the *lower end* of the aforementioned United Nation's estimate ends up being true, (2) the *higher end* of this study's projected maximum yield increase turns out to be the case, (3) we do not become even more enamored with biofuels and red meat, and (4) climate change does not do something to throw a wrench into all of this.

Let us assume we are not that lucky. For the sake of argument, assume yield increases fall closer to the low end of the above study—38% yield increases by 2050. To make up for the yield shortfall we are going to need anywhere between 200 million and 750 million additional hectares of land by 2050 (Schade & Pimentel, 2010). A variety of studies have settled on the figure of 1.5 billion as the number of additional hectares available to be brought under cultivation (Balmford, Green, & Scharlemann, 2005; Schade & Pimentel, 2010). Much needs to be accomplished, however, before land can be brought into production—land rights have to be settled, credit must be available, and infrastructure and markets must be in place. These constrains explain why arable land worldwide has grown by a net average of 5 million hectares per year over the last two decades (Rabobank, 2010). It also means it will be decades until a sizable amount of arable land is prepared for agriculture. More problematic still is the projected slowdown in the annual growth of arable land, as potential arable land becomes increasingly marginal (the land easiest to convert has already been brought into production). The annual growth of arable land will slow from 0.30% between 1961 and 2005 to 0.10% between 2005 and 2050. This calculates out to an average annual net increase of arable area of 2.75 million hectares per year between 2005 and 2050 (Rabobank, 2010). That is 120 million additional hectares, which is well below the most optimistic estimates that claim only 200 million hectares will be needed by mid-century to satisfy global food demand. At the same time, arable land in developed and transitional countries will continue to decline, losing an estimated 0.23% a year between 2005 and 2050 (Bruinsma, 2009).

Keeping up with *current rates of demand*—there is a sociologically interesting phrase. Just what exactly does it mean? We talk as if we need to keep up with these rates. Do we? I am often asked, "How much food do we need to feed future world populations?" The question is not an easy one to answer. Before anyone can answer it we need to define certain things, like "food," "we," "feed," and "future world populations." Too often and to my great frustration, people try answering the question without any thought to the *assumptions* underlying it. For instance, depending upon whether we are expecting future generations to eat largely grain-based diets, versus, say, diets centered on red meat will greatly alter one's answer to the question. Similarly, are we assuming, when talking about feeding future "populations," that cars (biofuels) are part of the equation?

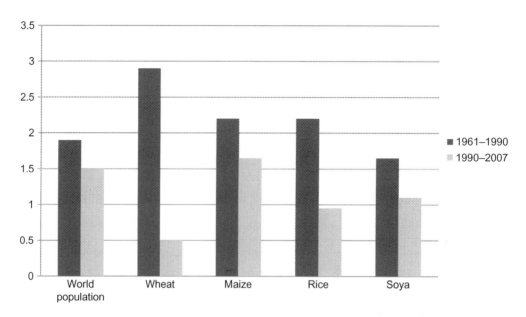

FIGURE 24.1 Annual average growth rates for world population and global yield increases. *Based on The Economist. (2011). The 9-billion people question: A special report on feeding the world. The Economist, February 26. <http://www.economist.com/surveys/downloadSurveyPDF.cfm?id = 18205243&surveyCode = %254e%2541&submit = View + PDF> Last accessed 03.04.15. (Economist, 2011)*

This chapter attempts to unpack pieces of these questions. It explores what it means to feed the world—does that assume, for example, feeding people healthily and sustainably? This inevitably gets us into issues of food security. But more specifically, as this book is about alternative proteins: What do we mean when envisioning sustainable protein food futures? Let us begin this journey by looking at the livestock sector.

24.2 LIVESTOCK: FACTS AND TRENDS

If everyone in the world were to consume meat at levels comparable to that found in Luxembourg and the United States—around 125–136 kg (276–300 lb) per person per year—there would only be enough grain remaining to support a global population of about 2.6 billion people (or 38% of the existing population) (Roberts, 2008). Table 24.1 takes this calculation further, estimating the global population that could be sustained if per capita meat consumption for the top 25 meat-consuming nations were replicated globally (assuming a beef, pork, and chicken ratio similar to that found in Luxembourg). As the table makes clear, no country comes close to having a per capita meat-consumption level that could be sustainably reproduced at the global level. In other words, if we are looking for countries to emulate—at least as far as meat consumption is concerned—we are not going to find any viable candidates in the table. Part of the reason driving current trends is the positive relationship between a country's gross domestic product (GDP) per capita and the average citizen's consumption of animal products, as illustrated in Fig. 24.2. Thus, as countries, most notably China, continue to climb the economic ladder, so too should we expect their appetite for meat to grow in equal fashion.

While global consumption of all basic foods will continue to increase—which is understandable given population growth alone—the consumption of meat in particular is expected to grow much faster than dairy, cereals, and starchy roots. Looking closer at that category "meat" reveals considerable variation in growth rates, when it comes to global consumption of sheep/goats, cattle/buffalo, chickens, and pigs from 1960 to 2010. These different rates are depicted in Fig. 24.3. As illustrated, the global consumption of chicken has increased 450% (or 4.5 times) relative to 1960 levels, compared with pigs, cattle/buffalo, and sheep/goats, which have increased 250%, 60%, and 50%, respectively.

Why do these trends in the consumption of animal proteins matter? Collectively, cattle, pigs, and poultry consume a significant amount of the world's corn, soybeans, and barley. And it is not just that livestock consume a lot of basic food that could otherwise be used to feed people directly. We also have to be mindful of how efficiently (or more accurately inefficiently) they convert feed into animal protein. Some animals are clearly better at this than others. Table 24.2 summarizes these conversion ratios, as they are called, for chickens, pigs, and cattle.

TABLE 24.1 Top 25 Per Capita Consumers of Meat (and Projected Global Population If Everyone in the World Consumed Meat at That Level)

Country	Total Per Person	Global Population That Could Be Supported
Luxembourg	136.5	2.5 to 3.49 billion
United States	125.4	2.5 to 3.49 billion
Australia	121.2	2.5 to 3.49 billion
New Zealand	115.7	2.5 to 3.49 billion
Spain	110.2	3.5 to 4.49 billion
French Polynesia	108.9	3.5 to 4.49 billion
Austria	103.1	3.5 to 4.49 billion
Israel	99.1	3.5 to 4.49 billion
Canada	98.7	3.5 to 4.49 billion
Bahamas	98.1	3.5 to 4.49 billion
Denmark	97.8	3.5 to 4.49 billion
Kuwait	97.4	3.5 to 4.49 billion
Saint Lucia	95.4	3.5 to 4.49 billion
Ireland	94.1	3.5 to 4.49 billion
Iceland	94.0	3.5 to 4.49 billion
Portugal	92.9	3.5 to 4.49 billion
Argentina	91.7	3.5 to 4.49 billion
Italy	91.4	3.5 to 4.49 billion
France	88.7	4.5 to 5.49 billion
Malta	88.5	4.5 to 5.49 billion
Germany	87.7	4.5 to 5.49 billion
United Kingdom	85.8	4.5 to 5.49 billion
Antigua and Barbuda	85.4	4.5 to 5.49 billion
Czech Republic	85.2	4.5 to 5.49 billion
Slovenia	83.8	4.5 to 5.49 billion

Source: Data obtained from the FAO.

Such conversion ratios, however, only apply to animals fed on grain. Professor John Webster at the University of Bristol (United Kingdom), and former President of both the Nutrition Society and the British Society for Animal Science, calculates that dairy cows on a 70–80% pasture-based diet give back more calories than they take in—quite a bit more, in fact (Webster, 2010). Webster places the return at 170%. Of course, this is due to a wonderful adaptive trait that allows ruminants to digest plant-based foods that we can not. Some regions of the world are well endowed with arable land, like Europe, Russia, and North America. Others are arable land-poor but rich in permanent pasture. In sub-Saharan Africa, for example, only 17% of land is arable, while 80.8% exists as permanent pasture (Peterson, 2009). In places such as this, raising livestock, from a food security perspective, truly makes sense, as livestock may well be the only thing that these lands can sustain.

394 PART | III Consumers, and Sustainability

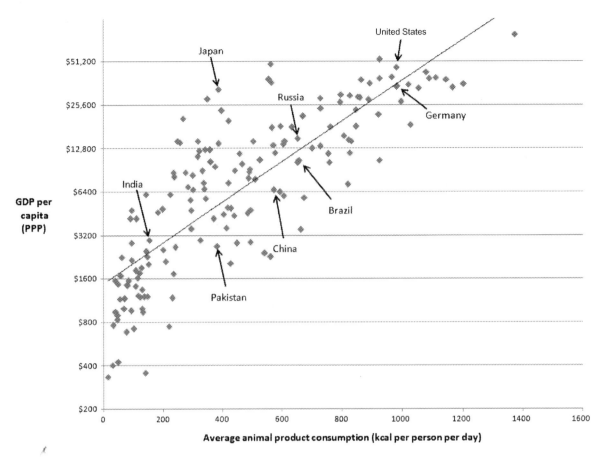

FIGURE 24.2 The relationship between GDP per capita and animal product consumption per capita.

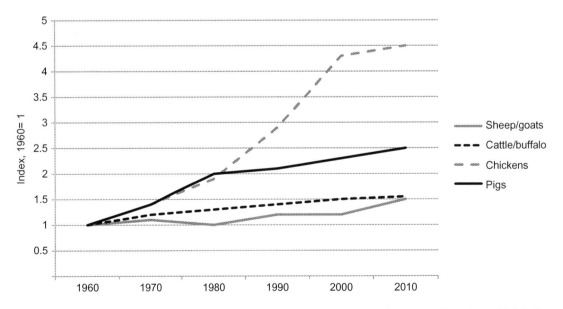

FIGURE 24.3 Changes in global consumption of animals since 1960. *Based on Godfray, H., Beddington, J., Crute, I., Hadded, L., Lawrence, D., Muir, J., ... Toulmin, C. (2010). Food security: The challenge of feeding 9 billion people.* Science, *327, 812−818. (Godfray et al., 2010)*

TABLE 24.2 Feed, Calories, and Protein Needed to Produce 1 kg of Chicken, Pork, and Beef

Grain (Calories/Protein in Grams) ⟶	Animal (Calories/Protein in Grams)
2 kg feed grain (6900/200)	1 kg chicken (1090/259)
4 kg feed grain (13,800/400)	1 kg pork (1180/187)
8 kg feed grain (27,600/700)	1 kg beef (1140/226)

Monogastrics too have a unique ability. Pigs and poultry are prized worldwide for their ability to thrive on food waste. By definition, food waste is no longer food, as by this state it is said to have exited the food system. Raising animals—poultry and pigs—at least partially on waste might make good sense from a food security perspective, particularly if there is a lot of organic waste that is going to, well, waste.

It is impossible to discuss the livestock sector without also mentioning its links to climate change. It has been calculated that producing a single kilogram of beef generates as much CO_2 as driving 250 kilometers in an average European car or using a 100-watt bulb continuously for 20 days (Ogino, Orito, Shimada, & Hirooka, 2007). Greenhouse gas emissions from agriculture are increased. The majority of this increase (54%) is accounted for in combined CH_4 and N_2O emissions from livestock manure management systems (reflecting the increased use of emission-intensive liquid systems over this time period) (EPA, 2015). Animal agriculture is also responsible for roughly 37% of all human-induced methane emissions, which has a global warming potential 23 times greater than that of CO_2 (EPA, 2015).

As the global demand for meat is expected to double from 2010 to 2050, the water footprint of livestock will only grow, particularly owing to the water-intensive crops (like corn, soybeans, and other coarse grains) that are fed to these animals (see Table 24.3). The relative thirstiness of ground beef ("bovine meat" in the table) is due in large part to the beef cow's consumption of grains. Even after factoring in for nutritional value, the (global average) confined beef cow requires 10.16 liters of water for every kcal produced. As a protein source, it fares better than only nuts and fruits on a liter per gram of protein basis (Hoekstra, 2015). In light of all this, it is not surprising that the United Nations (UN) concluded that water scarcity—not a lack of arable land—will be the number one constraint on food security in the decades ahead.

24.3 RETHINKING FOOD SECURITY

Reviewing the facts about livestock production makes many question how committed this sector is toward food security. As I have detailed elsewhere (Carolan, 2013), it all depends on how food security is defined.

The term "food security" was first used in a policy context at the 1974 World Food Congress. Later that year the Food and Agriculture Organization (FAO) came up with the following definition, where food security was said to involve "ensuring, to the utmost, the availability at all times of adequate world supplies of basic food stuffs, *primarily cereals*, so as to avoid acute food shortages in the event of widespread crop failures or national disasters, sustain a steady expansion of production and consumption, and reduce fluctuation in production and prices" (quoted in Shaw, 2007, p. 150; my emphasis). I will pick up on this definition momentarily, as there is plenty to question in a policy position that reduces "food security" to an "adequate" supply of rice, wheat, millet, and maze (a.k.a. cereals).

Its "spirit", if you will, can be traced back to at least the 1940s. For example, the Health Division of the League of Nations was charged in the 1930s with assessing the food situation among represented countries. The resulting publication, *Nutrition and Public Health*, released in 1935, represents arguably the first account of hunger in an international context (Shaw, 2007). The report offered a stark reminder that the so-called modern age, in terms of sheer numbers, was ushered in with as many hungry bodies (perhaps more) as any that had preceded it.

A few years later, in 1941, US President Roosevelt gave arguably the most consequential State of the Union Address of the 20th century. In this speech, Roosevelt identifies "four essential freedoms" that are shared "everywhere in the world": freedom of speech; of worship; from want; and from fear. The founding conference of the FAO of the United Nations in 1943 took Roosevelt's call to heart as it looked specifically "to consider the goal of freedom from want in relation to food and agriculture" (FAO, 1943, p. 1). One could locate the original spirit of food security within these four essential freedoms. In doing this, it is understood to be but a means to even more profound ends, namely, the enhancement of individual and societal freedom, prosperity, and wellbeing. This original spirit, however, was soon forgotten as means began to be mistaken for ends.

TABLE 24.3 The Global Average Water Footprint of Crop and Animal Products in Relation to Their Nutritional Value

Food Item	Water Footprint per Unit of Weight (L/kg)				Nutritional Content			Water Footprint per Unit of Nutritional Value		
	Green	Blue	Gray	Total	Calorie (kcal/kg)	Protein (g/kg)	Fat (g/kg)	Calorie (L/kcal)	Protein (L/g protein)	Fat (L/g fat)
Sugar crops	130	52	15	197	285	0	0	0.69	0	0
Vegetables	194	43	85	322	240	12	2.1	1.34	26	154
Starchy roots	327	16	43	387	827	13	1.7	0.47	31	226
Fruits	726	147	89	962	460	5.3	2.8	2.09	180	348
Cereals	1232	228	184	1644	3208	80	15	0.51	21	112
Oil crops	2023	220	121	2364	2908	149	209	0.81	16	11
Pulses	3180	141	734	4055	3412	215	23	1.19	19	180
Nuts	7016	1367	680	9063	2500	65	193	3.63	139	47
Milk	863	86	72	1020	560	33	31	1.82	31	33
Eggs	2592	244	429	3265	1425	111	100	2.29	29	33
Chicken meat	3545	313	467	4325	1440	127	100	3	34	43
Butter	4695	465	393	5553	7692	0	872	0.72	0	6.4
Pig meat	4907	459	622	5988	2786	105	259	2.15	57	23
Sheep/goat meat	8253	457	53	8763	2059	139	163	4.25	63	54
Bovine meat	14414	550	451	15415	1513	138	101	10.19	112	153

Source: Hoekstra, A. (2015). *The water footprint: The relation between human consumption and water use.* In: Antonelli, M., & Greco, F. (Ed.), The water we eat: Combining virtual water and water footprints (pp. 35–50). Springer: Switzerland.

The FAO and World Health Organization (WHO) compile food security indicator statistics on things like the prevalence of underweight children under the age of five and the proportion of the population below minimal levels of dietary energy consumption. Yet these data tell us absolutely nothing about the state of food security in high-income nations and at a minimum merely reinforce something we have long known: that incredibly impoverished countries are terribly food insecure. Or take a UN-sponsored book titled *Food Security*, which remarks that "the extent of hunger and food insecurity [in the US] is much less severe than in the developing world" (Dutta & Gundersen, 2007). In the space of a single sentence the affluent US is valorized, while the entire "developing" world is condemned on the basis of their respective levels of food security. Perhaps such pronouncements are empirically justified when food security is narrowly defined as, say, calories produced per capita. But would the statement still hold if food security were viewed through a lens more in tuned with the "spirit" mentioned above, where the aim is lifting societal wellbeing and not just global cereal yields?

Dominant food security discourse also shields certain actors from criticism. Again, take the case of the United States—frequently extoled as the most food-secure nation in the world (at least if you spend any time listening to US politicians). More than a third of its adults are defined as obese (CDC, n.d.). Avoidable annual food waste within this country amounts to over 55 million metric tons—nearly 29% of annual production—which if consumed could save from being emitted at least 113 million metric tons of carbon dioxide equivalents annually (Venkat, 2011). The annual total cost of pesticides alone in this nation, upon public health, the environment, and human communities, has been placed in the billions of dollars (Pimentel, 2005). And, as far as subjective wellbeing goes, the average citizen in the

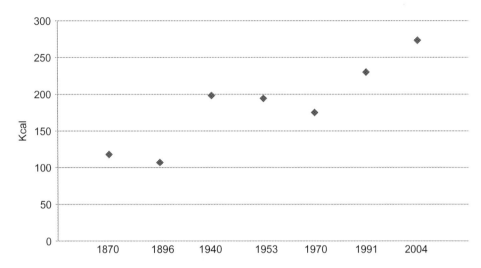

FIGURE 24.4 Total kcal per 100 grams of chicken for select years. Adapted from Wang, Y., Lehane, C., Ghebremeskel, K., & Crawford, M. (2009). *Modern organic and broiler chickens sold for human consumption provide more energy from fat than protein.* Public Health Nutrition, 13, 400–408. (Wang et al., 2009)

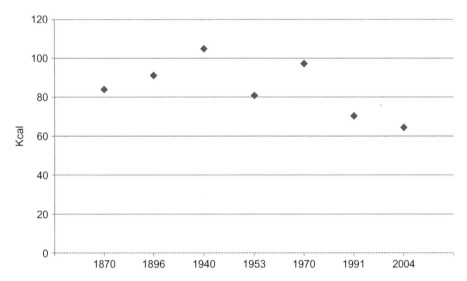

FIGURE 24.5 Kcal of protein per 100 grams of chicken for select years. Adapted from Wang, Y., Lehane, C., Ghebremeskel, K., & Crawford, M. (2009). *Modern organic and broiler chickens sold for human consumption provide more energy from fat than protein.* Public Health Nutrition, 13, 400–408.

US reports far lower levels of life satisfaction than her counterpart in countries with significantly lower income levels and much higher food costs (Carolan, 2013). We could not emulate this model globally if we tried, as it is entirely unsustainable. But even if we could, given the points just mentioned, why would we want to?

Additional deleterious effects of mistaking calorie security for food security can be found by looking at changes in the livestock industry—or, more accurately, changes to livestock themselves. Livestock today, for a variety of reasons, grow larger and faster than their ancestors. Chickens, for instance, now require 27 fewer days—and almost 50% less feed—to reach slaughter weight than was needed in 1950 (Catel, 2011). Yet how do today's highly efficient industrial chickens compare to their ancestors in terms of the quantity and type of calories yielded? Fig. 24.4 plots the total kcal per 100 grams of chicken from 1870 to 2004 (Wang, Lehane, Ghebremeskel, & Crawford, 2009). As the figure illustrates, chickens are becoming more calorically dense, an expected trend given agrifood policies' aforementioned emphasis on caloric output. Yet how can 100 grams of chicken contain almost 150% more calories today than it did in 1870? The answer is in the fat.

Today's conventional chicken is considerably fatter than its ancestors. Let us look first at how the animal's protein content has change. Kcal of protein per 100 grams of chicken from 1870 to 2004 is detailed in Fig. 24.5. Note the downward trend. The opposite can be said for the fat content of these birds. Not only do today's chickens carry less protein per 100 grams but, as shown in Fig. 24.6, they also carry remarkably more fat than in decades past. Moreover, while not shown in the latter figure, it is worth noting that the type of fat has also changed. Chickens today are not only fatter but possess a higher percentage of "bad" and a lower percentage of "good" fats than the chickens eaten by our ancestors.

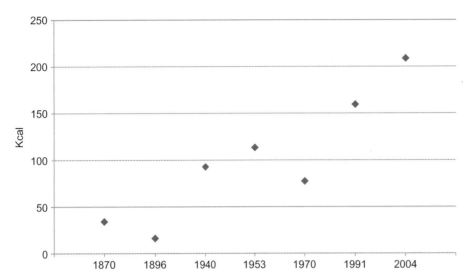

FIGURE 24.6 Kcal of fat per 100 grams of chicken for select years. Adapted from Wang, Y., Lehane, C., Ghebremeskel, K., & Crawford, M. (2009). Modern organic and broiler chickens sold for human consumption provide more energy from fat than protein. Public Health Nutrition, 13, 400–408.

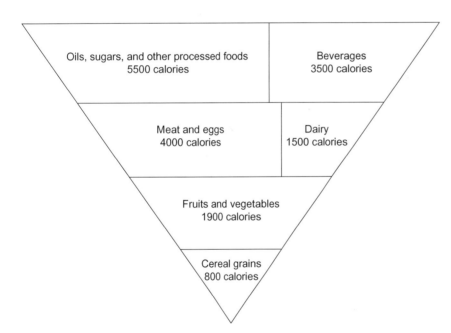

FIGURE 24.7 Breakdown of the 17,000 + calories (daily per capita) consumed by US food system. Based on Canning, P., Charles, A., Huang S., Polenske, K., & Waters, A. (2010). Energy use in the US food system. United States Department of Agriculture, Economic Research Service, Report number 94, March, Washington, DC. <http://ddr.nal.usda.gov/bitstream/10113/41413/1/CAT31049057.pdf> Last accessed 12.04.15; and Bomford, M. (2011). Beyond food miles. Post Carbon Institute, March 9, Santa Rosa, CA. <http://www.postcarbon.org/article/273686-beyond-food-miles#_edn9> Last accessed 12.04.15. (Canning, Charles, Huang, Polenske, & Waters, 2010; Bomford, 2011)

And let us not forget the subject of this book: *sustainable* proteins. Does food security presuppose sustainability? It would have to, right? It is a hard circle to square, to claim that a fundamentally unsustainable system is somehow nurturing security of any sort.

The current food regimen—and protein regimen—is capital-intensive, which is simply another (less pejorative) way of saying they it is *energy*-intensive (Carolan, 2011a). Things start getting really interesting once you begin breaking down energy use by food type. Data from the USDA tell us that the total energy used in producing, processing, and transporting food in the United States is over 17,000 calories (as a unit of energy) on a per capita daily basis. Breaking those energy units down according to specific food categories, we can see that over half go toward the making of highly processed foods; a third to the making of animal products including meat, eggs, and milk; and a sixth to grains, fruits, and vegetables (Fig. 24.7). Turns out, eating healthy is not just good for us but for future generations as well.

24.4 GROWING HOMOGENEITY IN GLOBAL FOOD SUPPLIES

A rule held throughout the sciences—from agroecology to nutrition, biology, and sociology—is that, at least within certain ranges, diversity enhances the health, functioning, and resiliency of systems. Yet modern agriculture and global food commodity chains have pointed us in the other direction, toward a *shrinking* of biodiversity, cultural diversity, knowledge diversity, and even taste diversity. A study recently published in the *Proceedings of the National Academy of Sciences* reveals an emerging standard global food supply consisting of such energy-dense foods as soybeans, sunflower oil, and palm oil, along with more historically familiar staples like rice and wheat (Khoury et al., 2014). Wheat was found to be a major staple in 97.4% of all countries and rice in 90.8%, whereas soybean has become significant in 74.3% of countries. Meanwhile, many crops with long-held regional and cultural importance—cereals like sorghum, millets, and rye as well as root crops such as sweet potato, cassava, and yam—are disappearing from fields and diets. For example, a nutritious tuber crop known as *Oca*, once grown throughout the Andean highlands, has declined significantly in this region both in cultivation and consumption. Fig. 24.8 illustrates these trends. As the figure details, soybean consumption has increased 282% in developing countries between 1969 and 2009, while the consumption of millet and sorghum has more than halved during that same time period. This is an interesting nutritional disparity between the foods at the top and bottom of the figure. Those being eaten at greater rates tend to be richer in macronutrients, while those disappearing are micronutrient-rich. Not only that, many of the crops near the bottom of the figure are stress-tolerant, which makes them particularly valuable when we talk about sustainably feeding future populations in the context of climate change.

Another way to visualize this move toward global diet homogeneity is through the following image constructed (and graciously provided to me) by the above study's lead author, Colin Khoury: Fig. 24.9. Notice the dietary "spread" that existed half a century ago around the world, by the dispersal of light-colored dots. And today: a clear "clumping" of darker dots near the middle of the figure.

In a later publication, researchers offer the following five policy recommendation to foster diversity in food production and consumption and thus improve nutrition and food security (Khoury & Jarvis, 2014).

- Continue to safeguard and improve major staple crops.
- Extend the benefits of emerging crops to more farmers in an eco-efficient manner.
- Aggressively promote the development of previously neglected crops that are resilient and nutritious.
- Address food security in a holistic manner through the development of ecologically sensitive and nutritionally diverse food systems.
- Better explain the relationships between food diversity and nutrition, while closely monitoring this diversity and advocating for its use to improve human health.

24.5 SOCIOLOGICAL PATHWAYS FOR MORE SUSTAINABLE PROTEIN OPTIONS

Based on the above, it could be argued (and is by many) that what we are doing, in terms of producing food and proteins in particular, might be working in the short term. The long-term consequences of these actions, however, to our health and the environment's, and to the livelihoods of future generations are unacceptable. What are we to do?

Changing behaviors and tastes takes time. I am not a fan of mandating diets or practices. Besides, such actions rarely work, as evidenced recently in Samoa when the government tried banning the sales of turkey tails, which merely lead to the creation of a black-market of this fatty food (Barclay, 2013). So: how do we encourage consumers to choose alternative protein pathways?

We need to first be mindful of cultural realities. When talking about proteins we have to realize meat's special status. And the redder the meat the "better." A number of cultural analyses have identified meat as the food with the highest status in the hierarchy of foods; a finding that appears to hold for developed (Twigg, 1984) and developing (Lokuruka, 2006) countries alike. Douglas and Nicod (1974) conducted a seminal study of meals among Britons and found meat to be at the center of practically every meal. Its cultural dominance can be seen by the fact that its presence signifies the dish, even when it is just one ingredient of many, whether salads (chicken cobb salad), soups (beef stew), or casseroles (tuna casserole). The dominant position of meat in Western cuisine is even reflected in Western vegetarian culture, as nonanimal products are made to appear as much like meat as possible (veggie hotdogs, soy hamburgers, etc.) (Gvion-Rosenberg, 1990).

In the past, substitution of one food or ingredient for another was the result of scarcity (Montanari, 1994). But the pathway to change is helped along considerably when the food doing the substituting is *similar* to the one it is replacing. Drawing lessons from an analysis of recent dietary changes in the United States, Wansink (2002) notes that for a novel food to become "accepted" it must (1) be available, (2) taste good, (3) be familiar, and (4) look, taste, and feel as in a way that is familiar. That last point helps explains what was described in the previous paragraph, about why, for instance, soy-proteins are made into the very foods they are looking to replace—hotdogs, patties, etc. Most Western

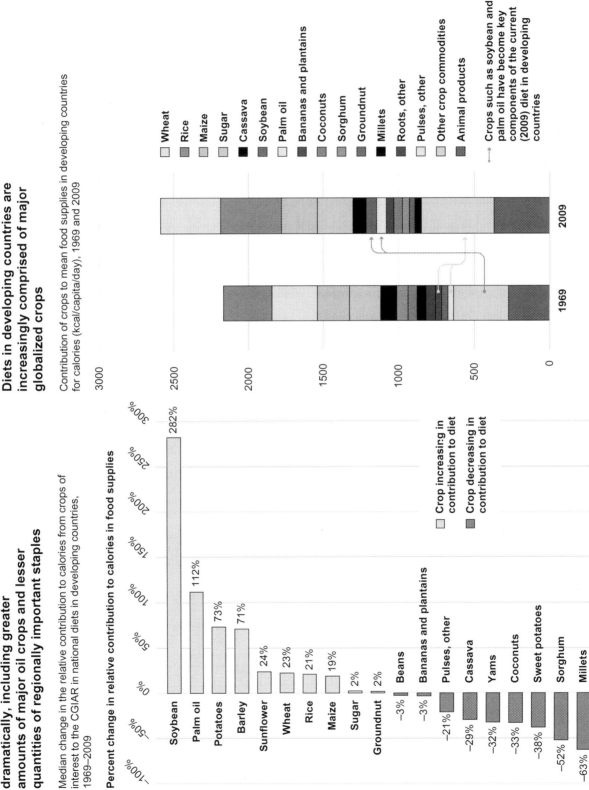

FIGURE 24.8 Adapted from Khoury, C., Bjorkman, A., Dempewolf, H., Ramirez-Villegas, J. Guarino, L., Jarvis, L., ... Stuik, P. (2014). Increasing homogeneity in global food supplies and the implications for food security. Proceedings of the National Academy of Sciences of the United States of America, 111(11), 4001–4006.

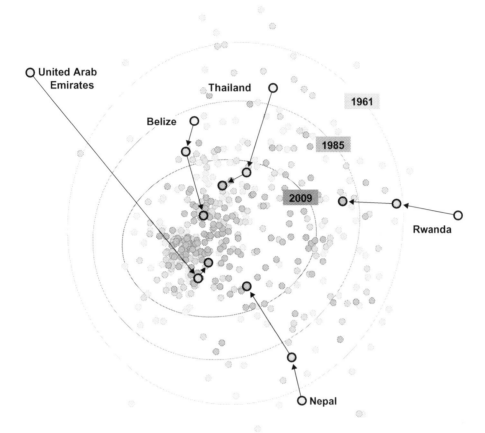

FIGURE 24.9 Adapted from Khoury, C., Bjorkman, A., Dempewolf, H., Ramirez-Villegas, J. Guarino, L., Jarvis, L., ... Stuik, P. (2014). Increasing homogeneity in global food supplies and the implications for food security. Proceedings of the National Academy of Sciences of the United States of America, 111(11), 4001–4006.

consumers (and increasingly consumers around the world), are familiar with hamburgers and hotdogs. This also explains why some, who are experimenting with edible insects, are placing them into foods like pizzas and grinding them up into hamburgers, soyburgers, and lentil burgers.

Therefore, one of the more significant barriers to overcome in the West will be existing meal formats and hierarchies. While the conventional hierarchy seems to be less followed by younger generations it does not look like it will entirely lose its cultural significance anytime soon (Schösler, De Boer, & Boersema, 2012). Acquaintance with "unconventional" meal structures, new cooking abilities, and an openness to experiment with foods are all variables that play into whether people are willing to explore meals without meat (Schösler et al., 2012).

A lower-hanging fruit, which might be employed to bridge consumers from one protein pathway to another, could be to not initially challenge existing meal formats and hierarchies. Instead, the aim could be to make more incremental changes towards the proteins consumed, allowing eaters time to become familiar with the foods, flavors, tastes, and mouth feels associated with them. A good example of this happening successfully is with soybeans. Thirty years ago soybeans were a terribly stigmatized food, at least in North America—so much so that soybean oil had to be called vegetable oil because no one would buy the former. Fast forward to today: the supply of edible soybeans can barely keep up with demand—though calling them "edamame" was initially strategic to avoid the term "soybean." The long-term aim of this technique: an intermediate step to acclimatize consumers to a new meal structure that does not

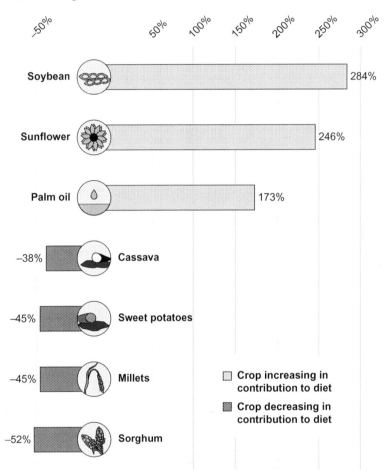

FIGURE 24.9 Continued

have red meat at the top. As noted, most meat substitutes fit well in this pathway as they do not require consumers to make any additional adjustments to meal patterns and they are designed to look, taste, feel, and even smell similar to the meat they are replacing (Schösler et al., 2012). Another piece that could be emphasized by these foods: they allow the easy preparation of a vegetarian component alongside with meat in households where some people eat meat and others do not. This could also act as a pathway to further adoption, as meat eaters in household see others eat alternative protein they will become more likely to try alternatives themselves (Carolan, 2011b).

Beyond taste, affordability, familiarity, and accessibility my own research suggests that policy needs to be better directed at giving people the requisite skill sets and knowledge to prepare and cook alternative foods, proteins included (Carolan, 2011b). Even if alternative proteins were to become *less expensive* than conventional proteins, without knowing how to eat those foods consumers will continue to eat what they know and what they know how to cook. Thought also has to be given to the types of materials that are needed to prepare these new proteins. If they are going to require new pots or pans, for instance, then that is another transaction cost that needs to be taken into consideration. Consumers are less likely to adopt new foods if such an act requires investments in new technologists and new materials.

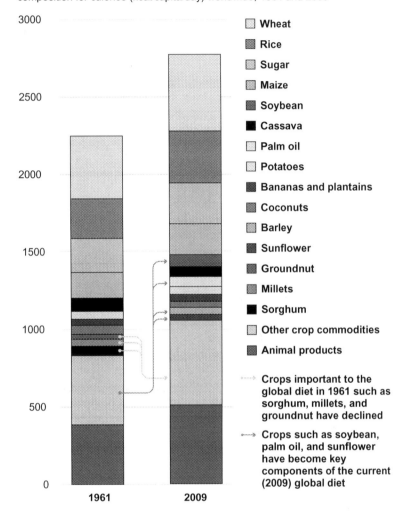

FIGURE 24.9 Continued

We should also look toward our healthcare systems to migrate from high meat consumption to lower and substitute with healthier alternatives; after all, the best (health care) defense is a strong (food care) offense. The annual minimum medical cost per case of undiagnosed diabetes in the United States is US$1744, US$6649 for diagnosed diabetes, and US$443 for prediabetes (CDC, 2014). Over a lifetime, those costs translate into tens if not hundreds of thousands of dollars. Thanks to the Affordable Care Act (also known as Obama Care), to quote Pollan (2009), "every can of soda or Happy Meal or chicken nugget on a school lunch menu will look like a threat to future profits" among insurance companies. It will not be long before Big Insurance—the one "Big" that can give Big Food a run for its money—sets its sights on addressing some of the underlying factors making *us* sick, like diet where the opportunities for healthcare cost reductions are high.

Of course, none of this is meant to replace the importance of education. Programs to educate consumers on dietary changes to mitigate major diseases, such as lowering animal fat intake, increasing, for instance, plant food intake, are essential. Yet I place this recommendation later in this section to emphasize the point that education will not solve anything by itself. While an important piece in all of this, it is but one solution among many that need to be adopted.

That is the consumer angle. What about producers? How do we get farmers, ranchers, and others to switch to raising alternative protein sources? It is the old chicken and egg question: which comes first, supply or demand? The history of food demand is littered with examples of consumer "choices" actually being *supply-driven* (Rivera-Ferre & Arce, 2009). An increasing demand at the consumer side has been presented as an illustration of the power of consumers to determine the trends in food production. This argument is then used to *justify* efforts in increasing production and productivity through the intensification of conventional protein systems, when in fact those systems are *responsible* for many of those consumer "choices." I mention this only to highlight the fact that the current protein regimen is not innocent; it is not, in other words, a blameless reflection of consumer demands. Those demands in part exist because the current food regime put them in place (Carolan, 2015).

Take agricultural subsidies. Modern agricultural subsidy policy emerged in the early decades of the 20th century. Initially, the policies were put into place to act as income redistribution measures. At this time farm incomes, on average, were considerably lower and less stable than those obtained in other sectors of the economy. We should also be mindful of the political realities at the time. The rural voting electorate in all countries was a sizable percentage of the total population. In the United States, in 1930, with 56% of the population classified as "urban" and 44% classified as "rural", the problem of rural poverty carried significant currency in Washington, DC. Similar demographics were also found in Europe, though some countries (eg, France) were significantly more rural than others (eg, England). Politicians no doubt wanted to be seen as sensitive to the plight of this sizable constituency.

This justification for subsidies no longer holds. Today, farm incomes in affluent countries are, on average, above those of the average (nonfarm) household. But this does not mean that farmers are on the whole better off than their nonfarming neighbors. What is different today, compared to the 1930s, is the level of income disparity that exists *within* the agricultural sector. Unlike three-quarters of a century ago, when subsidies served more as a safety net to protect those most in need, the overwhelming majority of farm subsidies today are going to the most wealthy.

Between 1995 and 2012, the US government paid out US$293 billion in farm payments. Of this, 75% (or US$178.5 billion) went to 10% of all farms. The top recipient: from 1995 to 2012, Riceland Foods, Inc. (Stuttgart, AR) received over US$554 million—that is more than what was paid to all the farmers in Alaska, Connecticut, Hawaii, Maine, Massachusetts, Nevada, New Hampshire, New Jersey, and Rhode Island combined. The top three recipients—Riceland Foods, Inc., Producers Rice Mill (Wynne, AR) and Farmers Rice Coop (Sacramento, CA)—collectively received during this period over *one billion* dollars.

What about the European Union (EU) and its Common Agricultural Policy? How is their €55 billion annual agricultural subsidy pie distributed? Turns out, the majority goes to large landowners and agribusinesses. The biggest "piece" has been going to the Dutch firm Campina (a Dutch dairy cooperative that merged with Royal Frieslands Foods in 2008). Between 1997 and 2009, Campina received €1.6 billion in taxpayer money. The Denmark-based firm Arla Foods Amba (formed by the 2000 merger between Sweden's Arla and Denmark's MD Foods) received the next-biggest subsidy. Between 1999 and 2009, their payments totaled €952 million. Rounding out the top three was the London-based company Tate and Lyle Europe, who received €826 million between 1999 and 2009.

In light of all the bad press agricultural subsides are getting these days, why are these policies allowed to continue? And how have we gotten to a place where the 30 most industrialized economies spend roughly a billion dollars a day on food and agricultural subsidies (Peterson, 2009)? There are no easy answers to questions like these. One could begin, however, by noting how the benefits of farm subsidies are concentrated, while their costs are relatively diffuse (spread across all taxpayers). Agricultural producers have more to lose than any other group would individually gain from the removal of subsidies. Consequently, those who gain from this arrangement will likely spend more to maintain the status quo than consumers and taxpayers, for whom subsidies cost them individually very little. And so while agricultural subsidies might change subtly from year to year, in any given country the policies themselves will likely not go away anytime soon.

Another useful concept as we think through why subsidies have proven so resilient is policy path dependency: the well-documented phenomenon whereby once a policy is enacted it tends to become "locked in." The greater the levels and history of support, the more dependent the farm and farm supply chain becomes on continuing levels of support, which creates tremendous resistance to the removal of these policies. As farm outputs today are utilized by not only traditional food manufacturers but also fuel, livestock, and industrial sectors of the economy, there are a lot of parties interested in maintaining the status quo.

There is considerable debate around whether to roll back subsidies entirely or to allow them to exist, just in a highly reformed state. At most, one-tenth of one percent of all domestic agriculture subsidies in the United States goes to supporting fruit and vegetable crops. What is keeping governments from doing more to subsidize healthy foods? Or, at the consumption end, why is additional money not spent on programs that help those of lower socioeconomic status buy fresh fruits and vegetables and alternative protein sources, like through what are commonly known as food stamps? Would not such a strategy also help transition consumers toward more sustainable, healthier diets?

Perhaps it is not a black-and-white question, of whether agricultural subsidies ought to exist or not. Maybe we should be more interested in who are being helped by subsides and the societal ends being served. In suggesting this I am thinking about the case involving the African nation of Malawi. For years, the country was starving, suffering from persistent famine. In 2005, after a disastrous corn harvest, five million of the country's 13 million residents needed emergency food aid. By 2007, the country was turning away food aid. What happened? Two words: fertilizer subsidies. Since the 1980s the World Bank was leaning on Malawi to eliminate its fertilizer subsidies. The removal of this subsidy, however, proved disastrous to poorer Malawian farmers. Without it, most could no longer afford fertilizer. Yet the gravely depleted soils in the country require inputs, artificial (eg, chemical fertilizer) and/or otherwise (eg, manure). Malawi's President, Bingu wa Mutharika, seeing other countries extensively subsidize their own farmers, decided after the 2005 harvest to bring back fertilizer subsidies.

The Malawi case also brings us back to the question, "Who benefits from subsidies?" Even with a fertilizer subsidy, Malawian farmers are at a significant disadvantage in the global marketplace when they have to compete against farms that can receive upwards of hundreds of thousands of dollars annually from their respective governments. Governments of affluent nations spend on average between US$6000 and $10,000 per farm laborer per year. For comparison, the typical African government spends less than US$10 per farm worker per year on agriculture. And as for the link between subsidies and the aforementioned changing structure of agriculture: a study by USDA economists implicates agricultural subsidies for having contributed directly to increases in the average size of US farms (Key & Roberts, 2007).

There are also cultural variables that need to be addressed when thinking about barriers to farmers switching to raising alternative protein sources. Research reveals that farmers may resist change on the basis of an anticipated change to their identity and/or to social/cultural rewards (such as status and respect) that were traditionally conferred through conventional farming practices. There are normative pressures to be a "good farmer," as defined by the social networks producers locate themselves within (Carolan, 2005). For example, agroforestry approaches that encourage farmers to also become foresters and leisure providers have been met with considerable resistance as they ask farmers to essentially become (identity-wise) something they are not, namely, foresters and leisure providers (Lloyd, Watkins, & Williams, 1995). Burgess, Clark, and Harrison (2000) sum up nicely this point, noting that "first and foremost, farmers saw themselves as food producers." Hence, to be a "good farmer" one need not be a "good forester." Indeed, in some networks, as long as food production remains a requisite of a farmer's identity, any actions that do not result in this end could ultimately diminish their status among other producers.

I mention this research to emphasize that the barriers to the adoption of certain production practices for farmers are not just economic in nature. In some instances, cultural barriers can be sufficient when it comes to keeping farmers from changing their practices and commodity profiles. Thus, for example, if macro livestock (eg, beef cow) producers do not feel that "real farmers" (or "good farmers") ought to raise micro livestock (eg, crickets), and their social networks do not believe this either, then it will matter little how profitable such an operation could be. Economic incentives, therefore, are only a piece of what is needed to transition producers over to alternative protein sources. Social norms need to be changed as well, a process that takes time, education, exposure to alternative operations already engaged in these practices, and often a willingness of community/farm leaders to take the risk of trying something new (in an attempt to create those changes in social norms among producers).

24.6 CONCLUSION

Looking ahead, the future of sustainable protein seems bright, regardless of whether we are championing these foods or not. The current protein regimen is simply not sustainable. The numbers just do not add up. Not even close.

The wise move would therefore be to plan for this future, rather than ignore it until we have no choice but to confront it—being proactive, in other words, rather than reactive. As detailed above, our eating preferences are dictated by more than just how something tastes and how much it costs. Culture, norms, meal structure expectations, knowledge, and skills all go into shaping why we eat the proteins that we do. Steps can be taken to shape consumer preferences so they ultimately choose alternative proteins. By waiting too long to have this conversation we risk finding ourselves in a situation where consumers are eating alternative protein not because they want to but because they have no choice. That is not a future we want to find ourselves in.

When we think about *sustainable* protein sources, therefore, we need to approach the term in the same spirit as we would anything with that adjective attached to it. Sustainability, *real* sustainability, ought to presuppose what is colloquially referred to as the triple bottom line, which is to say it should rest on principles that promote social, ecological, and economic sustainability. I mention this as a reminder that certain food policy scenarios, no matter how well intentioned, ecologically sound, or premised on seemingly just ethical postulates, will very likely fail if they appear too heavy-handed. I mention this to remind readers of the dangers of policies that are unmindful of the social and cultural realities that lie behind peoples' diets. This is not a call for cultural relativism—to let people eat whatever they want simply because "that's how they've always eaten." It is a call to be mindful of how, for certain populations, cultural and/or ethnic identities are wrapped up in the regular consumption of red meat. And then: find ways to work from that perspective to transition those diets in ways that fit with those pre-existing cultural practices. Whether those transitions involve meat-like substitutes (eg, cricket burgers) or new foods altogether (eg, sautéed crickets) will depend on a host of conditions. My point is that the most sustainable transitions must not be perceived as being imposed. For example, top-down directives from the government—such as the banning of certain meats—risk pushing foods into an informal ("black-market") economy. For a change in diet to be longlasting, *the* core principle of sustainability, it must feel self-directed. It must feel, in other words, as something eaters actually *want*, versus something they have to do.

I leave this as food for thought as we think about the "next steps." And fortunately there are plenty of options out there as we contemplate what these sustainable food futures ought to look like, as the following chapter explains.

REFERENCES

Balmford, A., Green, R., & Scharlemann, J. (2005). Sparing land for nature: Exploring the potential impact of changes in agricultural yield on the area needed for crop production. *Global Change Biology, 11*, 1594–1605.

Barclay, E. (2013). *Samoans await the return of the tasty turkey tail*. NPR May 9. <http://www.npr.org/sections/thesalt/2013/05/14/182568333/samoans-await-the-return-of-the-tasty-turkey-tail> Last accessed 04.06.15.

Bomford, M. (2011). *Beyond food miles*. Post Carbon Institute, March 9, Santa Rosa, CA. <http://www.postcarbon.org/article/273686-beyond-food-miles#_edn9> Last accessed 12.04.15.

Bruinsma, J. (2009). *The resource outlook to 2050: By how much do land, water and crop yields need to increase by 2050?* FAO Expert Meeting on How to Feed the World in 2050, Rome. <ftp://ftp.fao.org/docrep/fao/012/ak971e/ak971e00.pdf> Last accessed 03.06.15.

Burgess, J., Clark, J., & Harrison, C. (2000). Knowledges in action: An actor network analysis of a wetland agri-environment scheme. *Ecological Economics, 35*, 119–132.

Canning, P., Charles, A., Huang S., Polenske, K., & Waters, A. (2010). *Energy use in the US food system*. United States Department of Agriculture, Economic Research Service, Report number 94, March, Washington, DC. <http://ddr.nal.usda.gov/bitstream/10113/41413/1/CAT31049057.pdf> Last accessed 12.04.15.

Carolan, M. (2005). Barriers to the adoption of sustainable agriculture on rented land: An examination of contesting social fields. *Rural Sociology, 70*, 387–413.

Carolan, M. (2011a). *The real cost of cheap food*. New York: Earthscan/Routledge.

Carolan, M. (2011b). *Embodied food politics*. Burlington: Ashgate.

Carolan, M. (2013). *Reclaiming food security*. New York: Earthscan/Routledge.

Carolan, M. (2015). Affective sustainable landscapes and care ecologies: Getting a real feel for alternative food communities. *Sustainability Science, 10*, 317–329.

Catel, P. (2011). *Raising livestock*. Chicago: Heinemann-Raintree.

CDC. (2014). *National diabetes statistics report, 2014*. <http://www.cdc.gov/diabetes/data/statistics/2014statisticsreport.html> Last accessed 17.10.15.

CDC. (2015). *Adult obesity facts*. <http://www.cdc.gov/obesity/data/adult.html> Last accessed 29.05.16.

Douglas, M., & Nicod, M. (1974). Taking the biscuit: The structure of British meals. *New Society, 30*, 744–747.

Dutta, I., & Gundersen, C. (2007). Measures of food insecurity at the household level. In B. Guha-Khasnobis, S. Acharya, & B. Davis (Eds.), *Food Security* (pp. 42–61). New York: Oxford University Press.

Economist. (2011). *The 9-billion people question: A special report on feeding the world*. The Economist, February 26. <http://www.economist.com/surveys/downloadSurveyPDF.cfm?id=18205243&surveyCode=%254e%2541&submit=View+PDF> Last accessed 03.04.15.

EPA. (2015). *Sources of greenhouse gas emissions*. Environmental Protection Agency, Washington, DC. <http://www.epa.gov/climatechange/ghgemissions/sources/agriculture.html> Last accessed 15.07.15.

FAO (1943). *United nations conference on food and agriculture: Hot springs, virginia, May 18–June 3, final acts and section reports*. Washington, DC: United States Government Printing Office.

FAO (2012). *World agriculture towards 2030/2050: The 2012 revision*. ESA E Working Paper No. 12-03, Rome, Italy. <http://www.fao.org/fileadmin/user_upload/esag/docs/AT2050_revision_summary.pdf> Last accessed 03.06.15.

Godfray, H., Beddington, J., Crute, I., Hadded, L., Lawrence, D., Muir, J., ... Toulmin, C. (2010). Food security: The challenge of feeding 9 billion people. *Science, 327*, 812–818.

Gvion-Rosenberg, L. (1990). Why do vegetarian restaurants serve hamburgers?: Toward an understanding of a cuisine. *Semiotica, 80*, 61–79.

Hoekstra, A. (2015). The water footprint: The relation between human consumption and water use. In M. Antonelli, & F. Greco (Eds.), *The water we eat: Combining virtual water and water footprints* (pp. 35–50). Switzerland: Springer.

Key, N., & Roberts, A. (2007). *Commodity payments, farm business survival and farm size growth, economic research report, no ERR-51*. Economic Research Service, USDA, Washington, DC. <www.ers.usda.gov/Publications/ERR51/ERR51ref.pdf> Last accessed 11.08.15.

Khoury, C., Bjorkman, A., Dempewolf, H., Ramirez-Villegas, J., Guarino, L., Jarvis, L., ... Stuik, P. (2014). Increasing homogeneity in global food supplies and the implications for food security. *Proceedings of the National Academy of Sciences of the United States of America, 111*(11), 4001–4006.

Khoury, C., & Jarvis, A. (2014). *The changing composition of the global diet: Implications for CGIAR research*. CIAT Policy Brief International Center for Tropical Agriculture, Cali, Columbia, No 18. <http://ciat.cgiar.org/wp-content/uploads/2014/11/policy_brief_global_diets.pdf> Last accessed 22.01.15.

Lloyd, T., Watkins, C., & Williams, D. (1995). Turning farmers into foresters via market liberalization. *Journal of Agricultural Economics, 46*, 361–370.

Lokuruka, M. (2006). Meat is the meal and status is by meat. *Food and Foodways, 14*, 201–229.

Montanari, M. (1994). *The culture of food*. Oxford: Blackwell.

Ogino, A., Orito, H., Shimada, K., & Hirooka, H. (2007). Evaluating environmental impacts of the Japanese beef cow–calf system by the life cycle assessment method. *Animal Science Journal, 78*, 424–432.

Peterson, W. (2009). *A billion dollars a day: The economics and politics of agricultural subsides*. Malden: Wiley-Blackwell.

Pimentel, D. (2005). Environmental and economic costs of the application of pesticides primarily in the United States. *Environment, Development and Sustainability, 7*, 229–252.

Pollan, M. (2009). *Big food vs. big insurance*. New York Times, September 9. <http://www.nytimes.com/2009/09/10/opinion/10pollan.html?pagewanted=all&_r=0> Last accessed 18.10.15.

Rabobank (2010). *Sustainability and security of the global food supply chain*. The Netherlands: Rabobank Group.

Ray, D., Mueller, N., West, P., & Foley, J. (2013). Yield trends are insufficient to double global crop production by 2050. *PloS One, 8*, e66428. Available from http://dx.doi.org/10.1371/journal.pone.0066428.

Rivera-Ferre, M. G., & Arce, A. (2009). Supply vs. demand of agri-industrial meat and fish products: A chicken and egg paradigm? *International Journal of Sociology of Agriculture and Food, 16*, 90–105.

Roberts, P. (2008). *The end of food*. New York: Houghton Mifflin.

Schade, C., & Pimentel, D. (2010). Population crash: Prospects for famine in the twenty-first century. *Environment, Development and Sustainability, 12*, 245–262.

Schösler, H., De Boer, J., & Boersema, J. (2012). Can we cut out the meat of the dish? Constructing consumer-oriented pathways towards meat substitution. *Appetite, 58*, 39–47.

Shaw, D. (2007). *World food security: A history since 1945*. New York: Palgrave.

Twigg, J. (1984). Vegetarianism and the meanings of meat. In A. Murcott (Ed.), *The sociology of food and eating* (pp. 18–30). Aldershot: Gower Publishing.

Venkat, K. (2011). The climate change and economic impacts of food waste in the United States. *International Journal of Food System Dynamics, 2*, 431–446.

Wang, Y., Lehane, C., Ghebremeskel, K., & Crawford, M. (2009). Modern organic and broiler chickens sold for human consumption provide more energy from fat than protein. *Public Health Nutrition, 13*, 400–408.

Wansink, B. (2002). Changing eating habits on the home front. Lost lessons from World War II research. *Journal of Public Policy & Marketing, 21*, 90–99.

Webster, J. (2010). *The meat and dairy crisis*. Earthcast, 11 October, sponsored by Earthscan. <www.earthscan.co.uk/Earthcasts/tabid/101760/Default.aspx> Last accessed 01.11.14.

Chapter 25

Feeding the Globe Nutritious Food in 2050: Obligations and Ethical Choices

S.R. Nadathur[1], J.P.D. Wanasundara[2] and L. Scanlin[3]
[1]Givaudan Flavors, Cincinnati, OH, United States, [2]Agriculture and Agri-Food Canada, Saskatoon SK, Canada, [3]Colorado State University, Fort Collins, CO, United States

25.1 CLOSING COMMENTARY

The introductory chapter of this book has identified several challenges in front of us in the quest to feed a rapidly growing global population. In particular, the chapter proposed that consuming protein from plant and alternative sources would be more sustainable for the planet as compared to animal-derived protein, especially meat. An overburdened earth requires extensive exploitation of natural resources for activities including agriculture, transportation, and infrastructure. These activities contribute to deforestation and greenhouse gas (GHG) accumulation leading to climate change and a warming planet. Disparities in the developed and emerging economies include an unequal distribution of wealth and resources, which have increased socioeconomic inequality. We can continue on the same path of high meat consumption in developed and emerging economies, which will result in a warmer, inhospitable planet with little nutrition for all. Alternatively, we can change course, and choose a different path where humanity will share the responsibility for the greater good. "If we do not change our direction, we are likely to end up where we are headed" (Chinese Proverb). Sustainable living on the earth depends on multiple factors and one factor affects the other. One cannot talk about climate change without addressing population, food, transportation, and power. Our chosen path ought to include reducing meat consumption, driving less, harnessing solar and wind energy, and limiting population growth. Every one of these aspects is interlinked and their increase or reduction has global consequences. Each person has to do his or her part for a sustainable planet.

25.2 SUSTAINABLE PROTEIN SOURCES

Several sustainable protein sources have and will continue to provide valuable nutrition to humanity over the next several decades. These include cereals, pseudocereals, legumes and pulses, and protein-rich oilseeds. In addition, there are exciting new sources including algae, mycoprotein, and insect. These protein sources are sustainable and require fewer resources (land, water, and energy) compared to meat, while providing valuable nutrients and minerals. Table 25.1 summarizes the different sustainable sources discussed in this book along with their key nutrients. Combining cereal grains with legumes and pulses provides a complete amino acid profile similar to that provided by meat or dairy products. Utilizing land to produce these sources for direct consumption of these grains, nuts, and vegetables, will deliver needed nutrition as the population surges in the next 30 years.

25.2.1 Current State of Protein Production

Proteins provide energy and are the main source of nitrogen in our diet. Hence, it is vital that we view protein as an essential part of our diet and understand the key role they play within the human body. Without adequate protein in our diet, we will waste away as the body will break down internal proteins for its amino acid requirements. Plants require nitrogen to make protein, which animals consume in turn to produce meat, eggs, or milk. In an assessment of nitrogen loss along the food chain, Smil (2002) found that only 13% of initial nitrogen fertilizer inputs end up in plant and

TABLE 25.1 Summary of Sustainable Protein Sources and Their Key Nutrients

Source[a]	Protein (g)	Fat (g)	Carbohydrates (g)	Important Micronutrients	
				Vitamin	Mineral
Cereals					
Brown rice (195 g, cooked)	5.0	1.7	44.7	Niacin B3	Manganese
Millet (174 g, cooked)	6.1	1.7	41.1	Thiamin B1	Copper
Oats (39 g, dry)	13.2	5.4	56.5	Biotin B5	Manganese
Sorghum (100 g)	11.3	3.3	74.6	Thiamin B1	Phosphorus
Whole wheat (182 g, cooked)	5.6	0.4	33.8	Pantothenic acid B5	Manganese
Pseudocereals					
Amaranth (100 g)	14.0	7.0	66.0	Folate B9	Manganese
Chia (28 g)	4.4	9.1	12.0	Niacin B3	Phosphorus
Quinoa (1 cup cooked)	8.1	3.4	39.4	Thiamin B1	Manganese
Legumes and Pulses					
Black beans (172 g, cooked)	15.2	0.9	40.8	Thiamin B1	Molybdenum
Lentils (198 g, cooked)	17.9	0.8	39.9	Pantothenic acid B5	Molybdenum
Lupine (166 g, cooked)	26.0	4.9	16.4	Thiamin B1	Magnesium
Pea, split (196 g, cooked)	16.4	0.7	41.3	Thiamin B1	Molybdenum
Peanut, raw (36.50 g)	9.4	5.9	18.0	Biotin B7	Copper
Soybeans (172 g, cooked)	28.6	15.4	17.1	Niacin B3	Calcium
Oilseeds					
Canola, meal (100 g)[b]	36.0	3.5	5.0	Choline, B complex	Iron
Flaxseed, ground (14 g, ground)	2.6	5.9	4.0	Thiamin B1	Copper
Hemp, whole seed (100 g)	32.0	48.0	8.0	Riboflavin B2	Magnesium
Other					
Chlorella (algae) (100 g)	61.0	11.0	23.0	Vitamin A	Phosphorus
Mycoprotein (100 g)	11.0	2.9	9.0	Niacin B3	Selenium
Crickets (100 g cooked)	58.5	24.0	8.4	Riboflavin B2	Zinc
Animal Protein Sources					
Beef (115 g, grass-fed)	26.1	8.1	0	Cobalamin B12	Selenium
Milk (115 g, grass-fed)	3.8	3.6	5.9	Cobalamin B12	Iodine

[a]All data in as-it-is basis, not corrected for moisture. Weight of cooked protein source may vary.
[b]Canola seed or meal is not commonly used in food products. Carbohydrates are mostly free sugars (CCC; Assadi, Janmoammadi, Taghizadeh, & Alijani, 2011).
Source: Adapted from various sources: Assadi, E., Janmoammadi, H., Taghizadeh, A., Alijani, S., 2011. Nutrient composition of different varieties of full-fat canola seed and nitrogen-corrected true metabolizable energy of full-fat canola seed with or without enzyme addition and thermal processing. Journal of Applied Poultry Research 20, 95–101; CCC. Canola Council of Canada (www.canolacouncil.org/); The world's healthiest foods (http://www.whfoods.com/foodstoc.php); SELF Nutrition data (http://nutritiondata.self.com); Lupin nutrition (http://www.livestrong.com/article/459078-the-nutrition-in-lupine-seeds/); Amaranth nutrition (http://skipthepie.org/cereal-grains-and-pasta/amaranth-grain-cooked/#proteins); Algae nutrition (https://www.sunchlorellausa.com/chlorella-nutrition-analysis-table); Mycoprotein nutrition (http://www.mycoprotein.org/what_is_mycoprotein/nutritional_composition.html); and Cricket flours (http://www.cricketflours.com/cricket-nutritional-value/, http://www.precisionnutrition.com/eating-bugs).

animal foods. Approximately 70% of the nitrogen in harvested food crops becomes available for direct human consumption (accounting for processing and storage losses). However, on average, nearly 7 kg of feed nitrogen are needed to produce only 1 kg of nitrogen in meat, eggs, and dairy products. Animal production systems can be considered based on protein conversion efficiencies for the following: beef (5%) < pork (13%) < poultry (25%) < eggs (30%) < carp (30%) < milk (40%). It is evident that dairy, egg, and carp (and other aquacultured herbivore fish) are more efficient animal production systems relative to beef, pork, and poultry. Poultry has higher protein production efficiencies relative to beef and pork, but beef and pork together comprise nearly two-thirds of the industrial livestock production for the world meat market (http://www.fao.org/ag/againfo/themes/en/meat/background.html# Accessed 20.08.15.) By 2030, world aggregate consumption of cereals is expected to increase by 1 billion metric tons from 1.89 billion metric tons recorded in 1997/99. Nearly half of this cereal production is destined for feed to generate meat and other animal proteins (Bruinsma, 2003). A major shift is imperative. We must move away from inefficient, less sustainable meat protein production that amplifies industrialized farming and intensive animal control. The consequences of intensive animal farming also generate added costs to the health of both animals and humans.

25.2.2 Change in Consumption Patterns, Especially Meat and the Western Diet

Driven by urbanization, globalization, and economic development, world demand for meat continuously rose over the last 50 years. By 2011, meat became the main source for supplying the continued animal protein demand in countries with over 10 million inhabitants, with the exception of North Korea and South Africa (Sans & Combris, 2015). Cultural and social perception of economic prosperity equating to purchasing power and consumption of meat and animal proteins has been a major cause for this change. At current levels, average intake of animal protein among the world population is 39.4% of total calories, of which meat protein intake is 15 g/person/day. Among Organization for Economic Cooperation and Development (OECD) countries, ranges between low-income and high-income countries are 21.9–59.5% of total calories and 6–30 g protein/person/day. (The OECD brings together 39 countries that are responsible for 80% of world trade and investment.) Despite a rise in per capita GDP, India remains below the world average for animal and meat protein intake (Sans & Combris, 2015). China is currently increasing its meat consumption as affluence in the Chinese economy has afforded the ability to buy lands in other countries to satisfy their demand for natural resources (National Geographic, 2014a).

There are differing opinions on whether meat is essential for human existence. Some consumers believe that meat is a vital part of the diet and will not consider reducing meat consumption. Meat-based foods are marketed in Western societies as inexpensive, fast, and convenient. Hamburger meat (ground meat) is often a main source of food for the poor of Western society, while high-end customers value and savor the taste of a well-aged steak. According to food historians, a transition from bread (cereal protein) to meat (animal-derived protein) in Europe occurred after World War II. Consumers today obtain their meat from supermarkets, where it is presented in a way that avoids the link between industrialized, intensive animal rearing and processing (Schösler, de Boer, & Boersema, 2012). A study involving Dutch consumers showed a diminished concern regarding processes involved to produce the meat they consume. However, increasing people's involvement in various aspects of food production enables a better appreciation of dietary habits and their effects of such choices on the environment (de Boer, Boersema, & Aiking, 2009). The sheer volume and routine consumption of meat have become significant when addressing the changes needed in meat consumption patterns. Along with meat consumption and other influences migrating from the Western world, health issues have ensued. The prevalence of obesity, cancer, and diabetes has increased throughout the globe. Consequently, the associated costs of treating chronic diseases have soared, putting an enormous strain on people and institutions.

Globally, the percentage of people who practice a vegetarian or vegan diet is approximately 10%. Over 70% of vegetarians are in India, while vegan consumers in the United States doubled to 5% of the population in 2013 (http://www.huffingtonpost.com/2013/04/02/interest-in-vegan-diets-on-the-rise_n_3003221.html). Vegetarianism in India has its roots in nonviolence towards animals originating from ancient religious concepts. Yet, this dietary habit among this large section of the population is critical as India's surging economy is also creating a large number of affluent people. Typically, affluence increases the consumption of Western-style diets; hence, it is vital that this section of the populace in India stay with their original diets. Vegetarian diets have spread to other parts of Asia (including Sri Lanka, China, and South East Asia), in parallel with teachings of the Buddha that bring about nonviolence and environmental responsibility. In other parts of the globe, vegetarian or vegan habits have strengthened due to concerns for the environment and health. Europeans are more receptive to a reduction in meat consumption citing environment and health as chief reasons. Thus, consumers are becoming increasingly aware of the implications of their dietary habits and making appropriate choices for a more sustainable planet.

25.2.3 Are We Consuming Too Much Protein?

Protein requirements for an average, healthy adult men and women are 56 and 46 grams per day, respectively. These dietary requirements are satisfied from meals consumed throughout the day. In many developed economies, protein intake is higher than recommended requirements due to an overabundance of meat and dairy products. The recent trend in high-protein foods has increased the daily intake for some consumers. Long-term overconsumption of protein can have adverse effects on bone tissues, renal and liver functions, and coronary artery disease (Delimaris, 2013). High-protein diets generate more acids in body fluids as sulfates and phosphates, especially high levels from oxidation of sulfur amino acids (methionine and cysteine). When the body is challenged with a high load of dietary acid, kidneys need to excrete more acidic urine. Hence, bone tissues have to provide additional buffer ions leading to increased mineral loss and affecting bones and renal functions. Though higher protein may be required for some sections of the populace, adhering to the recommended protein requirements may be sufficient for most people. This in turn will put fewer burdens on producing animal-derived protein in the coming years.

25.2.4 Diet Change, Consumers, and Policies

Food choice is a complex function of both sensory and nonsensory factors. Among the nonsensory factors are included food-related attitudes and expectations, moods, health claims, price, ethical concerns, environmental, sustainability, and social aspects of food selection. Today's consumer understands that good eating habits are important to support a healthy lifestyle. Flavor and taste remain the top sensory attributes influencing food choices. In addition, several changes are shaping consumer choices. Many people understand that their dietary habits and other activities affect the environment. As a result, consumers have modified daily activities such as eating local, switching to plant-based diets, recycling, riding public transportation, and driving more fuel-efficient vehicles.

The United Nations has urged people to move to diets without meat or dairy (Guardian, 2010). Not only are plant-based diets more sustainable for the planet, they provide protein, phytonutrients and minerals that are protective for people's health. A large study of 73,000 ethnically diverse participants found that diet modifications towards a plant-based diet and away from animal proteins, can help mitigate climate change while improving longevity (Science Daily, 2014). Small changes within individual diets across a broad population base do contribute to meaningful reductions in GHG emissions. Considering several aspects (such as health, environmental, and socioeconomic elements), the implementation of plant-based diet policies is a suggested solution to ensure that the earth will have a sustainable food supply for future generations (Sabate & Soret, 2014). The implementation of such policy initiatives requires a broad understanding of the challenges ahead and the willingness of consumers to make necessary sacrifices. Consumers around the globe understand that human activities affect the planet and that changes are required to reduce their carbon footprint. The carbon footprint of a vegetarian diet is slightly higher than that of a vegan diet, while a meat-based diet has been shown to produce twice the carbon emissions of a vegan diet (Scarborough et al., 2014). An ovo-lacto vegetarian diet has been shown to use less natural resources (land, water, energy) and found to be more sustainable than a meat-based diet when comparing isocaloric diets (Pimentel & Pimentel, 2003).

Changing food habits or behaviors is not an easy task. Requiring people to reduce their meat consumption and tying such changes to global warming becomes a complicated topic. Some sections of the population do not believe that global warming is real and that the threat of a major catastrophe is overstated. Others are likely to question whether their reduced meat consumption would even make a meaningful impact on GHG reductions. Humankind can debate the veracity of climate change or claim that these changes are a natural weather cyclic phenomenon. However, with the addition of 3 billion people in the next 30 years, it is imperative that we consider the impact on future generations of taking no action today.

The recent agreement to cap the increase in global warming from the birth of the Industrial Age to 2°C over the next few decades, is a major step in shifting to an alternate path for the greater good of human civilization (http://www.wsj.com/articles/final-draft-of-global-climate-change-deal-is-complete-1449906731). The ramifications of the Climate Change Treaty illustrate the complexities in aligning the needs of various countries in the world. Not every country will feel the effects of climate change to the same degree. Emerging economies with higher populations will likely experience the greatest impact and will need to allocate additional resources towards feeding their citizens. Therefore, developing countries will require more assistance and leeway, while developed economies can better withstand disruptions in socioeconomic conditions. Finding common ground and educating consumers on food habits and water usage and its impact on climate change will be a step in the right direction. "When one tugs at a single thing in nature, he finds it attached to the rest of the world" (John Muir, 1838–1914). Thus, the act of reducing meat consumption in favor of plant-based diets can begin the process of better resource utilization. This is especially important in the case of water, which has become a precious commodity in a warmer planet.

25.2.5 Challenges With Diet Change

The scenario of consuming less animal protein is not without its challenges. The world cattle population is around 1.3 billion, while dairy cows account for 270 million (AHDB Dairy, 2015). Dairy products are an important source of protein for a variety of groups including vegetarians. In addition, dairy products are an excellent source of calcium, while fermented dairy products contain beneficial probiotics. Animal production also provides livelihood for countless ranchers, dairy cattle farmers, and processors. Adapting to a different livelihood would likely be extremely difficult; although this may be an option for some should animal production decrease. Although the prospect of change sounds ominous, animal producers would face similar consequence with a major drought or other disruptive weather event. The droughts of 2011 and 2012 resulted in the culling of over 50,000 cows in the American Midwest. Similar weather events will likely occur in the future, which reinforces the need to make a courageous shift in our path rather than repeat similar situations in the future. Producers that grow crops for animal feed may face less challenge when converting their lands to cultivate crops for direct human consumption. With an additional 3 billion people inhabiting the earth in the next 30 years, drought-tolerant plant-based protein sources will likely receive fair prices. Another hurdle to diet change is the fact that farmers in several countries rely on subsidies to grow certain crops. Hence, changes to agriculture policies would require political debate and actions in many countries for implementation.

25.3 ENVIRONMENTALLY FRIENDLY FOOD OPTIONS

25.3.1 Meat Alternates

In order to make effective changes to meat consumption, consumers who are willing to change their dietary patterns should have a range of meat-free products that align with their food practices. In addition, studies have indicated an understanding that self-indulgence (hedonism) of food has a strong positive association with tasty food (Schösler et al., 2012). With an increased understanding of health and environmental aspects of food production as well as a consumer demand for nonmeat alternatives, manufacturers have introduced meat alternates or substitutes that mimic the texture, appearance, and taste of meat. The market for meat substitutes or alternates is growing exponentially. Meat substitutes that are based on soy or wheat (seitan) date back to ancient Asian cultures. The very first commercial meat alternative in the Western world, developed by Dr. John H. Kellogg (US Patent 670,283, 1899), began with a "meat-like" canned product made from peanut as the main ingredient. It was soon followed by soy and wheat gluten-based products developed in 1922 (Shurtleff & Aoyagi, 2014). Today, most of the meat alternatives in the market are soy protein-based, while other sources such as wheat gluten can be used (Asgar, Fazilah, Huda, Bhat, & Karim, 2010). The soy proteins are converted to products that provide texture, bite, and sensation, similar to that of chewing meat. This provides sensory satisfaction to the consumer who has experienced meat products. Developed with an understanding of the health benefits of consuming a nonmeat diet, initial soy proteins used for meat alternatives were bitter and had strong beany overtones. This resulted in early acceptability challenges with consumers. Advances in protein processing together with knowledge gained on chemical interactions during protein processing have been able to provide products with much improved taste, texture, and overall acceptability.

Mimicking the texture of meat requires the creation of multiple S—S (disulfide) linkages enabling a close configuration of the protein and tissues that do not exist in nonmeat or plant proteins. Recent scientific advances have aided in the creation of protein matrices that can provide a meat-like texture. Thermal processes to recreate the required disulfide bridges were at the heart of the development work on meat substitutes by Hsieh and Huff (2012), at the University of Missouri. Thermal extrusion of plant protein mixtures under optimal conditions develops protein cross-links (IEEE Spectrum, 2013). This extrusion technology is now part of *Beyond Meat* and is utilized to produce chicken substitutes with some success (http://engineering.missouri.edu/2012/06/hsiehs-soy-chicken-research-moves-closer-to-consumer-kitchens/). The next introduction will be a red meat substitute, currently under development (http://www.foodnavigator-usa.com/Manufacturers/Beyond-Meat-unleashes-The-Beast-the-ultimate-burger-minus-the-beef).

In addition to texture and taste, introducing a blood-like feel to the product is part of the next generation of meat alternatives. This version of hamburger meat comes from *Impossible Foods* (http://impossiblefoods.com/) based in San Francisco. Dr. Patrick Brown and his team are developing meat-like alternates that also sizzle like burgers. Meat-like products made from cells in the lab are yet another development to counter environmental impacts of animal production. Dr. Mark Post and colleagues isolated and grew muscle cells with serum from a cow. This process increased cellular mass similar to that which occurs in livestock. This lab-made "cultured meat (beef)" (http://culturedbeef.net/) proves the concept of obtaining meat-like product through tissue culture. Since then, a company has formed to produce this alternate meat (MosaMeat). At this time, there are challenges of scaling up as an affordable replacement for meat, while careful monitoring is required to prevent microbial contamination in large fermenters. An entrepreneurial and research team in New York from *Modern Meadow* (led by the Forgasc family (http://www.modernmeadow.com/#home)), employs biofabrication and tissue engineering to culture meat and materials without animal slaughter (Roush, 2014). Their first commercial product they plan to launch is leather that is manufactured entirely from plant-based media.

Several companies that produce new meat alternates have the same goals in support of the environment and a sustainable food supply, while drawing upon investments from venture capitalists and wealthy individuals. Although there is clear resonance for meat alternatives from certain consumer segments, future growth and consumption of these products by a broad consumer base remains to be determined. As a potential hurdle to meat alternatives, whether plant-based or cultured, are their usual long ingredient statement as compared to meat, which typically has a "clean label" or short ingredient statement (without hard to read ingredient additives). A current trend in the United States is for consumer products with "clean labels." A broader question for consumers may be to rethink whether nonanimal foods have to taste like meat, or whether consumers can incorporate more good tasting, artisanal dishes made from protein-rich plants (and alternative protein sources), such as those prevalent in Asia, Africa, and Latin America.

25.3.2 Newer Sources of Protein

Novel protein sources extend beyond underutilized seed proteins. Generating protein-rich microbial (eg, algae, bacteria, fungi, yeast) biomass, while utilizing wastestream is a good example. The new venture, *Nutrinsic* (http://nutrinsic.com/), based in Denver (CO, United States) utilizes nutrients in the wastewater of the beer-making process to produce single-cell proteins (SCPs) after optimizing growth conditions. The early development phase of this venture will initially target animal and fish feed markets while proteins destined for human consumption are in the planning stages. Nasseri, Rasoul-Amini, Morowvat, and Ghasemi (2011) provided a comprehensive review of the use of agricultural wastes as substrates to generate SCP. Cellulose-rich waste plant material from food processing (eg, peels of banana, mango, pomegranate, sweet orange, and apple) can be used for producing *Saccharomyces cerevisiae* cells (Khan, Khan, Ahmed, & Tanveer, 2010). High nucleic acid content and low cell wall digestibility have been the main constraints inherent to SCP. Surmounting this obstacle can help SCP find a broader use as food protein. At present, a considerable amount of knowledge and knowhow is available in converting lignocellulosic biomass (crop and forestry residues) into suitable fermentable substrates for fuel ethanol and other valuable chemical generation (Kang, Appel, Tan, & Dewil, 2014). The potential exists for combining production of SCP and chemical streams, similar to an operation model for algae proteins.

Current research and market trends are to generate purified forms of protein from several plant-based sources including soy and pea (which are well-established), and newer protein sources such as oats, rice, and hemp. The growth of various current and newer protein sources is depicted in Fig. 25.1 and the future protein supply will be from diverse sources. Soy proteins are designated as first generation, while rice, pea, and canola form the second-generation ingredients. Proteins from plant sources including duckweed and moringa would form the third generation. Market research has indicated that the increase in soy protein consumption will come via its use in foods directly with a simultaneous reduction in animal feed use (Lux Research, http://www.luxresearchinc.com/news-and-events/press-releases/read/alternative-proteins-claim-third-market-2054 Accessed 27.10.15.). Proteins from algae, insects, those from agricultural

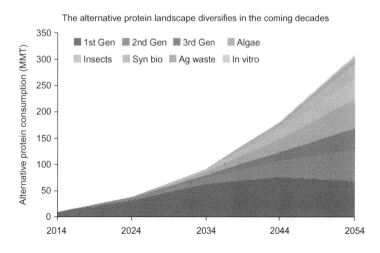

FIGURE 25.1 Forecast for plant and alternative protein consumption from now to 2054. *Adapted from Lux Research.*

waste (Ag waste), and generated via new biotechnological processes (Syn bio), are expected to increase exponentially in the next two to three decades (Fig. 25.1). In vitro proteins are similar to those generated by Modern Meadow, cultured beef product (MosaMeat) discussed earlier in this chapter.

Purified proteins are the main ingredients in products such as nutrition bars, beverages, exercise supplements, or those which provide needed nutrition for the elderly. One may contemplate, do all plant-based or animal-derived proteins need to be in a pure or isolated form to add to products and our food? Are not whole-food versions suitable as direct protein sources, alone or in combination? Obtaining purified protein from its native matrix requires process interventions that add to the cost of the final ingredient and to the post-farm GHG contribution. Generating a purified protein ingredient without objectionable color or taste is quite difficult, considering the myriad of naturally occurring chemical compounds found in living tissues. Scientific research continues to indicate the importance of consuming whole foods that are rich in protein and provide complementing macro- and microlevel components for nutrition and aid in slow release of calories. Technological interventions that are required to produce purified proteins are captured in the final price of the product, for which the consumer ultimately carries the cost burden. Eventually, economics will be the driving factor in whether consumers want purified protein or the associated whole food. It will be more practical to use purification approaches to obtain proteins from abundant sources that are rich in protein but not currently utilized for human consumption. For example, oil-extracted residue (a defatted protein-rich material and current byproduct) from canola/rapeseed, is a logical source for protein production rather than lentil, chickpea, beans, or quinoa, which can be directly consumed as protein-rich whole foods.

25.4 RELEVANCE OF BIG FOOD MANUFACTURERS

Global food manufacturers have recognized the importance of issues pertaining to human health, the environment, and the planet. Sustainability is a key platform for most food and ingredient manufacturers including sourcing of raw materials, energy and water usage, and packaging. Consumer trends in making planet-friendly food choices such as reducing one's own carbon footprint are making food manufacturers rethink their new product development. Health and wellness trends including consumption of plant-based diets and the current popularity of high-protein foods are also changing the type of new product introductions. Multinational mergers can introduce new foods from other regions, while acquisitions of smaller companies that produce eco-friendly foods, can support big-food manufacturers to achieve relevance in these changing environments. For example, *tofu* and *tofu*-products are traditional products from the Orient and a mainstay meat substitute. Greek-style yogurt took the high-protein trend to major heights, while *hummus*, a traditional side dish from the Middle East made from chickpea and sesame, has won over North America. Chips and snacks made from pulses (chickpea, lentil, beans) or kale are showing up in grocery aisles. The introduction and success of such "foreign" products will be very important to move diets away from being primarily meat-based in developed economies.

Large companies have been traditionally slow to react to trends. Yet when they do, they can turn regional trends into global mega trends. On the other hand, food start-ups originate from a "niche" consumer trend and usually include "healthy" and/or sustainability rationale. When market trends indicate signs of adoption by a larger consumer base, big food companies are known to have acquired start-ups that have conquered a niche space. Usually, these food start-ups have aggressively focused on finding solutions to provide sustainable foods.

Alternatives to eggs, milk, and cheese are either commercialized or in the process of being developed. However, regulations and consumer choices will be crucial for widespread acceptance. Again, it would behoove start-ups to deliberate for instance, whether a substitute for cheese has to be a highly formulated cheese imitation, or rather, a great tasting, nutritious food that is also functional. To be relevant, big food manufacturers need the courage to introduce products from around the globe as they have the resources and ability to withstand the downside risk with new product launches. Products or solutions need not imitate meat, eggs, or dairy to be successful. Billions of people around the globe eat foods which are meat-free but still satisfy daily nutrient requirements. Matching the taste of meat by providing a product with a long label of ingredients is contrary to current consumer trends for clean labels. Rather food manufacturers may aim to produce good-tasting, simple foods from nutritious plant and alternative protein sources, which are successful in other parts of the globe. These trends are evident in recent offerings in quick service restaurants (QSRs) such as dishes including ancient grains and pulses.

25.5 PRODUCTION OF MORE FOOD FROM THE SAME LAND (AND ALTERNATE FARMING METHODS)

World population growth puts a direct strain on global food supply, demanding agriculture intensification strategies other than deforestation to increase agriculture land area. Ideally, food crops should grow fast, fix nitrogen, and be high-yielding. Agriculture intensification could ensue from using available resources to maximize production, while maintaining environmental sustainability. Similar to zero or no-tilling, precision agriculture in combination with monitoring crop and soil conditions will allow maximizing yields. Managing nutrient supply to the plant, optimizing space, light, and water will be key factors. Abraham et al. (2014) showed how the learning from rice irrigation, of optimizing water and space, might be transferred to crops such as millet, wheat, and teff. These methods increased yields two- to threefold compared to that obtained using traditional practices in several countries including India, Ethiopia, Mali, and Nepal. Currently, a vertical method of growing crops is one of the innovative approaches in trials near Chicago, Illinois (http://farmedhere.com/). With this approach, plants are capable of multiple harvests per year while using one tenth of the water required as those grown in the field.

After water, nitrogen is the limiting factor for the grower and the environment. Nitrogen in fertilizers comes via the Haber–Bosch process of synthesizing ammonia and is dependent on fossil fuels. Leguminous crops produce protein-rich seeds, as well as aid in fixing atmospheric nitrogen leading to reduced fertilizer demand. This fixed nitrogen increases yields of the subsequent crop (Przednowek, Entz, Irvine, Flaten, & Thiessen-Martens, 2004) while less fertilizer addition improves the soil ecosystem. With reduced fertilizer addition, there is limited nitrogen run-off, leading to reduced occurrence of algal blooms in water bodies. Nitrogen fixation is affected by temperature, salinity, and moisture of the soil (Serraj & Adu Gyampi, 2004). Considering that these factors may alter with ongoing climate change, further understanding of nitrogen fixation would be beneficial to both farmers and policy officials.

25.5.1 Agriculture and Climate Change: Crop Adaptation

With continued change in weather patterns due to global warming, the ability of plants to thrive in changing environments may require adaptation. It is widely expected that with an increase in global temperatures, temperature latitudes will move up from current locations, and warmer weather will cover a larger area. C3 crops such as wheat, rice, and beans may likely suffer in extended periods of dry weather. Rice is the staple grain in Asia, while wheat is one of the major grains in the Americas, Europe, and parts of Asia. Thus, crops that are able to withstand such temperature shifts and regulate transpiration will be beneficial to farmers. Recent advances such as the inclusion of the submergence gene into rice seeds would aid the plant's survival in flood conditions (Xu et al., 2006). Typically, transplanted rice saplings die within a week of complete submergence. The sub1A gene helps rice saplings tolerate water and continue to grow when conditions are favorable. Other studies have shown that this gene also helps combat stress induced by leaf senescence (Fukao, Yeung & Bailey-Serres, 2012). In addition, inclusion of weed genes into plants is likely to help with the plant's survival in warmer climates. Red rice, a weedy plant, can take over when present in a rice plantation, especially in warmer climates with higher CO_2 levels present (Ziska et al., 2014). However, red rice seeds shatter on impact and the plant has very little use for agriculture today. The team at the United States Department of Agriculture (USDA) is working to transfer some of the positive attributes of red rice to regular rice to enable farmers to adapt to a warmer climate (Ziska, Tomecek, & Gealy, 2014).

25.5.2 Are GMO's Necessary to Feed the World?

Even small individual dietary changes from a primarily meat-based to a plant-based diet, by a large group of consumers, would help reduce resource utilization (land, energy, water) and slow down GHG emission. As discussed, this would involve converting land designated for animal feed to grow cereals, pulses, grains, and other plants for direct human consumption. In such a scenario, sustainable protein-rich crops would become available for more people globally. In addition, proper storage and utilization of such crops would further support large sectors of people who go hungry each day.

However, as the planet deals with climate change and unpredictable weather patterns, farmers do require plants to withstand harsh variations in temperatures, water, and CO_2 conditions. In these cases, both traditional and genetic engineering would be required to create new seeds or saplings. Introduction of genes such as sub1A raises the inevitable questions on genetic modification. This issue is very divisive and proponents argue that modification of genes is critical to develop higher-yielding and disease-resistant crops. However, opponents contend that some of the chemicals that the seeds are resistant for have harmful effects on critical organs. In addition, there is concern that these modified crops are monoculture-based and that genes can transfer to other nearby crops. Consumers, scientists, and policy officials must debate the topic of genetic modification. Advancements in science are critical in the broad goal to feeding the expanding global populace. We can turn to heirloom seeds or traditional grafting methods to develop new plants. Genetic modifications may be a necessary tool to produce varieties that are able to tolerate harsh weather conditions. Rather than viewing GMOs as negative, transparency by organizations that employ genetic modification or incorporate GMOs into products (with labeling as such), consumer education, and vigorous debates should occur as we enter a critical phase for the planet.

25.6 REDUCTION IN FOOD WASTE

Together with production intensification, sparing our perishable foods and crops is a critical element of sustainability and feeding a growing population. Food wastage at and post-farm accounts for a third of our outputs, which equates to about 1.3 billion tons annually, worldwide. Two hundred and thirty million tons of this waste is from developed countries (UNEP, 2013). In addition, 50% of the water used is lost due to food thrown away (FAO, 2011). Wastage contributes to inefficiencies with energy, land, fertilizer, labor, and all inputs at each stage of food production. A recent study found that the annual cost of food wasted in the United States is nearly $160 billion (Neff, Spiker, & Truant, 2015). Wasted food ends up in garbage dumps and contributes to the GHG emission from landfills. Rather, proper food management would reduce this waste and or/benefit those who currently suffer from hunger and malnutrition.

Wastage also occurs due to a variety of postharvest losses due to spoilage, pests, and improper or insufficient storage conditions. In the developing world, food waste occurs prior to processing. This is especially true in parts of Asia and southern Africa, regions that can ill afford to let food go to waste. Unless well controlled, temperatures and humidity in these regions are ideal for the growth of microorganisms or pests leading to loss of crops, produce and grains. In developed economies, adequate storage, refrigeration, packaging, and processing facilities ensure that there is more than enough food available. Food waste in these countries occurs mostly from processing and packaging issues with food that has already been prepared. Furthermore, large portion sizes, large volumes of inexpensive and unhealthy food, and potential lawsuits of donating unused foods to the needy, are contributory factors to todayontributory ffood wastage (Godfray et al., 2010).

Food waste can occur due to cosmetic defects at the farm level such as misshapen fruits and vegetables, considered unappealing to fussy consumers. A Canada-based organization, *Second Harvest* (http://www.secondharvest.ca/), revisits fields to recover crops left unharvested and distributes the would-be wasted crops to grocery retailers and restaurant outlets. Such missions also help population groups who may otherwise not have been able to afford nutritious food.

Unequal socioeconomic conditions exist even in developed countries. This situation can lead to poverty, the consequences of which for many are unhealthy food choices. In fact, many poor people are obese in the United States as foods with high calories from sugar and fat are often the main sources of sustenance (National Geographic, 2014b). Food deserts (defined by the USDA as urban neighborhoods and rural towns without ready access to fresh, healthy, and affordable food) exist in many areas. Populations in food deserts subsist on unhealthy food options. According to USDA estimates, nearly 23.5 million people in the United States live in food deserts, of which about 57% are low-income residents. Caught in a cyclic pattern, poverty increases food deserts, while food deserts increase unhealthy food choices and poor lifestyles. At the same time, the food situation is still dire in developing countries and emerging economies. Around 800 million people consume less than adequate food according to the United Nations World Food Programme (http://www.wfp.org/). As this number is likely to increase in the coming decades, progress in food production management and distribution, portion control, and reduction of food waste is even more critical.

Advances in science can help increase the shelf life of products, especially perishables, through improvements in packaging, processing, and natural preservatives. This will help reduce food wastage. Prudent buying of groceries, on an as-needed basis, is also in greater practice in several parts of the globe. Food deserts may be addressed by initiating community gardens and mobilizing markets and food storage units where needed. Resolving issues of food waste at the same time moving to healthier options will help to make food production more sustainable.

25.7 USING MICROBIOMES TO OUR ADVANTAGE

Our intestinal microbiome is comprised of various microorganisms. The inhabitants of this microbiome are highly diverse and dynamic in nature and assist in completing the digestion process. Five bacterial phyla including *Firmicutes*, *Bacteroidetes*, *Actinobacteria*, *Proteobacteria*, and *Verrucomicrobia* dominate gut microbial communities, with up to 90% of species belonging to the first two (Neis, Dejong, & Rensen, 2015). Western-style diets have been implicated in altering the type of microorganisms and consequently the metabolic activity in the gut. This altered activity is thought to contribute to chronic illnesses including obesity, insulin resistance, and inflammatory bowel diseases. Impaired short- and long-term memories have been correlated to an increase in Clostridiales and a reduction in Bacteriodales. The gut microbiome is vital for our normal functioning from an infant stage and maintaining the balance of good bacteria to bad bacteria is critical (Voreades, Kozil, & Weir, 2014). With the spread of Western diets to other parts of the globe, chronic illness may become rampant in the future (CNN, 2015; Popkin, Adair, & Ng, 2012).

Wu et al. (2011) showed diet dependence on the metabolites of gut microbiota. Depending on the type of diet, either *Bacteroides* (Western), or *Prevotella* (low protein) dominated the bowels. A recent study showed that the composition of the diet readily alters the human gut microbiome (David et al., 2014). When participants of the study went on an animal-protein-based diet and then switched to a plant-based diet, the microbial community structure changed. Bile secretions (which breakdown fats) increased with intake of foods rich in meat and dairy fats. *Bilophilia* and *Bacteroides* thrive in such environments and their numbers increase significantly resulting in a decrease in populations of *Firmicutes*, which can digest plant polysaccharides. Alteration of the microbiome with a reduction in friendly *Firmicutes* bacteria, and an increase in *Bilophilia* leading to inflammation in the bowel, can occur within a few days of switching diets. A recent study of mice found that high-sugar diets affect cognitive function (Magnusson et al., 2015). These results clearly illustrate the critical role of microorganisms in our gut for our health and well-being.

As a corollary, it would be a panacea if gut microbiomes influence our eating habits. For instance, weight loss-associated changes due to shifts in the dominance of gut bacterial community species have been demonstrated in both obese human subjects and animal studies. Rather than advocating to consumers to eat certain foods, can bacteria in the colon aid in the selection of healthy foods? Studies have found that bacteria can influence our food habits (Alcock, Maley, & Aktipis, 2014). Cravings for fried foods or high-sugar products can be mood-driven, and in fact, our moods affect the foods we eat (Harvard Health Publication, 2012). Thus, our microbiome can create signals via the nervous system to alter our moods and consequently our food choices. This mechanism provides an opportunity to harness the microbiome to shape our food choices. If the microbiome can affect our moods or cravings, can they alter our desire to like certain foods? Bacteria differ greatly in their requirements for food sources and nutrients. This requirement may be fully utilized in creating specific environments within the gut, which may harbor certain kinds of microbial population. Enriching certain foods with specific nutrients (prebiotics) that harbor and/or propagate specific, healthy microflora (probiotics) is one such possibility. A potential outcome of further developments in microbiomes may perhaps change people's dietary habits towards environmentally friendly food selections.

25.8 SUSTAINABLE FUTURE POPULATIONS

An equally critical step that would be required on our part would be to alter the projected increase in population. Global population was around 2 billion in the 1920s, and grew to 5 billion in the 1980s. The growth rate, aided by a reduction in infant mortality and advances in medicine, is adding to the populace at a staggering pace. Every 13–14 years, another billion people are beginning their lives on the planet. It is important that these new residents have adequate access to education, jobs, healthcare, and natural resources required to thrive.

"Population, when unchecked, increases in a geometrical ratio. Subsistence on the other hand increases only in an arithmetical ratio" (Thomas Malthus, 1766–1834). We are consuming global resources at an alarming rate, including water, land, and energy. Needs for infrastructure in emerging countries are skyrocketing beyond capabilities to build them. Several countries go without power, clean water, and many other facilities that people in developed countries take for granted. Without access to necessities, disparities in many aspects are increasing between developed and emerging countries. This chasm could reach a tipping point in the near future leading to major strife and revolution.

In order to have a sustainable planet, Western and other affluent countries will need to reduce meat consumption. Concurrently, it is imperative that emerging economies (especially South Asia, South East Asia, and sub-Saharan Africa), address the rapid population growth. Population projections suggest that the number of people inhabiting the earth will be 9.6–12.3 billion by 2100 (http://news.nationalgeographic.com/news/2014/09/140918-population-global-united-nations-2100-boom-africa/). People need food, resources, and necessities, which cause more GHG emissions. Consequently, it is vital to resolve this issue for a sustainable planet. We cannot leave population control to mere discussions and hope that things will work out. "We have been God-like in our planned breeding of our domesticated plants and animals, but we have been rabbit-like in our unplanned breeding of ourselves" (Arnold Toynbee, 1899–1975). An extensive modeling study indicated that even strict population controls and catastrophes would still leave the earth with a population between 5 and 10 billion people by 2100 (Bradshaw & Brook, 2014). The authors evaluated models ranging from "the current path we are on" to scenarios that included major calamities affecting the earth. None of the scenarios reduced the global population below 5 billion people. The authors concluded that since the population figures did not budge much, the best path forward would be to preserve our natural resources. Some recent papers though, have questioned the lumping of countries as equal that led to the modeling results. In reality, large-scale epidemics or major calamities may affect the world in unforeseen ways and regardless of challenges to this model the projected number of people remaining on earth in 2100 is unsustainable.

25.9 MORAL OBLIGATIONS AND QUESTIONS PEOPLE NEED TO DEBATE

The world population will reach 10 billion in the next 30 years barring a major catastrophe to strike the earth. Ten billion is 30% more than our current global population, which is already twice the number of people that the earth can support (Global Footprint Network: http://www.footprintnetwork.org/en/index.php/GFN/). Producing and feeding this many people will be an enormous task. Humanity will have to figure out whether one group can have an abundance of food, while other people go hungry. Numerous questions need to be considered and addressed. Can Western societies continue on a diet high in meat, or should land used for animal feed be shifted to cultivate protein-rich crops for a vast majority? Is genetic modification of crops essential for increasing yields? If more people in Western societies convert to predominately plant-based diets, will there be more food to supply all? Can we prevent the spread of Western diets to rapidly growing affluent economies? "No one saves us but ourselves. No one and no one may. We ourselves must walk the path" (Lord Buddha, 563−483 BCE).

Natural resources are depleting at a rapid rate, which will continue as another 3 billion people join in the coming decades. The use of these resources is a contributory factor for increased GHG from human activities including farming. The need for food management has never been greater, and fresh water is likely to become an invaluable commodity. As we grapple with this challenge, can research identify methods to grow more food using fewer resources? States in India are claiming ownership of water from their territories. Similar activism is rising in the Sacramento delta, United States, to question the need for water to flow into the southern valley. How will governments or countries handle such disputes as the planet becomes warmer? Will subsidies continue to influence farming?

There are huge disparities between developed and developing economies, although the former has been built upon the latter. A majority of the world's population will reside in the developing and emerging economies, which will likely have reduced access to a wide variety of facilities including education, jobs, healthcare, and infrastructure. Can the

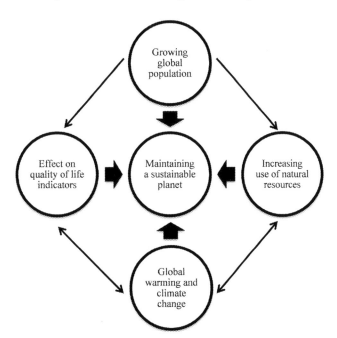

FIGURE 25.2 Depiction of the effects of population growth and their related effects.

earth sustain this vast proliferation of humanity? A report from the United Nations Organization (http://www.un.org/press/en/2013/dev3008.doc.htm) indicates that over 6 billion will reside in an urbanized setting by 2050. Will this continued inequality lead to strife? Will there be large migrations of people fleeing to "greener" pastures? Alternatively, will people come together and sacrifice for the common good? People in developed economies may be able to withstand disruptions to current behaviors as compared to those in emerging economies. If we continue on our current path of high meat consumption, rapid destruction of our natural resources, leading to a warmer earth and food production limitations, will the United Nations intervene to assist poorer countries? Will the global population be subject to broad mandatory guidelines? Will consumers make proper choices and sacrifice for the long-term sustainability of the planet? Each of these factors discussed above are interlinked (Fig. 25.2), and people need to change many of their current habits for the planet to be sustainable for future generations.

The authors who have contributed to this book have a common desire to make a difference for a sustainable planet. They have also dedicated their life's work to the considerate pursuit of feeding people. We have discussed the current state of the planet, especially with respect to issues with food and food proteins and their relationship to a future state. A spirited debate of these difficult issues will require action as the planet inches towards a critical stage. However, consequences of not changing our current path are likely to be grim. "The greater the obstacle, the more glory in overcoming it" (Moliere, 1622–73). Let us make a courageous choice to change course.

DISCLAIMER

The views and opinions expressed in this chapter are those of the authors and do not reflect the official policy or position of the affiliated organizations.

REFERENCES

Abraham, B., Araya, H., Berhe, T., Edwards, S., Gujja, B., Khadka, R. B., ... Verma, A. (2014). The system of crop intensification: Reports from the field on improving agricultural production, food security, and resilience to climate change for multiple crops. *Agriculture and Food Security*, *3*, 4. Available from http://dx.doi.org/10.1186/2048-7010-3-4.

AHDB Dairy. (2015). *World dairy cow numbers.* <http://dairy.ahdb.org.uk/market-information/farming-data/cow-numbers/world-cow-numbers/#.VgaWfMiISm4>.

Alcock, J., Maley, C. C., & Aktipis, C. A. (2014). Is eating behavior manipulated by the gastrointestinal microbiota? Evolutionary pressures and potential mechanisms. *Bioessays*, *36*, 940–949.

Asgar, M. A., Fazilah, A., Huda, N., Bhat, R., & Karim, A. A. (2010). Non-meat protein alternatives as meat extenders and meat analogs. *Comprehensive Reviews in Food Science and Food Safety*, *9*, S13–S30.

Assadi, E., Janmoammadi, H., Taghizadeh, A., & Alijani, S. (2011). Nutrient composition of different varieties of full-fat canola seed and nitrogen-corrected true metabolizable energy of full-fat canola seed with or without enzyme addition and thermal processing. *Journal of Applied Poultry Research*, *20*, 95–101.

Bradshaw, C. J. A., & Brook, B. W. (2014). Human population reduction is not a quick fix for environmental problems. *Proceedings of the National Academy of Sciences of the United States of America*, *11*(46), 16610–16615.

Bruinsma, J. (2003). *World agriculture towards 2015/2030: An FAO perspective.* London: EarthScan Publication Ltd.. p. 430. <ftp://ftp.fao.org/docrep/fao/005/y4252E/y4252e.pdf>.

CNN. (2015). *Step away from the burger: Why a "Western diet" is bad for your health.* <http://www.cnn.com/2015/07/07/health/western-diet-health/>.

David, L. A., Maurice, C. F., Carmody, R. N., Gootenberg, D. B., Button, J. E., Wolfe, B. E., ... Turnbaugh, P. J. (2014). Diet rapidly and reproducibly alters the human gut microbiome. *Nature*, *505*(7484), 559–563.

de Boer, J., Boersema, J. J., & Aiking, H. (2009). Consumers' motivational associations favoring free-range meat or less meat. *Ecological Economics*, *68*, 850–860.

Delimaris, I. (2013). Adverse effects associated with protein intake above the recommended dietary allowance for adults. *ISRN Nutrition*, . ID 126929, 6 p. http://dx.doi.org/10.5402/2013/126929

FAO. (2011). *Food wastage footprint. Impacts on natural resources.* <http://www.fao.org/docrep/018/i3347e/i3347e.pdf>.

Fukao, T., Yeung, E., & Bailey-Serres, J. (2012). The submergence tolerance gene SUB1A delays leaf senescence under prolonged darkness through hormonal regulation in rice. *Plant Physiology*, *160*, 1795–1807.

Godfray, H. C. J., Beddington, J. R., Crute, I. R., Haddard, L., Lawrence, D., Muir, J. F., ... Toulmin, C. (2010). Food security: The challenge of feeding 9 billion people. *Science*, *237*, 812–818.

Guardian. (2010). *UN urges global move to meat, and dairy free diet.* <http://www.theguardian.com/environment/2010/jun/02/un-report-meat-free-diet>.

Harvard Health Publication. (2012). *How stress can make us overeat.* <http://www.health.harvard.edu/healthbeat/>.

Hsieh, F. -H., & Huff, H. E. (2012). *Meat analog compositions and process*. US patent 20120093994 A1.
IEEE Spectrum. (2013). *The better meat substitute*. <http://spectrum.ieee.org/energy/environment/the-better-meat-substitute>.
Kang, Q., Appel, L., Tan, T., & Dewil, R. (2014). Bioethanolfrom lignocellulosic biomass: Current findings determine research priorities. *The Scientific World Journal*, . ID 298153. 13 p. http://dx.doi.org/10.1155/2014/298153
Khan, M., Khan, S. S., Ahmed, Z., & Tanveer, A. (2010). Production of single cell protein from *Saccharomyces cerevisiae* by utilizing fruit wastes. *Nanobiotechnica Universale*, *1*(2), 127−132.
Magnusson, K. R., Hauck, L., Jeffrey, B. M., Elias, V., Humphrey, A., Nath, R., ... Bermudez, L. E. (2015). Relationships between diet-related changes in the gut microbiome and cognitive flexibility. *Neuroscience*, *300*, 128−140.
Nasseri, A. T., Rasoul-Amini, S., Morowvat, M. H., & Ghasemi, Y. (2011). Single cell protein: Production and processes. *American Journal of Food Technology*, *6*, 103−116.
National Geographic. (2014a). *The next breadbasket* (pp. 29−49).
National Geographic. (2014b). *The new face of hunger* (pp. 51−71).
Neff, R. A., Spiker, M. L., & Truant, P. L. (2015). Wasted food: U.S. consumers' reported awareness, attitudes, and behaviors. *PLoS One*, *10*(6), e0127881. Available from http://dx.doi.org/10.1371/journal.pone.0127881.
Neis, E. P. J. G., Dejong, C. H. C., & Rensen, S. S. (2015). The role of microbial amino acid metabolism in host metabolism. *Nutrients*, *7*, 2930−2946.
Pimentel, D., & Pimentel, M. (2003). Sustainability of meat-based and plant diets and the environment. *American Journal of Clinical Nutrition*, *78* (Suppl.), 660S−663S.
Popkin, B. M., Adair, L. S., & Ng, S. W. (2012). Now and then: The global nutrition transition: The pandemic of obesity in developing countries. *Nutrition Reviews*, *70*(1), 3−21.
Przednowek, D. W. A., Entz, M. H., Irvine, B., Flaten, D. N., & Thiessen-Martens, J. R. (2004). Rotational yield and apparent N benefits of grain legumes in southern Manitoba. *Canadian Journal of Plant Science*, *84*, 1093−1096.
Roush, W. (2014). *Modern Meadow grazes on $10M to grow leather without cows*. Retrieved from: <http://www.xconomy.com/new-york/2014/06/18/modern-meadow-grazes-on-10m-to-grow-leather-without-cows/> Accessed November 2015.
Sabate, J., & Soret, S. (2014). Sustainability of plant-based diets. *American Journal of Clinical Nutrition*, *100*(Suppl.), 476S−482S.
Sans, P., & Combris, P. (2015). World meat consumption patterns: An overview of the last fifty years (1961−2011). *Meat Science*, *109*, 106−111.
Scarborough, P., Appleby, P. N., Mizdrak, A., Briggs, A. D. M., Travis, R. C., Bradbury, K. E., & Key, T. J. (2014). Dietary greenhouse gas emissions of meat-eaters, fish-eaters, vegetarians and vegans in the UK. *Climatic Change*, *125*(2), 179−192. Available from http://dx.doi.org/10.1007/s10584-014-1169-1.
Schösler, H., de Boer, J., & Boersema, J. J. (2012). Can we cut out the meat of the dish? Constructing consumer-oriented pathways towards meat substitution. *Appetite*, *58*, 39−47.
Science Daily (2014). *Vegetarian diets produce fewer greenhouse gases and increase longevity*. Loma Linda University Medical Center. June 25. <www.sciencedaily.com/releases/2014/06/140625145536.htm>.
Serraj, R., & Adu Gyampi, J. (2004). Role of symbiotic nitrogen fixation in the improvement of legume productivity under stressed environments. *West African Journal of Applied Ecology*, *6*(1), 95−109.
Shurtleff, W., & Aoyagi, A. (2014). *History of meat alternatives: 965 CE to 2014*. Laffayette, CA: Soy Information Centre, p. 1437.
Smil, V. (2002). Nitrogen and food production: Proteins for human diets. *Ambio*, *31*, 126−131.
UNEP. (2013). *Food waste facts*. <http://www.unep.org/wed/2013/quickfacts/>.
Voreades, N., Kozil, A., & Weir, T. L. (2014). Diet and the development of the human intestinal microbiome. *Frontiers in Microbiology*, *5*, 494. Available from http://dx.doi.org/10.3389/fmicb.2014.00494.
Wu, G. D., Chen, J., Hoffmann, C., Bittinger, K., Chen, Y.-Y., Keilbaugh, S. A., ... Lewis, J. D. (2011). Linking long-term dietary patterns with gut microbial enterotypes. *Science*, *334*(6052), 105−108. Available from http://dx.doi.org/10.1126/science.1208344.
Xu, K., Xu, X., Fukao, T., Canlas, P., Maghirang-Rodriguez, R., Heuer, S., ... Mackill, D. J. (2006). Sub1A is an ethylene-response-factor-like gene that confers submergence tolerance to rice. *Nature*, *442*, 705−708.
Ziska, L. H., Tomecek, M. B., & Gealy, D. R. (2014). Assessment of cultivated and wild, weedy rice lines to concurrent changes in CO_2 concentration and air temperature: Determining traits for enhanced seed yield with increasing atmospheric CO_2. *Functional Plant Biology*, *41*, 236−243.

Index

Note: Page numbers followed by "*f*" and "*t*" refer to figures and tables, respectively.

A

ABTS (2,2'-azino-bis(3 ethylbenzothiazoline-6-sulfonic acid)), 275
2-Acetyl-1-pyrroline (2-AP), 57–58
Acheta domestica, 345
Acheta domesticus, 343–344, 348–349
Acid detergent fiber (ADF) content, 346
Aflatoxin, 217
Africa Biofortified Sorghum project, 97
African legumes. *See* Bambara groundnut; Marama beans
Agricultural subsidies, 404
Agriculture and climate change, 416
AGT Foods, 187–188
Air classification technology, 187–188
Air impact blanching, 215
Air lift fermentation, 308–309, 308*f*
Air-classified pea protein, 149*f*
Air-classified pea starch, 150*f*
Albumins, 2–3, 242–243
    2S albumin, 125, 227–228, 296
    antioxidative activity, 59
    hemp seed, 124
    lentil, 187
    rice, 52
Alcalase hydrolysis, 247–248
Alkaloids, in lupins, 172–173
Allergenicity
    of bambara groundnut, 204
    of canola/rapeseed (C/RS) proteins, 296
    of flaxseed proteins, 139
    and food protein, 5
    of hemp seed, 125
    of lentil proteins, 189
    of lupin, 174
    of marama beans, 200–201
    of peanut, 219
    of pea proteins, 154
    of quinoa, 230
    of rice proteins, 55–57
    of wheat proteins, 73
Allergies, protein, 38–39
α-amylase, in rice, 54, 58–59
α-amylase inhibitor, 58
α-amylase/subtilisin inhibitor, 58–59
α-amylase/trypsin inhibitor, 58–59
α-galactosides, 178
Alphitobius diaperinus, 344, 349
Amaranth, 239, 410*t*
amaranth proteins and amino acids for human nutrition, 242–243
antioxidant capacities of amaranth peptides, 247–248
bioactive peptides related to antihypertensive functions, 244–247
food applications of, 262–263
genetic engineering of amaranth proteins, 249–251
main storage protein fractions, 242*t*
nutritional components in, 240–242
potential uses of amaranth proteins in food industry, 248–249
processing of, 260–262
    milling and fractionation, 260–261
    wet milling for production of starch-rich, fiber-rich, or protein-rich fractions, 261–262
proximate composition of, 245*f*
Amaranth hydrolysates, 249
Amaranth production, sustainability of, 257–260
    harvesting, 259
    land, water, and energy uses, 258–259
    origin and distribution, 257
    postharvest processing, 259–260
    production and yield, 257–258
    production cost, 260
    SEM picture of single amaranth grain, 261*f*
Amaranthus caudatus, 239, 240*t*, 257
Amaranthus cruentus, 239, 240*t*, 257
Amaranthus hypochondriacus, 239, 240*t*, 244–245, 249–250, 257
Amaranthus mantegazzianus, 262
Amaranthus mantegazzium, 244
Amaranthus manteggazianus, 247–248
Amarantin, 243
Amarantin gene, 250–251
Amino acid composition, 71–72
    of canola/rapeseed (C/RS), 292–293
    of commercial rice products, 56*t*
    of different amaranth species, 241*t*
    of flaxseed protein, 138*t*
    of flour and isolated globulin from chia seeds, 272*t*
    of lentil compared, 186*t*
    of lupin varieties, 170*t*
    of peanuts and peanut products, 218*t*
    of proteins in quinoa, 227*t*
    of soy protein products, 34*t*
Amino acids (AAs), 1–2, 240–242, 360
    in chia, 269–274
    in chia seeds, 271
    depiction of, 2*f*
    in edible insects, 345
    for human nutrition, 242–243
    in peanuts, 217–218, 218*t*
Anaphe panda, 344
Angiotensin I-converting enzyme, 60, 271–272
    inhibition, 298
Angiotensin-converting enzyme, 129–131, 244–247
Animal feeding experiments, 228
Animal Protein Sources, 410*t*
Antihypertensive functions, bioactive peptides related to, 244–247
Antinutrients, 84–86, 364
Antinutritional factors
    in canola/rapeseed (C/RS), 294–295
        carbohydrates and fiber, 295
        glucosinolates, 294–295
        phenolics, 295
        phytates, 295
    in lupin, 172–174
    in quinoa, 230
    in rice, 58–59, 173*t*
        enzyme inhibitors, 58–59
        enzymes, 58
Astringency, 379
    modulation, 384
Avenins, 107, 109

B

Bacteroides, 418
Bambara groundnut, 197, 202–206
    allergenicity, 204
    antinutritive factors, 204
    composition of, 203
    current and future uses and applications, 204–205
    issues and challenges, 205–206
    land use, 202–203
    nutritive value, 204
    off-tastes associated with, 205
    protein isolation, 203–204
    proteins, 199*t*, 203
    sustainability of, 202–203
    water use, 202–203

Batters, application of lupin protein concentrate in, 176
Beef, 27, 320, 409–411, 410t
β-conglycinin, 26
Bifidobacteria, 178, 364
Big food manufacturers, relevance of, 415
Bilophilia, 418
Bioactive peptides
  from chia seeds, 273f
  related to antihypertensive functions, 244–247
Bioethanol production, 95–96
Bitter taste, 379
  modulation, 384
Black beans, 410t
Black fonio, 81t, 82, 88t
Black soldier fly, 345
Blanching, 215
Blood glucose level, lupin and, 178–179
Blood pressure, reduction of
  chia and, 273–274
  lupin and, 179
Bloodwood apples, 342
Blue water, 13
Blue water footprint, 30, 32t
Body mass index (BMI), 364
Bowel function, lupin and, 178
Brachytrupes sp., 348
Branched-chain amino acids (BCAA), 71–72
Brassica juncea, 285, 296
Brassica napus, 285, 288, 294, 296, 298–299
Brassica rapa, 285, 296
Brassicaceae seeds, 296
Brewing and bioethanol production, 95–96
Broccoli, 382–383
Brown rice, 410t
Bush coconuts, 342
Buying point, 214

C

C3 crops, 416
C4 photosynthesis, 258
Calories, in peanuts, 216
Canola/rapeseed (C/RS), 283, 410t
  allergenicity of, 296
  amino acid composition of canola meal and protein products, 293t
  antinutritional factors of, 294–295
    carbohydrates and fiber, 295
    glucosinolates, 294–295
    phenolics, 295
    phytates, 295
  applications and current products, 297
    potential food applications as protein supplements or bulk proteins, 297
  chemical composition of the seed, 286–288
  functional properties of protein products, 296–297
    emulsifying properties, 296–297
    foaming properties, 297
    heat-induced gel formation ability, 297
    solubility, 296
  issues and challenges, 299
    new uses, 298–299
      bioactive peptides, 298–299
  nutritional value, 292–294
    amino acid composition, 292–293
    digestibility in human and animal models and the processing effects, 293–294
  off-tastes associated with using oilseed proteins, 299–300
  processes of protein product preparation, 289–292
    aqueous alkaline conditions, involving, 290–291
    chromatographic separation, 291
    combination of chemical and physical methods, 292
    processes targeting specific seed protein types/fractions, 291–292
    protein micelle mass formation, 291
    significant considerations, 289–290
    solubility-based separation, 291–292
  production of, 285–286
    energy use, 286
    land use, 286
    water use, 286
  protein types of, 288–289
    cruciferin, 288
    minor proteins, 289
    napin, 288
Carbohydrates, 240–242
  and fiber, 295
  in lupin, 170–171
  in peanuts, 216
  in quinoa, 229
Carbon footprint, 211t, 331f, 332
  of soy protein, 28–30
Carbon Reduction Label, 318
Carboxypeptidases, 58
Cardiovascular disease (CVD), 363
Cardiovascular health, soy protein and, 36–37
Caseinate, 30
Catalase (CAT), 275
Caterpillars, 342–343
Celiac disease, 73, 110
Cereals, 7, 68–69, 105–106, 201, 240t, 364, 410t
Chapul, 349
Chenopodin, 227–228
Chenopodium quinoa Willd. *See* Quinoa
Chia, 265, 410t
  antioxidant properties, 276
  consumption of, 267–268
  functional benefits, 276–277
  future of chia seeds, 277–278
  health benefits, 276
  main storage protein fractions of chia seeds, 270t
  nutritional value, 268–275
    fiber, 268
    lipids, 268
    phenolic compounds, 268
    polyphenols, oil, and peptides with antioxidant capacity, 274–275
    protein content and amino acids, 269–274
    obtaining bioactive peptides from chia seeds, 273f
  phenolic compounds' concentration in chia seeds, 269t
  sustainability of, 265–267
    energy use, 267
    land use, 266
    production, 265–266
    water use, 266–267
  world production of chia seed, 267t
Chicken, 320, 397
China-Cornell-Oxford Project, 8
Chitin, in edible insects, 346
Chlorella, 327, 333–335, 338, 410t
Chlorella protothecoides, 335
Chlorella pyrenoidosa, 335, 338
Chlorella vulgaris, 335, 338
Cholecystokinin (CCK), 298, 366
Cholecystokinin-1 (CCK-1) receptor, 298
Cholesterol reduction
  lupin and, 178
  rice protein extraction and, 59
  soy protein and, 37, 37f
Choline, 288
Chronic kidney disease (CKD)
  hemp seed proteins and, 128
Chymotrypsin inhibitors, 152
Climate change, 10–11, 14, 383, 386
  adaptation and resilience, 333
  and peanut production, 209–211
Climate Change Treaty, 412
CO_2 levels, effects of
  in atmosphere, 14
Cocoa powder, 384
Complex proteins. *See* Conjugated proteins
Conjugated proteins, 3
Consumer, 377–378
  acceptance, 336
  role of, 16
  trends, 415
Consumption patterns, change in, 411
Cooking, effect of
  on proteins, 92–93, 154, 360
Corn, proximate composition of, 240t
Corn soy blend, 97
Coronary heart disease (CHD), 363
Cradle to cradle approach, 323
Cradle-to-gate lifecycle assessment scope, 330f, 330t
Crickets (*Acheta domesticus* and *Brachytrupes* sp.), 348, 410t
Crop adaptation, 416
Cruciferin, 288, 291, 299
Crude protein content, 345
Cultural influence on food choices, 380–382
Cyanogenesis, 200
Cyanogenic glycosides, 200
Cyclodextrins, 384
Cysteine proteinases, in rice, 58
Cystococcus pomiformis, 342

D

Damage kernels (DK), 214
De Hobbit, 177

Deamidases, 113
Deamidation, 113, 385
Defatted flaxseed meal (DFM), 134–135
Defatted flour, 125–126
Defatted soy flour, manufacturing process of, 25f
Degree of milling (DM), 50
Dehuller, 148, 148f
Desalination, 13
Devitalized wheat gluten, 69
Diet change, challenges with, 413
Diet change, consumers, and policies, 412
Dietary fiber, 152, 158–159, 170–171, 229, 268, 314
Dietary patterns around the globe, 8–9
Dietary protein flow, 2f
Direct land use changes, 30
Dispensable amino acids, 4
Distillers' dried grains and solubles (DDGS), 95–96
Domestic house fly (*Musca domestica*), 345
DPPH (2,2-diphenyl-1-picrylhydrazyl), 274
DPPH radical scavenging, 129
Dry blanching, 215
Dry milling technology, 148

E

Eating habits, shifting, 386
Edestin, 123–124
Egg replacement in baked goods, 175–176
Egg white proteins, 6–7
Emulsification activity index (EAI), 128
Emulsifying capacity (EC), 296–297
Emulsion activity index (EAI), 296–297
Emulsion stability (ES), 296–297
Energy use, 30
    amaranth, 258–259
    canola/rapeseed (C/RS), 286
    chia, 267
    flaxseed production, 135
    hemp cultivation, 122
    lentil production, 187
    lupin production, 167
    oat production, 106
    pea production, 146–147
    quinoa production, 225
    rice production, 49
    soy protein, 31
    wheat production, 68
Entomophagy, 347
Environmentally friendly food options, 413–415
    meat alternates, 413–414
    newer sources of protein, 414–415
Escherichia coli, 244–245, 250–251, 345, 348
Essential amino acid (EAA), 3, 110t, 200t, 226–227
Expanded bed adsorption (EBA)-ion exchange chromatography (IEC), 291
Extruded snacks, application of pea in, 160–161

F

Farmer incentives, 69
Farming insects, 344–345
Fat mimetics, 313
Fats
    in edible insects, 346
    in lupin, 170
    in mycoprotein, 314
    in peanuts, 216
Fatty acid
    in edible insects, 346
    in mycoprotein, 315t
Fava bean isolate (FPI), 175
Feed conversion ratio (FCR), 15
Fertilizers, 13–14
Fiber
    in chia, 268
    in mycoprotein, 314
    in quinoa, 229
Fibrous proteins, 3
Finger millet, 81t, 82, 86, 88t
Finola, 122–123
Flavor and taste, 378–379
    physiology of taste, 378–379
        astringency, 379
        bitter taste, 379
Flavors, binding of
    by proteins, 384–385
Flavors' role in modulating off-notes in protein-based products, 384
    astringency modulation, 384
    bitter taste modulation, 384
Flavourzyme, 54
Flax, 133
Flaxseed, ground, 410t
Flaxseed proteins
    application and current products, 140
    calmodulin (CaM)binding activity, 141
    commercially available products, 136t
    extraction, 135–138, 137t
    nutritive value of, 138–139
        allergenicity of, 139
        amino acids and proteins, 138–139
    oil absorption capacities (OAC), 140
    potential new uses, issues, and challenges, 141–142
    uses and functionality of, 139–140
Flaxseeds, 133
    chemical composition, 134
    processing of proteins and types of products from, 135–138
    sustainability of, 134–135
        energy use, 135
        land use, 134
        water use, 135
Food Allergen Labeling and Consumer Protection Act (FALCPA), 9
Food and diet, proteins and their role in, 1–8
    defining proteins, 2–4
        classification of proteins, 2–4
        structural levels, 2
        plant-derived protein and alternate protein sources, 7–8
        protein as a macromolecule, 5–7
        protein as a macronutrient, 4–5
        allergenicity and food protein, 5
Food choices, cultural influence on, 380–382
Food habits, changing, 385
Food production and consequences, 10f
Food security, 15–16
Food security and policy, 391
    growing homogeneity in global food supplies, 398–399
    livestock: facts and trends, 392–395
    rethinking food security, 395–398
    sociological pathways for more sustainable protein options, 399–405
Food waste, reduction in, 417
Foods, sustainable protein sources in, 383–385
    binding of flavors by proteins, 384–385
    off-tastes associated with plant proteins, 383–384
    role of flavors in modulating off-notes in protein-based products, 384
        astringency modulation, 384
        bitter taste modulation, 384
Foreign material (FM), 214
Fossil energy, 13–14
Foxtail millet, 81t, 82, 88t
Frank Products, 175–176
Freedom foods, 9–10
"Free-from" foods, 9
Fresh water, 12–13
Functional benefits, of chia, 276–277
Functional properties of proteins, 5–7, 6t
Functionality of food proteins, 5
Fungal fermentation technology, 306–309
    air lift fermentation, 308–309, 308f
Fusarium graminearum, 305
Fusarium venenatum, 305–306, 308

G

Galleria melonella, 349
γ-conglutin, 178–179
Gas-fired revolving drum ovens, 215
Gelation, 249
Genetically engineered modified (GE M) soybeans, 42
Genetically modified (GM) food, 299
Genetically modified organisms (GMOs), 416–417
Genetics and food choices, 380
Giant mealworm, 349
Gliadins, 72, 74
Global warming and climate change, 14
Globular proteins, 3, 384–385
Globulins, 2–3, 242–243, 270
    7S globulin, 243
    11S globulin, 108, 227–228, 243, 249, 270
    antioxidative activity, 60
    hemp seed, 123–124
    oat, 107–108
    of rice, 52
Glucosinolates, 294–295
Glutamine, 72
Glutathione (GHS), 275
Glutathione peroxidase (GPx), 275
Glutathione reductase (GRd), 275

Glutelins, 51–52, 242–243
  antioxidative activity, 60
  in rice, 53
Gluten
  in bread application, 74–75
  extraction from wheat, 70
  intolerance, 73
Gluten proteins of wheat, 6–7
Gluten-free foods, 9
Gluten-free products, 262–263
Glutenins, 69–70, 74
Glycine max. *See* Soy protein
Glycinin, 26
"Good-for-you" items, 9
Granular comminute texture, creation of, 313
Gray water, 13, 211
Gray water footprint, 32, 32t
Green water, 13, 211
Green water footprint, 32, 32t
Greenhouse gases (GHG), 10–11, 10f, 14–16
  emissions, 28, 209, 331–332, 343
Gryllus bimaculatus, 344–345, 348

H

Hamburger meat, 411
Harvesting, of amaranth, 259
Health and wellness trends, 9
Healthy diet, affording, 382
Hemp, 121
  cultivation
    energy use and cost, 122
    land use, 122
    water use, 122
  fiber, 121–122
  growing regions and yield, 121–122
  plant and seed, 122–123
  seed composition and protein quality, 123
  whole seed, 410t
Hemp seed protein hydrolysate (HPH), 129–131
Hemp seed protein isolate (HPI), 123–124, 127–128
Hemp seed proteins, 123–125
  albumin, 124
  allergenicity, 125
  bioactive properties of, 128–131
    antihypertensive, 129–131
    antioxidant, 129
    renal disease modulation, 128
  digestion of, 129
  functional properties of, 125–128
    defatted flour, 125–126
    protein concentrates, 126
    protein isolates, 127–128
  globulin, 123–124
  sulfur-rich proteins, 124–125
Hermetia illucens, 345
Hermetia illuscens, 345
Heterotrophic cultivation, 328
Heterotrophic microalgae, 327
  Chlorella classification, 327
  consumer acceptance, 336
  future developments, 337–338
  nutritional value, 333–334
  production, 327–329
  properties and applications of whole algae protein, 335–336
  safety, 335
  sustainability profile, 329–333
    climate change adaptation and resilience, 333
    low environmental impact, 330–333
    Solazyme Inc. (case study), 329
Hexane in soy milling, 33
High-density lipoprotein (HDL) cholesterol, 363
High-protein diets, 412
Histones, 2–3
Homogeneity, growing
  in global food supplies, 398–399
Honey, 342
House cricket (*Acheta domesticus*), 343–344
Housefly (*Musca domestica*), 348
Human feeding experiments, 228
Hummus, 415
Hydrophobic interaction chromatography (HIC), 291
Hyperglycemia, suppression of, 59
Hypertension, 179
  reduction in, 60
Hyphae
  interaction between, 311
  orientation and dispersion of, 311–312
Hyphal morphology, 311
Hyphal pressure, 312

I

Ice cream, 382–383
Imbrasia belina, 342
Indirect land use changes (ILUCs), 30
Insects, edible, 341
  consumer attitudes, 347–348
  environment, 343–344
  ethno-entomology, 342–343
  farming insects, 344–345
  food safety, 348–349
  legislation, 350–351
  nutrition, 345–346
    chitin, 346
    fats and fatty acids, 346
    minerals, 346
    protein content and amino acids, 345
    vitamins, 346
  processing and marketing, 349–350
Insects as food, 350–351
Intergovernmental Panel for Climate Change (IPCC), 28
International Congress on Andean Food Crops, 223
International Platform of Insects for Food and Feed (IPIFF), 351
Intolerance mechanism of wheat proteins, 73
Introduction of new foods and changing consumer habits, 385–386
Isoflavones
  in lupin, 179
  in soy foods, 38
Isolated soy protein (ISP), 23, 26, 39–40
  carbon footprint of, 28
  land use footprint of, 30
  manufacturing, 33
  manufacturing process, 24–26
  water use footprint of, 30
Isolates, quinoa protein concentrates (QPCs) and, 231–233

K

Kafirin, 87, 92, 99

L

Lactic acid fermentation, 94–95, 96t
Land efficiency, 333
Land use
  amaranth, 258–259
  bambara groundnut, 202–203
  canola/rapeseed (C/RS), 286
  chia, 266
  flaxseed production, 134
  hemp cultivation, 122
  lentil production, 185–186
  lupin production, 166
  mycoprotein, 321–322
  oat production, 105–106
  peanut production, 212
  quinoa production, 225
  rice production, 48
  wheat production, 67
Land-use efficiency, 82
Lectins (hemagglutinins), 152–153
Legumes, 28–29, 83, 96–97, 360, 363–364, 410t
Leguminosae, 360
Leguminous crops, 125, 416
Lentil, 185, 410t
  amino acid composition of, 186t
    effect of different cooking methods on, 190t
  applications and current products, 191–192
  sustainability of, 185–187
    diseases affecting lentil plant, 187
    energy use, 187
    land use, 185–186
    water use, 186
Lentil flour, off-flavors associated with, 193
Lentil proteins, 185, 187–188
  antinutritional factors and protein digestibility, 190–191
  characterization, 187
  functionality, 192
  health properties, 192–193
    bioactive peptides, 192–193
    chronic diseases, 193
  off-flavors associated with, 193
  processing into protein concentrates or isolates, 187–188
  quality, 189–190
Lesser mealworm (*Alphitobius diaperinus*), 344
Lethocerus indicus, 342

Life cycle assessment (LCA), 26−27, 209−212, 330
Linatine, 141
Linoleic acid, 216, 219, 240−242
Lipids
　in chia, 268
　in quinoa, 229
Lipoxygenase, 159, 202, 383
Lipoxygenase enzyme oxidation (Lox) of lipids, 41−42
Livestock, 392−395
Locusta migratoria, 343−344
Loose shelled kernels (LSK), 214
Low-density lipoprotein (LDL) cholesterol, 363
　soy protein and, 37
Lupeh, 177
Lupin, 165
　allergenicity, 174
　antinutritive factors, 172−174
　　alkaloids, 172−173
　　phytates and lectins, 172
　　raffinose family oligosaccharides, 173−174
　application/current products, 175−176
　　in batters, 176
　　bakery applications, 175
　　egg replacement in baked goods, 175−176
　cultivation of *Lupinus* species, 165−166
　current food products, 176−177
　　nutritional applications, 176−177
　food (protein) dependence of the EU, 168
　health aspects of, 177−179
　　blood pressure, 179
　　bowel function, 178
　　cholesterol, 178
　　satiety and blood glucose level, 178−179
　nutritive value, 169−171
　　carbohydrates, 170−171
　　evaluation of protein quality and digestibility, 171
　　fats, 170
　　heavy metals, 171
　　minerals, 171
　　protein, 170
　off-tastes, 174
　processing of, 168−169
　　concentrate, 168−169
　　flour, 168
　　isolates, 169
　sustainability of, 166−167
　　energy use, 167
　　land use, 166
　　water use, 166−167
　uses and functionality, 174−175
　　lupin flour, 174−175
　　lupin protein concentrate, 175
　　lupin protein isolate, 175
Lupin Foods, 177
Lupin kernel fiber, 178−179
Lupin protein, 170
Lupin protein isolates (LPIs), 169, 175−176
Lupine, 410t
Lupinus angustifolius, 170
Lysine, 84, 109, 160−161, 292−293

M

Macrobrachium spp., 348
Macronutrient in food, protein as, 4−5
Maillard reaction products, 57−58, 228, 384
Main storage protein fractions
　of amaranth species, 242t
　of chia seeds, 270t
Malonaldehyde (MDA), 141
Malting, 93−94, 95t
Marama beans, 197−202
　allergenicity, 200−201
　antinutritive factors, 200−201
　composition of, 199
　current and future uses and applications, 201
　issues and challenges, 202
　marama proteins, composition of, 199, 199t
　nutritive value, 200−201
　off-tastes associated with, 202
　protein isolation, 199
Mealworms, 343, 346, 348
Meat alternates, 413−414
Meat and meat analogs, application of pea in, 161
Meat consumption, 12, 15−16, 318, 368−369, 385, 411
Meat replacement, 40, 367−369
　changing the diet of a nation, 368−369
　complexity of food choice, 367−368
　decreasing meat consumption, 369
Meat-based diets, 8, 12, 377, 412
Microalgae, 327−329, 334
Microbiomes, 417−418
Micronutrients
　in peanuts, 218−219
　in quinoa, 229−230
Migratory locust (*Locusta migratoria*), 343−344
Milk, 15, 201, 205, 410t
Millets, 79, 383−384, 410t
Minerals
　in edible insects, 346
　in lupin, 171
　in mycoprotein, 315−316, 315t
　in pea, 152
　in quinoa, 229
Minor proteins, 109, 289
Monogastrics, 395
Monounsaturated fatty acids (MUFAs), 346
2MRP (methionine-rich proteins), 242−243
Mucilage, 135−136, 139, 276
Musca domestica, 345, 348
Muscle protein synthesis (MPS)
　soy protein and, 35
Mycoprotein, 305, 410t
　amino acid analysis of, 314t
　cradle to cradle approach, 323
　creation of granular comminute texture, 313
　and creation of meat-like texture, 309−312
　　hyphal morphology, 311
　　hyphal pressure, 312
　　hypotheses on texture creation, 310−311
　　interaction between hyphae, 311
　　orientation and dispersion of the hyphae, 311−312
　　phase volume, 312
　cultivation and processing of, 306−313
　environmental impact, 318−322
　　land use, 321−322
　　product carbon footprint, 318−320, 319f
　　water footprint, 320−321
　fat mimetics, 313
　fatty acid composition of, 315t
　fermentation process for the production of, 307f
　filamentous and branched nature of, 309f
　food safety and the regulatory framework, 305−306
　fungal fermentation technology, 306−309
　　air lift fermentation, 308−309
　mineral content of, 315t
　nonstarch polysaccharide content of, 315t
　nutritional properties, 313−316
　　fat, 314
　　fiber, 314
　　minerals, 315−316
　　protein, 313
　　vitamins, 316
　nutrition research, 316−317
　　effects on glycemic response, 317
　　effects on satiety, 317
　　effects on total cholesterol, LDL cholesterol, and high-density lipoprotein cholesterol, 316−317
　origins and discovery of, 305
　process variables that impact quality, 312−313
　　fiber alignment, 312
　　freezing and frozen storage, 312−313
　　mixing, 312
　　thermal gel creation, 312
　protein quality of, 314t
　typical composition of, 306t
　vitamin content of, 316t
Myrosinase enzyme, 290, 294−295

N

Napin, 288
Natunola, 135−136
Natural resources for agriculture, 12−14
Neuronal nitric oxide synthase (nNOS), 141
Newer sources of protein, 414−415
Nitrogen, 13−14, 68, 416
Nitrogen fixation, 145−146, 187, 416
Nitrogen solubility index (NSI), 70, 71f
Nitrogenous food, 1−2
Nonessential amino acids, 4
Nonstarch polysaccharide content of mycoprotein, 315t
No-observed-adverse-effect-level (NOAEL), 294
Nutraceutical compounds, 247
Nutrition research, of mycoprotein, 316−317
　effects on glycemic response, 317
　effects on satiety, 317
　effects on total cholesterol, LDL cholesterol, and high-density lipoprotein cholesterol, 316−317

Nutritional applications, of lupin, 176–177
Nutritional components in amaranth, 240–242
Nutritional properties, in mycoprotein, 313–316
Nutritional quality, of quinoa, 226–230
Nutritive value, 3
   of bambara groundnut, 204
   of canola/rapeseed (C/RS), 292–294
   of chia, 268–275
   of flaxseed proteins. See Flaxseed proteins: nutritive value of
   of heterotrophic microalgae, 333–334
   of lentil, 188–189, 189t
   of lupin. See Lupin: nutritive value
   of marama beans, 200–201
   of pea. See Pea: nutritive value of
   of peanut, 216–219
   of soy protein. See Soy protein: nutritive value

O

Oat, 105–107, 410t
   applications of, 114–115
      baked products, 114
      extruded products, 114
      vegan products, 114–115
   energy use, 106
   functional characteristics of, 112–113
   future outlook, 115
   health aspects, 106–107
   land use, 105–106
   localization and structure of, 107–110
      globulins, 107–108
      minor protein fractions, 109
      nutritional properties and suitability for celiac patients, 109–110
      prolamins, 109
      protein in the oat grain, 107
   manufacture of, 111–112
      dry methods, 111–112
      wet methods, 111
   water use, 106
Oat protein concentrates (OPCs), 111, 114–115
Oat protein isolate (OPI), 112
Obesity, 382, 396–397
Off-flavors associated with lentil flour and lentil protein, 193
Off-tastes
   associated with bambara groundnut, 205
   associated with lupin, 174
   associated with marama beans, 202
   associated with peas, 154–155
   associated with plant proteins, 383–384
   associated with quinoa protein concentrate (QPC), 233–234
   associated with using oilseed proteins, 299–300
Oil extraction, 289–290, 292–293, 299
Oil-roasted peanuts, 216
Oilseeds, 7, 53–54, 410t
Oleic acid, 216
Oleosins, 109, 289
Olfaction, 378
Oligosaccharides, 173–174, 178, 364
ω-3 fatty acid, 276
ω-6 fatty acid, 276
Organization for Economic Cooperation and Development (OECD) countries, 411
Orthonasal olfaction, 378
Oryzacystatin-I, -II, and -III, 59
Oryzasin, 58
Oryzatensin, 60
Osborne classification system, 2–3
Osborne protein, 87
Osborne's method, 242
Oxalates, in soy foods, 38
4-Oxalocrotonate tautomerase, 1–2
Oxya spp., 342

P

Paddy rice, 48–50
Palm trees, 342–343
Pasta, 75, 159–160, 177
Patanga succinct, 342
Pea, 145
   applications and current products, 159–161
      baked goods, 159
      extruded snacks, 160–161
      meat and meat analogs, 161
      pasta and noodle, 159–160
   cultivars, 146
   cultivation, 145–146
   health benefits of, 161
   nutritive value of, 150–155
      allergenicity, 154
      antinutritive factors, 152–153
      bioavailability, 153–154
      major components, 150–152
      minerals and vitamins, 152
      off-tastes, 154–155
   processing of, 147–150
   sustainability, energy, and water use, 146–147
   uses and functionality, 155–159
      pea fiber, 158–159
      pea flour, 156
      pea proteins, 156–157
      pea starch, 157–158
      split peas, 156
      whole peas, 155
Pea, split, 410t
Pea protein isolate (PPI), 175
Peanut, raw, 410t
Peanut butter, 209, 215–216
Peanut production and processing, process flow diagram of, 210f
Peanut products, 209
   cultivation techniques, 213
   environmental impact and sustainability, 209–212
      climate change impacts, 209–211
      land use impacts, 212
      water use impacts, 211–212
   nutritional composition, 217t
   nutritional value, 216–219
      amino acids and protein, 217–218, 218t
      calories, fats, protein, carbohydrates, 216
      micronutrients, 218–219
      taste profiles and allergenicity, 219
   peanut candies, 216
   peanut milk, 216
   peanut processing, 214–215
      grading, 214
      peanut drying, 214
      product processing, 215
      shelling, 215
   production regions, 213
   uses, functionality, and current products, 215–216
Pearl millet, 79, 81–84, 81t, 88t
Penicillium, 305
Pennisetin, 87
Peroxidases (POD), 276–277
Phaseolus vulgaris L., 13, 360
Phenolic compounds, 201
   in canola/rapeseed (C/RS), 295
   in chia, 268, 269t
   in marama beans, 201
Phenylthiocarbamide (PTC), 380
Phylogenic tree, 328f
Physicochemical properties of proteins, 6t
Phytases, 54, 295
   and lectins, 172
   and soy foods, 38
Phytic acid, 73, 152
Phytochemicals
   in lentil, 189
   in quinoa, 229–230
Pin mill, 148, 149f
Plant protein sources, 7
   nutritional adequacy aspects, 360–362
Plant proteins, off-tastes associated with, 383–384
Plant-based foods, 10, 165, 204, 364
Plant-based protein sources
   health and wellbeing aspects, 363–367
      satiety and weight management, 364–367
      systemic and gut health impacts, 363–364
Plant-based protein supplementations, transition towards, 359–360
Plant-derived protein and alternate protein sources, 7–8
   fossil energy, nitrogen, and proteins, 13–14
   global warming and climate change, 14
   land for food, feed, and fuel, 12
   living on the earth in 2050, 10–12
   quality of life, 15
   water consumption, 12–13
Polyphenols, 153
Polyphenols, oil, and peptides with antioxidant capacity, 274–275
Polyunsaturated fatty acids (PUFAs), 268, 346
"Poor man's meat". See Lentil
Population increases and their effects, 11–12
Pork, 346, 409–411
Postharvest processing, of amaranth, 259–260
Poultry, 322, 395, 409–411
Prevotella, 418
Primary structure of protein, 2, 3f
Probenecid, 384
Processing

of amaranth, 260–262
of edible insects, 349–350
of lupin, 168–169
concentrate, 168–169
flour, 168
isolates, 169
peanut processing, 214–215
of peas, 147–150
of proteins and types of products from flaxseed, 135–138
of quinoa, 230–233
of rice and rice proteins, 49–55
sorghum and millet processing, 92–97
Product carbon footprint, 318–320, 319f
Product trends, 9–10
Prolamin fractions, 52–53, 106–107, 243
Prolamins, 2–3
antioxidative activity, 60
millet, 87, 92
of rice, 52–53
6-Propylthiouracil (PROP), 380
Proso millet, 81t, 82, 88t
Protein digestibility corrected amino acid score (PDCAAS), 93, 191, 228, 306, 313
protein digestibility corrected amino acid scores (PDCASS), 294, 334
Protein digestion, 4, 129–131
Protein dispersibility index (PDI), 159, 289–290
Protein efficiency ratio (PER)
of lentil, 191
of lupin, 171
Protein hydrolysates, 60, 128–129, 249
Protein micelle mass (PMM), 291
formation, 291
Pseudocereals, 258, 410t
Pulse proteins, 189–190
Pulses, 7, 171, 185, 360, 363–364, 410t
Purified proteins, 415

Q

Quality of life, 15
Quality of protein, 4–5, 109–110
Quaternary structure of protein, 2, 3f
Quick service restaurants (QSRs), 415
Quinoa, 223, 383, 410t
amino acid composition of the proteins in, 227t
flow diagram of a pilot-scale process for quinoa protein concentrate and coingredients, 232f
future research needs, 234–235
morphology, 225
nutritional quality, 226–230
allergenicity, 230
antinutritional factors, 230
carbohydrates, 229
fiber, 229
lipids, 229
macro- and micronutrients, 229–230
phytochemicals, 230
protein content, 226
protein digestibility, 228
protein quality, 226–228
vitamins and minerals, 229
processing methods, 230–233
quinoa protein concentrates (QPCs) and isolates, 231–233
quinoa seed from "farm to fork", 230–231
production of, 224–225
energy use and cost, 225
growing regions and yields, 224
land use, 225
water use, 225
quinoa protein functionality, off-tastes, and challenges, 233–234
quinoa seed structure and composition, 226f
Quinoa protein concentrate (QPC), 224, 233–234
Quorn Foods, 305, 318–319, 321, 323

R

Raffinose family oligosaccharides (RFOs), 173–174, 178
Raffinose-type sugars, 153
Red rice, 416
Renin, 129–131
Rhizobia, 145–146
Rhynchophorus ferrugineus, 344
Rice, production of, 47–49, 416
energy use, 49
land use, 48
water use, 48–49
Rice milling systems, 50–51
products of, 51t
Rice protein, 47, 49f
allergenicity, 55–57
antinutritional factors, 58–59
enzyme inhibitors, 58–59
enzymes, 58
flavor compounds and off tastes, 57–58
functional properties and applications, 55
potential new uses and emerging health benefits, 59–60
antioxidative activity, 59–60
ileum-contracting, antiopioid, and phagocytosis-promoting activities, 60
reduction in hypertension, 60
reduction of cholesterol and triacylglycerol levels, 59
suppression of hyperglycemia, 59
processing of, 49–55
albumins, 52
globulins, 52
glutelins, 53
prolamins, 52–53
protein localization, 51–52
protein types, 52–53
production of, 53–55
endosperm protein, 54–55
rice bran protein products, 53–54
proximate composition of, 240t
RNAi (RNA interference) technology, 97
RTRS (round table on responsible soy), 33, 42
Ruspolia nitidula, 342

S

Saccharomyces cerevisiae, 414
Salmonella, 348
Salvia genus, 265
Salvia hispanica, 274
Saponins, 153, 233–235, 364
Scleroproteins, 2–3
Secondary structure of protein, 2, 3f
Sedimentation coefficient, 3
Seitan, 75
Short-lived climate pollutants (SLCPs), 15–16
Simple proteins, 3
Sinapis alba, 296
Single-cell algae, 327
Single-cell proteins (SCPs), 414
Skimmed milk powder (SMP), 30
Soil micronutrient levels, 145–146
Solazyme Bunge Oils, 331–332
Solazyme Inc. (case study), 329
Solazyme production process, 329f
Solubility-based classification, 2–3
Solubilized wheat proteins, 69
Soluble dietary fiber (SDF) fraction, 295
Sorghum and millets, 79, 80f
grain proteins, composition and structures of, 88t
grain weight, protein and lysine content, 81t
indispensible amino acid composition of, 85t
potential applications for kafirin, 92
processing, 92–97
brewing and bioethanol production, 95–96
compositing with legumes, 96–97, 98t
effects of cooking on the proteins, 92–93
lactic acid fermentation, 94–95, 96t
malting, 93–94, 95t
milling, 93
production, 79–82, 81t
cost of grains, 83
cultivation with legumes, 83
land-use efficiency, 82
sustainable agriculture, 83
water efficiency, 82–83
prolamin proteins, 87
protein isolation and functionality, 87–92
protein nutritive quality, 83–87
antinutrients, 84–86
other nutrients, phytochemicals, and nutritional quality issues, 86–87
protein quality, 84
protein toxicity, 86
protein quality, developments in improving, 97–99
Sound mature kernels (SMK), 214
Sound splits (SS), 214
Soy protein, 21, 414–415
amino acid composition of, 34t
application and current products, 40
cholesterol-lowering effect of, 37, 37f
composition of, 24f
as a good source of protein across the lifespan, 39
nutritive value, 33–39
cardiovascular health, 36–37

Soy protein (*Continued*)
    muscle health, 34–35
    nutritional relevance of other seed constituents, 37–38
    protein allergies, 38–39
    protein nutrition, 33–34
    weight management and satiety, 35–36
  potential new uses, issues, and challenges, 40–42
    generational flavor improvements, 41–42
    genetic modified and identity preserved, 42
  production, 23–24
  recovery, 24–26
  sustainability of, 26–33
    attributional modeling, 27
    consequential modeling, 27
    cradle-to-gate life cycle impact assessment, 28–31
    energy use at farm level, 31
    ISP manufacturing, 33
    land use at farm level and deforestation, 32–33
    use of hexane in soy milling, 33
    water use at farm level, 32
  types and protein products, 26
  uses and functionality, 39–40
Soybean protein, 9–10, 33–34, 41–42, 410t
Soybean Sustainability Assurance Protocol (SSAP), 42
Spent flake, 24–25
Spin blanching, 215
Spinach, 38
Spirulina, 327, 333–334, 338
Split lentils, 191
Split peas, 148, 156, 156f
Stress-tolerant species, quinoa as, 224
Structure of protein, 2, 3f
Structure-based classification systems, 4
Structure–function relationships of food protein, 6–7
Sub1A gene, 416
Sulfur-rich proteins
  hemp seed, 124–125
Supercritical carbon dioxide (SC-CO$_2$), 112
Superoxide dismutase (SOD), 129
Sustainability
  of amaranth production, 257–260
  of bambara groundnut, 202–203
  of chia, 265–267
  of flax, 134–135
  of lentil, 185–187
  of lupin, 166–167
  of lupin, 166–167
  of pea, 146–147
  of peanut products, 209–212
  of soy, 31–33
  of wheat, 68–69
Sustainable diet, 359
Sustainable future populations, 418–419
Sustainable Technologies Promotion Center, 231

T

Tannin sorghums, 84
Tannins, 84, 153
Taste, physiology of, 378–379
  astringency, 379
  bitter taste, 379, 384
Taste preferences and influences, 379–383
  affording a healthy diet, 382
  cultural influence on food choices, 380–382
  genetics and food choices, 380
  ice cream, broccoli, and nuts, 382–383
Teff, 81t, 82, 88t
Tenebrio molitor, 343–344, 348–349
TeuTexx Proteins, 297
Textured soy proteins, 40
Texturized vegetable proteins, 205
Texturized wheat proteins, 76
Tofu, 317, 415
Total sound mature kernels (TSMK), 214
Transglutaminase, 113, 156–157
Triglycerides, 363
Trypsin, 152
Trypsin inhibitors, in soy foods, 37–38
Tryptophanins, 109

V

Vanillin, 57–58
Vegetable-based meat alternatives and new developments, 75–76
Vegetarian Butcher, 177
Vegetation, 14
Vicilins, 243
Viscozyme L, 54, 136
Vitamins
  in edible insects, 346
  in mycoprotein, 316, 316t
  in pea, 152
  in quinoa, 229
Vivera, 177
Volatile organic compounds (VOCs), 233–234

W

Wagon drying, 214
Water blanching, 215
Water classification, 13
Water consumption, 13, 106, 332
Water efficiency, 82–83
Water footprint, 32, 211–212, 212t
Water Footprint Network (WFN), 211
Water stress, 13
Water use
  amaranth, 258–259
  bambara groundnut, 202–203
  canola/rapeseed (C/RS), 286
  chia, 266–267
  flaxseed production, 135
  hemp cultivation, 122
  lentil production, 186
  lupin production, 166–167
  oat production, 106
  peanut production, 211–212
  pea production, 146–147
  quinoa production, 225
  rice production, 48–49
  wheat production, 68
Water-insoluble oat bran concentrate (WIS-OBC), 114
Water-soluble oat bran concentrate (WS-OBC), 114
Weight management and satiety
  soy protein and, 35–36
Western diet, 8–10, 385, 411
Wet fractionation technology for peas, 150, 151f
Wheat
  agricultural production, 67
  energy use, 68
  land use, 67
  proximate composition of, 240t
  sustainability of, 68–69
  water use, 68
Wheat gluten, 69–70, 70f, 74–75
Wheat proteins, 67, 69–70
  allergenicity and intolerance mechanism, 73
  amino acid composition, 71–72
  antinutritive factors, 73
  applications in food and feed, 74–76
    animal nutrition, 75
    breakfast cereals and pasta, 75
    gluten in bread application, 74–75
    new product and technology for wheat-based meat, 76
    protein-enriched foods, 75
    vegetable-based meat alternatives and new developments, 75–76
  digestibility data and mechanism, 72–73
  functionality, 74
    emulsification, 74
    foaming, 74
    satiety, 74
    solubility, 74
  gluten extraction from wheat, 70
  protein hydrolysis, 70
Wheat-based meat, new product and technology for, 76
White flakes, 24–25
White fonio, 81t, 82, 88t
Whole algae protein, 330–332
  properties and applications of, 335–336
Whole peas, 150, 155
Whole seed quinoa flour, 232–233
Whole wheat, 410t

Y

Yellow mealworm, 343–344
Yellow peas, soaking quality of, 155f

Z

Zophobas atratus, 349

Printed in the United States
By Bookmasters